Pediatric Toxicology

Pediatric Toxicology
Diagnosis and Management of the Poisoned Child

Timothy B. Erickson, MD, FACEP, FACMT, FAACT
Associate Professor
Department of Emergency Medicine
Director, Division of Clinical Toxicology
Emergency Medicine Residency Program Director
University of Illinois at Chicago
Chicago, Illinois

William R. Ahrens, MD
Associate Clinical Professor
Department of Emergency Medicine
Department of Pediatrics
University of Illinois at Chicago
Chicago, Illinois

Steven E. Aks, DO, FACMT, FACEP
Associate Professor
Department of Emergency Medicine
Cook County Hospital
Section of Clinical Toxicology
Director, The Toxikon Consortium
Chicago, Illinois

Carl R. Baum, MD, FAAP, FACMT
Department of Pediatrics
Yale University
Director, Center for Children's Environmental Toxicology
Yale-New Haven Children's Hospital
New Haven, Connecticut

Louis J. Ling, MD, FACEP, FACMT
Professor
Department of Emergency Medicine
Medical Director, Hennepin Regional Poison Center
University of Minnesota
Hennepin County Medical Center
Minneapolis, Minnesota

McGraw-Hill
Medical Publishing Division

New York   Chicago   San Francisco   Lisbon   London   Madrid   Mexico City   Milan
New Delhi   San Juan   Seoul   Singapore   Sydney   Toronto

The McGraw-Hill Companies

Pediatric Toxicology: Diagnosis and Management of the Poisoned Child

1 2 3 4 5 6 7 8 9 0   DOC/DOC   0 9 8 7 6 5 4

ISBN 0-07-141736-2

This book was set in Times Roman by MidAtlantic Books and Journals.
The editor was Andrea Seils.
The production supervisor was Richard Ruzycka.
Project management was provided by Jennsin Services.
RR Donnelley was printer and binder.

This book is printed on acid-free paper.

Library of Congress Cataloging-in-Publication Data

Pediatric toxicology : diagnosis & management of the poisoned child / edited by Timothy
    Erickson ... [et al.].— 1st ed.
       p. ; cm.
    Includes bibliographical references and index.
    ISBN 0-07-141736-2
    1. Pediatric toxicology. I. Erickson, Timothy (Timothy Bruce), 1960–
[DNLM: 1. Poisoning—diagnosis—Child. 2. Poisoning—therapy—Child. 3.
Emergencies—Child. QV 600 P3713 2004]
RA1225.P43 2004
615.9′083—dc22

                                                                      2004040323

To my wife Valerie for her love, support and patience, my children Camille, Isabelle, Celeste and Julian, my parents Robert, Gladys and Janine, as well as my siblings; to my co-editors and authors for all their dedicated work and expertise; to Gary Strange and Dan Hryhorczuk for their years of mentorship and wisdom, and my peers in Emergency Medicine at UIC and Toxikon; Steve Goldberg who taught me pediatrics and continues to care for my children; to modern-day Fathers of Toxicology Barry Rumack and Lewis Goldfrank for their help and advice with the book, along with special thanks to Paracelsus.

Timothy B. Erickson

To Doctors Jane Bleusbach and Mary Lou Daoust, and to Sister Silvia Pacheco, for allowing us to participate in their decades of service to the children of Guatemala.

William R. Ahrens

To my parents Gloria and Franklin for their unwavering support and direction, To Julie and Jake for providing me with support, perspective, love, and happiness, and finally to the members and trainees of The Toxikon Consortium for being the ideal model of collaboration for service, and education in toxicology.

Steven E. Aks

To all children, who need their own books. To my colleagues in poison centers and emergency rooms, unwavering in their care for children. To my family, accomplished in art and science. To Eli and Sophie, intrepid every day. To Diane, my best friend, for her love and patience.

Carl R. Baum

For children everywhere and to the dedicated professionals who care for them. This includes my own children, Amanda, Ali, and Eric, who make it all worthwhile. For the staff of the Hennepin Regional Poison Center who are always alert and helping the children of Minnesota, North Dakota, and South Dakota every minute of every day.

Louis J. Ling

CONTENTS

CONTRIBUTORS

William R. Ahrens, MD
Associate Clinical Professor
Department of Emergency Medicine
Department of Pediatrics
University of Illinois at Chicago
Chicago, Illinois

Steven E. Aks, DO, FACMT, FACEP
Associate Professor
Department of Emergency Medicine
Cook County Hospital
Section of Clinical Toxicology
Director, The Toxikon Consortium
Chicago, Illinois

Yona Amitai, MD
Mother, Child, and Adolescent Health
Ministry of Health
Jerusalem, Israel

Angela Anderson, MD
Hasbro Children's Hospital
Pediatric Emergency Medicine
Providence, Rhode Island

Deborah L. Anderson, PharmD
Director, Hennepin Regional Poison Center
Minneapolis, Minnesota

Paul S. Auerbach, MD
Clinical Professor
Department of Emergency Medicine
Stanford University Medical Center
Stanford, California

Alexander B. Baer, MD
Assistant Clinical Professor
Blue Ridge Poison Center
Associate Professor
University of Virginia Health System
University of Virginia
Charlottesville, Virginia

Stacey Bangh, MD
Hennepin Regional Poison Center
Hennepin County Medical Center
Minneapolis, Minnesota

William Banner, Jr, MD, PhD, FAACT, FACMT
The Children's Hospital at Saint Francis
Tulsa, Oklahoma

Fermin Barrueto, Jr, MD
New York City Poison Control Center
New York, New York

R. Philip Barton, MD
Co-Director
Pediatric Intensive Care Unit
The Children's Hospital at Saint Francis
Tulsa, Oklahoma

Carl R. Baum, MD, FAAP, FACMT
Department of Pediatrics
Yale University
Director, Center for Children's Environmental Toxicology
Yale-New Haven Children's Hospital
New Haven, Connecticut

Elisabeth F. Bilden, MD
Hennepin Regional Poison Control Center
Minneapolis, Minnesota

Kenneth Bizovi, MD
Assistant Professor, Emergency Medicine
Oregon Health and Science University
Emergency Services
Oregon Poison Control Center
Portland, Oregon

G. Randall Bond, MD, FACMT
Cincinnati Children's Hospital Medical Center
Cincinnati, Ohio

Jeffrey Brent, MD, PhD, FAACT, FACMT
Professor
Toxicology Associates
University of Colorado
Denver, Colorado

Sean M. Bryant, MD
Assistant Professor
Cook County Hospital
Department of Emergency Medicine
The Toxikon Consortium
Chicago, Illinois

Anthony M. Burda, PharmD, DABAT
Poison Control Specialist
Illinois Poison Control Center
Chicago, Illinois

Diane P. Calello, MD
The Children's Hospital of Philadelphia
Division of Emergency Medicine
Philadelphia, Pennsylvania

Andrea G. Carlson, MD
Assistant Professor
Christ Medical Center
The Toxikon Consortium
Chicago, Illinois

Dominic Chalut, MD, FRCPC
McGill University Health Center
Montreal Children's Hospital
Montreal, Quebec, Canada

Peter Chyka, PharmD, DABAT, FAACT
Professor, Department of Pharmacy
University of Tennessee Health Science Center
Memphis, Tennessee

Richard F. Clark, MD, FACMT, FAACT, FACEP
Professor of Medicine
Toxicology Fellowship Director
Director, Division of Medical Toxicology
University of California-San Diego Medical Center
San Diego, California

Kirk L. Cumpston, DO
Medical Director
Poison Control Center
Department of Emergency Medicine
University of New Mexico
Albuquerque, New Mexico

Timothy B. Erickson, MD, FACEP, FACMT, FAACT
Associate Professor
Department of Emergency Medicine
Director, Division of Clinical Toxicology
Emergency Medicine Residency Director
University of Illinois at Chicago
Chicago, Illinois

Michele Burns Ewald, MD
Children's Hospital Boston
Boston, Massachusetts

Yaron Finkelstein, MD
Children's Hospital Toronto
Toronto, Ontario, Canada

Connie Fischbein, PharmD
Poison Control Specialist
Illinois Poison Center
Chicago, Illinois

Rotem Freide, MD
Attending, Intensive Care Medicine
Rush Presbyterian St. Luke's Medical Center
Chicago, Illinois

Gregory Gaar, MD, FAAP, FAACT
Medical Toxicology Consultants
Tampa General Hospital
University of South Florida
Tampa, Florida

Gary Lee Geis, MD
Fellow, Pediatric Emergency Medicine
Cincinnati Children's Hospital Medical Center
Cincinnati, Ohio

Rachel Goldstein, DO, MSc
Toxicology Fellow
University of Connecticut School of Medicine
Farmington, Connecticut

Michael I. Greenberg, MD, MPH
Professor of Emergency Medicine
Professor of Public Health
Drexel University College of Medicine
Philadelphia, Pennsylvania

Howard A. Greller, MD
New York City Poison Control Center
New York, New York

David D. Gummin, MD
Infinity HealthCare
Emergency Medicine/Clinical Toxiclogy
Milwaukee, Wisconsin

Leon Gussow, MD, FACEP, FACMT
Assistant Professor of Emergency Medicine/Rush
  Medical College
Cook County Hospital
Department of Emergency Medicine
Chicago, Illinois

In-Hei Hahn, MD
St. Luke's Roosevelt Hospital Center
Department of Emergency Medicine
Clinical Toxicology
New York, New York

Christina E. Hantsch, MD
Medical Director
Illinois Poison Control Center
Loyola University
Chicago, Illinois

Carson R. Harris, MD
Emergency Medicine Department
Regions Hospital
University of Minnesota Medical School
St. Paul, Minnesota

Vivian Harris, MD
Stroger Cook County Hospital
Department of Radiology
Chicago, Illinois

Rachel Haroz, MD
Toxicology Fellow
Drexel University College of Medicine
Philadelphia, Pennsylvania

Fred M. Henretig, MD
The Children's Hospital of Philadelphia
Division of Emergency Medicine/Clinical Toxicology
Philadelphia, Pennsylvania

Robert J. Hoffman, MD
Department of Emergency Medicine
Beth Israel Medical Center
New York, New York

Robert S. Hoffman, MD, FACMT, FAACT
New York City Poison Control Center
Medical Director
New York, New York

Christopher P. Holstege, MD
Department of Emergency Medicine
University of Virginia Health System
Charlottesville, Virginia

Susan Hou, MD
Division of Nephrology
Loyola University Medical Center
Maywood, Illinois

Daniel Hryhorczuk, MD, ABMT, MPH
Director, Great Lakes Centers
University of Illinois at Chicago School of Public Health
The Toxikon Consortium
Chicago, Illinois

Marianne Ingels, MD
Emergency Physician
Integris Baptist Medical Center
Oklahoma City, Oklahoma

Susan A. Kecskes, MD
Pediatric Intensive Care Unit Director
Department of Pediatrics
University of Illinois at Chicago
Chicago, Illinois

Mark A. Kirk, MD, FACMT
Assistant Professor of Emergency Medicine and
  Clinical Toxicology
Department of Emergency Medicine
University of Virginia Health System
Charlottesville, Virginia

Anne Krantz, MD, ABMT, MPH
Chief, Section of Clinical Toxicology
Division of Occupational Medicine
Stroger Hospital of Cook County
Chicago, Illinois

Edward P. Krenzelok, PharmD, FAACT
Director
Pittsburgh Poison Control Center
Pittsburgh, Pennsylvania

Ken Kulig, MD, FAACT, FACMT
Toxicology Associates, LLC
Associate Professor
Division of Emergency Medicine and Trauma
University of Colorado
Denver, Colorado

Ruth A. Lawrence, MD, FAACT
University of Rochester
Department of Pediatrics
Finger Lakes Poison Center
Rochester, New York

Jerrold B. Leiken, MD, FACEP, FACMT, FACP
OMEGA
Glenbrook Hospital
Glenview, Illinois
The Toxikon Consortium
Chicago, Illinois

Erica L. Liebelt, MD, FACMT
Associate Professor of Pediatrics and
  Emergency Medicine
University of Alabama at Birmingham School
  of Medicine
Director, Medical Toxicology Services
Children's Hospital and University Hospital
Co-Medical Director
Regional Poison Control Center
Birmingham, Alabama

Louis J. Ling, MD, FACEP, FACMT
Professor
Department of Emergency Medicine
Medical Director, Hennepin Regional Poison Center
Hennepin County Medical Center
University of Minnesota
Minneapolis, Minnesota

Jack W. Lipscomb, PharmD
TAP Pharmaceutical Products, Inc.
Poison Control Specialist
Illinois Poison Center
Lake Forest, Illinois

Toby L. Litovitz, MD
Executive and Medical Director
National Capital Poison Center
Washington, DC

Heather Long, MD
New York City Poison Control Center
New York, New York

Rebekah Mannix, MD
Fellow, Pediatric Emergency Medicine and Toxicology
Children's Hospital Boston
Boston, Massachusetts

Andrea Marmor, MD
Department of Pediatrics
San Francisco General Hospital
San Francisco, California

Suzanne Mazor, MD
Division of Emergency Medicine
Department of Pediarics
Seattle Children's Hospital
Seattle Poison Control Center
Seattle, Washington

Charles A. McKay, MD, FACMT, FACEP, ABIM
Associate Medical Director
Connecticut Poison Control Center
Associate Professor of Emergency Medicine
University of Connecticut School of Medicine
Farmington, Connecticut
Director, Toxicology Service
Department of Traumatology and Emergency Medicine
Hartford Hospital
Hartford, Connecticut

Bonnie McManus, MD
Department of Emergency Medicine
Elmhurst Hospital
Elmhurst, Illinois
The Toxikon Consortium
Chicago, Illinois

Gregory M. Mueller, PhD
Mycologist
Departmental Chair
The Field Museum
Chicago, Illinois

Mark Mycyk, MD
Assistant Professor
Northwestern Memorial Hospital
Division of Emergency Medicine
The Toxikon Consortium
Chicago, Illinois

Lewis S. Nelson, MD, FACMT
Toxicology Fellowship Director
New York City Poison Control Center
New York, New York

Michele K. Nichols, MD
Associate Professor of Pediatrics
University of Alabama at Birmingham School
 of Medicine
Co-Medical Director
Regional Poisom Control Center
Birmingham, Alabama

Steve R. Offerman, MD
Assistant Clinical Professor
Division of Emergency Medicine and Toxicology
University of California Davis School of Medicine
Sacramento, California

Janis M. Orlowski, MD
Nephrologist
Senior Vice President and Medical Director
Washington Hospital Medical Center
Department of Medical Affairs
Washington, DC

Kevin C. Osterhoudt, MD, MSCE
Section of Medical Toxicology
Division of Emergency Medicine
Children's Hospital of Philadelphia
Philadelphia, Pennsylvania

Frank P. Paloucek, PharmD, DABAT
Director, Residency Programs
Clinical Associate Professor in Pharmacy Practice
Department of Pharmacy Practice
College of Pharmacy University of Illinois at Chicago
Chicago, Illinois

Alberto Perez, MD
Department of Emergency Medicine
Hartford Hospital
Hartford, Connecticut

Holly Perry, MD
Assistant Professor of Pedicatrics
Attending Physician
Department of Emergency Medicine
University of Connecticut School of Medicine
Connecticut Children's Medical Center
Hartford, Connecticut

William H. Richardson, MD
Medical Director, Palmetto Regional Poison Center
Department of Emergency Medicine
Palmetto Health-Richland Memorial Hospital
Columbia, South Carolina

Joshua G. Schier, MD
Fellow, Medical Toxicology
New York City Poison Control Center
New York, New York

Aaron B. Schneir, MD
Assistant Professor
Division of Medical Toxicology
Department of Emergency Medicine
University of California San Diego Medical Center
San Diego Division California Poison Control System
San Diego, California

Donna Seger, MD, FAACT
Department of Emergency Medicine
Clinical Toxicology
Vanderbilt University Medical Center
Nashville, Tennessee

Michael Shannon, MD, FACMT, FAAP, MPH, FAACT
Children's Hospital Boston
Division of Emergency Medicine
Boston, Massachusetts

Curtis P. Snook, MD
Associate Professor
Division of Toxicology
University of Cincinnati College of Medicine
Department of Emergency Medicine
Cincinnati, Ohio

Gary R. Strange, MD, FACEP
Professor
Chair
Department of Emergency Medicine
Uniersity of Illinois
Chicago, Illinois

Ernest Stremski, MD
Children's Hospital of Wisconsin Poison Center
Associate Professor
Department of Pediatrics
Medical College of Wisconsin
Milwaukee, Wisconsin

Mark Su, MD
Assistant Professor of Emergency Medicine
SUNY Downstate Medical Center
Brooklyn, New York

Matthew D. Sztajnkrycer, MD, PhD
Assistant Professor
Department of Emergency Medicine
Mayo Clinic
Rochester, Minnesota

Asim Tarabar, MD
New York Poison Center
New York, New York

Milton Tennenbein, MD, FAAP, FAACT
Emergency Medicine

Children's Hospital
Winnipeg, Manitoba, Canada

Mark Thoman, MD, FAACT, FACMT, FAAP
University of Missouri School of Medicine
Kansas City, Missouri

Tri C. Tong, MD
Assistant Clinical Professor
University of California San Diego Medical Center
Clinical Toxicology
San Diego, California

Michael S. Wahl, MD, FACEP, FACMT
Medical Director
Illinois Poison Center
Chicago, Illinois

Frank G. Walter, MD, FACMT, FAACT
Department of Emergncy Medicine
University of Arizona
Tucson, Arizona

Sage W. Weiner, MD
Senior Fellow, Medical Toxicology
New York City Poison Control Center
New York, New York

Suzanne R. White, MD
Associate Clinical Professor
Department of Emergency Medicine
Detroit Receiving Hospital
Detroit, Michigan

James F. Wiley II, MD, FAC MT, FACEP, FAAP
University of Connecticut School of Medicine
Connecticut Children's Medical Center
Hartford, Connecticut

Alan Woolf, MD, MPH
Professor
Harvard University
Children's Hospital Boston
Massachusetts Poison Center
Boston, Massachusetts

Michele Zell-Kanter, PharmD, DABAT
Section of Clinical Toxicology
Division of Occupational Medicine
Stroger Hospital of Cook County
Chicago, Illinois

FOREWORD

Poison centers in the United States manage over 2 million exposures to toxic substances and over 1 million information calls per year. A recent Institute of Medicine report estimated episodes (actual or suspected exposures) to be over 4 million per year and concluded that poisoning was the second leading cause of death, with 30,800 in 2001 behind automobile-related deaths of 42,443 in the same year. Gun-related deaths were a close third, with 29,573. Whether poisoning will maintain second place or improve in the future is unclear. The report *Healthy People 2010* set a 2010 goal of reducing nonfatal poisonings to 292 per 100,000 from a baseline of 349 in 1997 and deaths from 6.8 per 100,000 in 1997 to 1.5 per 100,000. The Institute of Medicine, however, calculated 530 per 100,000 in 2001 and 8.5 deaths per 100,000 in that same year, making the 2010 goals unlikely.

Half of all poison exposures occur in children age 5 and younger. The focus on these children has been accidental exposure primarily in and around the home. In this age group, there are a small number of intentional cases such as in Munchausen syndrome by proxy; additionally there are errors in drug dosing throughout all age groups. The number of exposures drops rapidly between ages 6 and 10. However, the rate increases once again in children older than 10, who may attempt suicide or engage in a manipulative episode or, less commonly, have an accidental exposure. The mortality rate in these intentional episodes is very high and deserves increased attention.

Children age 5 and younger have been likened to "grazing animals" with a propensity to put anything they encounter into their mouth. Whereas in general we have believed that taste is not a deterrent, some data indicate that effervescence and extreme bitterness may indeed deter a significant ingestion in children ages 3 to 5. Why a child will spit out asparagus while happily sucking on a permanent marker or tasting a tablet or pesticide contin-

ues to be a mystery. However, most exposures in children 5 and younger are generally minimal because they rarely consume much volume. Caregivers become quite concerned and sometimes hysterical as children come into contact with potentially toxic drugs, chemicals, and plants. Fortunately, over time, poison centers have developed a rigorous approach to evaluating such a child and the majority may remain in the home with reassurance and follow-up calls.

Twenty to thirty years ago, the standard treatment for most ingestions was administration of syrup of ipecac. Although ipecac produces emesis in almost every instance, the question remained as to whether it changed the outcome of a case. True, ipecac is effective; true, it was usually safe; but, false, it was effective in reducing toxicity of the primary ingestant. We did argue about whether to induce emesis with hydrocarbons and decided that if the hydrocarbon was toxic we would use ipecac but if not, we would not. The full logic of that argument from 30 years ago escapes me at this point. Ipecac administration has, however, been abandoned as a barbaric throwback and no longer has a place in treatment. Gastric lavage was frequently used but was shown in several studies to be of little use and has been largely abandoned. Gastric lavage does leave a memorable impression on the patient as can be attested to by the writer of this foreword, who experienced the procedure in 1946 following a taste of rat poison. There are probably better methods to encourage people to become clinical toxicologists.

Poison prevention programs, publicity from poison prevention week, and a variety of other educational efforts unfortunately do not produce any evidence-based results. However, it does make intuitive sense that messages such as keeping medicines out of reach, and so on, have prevented some exposures and probably prevented morbidity and death. Where data do exist is in the reduction of the number of deaths following restriction of tablets available in bottles of children's aspirin to 36. This strategy was used to determine the number of iron tablets per bottle with notable success. The introduction of safety closures continues to be the most important contribution to a reduction in morbidity and mortality from accidental exposures. It is estimated that a reduction of 460 deaths or more and a mortality rate reduction of 45% was a direct result of this packaging. Both of these methods are passive in that there is no direct action required from caregivers to take advantage of these life-saving implementations. There is clearly benefit to further work in the area of passive prevention, which has not produced any new developments since the very early 1970s.

There are specific differences between adults and children following ingestion of some toxic substances and even between different ages of children. One early observation related to the accidental ingestion of Lomotil. A series of cases demonstrated that children who ingested even a few tablets of this drug might seem normal for as long as 8 hours after ingestion before suffering life-threatening problems. Some children sent home early after observation died. No such pattern occurred in adults. The differences in acetaminophen metabolism between children younger than age 9 to 12 with older children as well as other changes helps to explain the relative resistance in young children to quantities of this drug that are toxic in older children and adults.

The recent introduction of an intravenous form of N-acetylcysteine was marred by the potential for fluid overload if the product insert was followed for young children. This is primarily related to the difficulty of performing research that involves children. Although the United States Food and Drug Administration provides incentives for pharmaceutical manufacturers to study children, this has only been done for a handful of drugs. The remaining drugs, including those used in the treatment of poisoned patient, may contain the admonition that the "safety and efficacy of drug X has not been shown in children under the age of Y." There is a clear need for an authoritative source for dosage recommendations in these instances.

Physicians who treat children have frequently been in the position of having to determine the dosage of a critical therapeutic agent from the literature due to lack of data in the package insert. Having those calculations in one place will undoubtedly benefit our young patients. The authors of this book have carefully developed both diagnostic and therapeutic information to ensure that the correct treatment and the correct dosing will be rapidly and reliably available.

Barry H. Rumack, MD
Director Emeritus, Rocky Mountain Poison
and Drug Center
Clinical Professor of Pediatrics,
University of Colorado School of Medicine
Denver, Colorado
May 14, 2004

PREFACE

There is perhaps nothing more anxiety provoking to the health care professional than caring for a critically ill child. Figures 1 and 2 are classic works depicting sick children prior to the age of antibiotics, antidotes, chemotherapy, and pediatric intensive care units, when mortality from childhood illnesses was considerable. Fortunately, in present-day society, the majority of sick pediatric patients suffer minor morbidity and rarely mortality; however, many clinicians have limited experience in treating critically ill children, especially poisoned children. In addition, there are many uncommon and potentially dangerous poisons that a busy practitioner may encounter only once or twice during his or her entire career. This has led to the development of the field of toxicology, and in particular, pediatric toxicology.

Ironically, despite the fact that nearly two thirds of all poisoning cases reported to nation-wide poison control centers involve children, few reference sources are available to the practitioner that specifically address the care of the poisoned child. Most clinical trials in toxicology studies involve adult patients or adult volunteers. There are few well-designed investigations involving pediatric patients. Given obvious ethical considerations, and Institutional Review Board and Food and Drug Administration regulations, large clinical trials with children are not likely to become common. Thus, many recommendations involving poisoned children are based on retrospective case series with limited numbers, epidemiologic poison center data, anecdotal case reports, or studies in adults.

A number of textbooks have evolved to meet the demands of the growing subspecialty of toxicology. Most cover general concepts and specific toxins; some have an environmental or occupational focus. Recent outstanding reference books have discussed care in poisoned adult patients, with brief sections devoted to pediatric concerns. No recent textbook, however, has been devoted to pediatric toxicology. As a result, we sought to offer a new reference book focusing on the diagnosis and management of poisoned children.

Our goal was to organize a book that is uniform in its presentation, easy to access, and reasonably priced, to

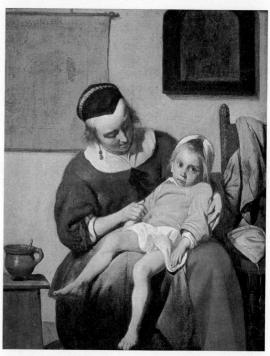

Fig. 1. *The Sick Child* by Gabriel Metsu (1660), Rijksmuseum, Amsterdam. (*Source:* Art Resource, Inc. www.artres.com. New York: 2004.)

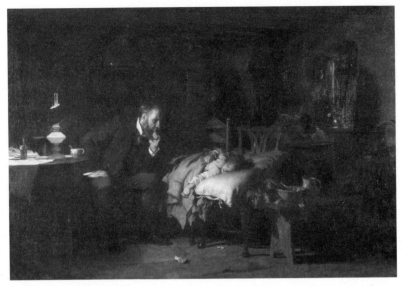

Fig. 2. *The Doctor* by Sir Samuel Luke Fildes (1891), Tate Gallery, London. (*Source:* Lyons AS, Petrucelli RJ: *Medicine: An illustrated history.* New York: Abradale Books, Harry Abrams In; 1987, pp 460–461.)

give the health care provider in the office, poison control center, emergency department, pediatric ward, or intensive care unit ready access to information regarding poisoned children. With treatment options and disposition issues, we thoroughly reviewed the literature and referenced well-designed studies whenever possible. If these were not available, we relied on poison center data and retrospective case series. With uncommon poisonings, we reviewed cases reports involving children, not adults. In addition, we recruited academic experts in the fields of toxicology and pediatrics from all over the country. Many authors have done original research on the chapters they wrote; most are active in treating poisoned children on a daily basis. Finally, if there existed minimal sound data regarding a specific or controversial issue, we would consult one another and frequently pose the question: "If this was one of our children, what would we do?" Having ten children among us with ages ranging from 2 to 19 years, we felt somewhat qualified to have this discussion. We attempted to make definitive suggestions regarding treatment and disposition decisions to help the clinician managing a poisoned child in real time, at the bedside. We also tackled recent controversial issues such as gastrointestinal decontamination with syrup

of ipecac, the use of hyperbaric oxygen therapy in carbon monoxide poisoning, and unsettling topics such as teen suicide and pregnancy, drug abuse, eating disorders, date rape, and child abuse.

Pediatric Toxicology: Diagnosis and Management of the Poisoned Child is set up at the beginning with general pediatric chapters highlighting special considerations in the poisoned pediatric patient, poison prevention, and the role of poison control centers. This is followed by special considerations regarding toxicology in the fetus, premature infant, neonate, toddler, and adolescent. Specific chapters on over-the-counter medications, prescription drugs, household products, illicit drugs, heavy metals, and environmental toxins are also presented. Each of these chapters begins with a case, and ends with a case outcome to highlight the important clinical points discussed in the chapter. We also tried to enhance the visual quality of the book with figures, tables, as well as a color plate section. We conclude the textbook with over 200 multiple-choice questions for review, test preparation, or continuing medical education.

We would like to acknowledge the guidance and wisdom of Andrea Seils, senior medical editor at McGraw-Hill. Andrea kept us in line and on schedule, and prevented our conference calls from going off track. We also thank her assistants Marta Colon and Jennifer D'Inzeo for valuable assistance with manuscript preparation. Thanks also to each of our personal staff members for their role in making this book possible. Most important, we graciously acknowledge our immediate family members who endured our long hours of obsession in trying to make this most informative and accurate textbook possible.

Finally, we sincerely believe that if this textbook assists one clinician in saving the life of one child, all the work was worthwhile.

Timothy B. Erickson
William R. Ahrens
Steven E. Aks
Carl R. Baum
Louis J. Ling

1

General Principles

Carl R. Baum
William R. Ahrens

After World War II, unprecedented numbers of new products became available. Some of these presented new hazards, and in the post-war era, between 400 and 500 children under the age of 6 years died annually as a result of poisoning. The visionary Chicago pharmacist Louis Gdalman, who had maintained a poison information service for over a decade at St. Luke's Hospital, inspired the American Academy of Pediatrics (AAP) to initiate a national campaign in 1948 that was intended to reduce the number of unintentional childhood poisonings. With assistance from the AAP and pediatrician Edward Press, MD, of the University of Illinois, Gdalman went on to establish the nation's first poison control center in 1953. Half a century later, progress has been made. However, despite their early involvement in establishing poison control initiatives, pediatricians represent a minority among toxicologists. Fifty years after the establishment of the first poison control center, the American Board of Pediatrics had certified only 27 pediatricians in medical toxicology.

HOW CHILDREN ARE DIFFERENT FROM ADULTS

Although case reports of pediatric poisonings abound, obvious ethical and clinical considerations have precluded the rigorous study of many toxicology-related issues in children. It is also evident that knowledge derived from the study of adults may not translate to the care of children. An example is gastric lavage: an orogastric tube that may be effective in removing pills from the stomach of an adult or adolescent would not be physically practical for a 15-month-old child. To recommend this form of gastric evacuation in toddlers and children based on the study of individuals several times their size

is unrealistic. Thus, one of the goals of this text is to acknowledge that data in children are often lacking or suboptimal, rather than recommending treatments be based solely on what is known in adults. Whenever possible, clinical decision-making discussions will be based on documented experience with poisoned pediatric patients.

DEVELOPMENTAL ASSESSMENT

A number of chapters in this book focus on the relationship between toxins and specific developmental stages of childhood. Newborn infants, particularly those born prematurely, are vulnerable to some toxins in light of their incompletely developed metabolic capabilities. Breastfed infants may be exposed to drugs or environmental toxins excreted in the breast milk.

As children become more mobile and curious, normal developmental milestones may bring them into contact with a variety of toxins. Hand-to-mouth activity in the older infant, for example, may cause exposure to lead-contaminated dust, and the fine pincer grasp of the toddler presents a potential hazard when tablets are left unsecured. As cognitive powers grow, older children and adolescents may gain a better comprehension of the dangers of their environment, but impulsive behaviors may increase the risk for toxin exposure. Adolescents who enter the workplace frequently encounter hazardous chemicals, but may not have access to appropriate protective equipment or education.

PHYSICAL ASSESSMENT

There are important differences between pediatric and adult patients in regards to vital signs, which reflect the

Table 1–1. Normal Vital Signs in Children

Temperature	
<38.0°C (100.4°F)	
Pulse rate (beats per minute)	
Neonate	95–160
1 wk–6 mo	105–180
6 mo–1 y	110–170
1–3 y	90–150
4–8 y	60–135
9–16 y	60–110
>16 y	60–100
Respiratory rate (breaths per minute)	
Neonate	30–50
1–6 mo	20–40
6 mo–2 y	20–30
2–12 y	16–24
>12 y	12–20
Blood pressure (systolic/diastolic, mm Hg, 50th percentile)	
Neonate	72/55
2 y	96/60
6 y	98/68
10 y	108/70
14 y	118/75
18 y	125/78

evolution of physiology from infancy to adulthood (Table 1–1). The higher heart rate and respiratory rate of infancy and early childhood reflect a higher basal metabolic rate. Infants have limited ability to increase stroke volume, and therefore must increase heart rate to increase cardiac output. Pediatric patients increase systemic vascular resistance to maintain blood pressure until late in many illnesses such as septic shock; however, precipitous cardiovascular collapse may then occur. Children have smaller airways than adults and have less respiratory reserve. Infants have limited ability to recruit alveoli, and thus depend on respiratory rate to increase minute ventilation. Many toxins cause alterations in temperature, and so it is important to remember that a rectal temperature of only 38.0°C (100.4°F) in infants younger than 2 to 3 months is significant and may be associated with life-threatening infection or poisoning.

PEDIATRIC DRUG SAFETY

The concept of dose, which is central to medical toxicology, has its roots in the sixteenth-century thinking of Paracelsus (Figure 1–1), where a sufficient dose of any substance renders it toxic. But what is the "correct" dose for a child? Trial and error often determine the dose of a particular drug used. As a result, up to 75% of drugs that pediatricians have historically prescribed lack appropriate testing for safety and efficacy in the pediatric population. Pharmaceutical companies have shied away from the complexities inherent in pediatric studies, and the financial returns have been rarely worth the effort. Harry Shirkey, MD, coined the term *therapeutic orphan* in 1963 to describe the plight of children who were pre-

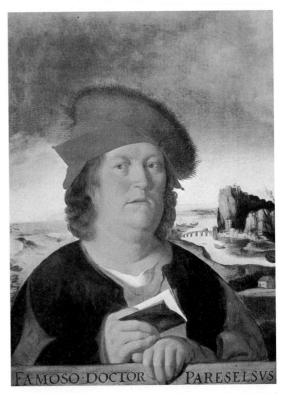

Fig. 1–1. Paracelsus, the father of toxicology, stated in his *Third Defense*, "What is there that is not poison? All things are poison and nothing [is] without poison. Solely, the dose determines that a thing is not a poison." Painting by Jan van Scorel: The Louvre, Paris.

scribed medications that were inadequately investigated. It was not until 1991, in fact, that succimer (Chemet), an oral lead chelator, became the first drug approved first for children, and later for adults. Beginning in the late 1990s, however, a series of events began to facilitate the pediatric drug investigation process. In 1997, Congress passed the Food and Drug Administration Modernization Act (FDAMA), which promised extended marketing exclusivity to companies that voluntarily developed pediatric pharmaceuticals. In 1998, the federal government adopted the *Pediatric Rule,* which ordered pharmaceutical companies to conduct clinical trials in children. In 2002, the Best Pharmaceuticals for Children Act allowed marketing exclusivity similar to that under the FDAMA. The U.S. District Court for the District of Columbia, however, rejected the Pediatric Rule on the grounds that the FDA lacked statutory authority to require pediatric trials. Rather than appealing the decision, the FDA and the AAP lobbied Congress to pass Senate bill S650, the Pediatric Research Equity Act, which was signed into law in 2003. The act grants the FDA authority to require pediatric trials to ensure safety and efficacy for use in children. A recent study reveals that the FDAMA has indeed stimulated pediatric clinical studies, with significant new dosing and safety information identified for numerous drugs.

SUMMARY

Pediatricians are among many child advocates in society. In addition to attending to medical and surgical problems that arise, pediatricians must assess a multitude of potential hazards in the environment of children. Effective advocacy extends to enlightening adult-oriented colleagues about the pitfalls of extrapolating principles of adult care to the pediatric patient. This is particularly true in the case of a poisoned child.

Children are the subjects of two thirds of all calls made to poison control centers, yet the old adage, "children are not little adults," reflects the concern that they are often viewed peripherally in an adult-centered world. Risk assessment of the poisoned child must consider the developmental stage and the dose involved in an exposure; physical evaluation should consider pediatric aspects of airway, breathing, circulation, as well as vital signs. Perhaps it is time for a new, child-centered paradigm: "Adults are not big children."

SUGGESTED READINGS

American Board of Pediatrics: *Pediatric Diplomates* (newsletter). Chapel Hill, NC: American Board of Pediatrics; Fall 2003.

Athreya BH, Silverman BK: *Pediatric Physical Diagnosis.* Norwalk, CT: Appleton-Century-Crofts; 1985.

Burda AM, Burda NM: The nation's first poison control center: taking a stand against accidental childhood poisoning in Chicago. *Vet Hum Toxicol* 39:115–119, 1997.

Deichmann WB, Henschler D, Holmstedt B, et al: What is there that is not poison? A study of the Third Defense by Paracelsus. *Arch Toxicol* 58:207–213, 1986.

Gunn VL, Nechyba C, eds: *The Harriet Lane Handbook.* 16th ed. Philadelphia: Mosby; 2002.

Liebelt EL, De Angelis CD: Evolving trends and treatment advances in pediatric poisoning. *JAMA* 282:1113–1115, 1999.

Lyons AS, Petrucelli RJ: *Medicine: An Illustrated History.* Albany, NY: Abradale Books, Harry N. Abrams, Inc; 1987: 376–377.

Roberts R, Rodriguez W, Murphy D, Crescenzi T: Pediatric drug labeling: improving the safety and efficacy of pediatric therapeutics. *JAMA* 290:905–911, 2003.

Shirkey H: Therapeutic orphans. *J Pediatr* 72:199–120, 1968.

Tenenbein M: Poisoning pearls regarding the very young. *Clin Pediatr Emerg Med* 1:176–179, 2000.

Watson WA, Litovitz L, Rodgers GC, et al: 2002 Annual report of the American Association of Poison Control Centers Toxic Surveillance System. *Am J Emerg Med* 21:353–421, 2003.

2

Pediatric Poison Prevention

Andrea Marmor

HIGH-YIELD FACTS

- The natural curiosity and exploratory behavior of young children, combined with risk factors such as improper storage of toxic substances and transient lack of supervision, make the pediatric population vulnerable to a majority of human poison exposures.

- Of the more than 2 million toxic exposures reported annually to the Toxic Exposure Surveillance System, children younger than 6 years old persistently account for 50% to 60% of reported cases.

- Although children are responsible for more than one half of all toxic exposures, they account for only a small minority of poisoning deaths.

- The majority of pediatric poisonings occur in the home, with around 15% occurring at outside locations such as a school, daycare center, or caretaker's residence.

- Efforts to reduce the incidence and impact of childhood poisonings have included primary (pre-event), secondary (event), and tertiary (post-event) prevention strategies.

Each year, more than 1 million children under age 6 years experience a toxic exposure. Although advances in poisoning prevention and treatment over the last 50 years have dramatically reduced the mortality of pediatric toxic ingestions, the high frequency of poisonings in children continues to exact a significant toll on children's health and on the health care system. To reduce this impact, the clinician's role must encompass prevention as well as management of childhood poisonings. This comprehensive approach demands an appreciation of the scope of pediatric poisonings and prevention strategies, familiarity with the unique presentations and effects of poisonings in children, and knowledge of the safest and most effective treatments.

This chapter describes the clinical and economic impacts of childhood poisoning and reviews the history and effectiveness of various primary, secondary, and tertiary prevention strategies.

IMPACT OF PEDIATRIC POISONINGS

The natural curiosity and exploratory behavior of young children, combined with risk factors such as improper storage of toxic substances and transient lack of supervision, make the pediatric population vulnerable to a majority of human poison exposures. Our understanding of the scope and pattern of pediatric toxic exposures has increased over the last 30 years, due to the development of the American Association of Poison Control Centers' (AAPCC) Toxic Exposure Surveillance System (TESS). Since its creation in 1983, TESS has grown dramatically, with its most recent report estimated to include 98.8% of human poison exposures reported to poison control centers (PCC). Data from the TESS have not only resulted in a greater understanding of the epidemiology of pediatric toxic exposure, they have been used to initiate successful educational and legislative efforts, as well as support research and training in toxicology. Of the more than 2 million toxic exposures reported annually to TESS, children younger than 6 years persistently account for 50% to 60% of reported cases. In 2002, American poison centers reporting to the AAPCC's TESS system responded to 2,380,028 human exposures. Approximately 46% of exposures involved children under the age of 3, and 52% involved children under the age of 5 (Table 2–1).

Pediatric poisoning prompted an average of 19,000 calls per poison center in 2001, and resulted in at least 120,000 visits to a health care facility. Fortunately, the vast majority of pediatric poisonings have either no or a minor clinical effect, and can be safely managed at home. In adolescents, however, for whom nearly half of toxic ingestions are intentional, 25% result in a moderate or major clinical effect. In general, when compared to ingestions in adults, events in young children are more likely to be accidental, less likely to be managed in a health care facility, and less likely to result in clinically significant effects including death.

Mortality

Although children are responsible for more than half of all toxic exposures, they account for only a small minority of poisoning deaths. In fact, whereas the overall fatality rate from poison exposures has remained relatively constant over the last 20 years, the proportion of these deaths due to children has declined, from 10.5% in 1983 to 2.4% in 2001. The absolute number of pediatric poisoning deaths has dramatically declined as well, from an

Table 2–1. Impact of Pediatric Poisonings (TESS Data)

Morbidity and mortality

Total human exposures in 2002	2,380,028
• Percent of 2002 exposures involving children <3	46
• Percent of 2002 exposures involving children <5	52
• Percent of exposures involving teens	<10
Proportion of all poisoning deaths in 1983 due to children	10.5
Proportion of all poisoning deaths in 2001 due to children	2.4
Proportion of poisoning deaths in 2001 due to teens (age 13–19)	7.2

Most common sources of pediatric toxic exposure in 2001

1. Cosmetics and personal care products (13.2%)
2. Cleaning substances (10.5%)
3. Analgesics (7.1%)
4. Plants
5. Cough and cold preparations

estimated 500 deaths per year in the 1940s to only 26 reported to TESS in 2001. This decrease is likely due to multiple factors, including successful prevention efforts targeted at the substances most likely to cause mortality, as well as improved management of pediatric poisoning victims. In contrast, poisoning deaths in the 13- to 19-year-old age group have increased steadily in the last 4 years. Although teenagers are responsible for fewer than 10% of reported poisonings overall, the substances and intent involved make them much more likely to be fatal. Teens accounted for 7.2% of total fatalities in 2001, with 75% of these ingestions being intentional, and nearly half attributed to suicide.

Although the TESS system is our most comprehensive source of data on poisoning epidemiology, several authors have pointed out that its estimates of mortality may have some limitations, because deaths that are later found to be due to poisoning may not be reported to a poison center. One study, conducted by Hoppe-Roberts in 2002, showed significant differences between TESS mortality data and that from the National Center for Health Statistics in both the overall number of pediatric poisoning deaths in 1994, and in the proportion of total poisoning deaths in children. The authors of this study urge that these differences be considered when proposing initiatives for education, policy, and research. However, because mortality among children is now so rare, current preventive and educational efforts tend to focus on modulating the still common but less fatal causes of pediatric poisoning.

Location

The majority of pediatric poisonings occur in the home, with around 15% occurring at outside locations such as a school, daycare center, or caretaker's residence. Non-pharmaceutical household products are the most frequently implicated substances in pediatric poisonings. In 2001 the most common sources of pediatric toxic exposure included cosmetics and personal care products (13.2%), cleaning substances (10.5%), and analgesics (7.1%), which along with plants and cough and cold preparations have consistently been responsible for the majority of pediatric poisonings for the past 10 years. Among pharmaceuticals, the most likely to cause significant morbidity and mortality in children include iron supplements, tricyclic antidepressants, cardiovascular medications, oral hypoglycemics, and narcotic analgesics. Due to successful prevention efforts targeted toward pharmaceuticals, most pediatric poisoning deaths in recent years have been caused by nonpharmaceutical and household products, with carbon monoxide, hydrocarbons, and caustics leading the list. In adults, however, analgesics are the most commonly ingested substance, as well as the leading cause of fatality.

Therapeutic errors are responsible for a small proportion (~4%) of poisonings in children, although in 2001 they were the reason behind 8 of the 26 pediatric deaths reported to TESS. The most common reasons for therapeutic errors in children were incorrect dosing, including taking a medication dose twice, and administration of an incorrect formulation or concentration.

Prevention

Efforts to reduce the incidence and impact of childhood poisonings have included primary (pre-event), secondary (event), and tertiary (post-event) prevention strategies (Table 2–2). The development of a national system of PCCs represents perhaps the most significant event in the history of pediatric poisoning prevention, and one that has impacted all areas of poisoning prevention. Pediatricians and pharmacists organized the first PCC in Chicago in the early 1950s, in response to an AAP report that its members lacked sources of information on the composition of medications and household products that at the time were causing a majority of childhood accidents. In the last 50 years, PCCs have evolved into a sophisticated information resource for both families and physicians. PCC use has been

shown to directly reduce health care costs, and data from PCC databases have been instrumental in identifying important causes of pediatric poisoning and initiating safety and educational measures that have had significant impact on childhood poisonings. Unfortunately, despite these multiple benefits, many of these centers are currently at risk for closure, due to insufficient funds.

Primary Prevention

Primary prevention efforts have focused on promoting actions to improve safety of the products most often implicated in pediatric poisoning, and on educational campaigns to promote awareness of poison centers and poisoning prevention strategies.

Protective packaging is a particularly successful example of passive injury prevention, and a model of collaboration between physicians, manufacturers, and legislative policy makers. Since Congress enacted the Poison Prevention Packaging Act in 1970, child-resistant closures are now required by law on all prescription drugs and dangerous household products. Several studies have confirmed the significant impact protective packaging has had on childhood poisonings. Most recently, Rodgers reported that the use of child-resistant packaging for oral prescription drugs since 1974 has reduced mortality by 45% from that projected without protective packaging, controlling for overall changes in prescription drug con-

Table 2–2. Strategis for Poisoning Prevention

	Strategy	**Examples**
Primary	Reduce the occurrence of pediatric poisonings	*Passive* –Protective packaging –Reduced alkali concentrations in household products *Active* –Warning labels on poisonous products –Home safety educational campaigns –Education during primary care visits
Secondary	Reduce the impact of a poisoning event on the child, once it has occurred	–Promotion of PCC use –Improved availability of accurate product information –Improved access to trained poison professionals –Home decontamination strategies (activated charcoal)
Tertiary	Minimize the impact of pediatric poisonings on the child and health care system	–Support for education and research regarding decontamination and management –Building of PCC databases –Growth of specialty field of toxicology

Abbreviation: PCC, Poison Control Center.

sumption and unintentional death rates in children. The U.S. Consumer Product Safety Commission has estimated that 800 children's lives have been saved since requirements for child-resistant packaging of aspirin and oral prescription medications in 1974. Deaths from salicylate overdose, formerly a major cause of mortality in children, have decreased by more than 80% since the 1960s. However, difficulty using child-resistant containers and failure to comply with regulations allow pharmaceuticals to remain a significant cause of childhood poisonings. A survey by the Centers for Disease Control and Prevention found that child-resistant containers had been replaced in nearly 20% of homes in which poisonings occurred in young children, and that nearly 20% of the drugs ingested belonged to grandparents, who often have difficulty opening child-resistant containers. Additional examples of successful passive primary prevention include the use of strip packaging to reduce the number of tablets ingested by a child, and reduced alkali concentrations from 30% to 5% in caustic household products.

Active primary preventions strategies such as education and awareness campaigns have not proven as effective. For example, warning labels campaigns, such as *Mr. Yuk* stickers, although highly recognizable by parents, have not been shown to significantly reduce childhood poisonings. In general, legislative and engineering actions such as safety packaging have made the most measurable impact on childhood poisoning; educational efforts have proven more difficult to assess. Despite the lack of proven efficacy, reviewing home poisoning prevention strategies continues to be a focus of the pediatric primary care visit, and the physician treating a poisoned child has a unique opportunity to review and reinforce these measures. The following items relevant to pediatric poisoning are suggested by the AAP as part of a home safety checklist for parents, which can be found on their web site (http://www.aap.org).

- Are there child-resistant caps on all medications, including vitamins, and are all medications stored in their original containers?
- Do you need a doorknob cover to prevent your child from going into the bathroom when you are not there?
- Are there child-resistant safety latches on all cabinets containing potentially harmful substances (cosmetics, medications, mouthwash, cleaning supplies)?
- Are dangerous products stored out of reach in cabinets with safety latches or locks or on high shelves, and in their original containers in the utility room, basement, and garage?

- Are the numbers of the Poison Control Center and your pediatrician posted on all phones?
- Teach your child to never pick and eat anything from a plant.
- Be sure you know what is growing in your yard so, if your child accidentally ingests a plant, you can give the proper information to your local Poison Control Center.

Secondary Prevention

Secondary prevention strategies include promoting the use of the PCC, improving the availability of accurate product information and trained poison professionals, and home decontamination.

Because most pediatric toxic exposures result in no or minor symptoms, the majority can be managed at home with proper consultation. Use of a PCC, therefore, can prevent unnecessary visits to a health care facility, and may help to minimize clinical impact by allowing a parent to begin therapeutic intervention early. Studies have firmly established that PCCs are effective in reducing hospital use and health expenditures, without an accompanying increase in morbidity. In one study by Miller, for example, use of a PCC reduced the number of patients of all ages requiring medical treatment by 24%, and saved approximately $175 per call in other medical expenditures. The cost effectiveness of PCCs has also been consistently shown, with savings far exceeding the operating budget of the center. The impact of PCC use on morbidity and mortality has been more difficult to quantify, because most childhood poisonings result in minimal clinical effects. However, avoiding unnecessary procedures and trauma associated with a visit to a health care facility must be considered a potential clinical benefit of the use of a PCC.

Owing to the clear economic benefits and theoretical clinical benefits of PCC use in childhood poisonings, increasing awareness and utilization among parents has been a major secondary prevention strategy. Most efforts have focused on educational campaigns. Poison center phone numbers are now found in the front of most telephone books, and certified centers are required to be available 24 hours a day, 7 days a week (Fig. 2–1). Studies of parental awareness have helped to identify groups of parents with barriers to awareness and use of poison centers. Low-income, minority, and non–English-speaking parents appear to be at particularly high risk, and at least one intervention targeting one of these high-risk groups—an instructional video in Spanish for parents attending educational

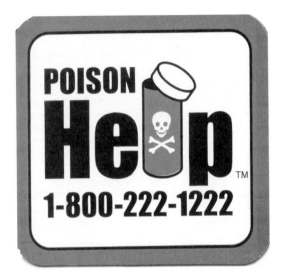

Fig. 2–1. Regional poison control centers are now easily contacted using a national toll-free telephone number.

classes—was shown to be highly effective in changing knowledge, attitudes, and behavioral intentions in parents. However, additional study is needed to further characterize the most effective methods for identifying and reaching target groups of parents.

Another focus of secondary prevention is on increasing availability of accurate information and qualified professionals in the event of a poisoning. The development of the POISINDEX computerized information resource system has been a major step toward this goal. The system allows PCCs to access product information and treatment protocols developed by toxicologists, and is integrated with TESS for collection of product event data. Success rate in retrieving product information from POISINDEX is estimated at 95%. Recent growth of the field of toxicology has resulted in a marked increase in the training and availability of certified specialists. The impact of these efforts to provide quality care was estimated in one study, which found that a regionalized PCC staffed by certified professionals was nine times as likely as a nonregionalized center to dispense accurate information.

Home Decontamination

Home decontamination as a secondary prevention strategy has encountered considerable controversy in recent years. Among the most notable evolving trends in pediatric poisoning prevention has been an increasing emphasis on expectant management, with an accompanying reexamination of the role for home gastrointestinal decontamination. Although syrup of ipecac has historically been one of the most widely and successfully promoted poisoning prevention strategies, its use is no longer recommended in health care facilities, and it has recently fallen out of favor for home use as well. As of 2003, the AAP no longer recommends the use of ipecac in the prehospital or emergency department setting. Since 1983 the reported use of decontamination with either ipecac or activated charcoal (AC) has dropped by more than 50%, mostly attributable to a marked decrease in the use of ipecac from 14% to less than 1%. With AC replacing ipecac as the recommended decontamination choice in health care facilities, the benefits of home decontamination and the question of whether guidance and educational efforts should focus on replacing ipecac with AC for home use has been hotly debated. Although some studies have demonstrated that syrup of ipecac or AC can be safely and effectively administered at home, thereby lowering time to decontamination and the need for referral to the ED, some authors propose a more selective role for home decontamination. They point out that the majority of pediatric poisonings do not require decontamination at all, and that in cases where decontamination is recommended, time to administration of AC is short even when purchased in a pharmacy. In addition, evidence is lacking for any positive effect of home decontamination on clinical outcome. The controversy will likely continue until additional evidence clarifies the role of home decontamination in pediatric poisoning.

Tertiary Prevention

Tertiary prevention seeks to minimize the effects of a poisoning on both the child and the health care system once it has occurred. Strategies include support for education and research regarding effective decontamination and management strategies.

The growth of PCC databases has been an important tool in improving our understanding of rare toxic events, and lends support to initiatives for investigation and training. Additionally, the training of specialized professionals in toxicology has resulted in a considerable increase in quantity and quality of information and research in this growing field. For example, research into management of the most common and dangerous ingestions have led to the development of individual antidotes, such as *N*-acetylcysteine for acetaminophen poisoning, Fab antibodies for digoxin, and fomepizole for toxic alcohols. Appreciation for the complexities of toxicology has led to increased training of students, residents, and faculty in the diagnosis and management of toxic ingestion, and the creation of a board-certified specialty. This greater number of physicians with training and interest in this important area is essential in promoting further advancement in all areas of prevention and management of childhood poisoning.

ROLE OF THE TREATING PHYSICIAN IN POISONING PREVENTION

The physician treating a child with a toxic ingestion has a valuable opportunity, as well as a duty, to prevent future poisonings. Once the child is medically stable, the physician should probe the circumstances surrounding the poisoning, as well as the overall social environment of the child. Risk factors such as lack of supervision, poor understanding of the child's capabilities, or inadequate storage of potentially toxic substances may be addressed with parental education or, if needed, social services. If the parent appropriately accessed the PCC this action should be reinforced; if not, find out what barriers were present and address them. Although its benefits are somewhat controversial, the physician may want to recommend the presence of AC at home, for use only if advised by the PCC. Whenever possible, the child's primary care physician should be notified so that he or she may continue the process of assessing home safety and parental educational needs.

The physician must also support the continued growth and availability of poison information resources, including PCCs and continued research efforts. Certified PCCs, despite proven cost-effectiveness, are threatened by lack of funding, and several large state centers have already closed. Physicians can advocate at the local and national levels for continued funding of these important resources. Areas that require further research by interested and qualified physicians include clarifying the impact of education, home decontamination, and other prevention strategies on clinical outcomes. This information is essential to continued development and support of effective poisoning prevention efforts.

SUGGESTED READINGS

American Academy of Pediatrics: *Home Safety Checklist.* Elk Grove Village, Ill: AAP Publications; 1999.

American Academy of Pediatrics, Committee on Injury, Violence, and Poison Prevention: Poison treatment in the home. *Pediatrics* 112:1182–1185, 2003.

American Academy of Clinical Toxicology, European Association of Poison Centres and Clinical Toxicologists: position statement: single dose charcoal. *Clin Toxicol* 35:721–774, 1997.

American Academy of Clinical Toxicology, European Association of Poison Centres and Clinical Toxicologists. Position statement: ipecac syrup. *Clin Toxicol* 35:699–709, 1997.

Bond GR: Home use of syrup of ipecac is associated with a reduction in pediatric emergency department visits. *Ann Emerg Med* 25:338–343, 1995.

Bond GR: Activated charcoal in the home: helpful and important or simply a distraction? *Pediatrics* 109:145–146, 2002.

Bond GR: The role of activated charcoal and gastric emptying in gastrointestinal decontamination: a state-of-the-art review. *Ann Emerg Med* 39:273–286, 2002.

Hoppe-Roberts JM, Lloyd LM, Chyka PA: Poisoning mortality in the United States: comparison of National Mortality Statistics and poison control center reports. *Ann Emerg Med* 35:440–448, 2000.

Kelly NR: Assessing parental utilization of the poison center: an emergency center-based survey. *Clin Pediatr* 36:467–473, 1997.

Kelly NR: Effects of a videotape to increase use of poison control centers by low-income and Spanish-speaking families: a randomized, controlled trial. *Pediatrics* 111:21–26, 2003.

Liebelt EL: Evolving trends and treatment advances in pediatric poisoning. *JAMA* 282:1113–1115, 1999.

Litovitz TL, Klein-Schwartz W, Rodgers GC, et al: 2001 annual report of the American Association of Poison Control Centers' Toxic Exposure Surveillance System. *Am J Emerg Med* 20:391–452, 2002.

Litovitz TL, Watson WA, Rodgers Jr GC, et al: 2002 annual report of the American Association of Poison Control Centers Toxic Exposure Surveillance System. *Am J Emerg Med* 21:353–421, 2003.

Lovejoy Jr FH: Poison centers, poison prevention, and the pediatrician. *Pediatrics* 94:220–224, 1994.

Miller TR, Lestina DC: Costs of poisoning in the United States and savings from poison control centers: a benefit-cost analysis. *Ann Emerg Med* 29:239–245, 1997.

Miller T, Lestina D: The costs of poisoning in the U.S. and the savings from poison control centers: A benefit–cost analysis. In *Government Financial Options to Preserve and Expand Poison Control Centers: A Report to Congress.* Landover, Md: National Public Services Research Institute; 1995.

Rivara FP, Grossman D: Injury control. In: Behrman RE, Kliegman RM, Jenson H, eds: *Nelson Textbook of Pediatrics.* 16th ed. Philadelphia: Saunders; 2000:231–237.

Robertson WO: Conflicting views in poison treatment (letter). *Pediatrics* 110:199–200, 2002.

Rodgers GB: The safety effects of child-resistant packaging for oral prescription drugs. Two decades of experience. *JAMA* 275:1661–1665, 1996.

Spiller HA: Conflicting views in poison treatment (letter). *Pediatrics* 110:199–200, 2002.

Spiller HA, Rodgers GC: Evaluation of administration of activated charcoal in the home. *Pediatrics* 108:E100, 2001.

Thompson DR, Trammel HL, Robertson NJ, et al: Evaluation of regional and nonregional poison centers. *N Engl J Med* 308:191–194, 1983.

Wan C, Cardus L, McGreevy B, et al: Content audit of POISINDEX. *Vet Hum Toxicol* 35:168–169, 1993.

3

Poison Control Centers

Michael S. Wahl
Jerrold B. Leikin
Mark Thoman

HIGH-YIELD FACTS

- Poison control centers are staffed primarily by health care personnel who have received training in toxicology.
- In 2002, 2,380,028 human exposures were reported to the American Association of Poison Control Center Toxic Exposure Surveillance System by 64 poison control centers nationwide.
- Approximately 46% of exposures involved children under the age of 3, and 52% involved children under the age of 5.
- It is estimated that for every $1 spent on poison control services, $7 dollars are saved by preventing unnecessary utilization of health care services.
- Poison control centers can provide health care professionals with treatment recommendations necessary to treat severely poisoned patients.

In the early 1900s, toxicology was viewed as an esoteric field of medicine. It was essentially ignored in medical schools and not regarded as a separate discipline. However, since 1953, when the first poison information hot line opened in Chicago, poison control centers have emerged as an integral part of the nation's health care system, and toxicology has developed into a recognized medical specialty.

As poison control centers began to flourish, the American Association of Poison Centers (AAPCC) was cre-

ated in 1958 for the purpose of developing educational programs for health care providers and, more importantly, standardizing the operation of poison control centers. Currently, criteria for AAPCC designation as a regional poison control include:

- A geographically defined region with a population base of 1 to 10 million people.
- Twenty-four hour a day availability to the general public and health care providers.
- Written protocols to guide staff on triage criteria.
- The availability of specialists, including a medical director in toxicology, who have passed a AAPCC certifying examination.
- Regional data collection to be reported to Toxic Exposure Surveillance System (TESS) for identifying trends, epidemiology, and new and emerging poisoning hazards.
- Educational programs for the general public and health care professionals (Table 3–1).

In the 1980s and 1990s there was a decline in the number of poison control centers, from 104 in 1991 to 64 in 2002 in the United States (52 of which were certified by the AAPCC). An updated list of poison control centers can be obtained from the AAPCC web site, www.aapcc.org.

In 2002, poison centers responded to an average 8.2 human exposures per 1000 population served. In 2002, American poison centers reporting to the AAPCC's TESS system responded to 2,380,028 human exposures. In addition to human exposure calls, poison centers also manage cases involving animal exposures, and supply information on poisons, poison prevention, drugs and drug identification, teratogenicity, as well as occupational, medical, and environmental concerns.

Table 3–1. American Association of Poison Control Centers Criteria for Regional Poison Center Certification

- The center must maintain comprehensive reference sources on poisonings.
- The center must serve a geographic area with a population base of optimally less than 10 million people.
- The center must operate 24 hours a day/365 days per year and be readily accessible by telephone.
- The center must participate in AAPCC's national data collection system, the Toxic Exposure Surveillance System (TESS).
- The center must be staffed at all times by licensed pharmacists, nurses, and/or physicians who attained additional training in clinical toxicology.
- The center must utilize and maintain protocols, follow-up guidelines, and quality assurance strategies that provide consistent approaches in the evaluation and treatment of the poisoned patient.
- The center must have a medical director and a managing director, and these directors must have specific qualifications.
- The center must have an ongoing quality improvement program.
- The center must provide education for the public and for health care professionals.

The administrative structures of a regional poison control center vary. Each center must have a managing director and a medical director; in some centers, a single individual fulfills both requirements. About half of the AAPCC-certified poison centers have a managing director certified by the American Board of Applied Toxicology (ABAT). Similarly, the medical director in an AAPCC-certified regional poison control center is usually certified in medical toxicology, either by the former American Board of Medical Toxicology, which has been replaced by the current American College of Medical Toxicology. Subspecialty certification in medical toxicology is sponsored jointly by the American Boards of Emergency Medicine, Pediatrics, and Preventative Medicine. In addition, most poison control centers maintain a list of non-physician consultants, who may include botanists, mycologists, zoologists, entomologists, and herpetologists.

In the United States, poison control centers are primarily information providers and do not provide direct treatment or stock antidotes. However, these centers are aware of the location of important antidotes stocked by hospitals and medical centers. Although the Joint Commission on Accreditation of Health Care Organizations does not address the specific criteria regarding antidote storage and availability, guidelines have been developed by the American Academy of Clinical Toxicology regarding recommended antidote availability. Suggested minimum stock quantities of antidotes are listed in Table 3–2.

The cost effectiveness of poison control centers has been evaluated in several studies. Because approximately 75% of reported toxic exposures are treated at home, poison control centers truly represent the nation's first successful attempt at home health care services. An economic analysis performed for the U.S. Department of Health and Human Services found that for every $1 spent on poison control services there was a result of $7 in medical savings. When compared with other cost-saving preventive health measures for children, only immunizations afford more cost savings (Fig. 3–1). Another analysis compared 1992 data on incidence, medical spending, and payment sources for poisoning in jurisdictions with and without poison control center services. The study found that access to a poison control center reduced the number of patients receiving medical treatment for poisoning by 24%; hospitalization was reduced by 12%. Each call from the public into a poison control center actually saved an estimated $175 in other medical spending in 1992. Because the average call cost to a poison center, including indirect costs, was approximately $28, this resulted in about $6.50 saved in medical care payments for each dollar spent on poison center services (Table 3–3). This amounted to an estimated reduction of $355 million nationally in medical spending. Increasing regional poison control center coverage to the entire U.S. population would be expected to result in a significant cost saving. In spite of these obvious financial benefits, poison control centers have continued to struggle for survival. However, government agencies are becoming increasingly aware of the benefits of these centers, and the potential dilemma facing the nation if more poison control centers close.

Poison control centers are essential to the future of clinical toxicology (Table 3–3). The poison center can play a central role in diagnosis, management, and resource coordination in the wake of a biological, chemical, or nuclear mass casualty disaster. Advances in telemedicine and digital photography can make poison referral more complete, which in turn can maximize the effectiveness of recommendations. In addition to providing outpatient assessment of exposures or sophisticated

Table 3–2. Uses and Suggested Minimum Stock Quantities for 25 Selected Antidotes

Antidote	Suggested Minimum Stock Quantity
N-Acetylcysteine (Mucomyst)	600 mL in 10- or 30-mL vials of 20% solution
Amyl nitrite, sodium nitrite, sodium thiosulfate (cyanide antidote kit)	Three antidote kits
Antivenin polyvalent (Crotalidae)—equine origin	10 vials (*Note:* 30 vials or more may be needed in serious cases)
Atropine sulfate	Five vials, 20 mL/vial (0.4 mg/mL) and twenty 10-mL (0.1 mg/mL) ampules. Total: 60 mg
Black widow spider antivenin (*Latrodectus mactans* antivenin)	One vial
Calcium disodium EDTA (Versenate)	Two 5-mL ampules, 200 mg/mL
Calcium gluconate, calcium chloride	10% calcium gluconate: Five 10-mL vials 10% calcium chloride: Five 10-mL vials
Deferoxamine mesylate (Desferal)	Twelve 500-mg vials
Digoxin immune Fab (Digibind)	20 vials
Dimercaprol (BAL in oil)	Ten 3-mL (100 mg/mL) ampules
Ethanol	8 L of 10% EtOH in D_5W and 1 pint 95% ethanol
Flumazenil (Romazicon)	Twenty 5-mL vials or ten 10-mL vials. Each has 0.1 mg/mL. Total: 10 mg
Folinic acid (Leucovorin), folic acid	Folinic acid: six 50-mg vials Folic acid: six 50-mg vials
Fomepizole (Antizol)	1.5 g/vial, 4 vials
Glucagon	Fifty 1-mg vials (may offer only 5–10 h of treatment in serious cases). A 10-mg/10-mL vial is no longer available from the manufacturer.
Hyperbaric oxygen (HBO)	Post the location and phone number of nearest HBO chamber.
Methylene blue	Ten 10-mL (10 mg/mL) ampules
Naloxone (Narcan)	Naloxene: fifty 1-mL ampules (0.4 mg/mL)
D-Penicillamine (Cuprimine)	Bottle of 100 capsules: 125 mg or 250 mg/capsule
Physostigmine salicylate (Antilirium)	Ten 2-mL (1 mg/mL) ampules
Phytonadione, vitamin K_1 (AquaMEPHYTON, Mephyton)	Two 0.5-mL ampules (2 mg/mL) and two 5-mL ampules (10 mg/mL)
Pralidoxime chloride, 2 PAM (Protopam)	1 g/kit, five kits
Pyridoxine hydrochloride, vitamin B_6	Twenty-five 10-mL (1 g) vials or eight 30-mL (3 g) vials
Sodium bicarbonate	Twenty-five 20-mEq vials
Succimer (Chemet)	Bottle of 100 capsules; 100 mg/capsule

Source: Modified from Burda AM: Poison antidotes: Issues of inadequate stocking with review of uses of 24 common antidotal agents. *J Pharm Pract* 10:235–248, 1997.

toxicology expertise to health care personnel, poison control centers serve as a training site for students, residents, pharmacists, physicians, and medical toxicology fellows. Fellowship-trained physicians are certified in medical toxicology through the medical toxicology subboard administered by the American Board of Emergency Medicine. Pharmacists and other qualified individuals in related specialties can be certified in toxicology by the ABAT. Medical Review Officer training and certification for Department of Transportation drug analysis can be obtained through the American College of Occupational and Environmental Medicine or the American Association of Medical Review Officers. As a focal point for these activities, the poison control center is critical to the training of all aspiring toxicologists and provides a venue to practice this specialty.

Table 3–3. Summary of Health and Economic Benefits of a Regional Poison Control Center

- Reduction of unnecessary emergency department visits and inappropriate use of medical resources.
- Decreased burden on a region's emergency medical transportation system.
- Reduction in adverse effects resulting from the use of outdated or hazardous first aid procedures in the home.
- A reduction in the time required to diagnose and establish definitive care for the poisoned victim.
- Minimizing public health effects of community exposure to toxic materials.
- Early detection and elimination of unusually hazardous commercial products through regulatory notification, recall, repackaging, reformulation, or product discontinuation.
- Improved care of poisoning victims, decreasing disabilities and costly long-term medical care.
- Reduced incidence of unintentional poisoning in the home and workplace.

- Enhanced management of drug-addicted patients by providing recommendations, referrals, and assistance.
- Reduced exposure to potential toxins during pregnancy.
- Improved patient care by educating physicians, nurses, paramedics, and other health care professionals in poison management and medical toxicology.
- Public education on poison prevention and injury prevention in the home and workplace.
- Toxicosurveillance on data collected by poison centers, which can identify hidden epidemics such as food poisoning or new emerging adverse drug effects.
- Resource for hospitals and general public for mass disaster from biological, chemical, or nuclear incidents or release.

SUGGESTED READINGS

American Academy of Clinical Toxicology: Facility assessment guidelines for regional toxicology treatment centers. *J Toxicol Clin Toxicol* 31:211–217, 1993.

Bindl L, Ruchardt J, Pfeiffer A, et al: Effect of a German poison control center on health care cost reductions in harmless exposure cases. *Vet Hum Toxicol* 39:48–50, 1997.

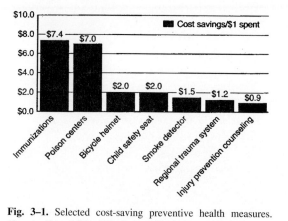

Fig. 3–1. Selected cost-saving preventive health measures. (*Source:* From Miller TR: Government Options to Preserve and Expand Poison Control Centers: A Report to Congress.)

Botticelli JT, Pierpaoli PG: Louis Gdalman, pioneer in hospital pharmacy poison information services. *Am J Hosp Pharm* 49:1445–1450, 1992.

Burda AM: Poison antidotes: issues of inadequate stocking with review of uses of 24 common antidotal agents. *J Pharm Pract* 10:235–248, 1997.

Burda AM, Burda NM: The nation's first poison control center: taking a stand against accidental childhood poisoning in Chicago. *Vet Hum Toxicol* 39:115–119, 1997.

Chyka PA, Conner HG: Availability of antidotes in rural and urban hospitals in Tennessee. *Am J Hosp Pharm* 51:1346–1348, 1994.

Dart RC, Stark Y: Insufficient stocking of poisoning antidotes in hospital pharmacies. *JAMA* 276:1508–1510, 1996.

Davis NM: Insufficient stocking of poisoning antidotes. *Hosp Pharm* 32:1078–1103, 1997.

de Garbino JP, Haines JA, Jacobsen D, et al: Evaluation of antidotes: activities of the International Programme on Chemical Safety. *J Toxicol Clin Toxicol* 35:333–343, 1997.

Felberg L, Litovitz TL, Morgan J: State of the nation's poison centers: 1995 American Association of Poison Control Centers survey of U. S. poison centers. *Vet Hum Toxicol* 38:445–453, 1996.

Freeman G: Is your pharmacy sufficiently stocked? Lack of key supplies is a liability risk. *Healthcare Risk Manage* 19:1–12, 1997.

Geller RJ, Fisher JG III, Leeper JD, et al: American poison control centers: still the same? *Ann Emerg Med* 17:599–603, 1988.

Harrison DL, Draugalis J, Slack MK, et al: Cost effectiveness of regional poison control centers. *Arch Intern Med* 156:2601–2608, 1996.

Howland MA, Weisman R, Sauter D, et al: Non-availability of poison antidotes. *N Engl J Med* 314:927–928, 1986.

Joint Commission on Accreditation of Healthcare Organizations (JCAHO): *1994 Accreditation Manual for Hospitals.* Oakbrook Terrance, IL: JCAHO; 1994:162.

Kanatani MS, Kearney TE, Levin RH, et al: Treatment of toxicologic emergencies—antidote preparedness: an evaluation of Bay area hospital pharmacies and its impact on emergency planning. *Vet Hum Toxicol* 34:319, 1992.

Kelly NR, Ellis MD, Kirkland RT, et al: Effectiveness of a poison center: impact on medical facility visits. *Vet Hum Toxicol* 39:44–48, 1997.

Litovitz T, Kearney TE, Holm K. et al: Poison control centers: is there an antidote for budget cuts? *Am J Emerg Med* 12:585–599, 1994.

Litovitz TL, Watson WA, Rodgers Jr GC, et al: 2002 Annual report of the American Association of Poison Control Centers Toxic Exposure Surveillance System. *Am J Emerg Med* 21:353–421, 2003.

Miller TR: Government Financial Options to Preserve and Expand Poison Control Centers: A Report to Congress.

Miller TR, Lestina DC: Costs of poisoning in the United States and savings from poison control centers: a benefit-cost analysis. *Ann Emerg Med* 29:239–245, 1997.

Parker DP, Dart RC, McNally JJ: Critical deficiencies in the treatment of toxicologic emergencies: antidote stocking in Arizona hospitals. *Vet Hum Toxicol* 32:376, 1990.

Scherger DL, Wrik KM, Dart RC: Disaster planning: how poison centers can prepare. *J Toxicol Clin Toxicol* 40:672, 2002.

Scherz RG, Robertson WO: The history of poison control centers in the United States. *J Toxicol Clin Toxicol* 12:291–296, 1978.

Spoeke DG: Guide to the acquisition, storage, and use of antidotes. *Am J Hosp Pharm* 38:498–506, 1981.

U.S. Consumer Product Safety Commission: *Poison Prevention Packaging: A Text for Pharmacists and Physicians.* Washington, DC: USCPSC;1993:5–7.

Vicas I, Kaczowowka R, Cull M, et al: Teletoxicology: A feasibility study. *J Toxicol Clin Toxicol* 40:671, 2002.

Williams RM: Are poison control centers cost-effective? *Ann Emerg Med* 29:246–247, 1997.

Woolf AD, Chrisanthus K: On site availability of selected antidotes: results of a survey of Massachusetts hospitals. *Am J Emerg Med* 15:62–66, 1997.

4

Maternal–Fetal Toxicology

Kirk L. Cumpston
Timothy B. Erickson

HIGH-YIELD FACTS

- Appropriate treatment of the mother will result in optimal treatment of the fetus.

- A one-time exposure to most drugs is unlikely to cause a teratogenic effect.

- If the fetus is exposed to a toxin between 20 and 60 days of gestation most often it will either spontaneously abort, or survive without abnormalities.

- Because of decreased gastrointestinal (GI) motility, gastric decontamination may be effective longer following an ingestion in the pregnant patient.

- Ipecac is contraindicated in the pregnant patient.

- Because of the oxygen-binding properties of fetal hemoglobin, the fetus is more susceptible to hypoxia in an acidotic state.

- Every female overdose patient of child-bearing age should have a pregnancy test.

As a general rule, the management of any pregnant patient that is exposed to a toxin is: "Treat the mother and you will treat the fetus." Despite this simplistic statement, there are well-described intricacies to a number of obstetric poisons that require a more in-depth review. There are some scenarios, such as the safety and utility of antidotes, which are unique to the pregnant patient. This chapter includes discussions of teratology, general management, abortifacients, common pharmaceuticals, environmental toxins, and drugs of abuse to which the pregnant patient may be exposed.

Exposure to a toxin can occur in different settings. The first involves the mother desiring to inflict harm upon herself by overdosing on medications. In another, the pregnant individual wants to harm the fetus or induce an abortion. A third setting involves accidental exposure of the pregnant mother to an environmental toxin such as lead or carbon monoxide. The final scenario is the pregnant patient abusing recreational drugs.

Statistically, overdose in pregnancy is a more common method of suicide attempt than gun shot wounds, self-mutilation, and jumping from high places. The mortality of the mother is relatively low, at 1% to 5%. However, the morbidity suffered by the mother and the fetus can be significant. Specifically, the surviving fetus may suffer lifelong effects from a prenatal exposure.

TERATOLOGY

The United States Food and Drug Administration (FDA) has developed a well-known system that categorizes the potential risk of teratogenicity to the fetus when the mother is exposed to a drug (Table 4–1.) These classifications must be interpreted with caution. Category A simply means that controlled studies in women fail to demonstrate a risk to the fetus. Category B means either animal studies have or have not demonstrated a risk to the fetus, and there are no controlled studies in women. Category C means either adverse effects have been discovered in animals, and there are no controlled studies in humans, or there are no studies in women or animals. Category D states there is a risk of teratogenicity to the human fetus, but if the therapeutic benefits of the drug to the pregnant woman outweigh the risks of teratogenicity

Table 4–1. Pregnancy Categories for Medications

A Controlled studies in pregnant women fail to demonstrate a risk to the fetus in the first trimester with no evidence of risk in later trimesters. The possibility of fetal harm appears remote.

B Either animal reproduction studies have not demonstrated a fetal risk, but there are no controlled studies in pregnant women, or animal reproduction studies have shown an adverse effect (other than a decrease in fertility) that was not confirmed in controlled studies in women in the first trimester and there is no evidence of a risk in later trimesters.

C Studies in animals have revealed adverse effects on the fetus (teratogenic or embryocidal effects or other). These agents should be used only if the potential benefits justify the potential risk to the fetus.

D There is positive evidence of human fetal risk, but the benefits from use in pregnant women may be acceptable despite the potential risk to the fetus.

X Studies in animals or human beings have demonstrated fetal abnormalities, or there is evidence of fetal risk.

Table 4–2. Physiologic Changes in Pregnancy

General
    Increased body mass (25% by term)
    Increased body water by 7–8 L
    Increased total body fat 3–4 kg (25%)
    Increased body temperature by 0.5°C

Gastrointestinal
    Increased nausea and vomiting
    Increased gastrointestinal reflux
    Decreased gastric acidity
    Decreased gastric motility
    Decreased small bowel motility
    Increased stomach emptying time

Cardiovascular
    Increased cardiac output (35% by 10 weeks; 50% by 25 weeks)
    Increased heart rate by 20%
    Decreased peripheral vascular resistance
    Increased peripheral blood flow
    Increased oxygen consumption by 20%
    Decreased oxygen extraction

Pulmonary
    Increased ventilatory response to CO_2
    Increased arterial Po_2 by 10 mmHg
    Decreased arterial Pco_2 by 10 mmHg
    Increased minute ventilation by 50%
    Increased respiratory rate by up to 15%

Renal
    Decreased urine concentration
    Increased ADH secretion
    Increased aldosterone secretion
    Increased plasma volume by 50%
    Increased extracellular fluid space by 70%
    Increased renal plasma flow
    Decreased serum creatinine and BUN

Urogenital
    Increased weight of uterus by 400% at 10 weeks and 2000% by term

Blood
    Increased blood volume by 40%
    Increased plasma volume by 50%
    Decreased hematocrit by 15%
    Decreased serum iron
    Increased WBC count by 66%
    Decreased serum albumin and protein
    Decreased plasma cholinesterase by 20%

Source: Adapted from Erickson T, Neylan V: Management principles of overdose in pregnancy. In: Haddad LM, Winchester JF, Shannon MW, eds: *Clinical Management of Poisoning and Drug Overdose.* 3rd ed. Philadelphia: Saunders; 1998:266–267.

to the fetus, its use is acceptable. Category X clearly states these drugs are contraindicated in pregnancy due to demonstrated fetal abnormalities in humans. The most challenging category is C. A majority of pharmaceuticals fall into this classification. The "safety" of category C may be based more on the absence of data than on the absence of proven teratogenic effects.

The potential for teratogenicity is often a concern even in a one-time exposure to a drug. According to studies by Czeizel and co-workers, when 1400 acute overdoses in pregnant women were followed over 30 years, there was no increase in congenital abnormalities when compared to women who did not overdose. If the fetus is exposed between 20 and 60 days of gestation, it either spontaneously aborts or survives without abnormalities.

Physiology of Pregnancy

Maternal Physiology

The hormonal effects of pregnancy cause delayed gastric emptying, decreased GI motility, and prolonged transit time, which may delay absorption but allow for an increased total absorption of an ingested toxin. This may theoretically permit increased decontamination of the drug before absorption, or allow delayed decontamination. However, when a patient presents late after an ingestion, a greater amount of the drug may have been absorbed in the pregnant verses a nonpregnant patient.

The minute ventilation increases in the pregnant patient by up to 50%. This may be beneficial in some overdoses, and detrimental in others. Pregnancy increases the glomerular filtration rate, allowing rapid elimination of drugs excreted in the urine, such as lithium. Dermal absorption is increased because of increased body surface area and blood flow. An increase in serum concentration of a drug can result from an increased volume of distribution (V_d) secondary to increased body fat and plasma volume. A lower serum albumin will also increase the amount of free drug. Therefore, accurately predicting toxicity in a pregnant patient can be difficult (Table 4–2).

Placental Physiology

The placenta is a semipermeable membrane that allows substances weighing less than 1000 D to flow across according to the concentration gradient. In general, particles are more likely to cross if they have a small molecular weight, low lipid solubility, neutral charge, and low protein binding. Iron is unique in that it moves across the placenta by receptor-mediated endocytosis.

Fetal Physiology

The main physiologic concern in the fetus is hypoxia. The fetal oxyhemoglobin disassociation curve lies to the left of the maternal oxyhemoglobin disassociation curve (Figure 4–1). Fetal hemoglobin has a higher affinity for oxygen than the maternal hemoglobin at the same partial pressure of oxygen. This allows oxygen to transfer from the maternal hemoglobin to the fetal hemoglobin under normal circumstances. When the mother has ingested a toxin causing cardiovascular instability or respiratory depression, the fetal circulation is influenced by the maternal hypoxia and acidosis. The fetus suffers from the same circulatory shock as the mother, resulting in a shift of the fetal oxyhemoglobin dissociation curve to the right. Because the fetal oxyhemoglobin dissociation curve has a hyperbolic shape, there is an exaggerated decrease in the binding of oxygen to fetal hemoglobin at lower partial pressures of oxygen, and an earlier release of oxygen at higher partial pressures.

The fetal response to hypoxia is vagally mediated apnea, bradycardia, systolic hypertension, peripheral vasoconstriction, and lactate production. The peripheral vasoconstriction shunts the majority of the blood flow to the critical organs such as the brain and heart, which theoret-

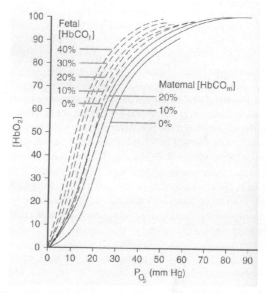

Fig. 4–1. Oxygen dissociation curve of maternal and fetal hemoglobin showing effects of carbon monoxide (CO). (Adapted from Longo [1977].)

ically increases the amount of toxin carried to these critical organs. Unfortunately the effects of toxicity exhibited in the mother may be magnified in the fetus.

GENERAL MANAGEMENT OF POISONINGS IN PREGNANCY

Support of the maternal airway, breathing, circulation, and neurologic status improves the ability of the fetus to survive a toxic insult. Treatment of hypotension in the pregnant patient differs than in the nonpregnant patient. The first step is to move the patient to the left lateral decubitus position to move the fundus of the gravid uterus off of the inferior vena cava. This may increase central venous pressure, resulting in increased circulatory perfusion. After this, resuscitation with isotonic fluids should proceed. Treatment of dysrhythmias with cardiac medications or unsynchronized cardioversion are indicated as with the nonpregnant patient. Mental status depression is empirically treated with oxygen, dextrose, and naloxone. Although fetal opioid withdrawal may occur, the benefits of reversing the mother's hypoxia from opioid overdose are greater than the risks. Fetal monitoring should be initiated as soon as possible. Emergent cesarean section may be necessary if monitoring indicates fetal compromise in the late stages of pregnancy.

Decontamination

Decontamination is tailored specifically for each patient and the specific exposure. Syrup of ipecac is specifically contraindicated in pregnancy because of increased abdominal and thoracic pressure during protracted emesis.

Gastric lavage and activated charcoal have the same indications and contraindications as in the nonpregnant patient. Because gastric motility is slowed in pregnancy, delayed administration of charcoal, gastric lavage, and whole bowel irrigation may be useful for decontamination. The usefulness of cathartics for GI decontamination has never been well documented; therefore, their addition to general decontamination measures is not mandatory. Multiple doses of a cathartic can cause electrolyte abnormalities, dehydration, and potentially induce premature labor.

Enhanced Elimination

Multiple-dose activated charcoal is indicated for the same toxic overdoses as in the nonpregnant patient: theophylline, phenobarbital, carbamazepine, dapsone, and quinine. Enhanced elimination of these drugs occurs because their physical properties or enterohepatic circulation allow for gut dialysis of the drug from the circulatory system into the GI tract, where it is adsorbed to the charcoal.

Hemodialysis appears to be safe for the mother and fetus during pregnancy. The use of chronic hemodialysis is described in pregnant women. One study related premature labor and intrauterine growth retardation in pregnant dialysis patients to their chronic diseases. Another study found none of the offspring of mothers on chronic dialysis had fetal abnormalities, and all were spontaneously delivered at term. Most of the toxicology cases of dialysis used in pregnancy are cited in case reports. In general, it should be assumed that the risks and benefits of hemodialysis in the pregnant patient should be the same as in the nonpregnant patient.

Antidotes

The effects of antidotes on the fetus are not well-studied. Case reports predominantly provide information on the maternal effects of antidotes. It is not known definitively, but it is unlikely that one fetal exposure to an antidote will cause harm. However, there are documented cases such as iron overdose in pregnancy in which withholding the antidote has caused maternal and fetal mortality.

ABORTIFACIENTS

An *abortifacient* is any substance used to terminate a pregnancy (Table 4–3). Historically, lead and quinine have been used as abortifacients, but now over-the-counter preparations such as acetaminophen, aspirin, iron, and herbal preparations are more commonly reported. The greatest dangers of abortifacients are the effect of the toxin on the mother, the potential teratogenic effect on the fetus, and the complications from delaying a physician-assisted abortion.

Most attempts to chemically abort a fetus are made in the first trimester. Acetaminophen and multidrug ingestions are the most common exposures, with minor maternal toxicity reported in most cases.

As a result of the serious nature of an abortifacient attempt and the often nonspecific clinical manifestation of the ingestion, a high index of suspicion is required to discover if this has occurred in the gravid patient. Therefore, every female overdose patient of child-bearing age should have a pregnancy test. In addition, women who present with significant vaginal bleeding should be historically screened for possible abortifacient use.

Table 4–3. Abortifacients

Angelica root (*Angelica archangelica*)
Black cohosh (*Cimicifuga racemosa*)
Blue cohosh (*Caulophyllum thalictroides*)
Buckthorn bark (*Rhamnus cathartica, frangula, alnifolia*)
Diethylcarbamazine
Ergotamine
Mifepristone (approved in France as an abortifacient in 1988)
Mistletoe (*Phoradendron falvescens, macrophyllum rubrum, serotinum, tomentosum; Viscum album*)
Poison hemlock (*Conium maculatum*)
Sodium chloride 20% by transabdominal intra-amniotic injection
Misoprostol
Pennyroyal (*Mentha pulegium/Hedeoma pulegioides*)
Windflower (*Anemone pulsatilla*)
Quinine
Rue (*Ruta graveolens*)
Savun/juniper (*Juniperus sabina*)
Mandrake (*Podophyllum peltatum*)
Tansy (*Tanacetum/Chrysanthemum vulgare*)

PHARMACEUTICALS

Acetaminophen

Acetaminophen is a common overdose in pregnancy. Although it does cross the placenta, a primary concern in acetaminophen toxicity is the formation of the toxic metabolite *N*-acetyl-*p*-benzoquinoneimine via the cytochrome P450 system. The fetus is relatively protected from hepatotoxicity in the first trimester because the fetal liver does not begin to activate cytochrome P450 activity until the 14th week of gestation.

N-acetylcysteine (NAC) is the antidote for acetaminophen-poisoned patients. Spontaneous abortion is increased when NAC is delayed in treating acetaminophen overdose in pregnant patients. There has been controversy over the ability of NAC to cross the placenta in humans. One study, using sheep to determine if NAC crossed the placenta, concluded that it did not undergo placental transfer. Another study, with a rat model, demonstrated that NAC could cross the placenta. NAC has been measured in fetal cord blood from human neonates born to mothers who received NAC as treatment for acetaminophen overdose. The level found in the cord blood was within the therapeutic range. An explanation for the discrepancy between animal species could be the number of layers of the different placentas. The human and rat placenta are both comprised of three layers while the sheep has five layers.

Oral administration of NAC is the most widely used route of administration, but the intravenous (IV) route can be used. Theoretically, the IV route may avoid the first-pass effect of the maternal liver, therefore increasing the amount of NAC that will reach the fetus.

In acetaminophen toxicity in the third trimester, an increase in infratentorial hemorrhage, fetal demise, and maternal death have been reported. For this reason, emergent delivery of the fetus by vaginal or cesarean section has been advocated in the third trimester in mothers suffering from fulminant hepatic failure secondary to acetaminophen overdose.

Acetaminophen toxicity in pregnancy does not automatically result in fetal death or malformations. Therefore, acetaminophen overdose does not necessitate an elective abortion.

Salicylates

Like acetaminophen overdose, salicylate overdose in pregnancy is common. The fetus is relatively vulnerable to salicylate toxicity in the third trimester. The fetus will have a greater serum concentration of salicylate than the mother, a larger portion will enter the fetal nervous system, and the fetus has decreased buffering capacity for metabolic acidosis. At any gestational age, the fetus metabolizes salicylate at a much slower rate because it has decreased glucuronidation.

An acute salicylate overdose prior to delivery can lead to maternal and fetal platelet dysfunction. This is of great concern in the fetus because of the possibility of intracranial bleeding. Chronic salicylate use during pregnancy can cause hyperbilirubinemia, lower birth weight, and increased mortality in the fetus. The mother may have a longer gestational period, prolonged labor, increased risk of hemorrhage, and a higher likelihood of requiring a cesarean section.

Treatment of salicylate overdose in pregnancy should proceed with the same decontamination, enhanced elimination, and supportive care as in the nonpregnant patient, including the criteria for hemodialysis (see Chapter 30). The main difference in the pregnant patient is the need for earlier and more aggressive treatment. Treatment of the mother should be initiated early at levels as low as 25 mg/dL. If the overdose occurs near the delivery date, emergent delivery of a fetus may be optimal in a severely toxic mother.

Iron

Iron supplementation during pregnancy is routine, which increases the possibility of a toxic exposure. Iron is different from acetaminophen and salicylates because the placenta provides a relatively effective barrier to iron penetration. Iron crosses the placenta by receptor-mediated endocytosis. As a result, the receptors can become saturated, limiting the rate of transport. A study done in sheep showed that maternal levels of iron did not correlate with fetal levels. This is also supported in human case reports. Consequently, the survival of the fetus depends on the treatment of maternal toxicity.

Activated charcoal is ineffective at binding iron. Whole-bowel irrigation can be effective if there opacities are seen on an abdominal radiograph (Figure 4–2). The amount of radiation risk to the fetus from a single radiograph to document the presence of iron tablets is minimal compared to the potential toxicity of a maternal iron overdose.

Deferoxamine (DFO) is the antidote for iron poisoning. It binds to free iron and the complex is eliminated in the urine. Indications for using DFO depend on a constellation of clinical signs. Hypotension, metabolic acidosis, GI bleeding, shock, and an iron level >500 μg/dL are all signs of severe iron poisoning and are indications for DFO administration. Some believe that the threshold for treatment with DFO in the pregnant patient should be

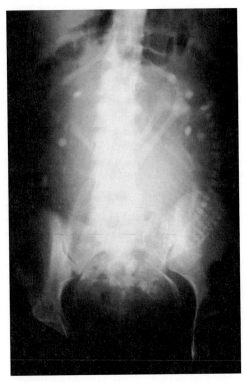

Fig. 4–2. Abdominal radiograph demonstrating radiopaque iron tablets ingested by a pregnant patient.

lowered to an iron level 350 μg/dL. The dose of DFO is the same as in the nonpregnant patient (see Chapter 68).

Because previous studies in animals have shown skeletal abnormalities in the fetus when the mother was exposed to high doses of DFO, this life-saving antidote has been withheld in pregnant women resulting in maternal and fetal death. However, multiple reviews of teratogenicity caused by DFO utilized for iron toxicity in pregnancy have not shown convincing evidence of any cause and effect relationship. DFO does not cross the placenta when studied in the sheep model.

ENVIRONMENTAL TOXINS IN PREGNANCY

Lead

Lead has no biological value to the human body. Removal of lead from gasoline has caused a dramatic reduction in the average blood lead level of children in the United States from 15 μg/dL in 1978 to 2 μg/dL in 1999. Des-

pite this advancement, lead poisoning is still a major health concern for children.

There are limited case reports describing lead poisoning in the pregnant patient. Most involve the mother exhibiting pica behavior. A study of lead exposure of pregnant women in their first trimester in New York City found that blood lead levels were inversely related to maternal age and length of time in the United States, and directly related to gestational age and pica behavior. Another study found that endogenous lead sources in bone continues to influence blood lead levels of immigrants in the United States during and after pregnancy.

Because almost 95% of the body's lead burden is stored in bones, bone resorption during pregnancy mobilizes lead and increases toxicity. Lead transfer across the placenta has been described at 12 to 14 weeks' gestation, and lead continues to accumulate in fetal tissue. An epidemiologic study performed in Turkey found that umbilical cord lead levels, which correlated significantly with maternal levels, were approximately 70% of the latter. A case report describing the radiographic findings seen in congenital lead poisoning described a dense cranial vault, lead lines in the distal ends of long bones, and delayed emergence of dentition. The authors recommend using these findings as a screen for subtle presentations of congenital lead poisoning.

Lead poisoning in pregnancy can lead to multiple effects on the mother and the fetus. Maternal hypertension, spontaneous abortion, and developmental impairment have a direct relationship to maternal lead burden. Another study found a dose-related relationship between blood lead level and congenital hemangiomas, lymphangiomas, hydrocele, skin tags, and undescended testicles.

Treating lead toxicity in the nonpregnant patient can involve chelation with a variety of agents. The traditional agents used for lead chelation are 2,3 dimercaptopropranol (British Anti-Lewisite [BAL]), ethylenediaminetetraacetate (EDTA), dimercaptosuccinic acid (DMSA, Succimer), and D-penicillamine. All of the chelators are known teratogens in animals, and are to be avoided in pregnancy unless the benefit of administration outweighs the risk.

DMSA has been shown to cause prenatal death, reduction in body weight, soft tissue abnormalities, and skeletal anomalies in mice when administered subcutaneously at doses greater than 400 mg/kg/d. There were no fetomaternal toxic effects noted after oral DMSA <100 mg/kg/d were administered. Because DMSA has not been studied in humans in controlled trials it is listed in pregnancy Category C. It has been used in pregnancy in the maximum human dose of 30 mg/kg/d without fetal abnormalities. Nevertheless in one case report, the blood lead level remained essentially unchanged from 44.0 μg/dL to 43.9 μg/dL after 18 days of chelation.

EDTA chelates calcium and zinc and is a known teratogenic agent when administered in pregnant rats. In two case reports, pregnant women received EDTA, 2 g/d IV dose, and 75 mg/kg/d IV dose, respectively. Both mothers delivered a normal fetus posttherapy. BAL is known to cause skeletal abnormalities in mice at doses >125 mg/kg/d when given subcutaneously.

Penicillamine has been found to be a teratogen in both humans and animals. It has been implicated as the cause of congenital connective tissue and other abnormalities in neonates born to women chelated during pregnancy for cysteinuria, rheumatoid arthritis, and Wilson disease. The dose used in pregnant women is 0.25 to 0.50 g/d. Because safer chelators such as DMSA are available, penicillamine should be avoided when chelating the pregnant patient.

Nutritional supplementation is a safe adjunct for treatment of lead toxicity. Many lead toxic patients are deficient in iron, zinc, and calcium. Women taking iron and folic acid have been found to have lower lead levels than matched cohorts. Alcohol and tobacco use have been found to correlate with higher lead levels, so abstinence from their use has multiple benefits.

It is unknown if chelation during pregnancy is effective at decreasing the fetal or maternal body lead burden, or improving the outcome of the fetus exposed to lead. The small amount of data on the risk of chelators to the fetus and the mother are provided in animal studies and human case reports. In the literature, a few cases reports have documented maternal chelation therapy for lead poisoning during pregnancy. The chelators used were EDTA, BAL, and DMSA. After birth, the blood lead levels were consistently higher in the neonate than the mother. None of these children were born with birth defects. At this time, nutritional supplementation along with analysis of the risk verses benefit of a chelation agent appears to be sound approach for treatment of gestational lead poisoning.

Carbon Monoxide

Carbon monoxide (CO) naturally occurs in the human body as a byproduct of hemoglobin catabolism. It remains the number one cause of poisoning mortality in the United States.

Carboxyhemoglobin (COHb) concentration increases during pregnancy because of both maternal and fetal contributions. In the mother, progesterone causes increased metabolism of hemoglobin leading to increased production of CO. The pregnant woman also is at increased risk of toxicity when exposed to environmental CO because of increased minute ventilation.

In an acute exposure, CO crosses the placenta by passive diffusion. The fetal COHb concentration equilibrates with the maternal COHb concentration 2 hours after exposure, and eventually doubles the maternal concentration. In chronic CO poisoning, fetal COHb concentration reaches maternal levels at a slower rate than in the acute scenario. The COHb concentration reaches equilibrium in 36 to 48 hours, with the percent fetal COHb 15% to 20% greater than the maternal levels (Figure 4–1). The fetus eliminates CO at a slower half-life of 7 hours on room air compared to 4 to 5 hours in the mother.

The combination of fetal hemoglobin physiology, delayed peak in fetal COHb concentration, elevated concentration of COHb compared to the maternal concentration, and prolonged elimination half-life increase the chance of significant morbidity and mortality in the fetus exposed to CO, even when the mother is relatively asymptomatic. Unfortunately, the maternal hemoglobin is the only CO concentration obtainable, and this level does not correlate well with maternal or fetal toxicity. Maternal symptoms of altered mental status, neurologic deficits, and seizures are better predictors of fetal toxicity than COHb concentrations.

The result of fetal CO exposure can lead to different effects on the fetus depending on the stage at which it is exposed. In the embryonic stage neurologic, skeletal, and cleft palate deformities can be seen. In the fetal stage, anoxic encephalopathy and growth restriction can result. In the third trimester, premature delivery, decreased immunity, right-sided cardiomegaly, and sodium channel and myelin defects have been reported.

Aggressive treatment of the CO-exposed mother is critically important for the fetus. Treatment of the pregnant woman exposed to CO is immediate removal from the source and application of 100% oxygen. Fetal and maternal outcome with or without HBO therapy has not been well studied at any COHb concentration. However, indications for HBO therapy in the pregnant patient have been suggested to be a COHb concentration greater than 15%, regardless of symptoms, or maternal mental status depression, seizures, acidosis, or evidence of fetal distress (Table 4–4).

Because of the delayed fetal accumulation of COHb, higher fetal COHb levels, and decreased elimination half-life of COHb in the fetus, there is variation from conventional therapy of CO poisoning. Continuation of

Table 4–4. Indications for Hyperbaric Oxygen Therapy in the Pregnant Patient

COHb level $\geq 15\%$
Mental status depression
Seizures
Metabolic acidosis
Fetal distress

100% oxygen five times longer than standard therapy in nonpregnant patients may be necessary to ensure greater elimination of the fetal COHb. Additional HBO therapy may also be needed if fetal signs of distress are demonstrated 12 hours after initial HBO therapy. One source suggests that if cesarean delivery is being considered, delivery of the fetus before HBO therapy can lead to a greater probability of fetal death. However, this opinion is not a result of clinical trials. Despite studies in animals linking HBO therapy with retinopathy, cardiovascular defects, and premature closure of the ductus arteriosus, human case reports and a prospective study have not shown significant morbidity or mortality in the mother or the fetus after HBO therapy.

Organophosphates

An organophosphate exposure in the pregnant patient is possible in certain environmental or occupational scenarios. A study of an Ontario farm population exposed to a variety of pesticides found that the timing of the exposure during gestation could predict the toxicity of a pesticide, including organophosphates. There is a significant risk of morbidity and mortality in the mother and the fetus exposed to organophosphates, but the relationship between chronic exposure and risk of effects is still uncertain. Organophosphates cross the placenta. Fetal organophosphate levels have been detected on autopsy of fatalities from organophosphate poisoning. The fetus may also be more susceptible to the effects of cholinesterase inhibition; studies have found 50% to 70% reduction of fetal red blood cell cholinesterase in normal neonates.

Access of terrorists to chemical weapons opens the possibility of a pregnant women being exposed to nerve gas agents like Sarin, Soman, Tabun, and VX. All of these agents inhibit acetylcholinesterase, causing cholinergic signs of toxicity such as bronchospasm, bradycardia, bronchorrhea, salivation, lacrimation, urinary and fecal incontinence, abdominal pain, and miosis. They may also cause nicotinic signs because of inhibition of the metabolism of acetylcholine at these receptors. Nicotinic symptoms include tachycardia, hypertension, muscle fas-

ciculations, weakness, and mydriasis. In 1995 a Japanese terrorist group released Sarin gas into a subway system. Five toxic pregnant women were treated with atropine only. No fetal malformations were reported 1 month and 1 year after the attack.

Management of organophosphate toxicity should proceed in the same manner as in the nonpregnant patient. Atropine should be used for cholinergic symptoms and pralidoxine should be used for nicotinic symptoms. The atropine serum level in the fetus is half the maternal level in 20 minutes in early pregnancy. In late pregnancy, fetal serum atropine reaches 93% of the maternal level in 5 minutes. There are case reports of both of these agents used in pregnant patients in which normal term babies were delivered.

A dose-related protective effect of pralidoxine against teratogenicity has been shown in a chick embryo model exposed to parathion and dicrotophos. Fetal tachycardia has been described in another case report in which a pregnant mother received atropine for organophosphate poisoning. However, it is unclear if the tachycardia developed from the atropine directly or the effects of fetal hypoxia. The fetus was delivered and both patients recovered after several days of intubation and atropine therapy. If the fetus is at a viable gestational age, emergent delivery allows treatment of both the mother and the neonate.

Cyanide

Cyanide exposure can occur as a result of dwelling fires, iatrogenic sodium nitroprusside toxicity, and chemical weapon attacks. Cyanide is a cellular asphyxiant, which binds to cytochrome a3 of the electron transport chain, uncoupling oxidative phosphorylation. This leads to decreased production of ATP and increased production of NADH. The result is multisystem cellular poisoning, cardiovascular instability, and metabolic acidosis.

The antidotes for cyanide poisoning are amyl nitrite, sodium nitrite, and sodium thiosulfate. They vary in potential teratogenicity, from amyl nitrite, which is in pregnancy category X, to sodium thiosulfate, which is in Category C; sodium nitrite is most likely in Category C. Epidemiologic studies have not evaluated these antidotes in humans or animals during pregnancy. Despite uncertainty of the risk of teratogenicity, these antidotes should not be withheld in pregnant patients with cyanide toxicity, although in the hospital setting, amyl nitrite should not be used.

Cyanide toxicity can result from prolonged use of sodium nitroprusside, which has been used to control severe hypertension in the pregnant patient with pre-eclampsia. The use of a thiosulfate drip in addition to nitroprusside drip for hypertension has been shown to prevent cyanide toxicity in gravid ewes. However, the follow-up study to this showed the antidote sodium thiosulfate did not cross the placenta. (Table 4–5). It was hypothesized that the fetal cyanide crosses the placenta down a concentration gradient and becomes bound to thiosulfate in the maternal circulation. These studies demonstrated that sodium thiosulfate was an effective prophylactic antidote to cyanide toxicity, and this was achieved without the antidote reaching the fetus. In the setting of acute exposure to cyanide, it seems intuitive that these studies support aggressive treatment of the pregnant mother.

DRUGS OF ABUSE IN PREGNANCY
Cocaine

Cocaine use is a common drug of abuse in women of childbearing age. One study found that 17% of urban women enrolled in prenatal care admitted to using cocaine once in their pregnancy. Smoking crack cocaine is the most common route of exposure, and many of the pregnant women who use this substance do not receive any prenatal care. Some mothers do not realize they are pregnant, whereas others surmise the pregnancy is lost and decide to continue using cocaine. Still others falsely

Table 4–5. Placental Permeability of Toxins and Antidotes

	Placental Permeability	
	Yes	No
Acetaminophen	X	
N-acetylcysteine	X	
Iron	X (receptor-mediated endocytosis)	
Deferoxamine		X
Lead	X	
Carbon monoxide	X	
Oxygen	X	
Organophosphate	X	
Atropine	X	
Cyanide	X	
Sodium thiosulfate		X

think that cocaine speeds labor. However, cocaine can actually lengthen labor and exacerbate pain. Infants born to mothers who abused cocaine during pregnancy may develop neurologic problems later in childhood. One recent study by Singer and associates showed that infants of 66 mothers who reported heavy cocaine use during pregnancy already had evidence of delays in auditory comprehension and language development by 1 year of age.

Cocaine toxicity can cause many different signs and symptoms. All are related to a sympathomimetic toxidrome. Hyperthermia, hypertension, tachycardia, agitation, seizures, stroke, myocardial infarction, intracerebral hemorrhage, and aortic dissection are possible results of cocaine use. The unique complications associated with cocaine use in pregnancy are abruptio placentae, decreased fetal growth, preterm labor, urinary congenital abnormalities, neurobehavioral abnormalities, and fetal demise.

The pregnant patient is theoretically at enhanced susceptibility to cocaine poisoning owing to reduced cholinesterase levels, causing her to have decreased ability to metabolize cocaine. The fetus also has reduced levels of cholinesterase, but the placenta has sufficient activity to allow metabolism of some of the cocaine before it crosses the placenta and affects the fetus. Cocaine experimentally administered to the pregnant ewe caused increased vascular resistance, decreased uterine flow, increased fetal heart rate and blood pressure, and lower fetal oxygen content. Progesterone may have an additive effect toward increasing cardiovascular toxicity in the pregnant patient.

Benzodiazepines are the medication of choice for treatment of cocaine-induced agitation, seizures, or tachycardia. Diazepam and lorazepam are both designated as Category D in pregnancy, and in some sources lorazepam is classified as Category X. However, one source states that no fetal malformations have been attributed to the administration of benzodiazepines during pregnancy. If a pregnant woman suffers cocaine-related seizures, agitation, and hyperthermia, the use of benzodiazepines may decrease morbidity and mortality. There may be respiratory depression on delivery of a fetus from a mother treated with benzodiazepines, but the benefits outweigh the risks. If efforts to halt seizures are refractory to benzodiazepines, phenobarbital is recommended over phenytoin, due to the latter's known teratogenic effects on the fetus. Rapid external cooling for hyperthermia is essential. In the setting of chest pain, investigation and treatment of possible myocardial ischemia is warranted. If abruptio placenta occurs, emergent cesarean delivery is likely to be required.

Heroin

Heroin overdose presents with the triad of respiratory depression, neurologic depression, and miosis. The antidote naloxone is administered in the pregnant patient with a heroin overdose. Concern about the possibility of fetal and neonatal withdrawal syndrome in heroin-dependent mothers given naloxone is outweighed by the benefit from reversing maternal and fetal hypoxia.

CONCLUSION

Screening for pregnancy is important in every female overdose patient of childbearing age. Fortunately, most acute overdoses will not have a teratogenic effect. Evaluation and treatment of the poisoned pregnant patient can be a challenge when considering which therapy will benefit both the mother and fetus, and harm neither. Aggressive supportive care of the airway, circulation, neurologic status, and general decontamination measures should be the primary goals in treatment. For the most part, administration of antidotes will have the same indications and contraindications as with nonpregnant patients. When the risk versus benefit is unknown regarding a specific therapeutic intervention, appropriate treatment of the mother will most often result in optimal management of the fetus.

SUGGESTED READINGS

Ansai N, Kimura T, Chida S, et al: Studies on the metabolic fate of *N*-acetylcysteine in rats and dogs *Pharmacometrics* 26: 249–260, 1983.

Arbuckle TE, Lin Z, Mery LS: An exploratory analysis of the effect of pesticide exposure on the risk of spontaneous abortion in an Ontario farm population. *Environ Health Perspect* 109:851–857, 2001.

Astroff BA, Young AD: The relationship between maternal and fetal effects following maternal organophosphate exposure during gestation in the rat. *Toxicol Ind Health* 14:869–889, 1998.

Aubard Y, Magne I: Carbon monoxide poisoning in pregnancy. *Br J Obstet Gynaecol* 107:833–838, 2000.

Bailey B: Organophosphate poisoning in pregnancy. *Ann Emerg Med* 29:299, 1997.

Canfield RL, Henderson CR, Cory-Slechta DA, et al: Intellectual impairment in children with blood lead concentrations below 10 µg per deciliter. *N Engl J Med* 348:1517–1526, 2003.

Curry SC, Bond GR, Raschke R, et al: An ovine model of maternal iron poisoning on pregnancy. *Ann Emerg Med* 19:632–638, 1990.

Curry SC, Carlton MW, Raschke RA: Prevention of fetal and maternal toxicity from nitroprusside confusion with sodium thiosulfate in gravid ewes. *Anesth Analg* 84:1121–1126, 1997.

Czeizel A, Szentesi I, Molnar G: Lack of effect of self-poisoning on subsequent reproductive outcome. *Mutat Res* 127: 175–182, 1984.

Czeizel AE, Tomcsik M, Timar L: Teratologic evaluation of 178 infants born to mothers who attempted suicide by drugs during pregnancy. *Obstet Gynecol* 90:195–201, 1997.

Domingo JL: Developmental toxicity of metal chelating agents. *Reprod Toxicol* 12:499–510, 1998.

Farrow JR, Davis GJ, Roy TM, et al: Fetal death due to nonlethal carbon monoxide poisoning. *J Forensic Sci* 35:1448–1452, 1990.

Fine JS: Reproductive and perinatal principles. In: Goldfrank LR, Flomenbaum NE, Lewin NA, Howland MA, Hoffman RS, Nelson LS, eds: *Goldfrank's Toxicologic Emergencies.* 7th ed. New York: McGraw-Hill; 2002.

Frank DA, Amaro H, Bauchner H, et al: Cocaine use during pregnancy: prevalence and correlates. *Pediatrics* 82:888–895, 1988.

Furman A: Maternal and umbilical cord blood lead levels: an Istanbul study. *Arch Environ Health* 56:26–28, 2001.

Garcia SJ, Seilder FJ, Qiao D, et al: Chlorpyrifos targets developing glia: effects of glial fibrillary acidic protein. *Dev Brain Res* 133:151–161, 2002.

Gbolade BA: Overdose and termination of pregnancy (letter). *Br J Gen Pract* 47:184, 1997.

Gomaa A, Hu H, Belinger D, et al: Maternal bone lead as an independent risk factor for fetal neurotoxicity: a prospective study. *Pediatrics* 110:110–118, 2002.

Graeme KA, Curry SC, Bikin DS, et al: The lack of transplacental movement of the cyanide antidote thiosulfate in the gravid ewe. *Anesth Analg* 89:1448–1452, 1999.

Hamilton S, Rothenberg SJ, Khan FA, et al: Neonatal lead poisoning from maternal pica behavior during pregnancy. *J Natl Med Assoc* 93:317–319, 2001.

Hertz-Picciotto I: The evidence that lead increases the risk for spontaneous abortion. *Am J Ind Med* 38:300–309, 2000.

Horowitz RS, Dart RC, Jarvie DR, et al: Placental transfer of *N*-acetylcysteine following human maternal acetaminophen toxicity. *J Toxicol Clin Toxicol* 35:447–451, 1997.

Horowitz RS, Mirkin DB: Lead poisoning and chelation in a mother–neonate pair. *J Toxicol Clin Toxicol* 39:727–731, 2001.

Houston H, Jacobson L: Overdose and termination of pregnancy: an important association? *Br J Gen Pract* 46:737–738, 1996

Jones JS, Dickson K, Carlson S: Unrecognized pregnancy in the overdosed or poisoned patient. *Am J Emerg Med* 15:538–541, 1997.

Karlowicz MG, White LE: Severe intracranial hemorrhage in a term neonate associated with maternal acetylsalicylic acid ingestion. *Clin Pediatr* 32:740–743, 1993.

Klitzman S, Sharma A, Nicaj L, et al: Lead poisoning among pregnant women in New York city: risk factors and screening practices. *J Urban Health* 79:225–237, 2002.

Kopelman AE, Plaut TA: Fetal compromise caused by maternal carbon monoxide poisoning. *J Perinatol* 18:4–77, 1998.

Koren G: *Maternal-Fetal Toxicology: A Clinician's Guide,* 2nd ed. New York: Marcel Dekker; 1994.

Koren GK, Sharav T, Garrettson LK, et al: A multicenter prospective study of fetal outcome following accidental carbon monoxide poisoning in pregnancy. *Reprod Toxicol* 5: 397–403, 1991.

Kozer E, Koren G: Management of paracetamol overdose: current controversies. *Drug Saf* 24:503–512, 2001.

Litovitz TL, Klein-Schwartz W, White S, et al: 2001 Annual report of the American Association of Poison Control Centers Toxic Exposure Surveillance System. *Am J Emerg Med* 20: 391–452, 2002.

Little DR: Cocaine addiction and pregnancy: education in primary prevention. *Res Staff Physician* 39:79–81, 1993.

Longo LD: The biological effects of carbon monoxide on the pregnant woman, fetus and newborn infant. *Am J Obstet Gynecol* 129:69–103, 1977.

Manoguerra AS: Iron poisoning: report of a fatal case in an adult. *Am J Hosp Pharm* 59:1088–1090, 1976.

Martinez-Frias ML, Rodriguez-Pinilla E, Bermejo E: Prenatal exposure of penicillamine and oral clefts. *Am J Med Genet* 76:274–275, 1998.

McElhatton PR, Sullivan FM, Volans GN: Paracetamol overdose in pregnancy: analysis of the outcomes of 300 cases referred to the Teratology Information Service. *Reprod Toxicol* 11:85–94, 1997.

Netland KE, Martinez J: Abortifacients: toxidromes, ancient to modern—A case series and review of the literature. *Acad Emerg Med* 7:824–829, 2000.

O'Hara TM, Bennett L, McCoy CP: Lead poisoning and toxicokinetics in a human fetus treated with CaNA2EDTA and thiamine. *Vet Diagn Invest* 7:531–537, 1995

Pearl M, Boxt LM: Radiographic findings in congenital lead poisoning. *Radiology* 136:83–84, 1980.

Perrone J, Hoffman RS: Toxic ingestions in pregnancy: abortifacient use in a case series of pregnant overdose patients. *Acad Emerg Med* 4:206–209, 1997.

Rayburn W, Aronow R, DeLancey B, et al: Drug overdose during pregnancy: an overview from a metropolitan poison control center. *Obstet Gynecol* 64:611–614, 1984.

Riggs BS, Bronsteine AC, Kulig KW, et al: Acute acetaminophen overdose during pregnancy. *Obstet Gynecol* 74:247–253, 1989.

Roberts I, Robinson MZ, Mughal JG, et al: Paracetamol metabolites in the neonate following maternal overdose. *Br J Pharmacol* 18:201–206, 1984

Rothenberg SJ, Khan F, Manalo M, et al: Maternal bone lead contribution to blood lead during and after pregnancy. *Environ Res* 82:81–90, 2000.

Rothenberg SJ, Kondrashov V, Manalo M, et al: Increases in hypertension and blood pressure during pregnancy with increased bone lead levels. *Am J Epidemiol* 156:1079–1087, 2002.

Selden BS, Burke TJ: Complete maternal and fetal recovery after prolonged cardiac arrest. *Ann Emerg Med* 17:346–349, 1988.

Seldon BS, Curry SC, Clark RF, et al: Transplacental transport of *N*-acetylcysteine in an ovine model. *Ann Emerg Med* 20:1069–1072, 1991.

Shannon M: Severe lead poisoning in pregnancy. *Ambul Pediatr* 3:37–39, 2003.

Silverman RK, Montano J: Hyperbaric oxygen treatment during pregnancy in acute carbon monoxide poisoning. *J Reprod Med* 42:309–311, 1997.

Singer LT, Arendt R, Minnes S, et al.: Developing language skills of cocaine-exposed infants. *Pediatrics* 107:1057–1064, 2001.

Singer ST, Vichinsky EP: Deferoxamine treatment during pregnancy: is it harmful? *Am J Hematol* 60:24–26, 1999.

Strom RL, Schiller P, Seeds AT, et al: Fatal iron poisoning in a pregnant female. *Minn Med* 59:483–489, 1976.

Tait PA, Vora A, James S, et al: Severe congenital lead poisoning in a preterm infant due to a herbal remedy. *Med J Aust* 177:193–195, 2002.

Tenebein M: Poisoning in pregnancy. In: Koren G, ed: *Maternal-Fetal Toxicology: A Clinician's Guide.* 2nd ed. New York: Marcel Dekker; 1994:223–252.

Thorp JM: Management of drug dependency, overdose, and withdrawal in the obstetric patient. *Obstet Gynecol Clin North Am* 22:131–142, 1995.

Tran T, Wax JR, Philput C, et al: Intentional iron overdose in pregnancy—management and outcome. *J Emerg Med* 18:225–228, 2000.

Tran T, Wax JR, Steinfeld JD, et al: Acute intentional iron overdose in pregnancy. *Obstet Gynecol* 92:678–679, 1998.

Turk J, Aks SE, Ampuero F, et al: Successful therapy of iron intoxication in pregnancy with intravenous deferoxamine and whole bowel irrigation. *Vet Human Toxicol* 35:441–444, 1993

Van Ameyde KJ, Tennebein M: Whole bowel irrigation during pregnancy. *Am J Obstet Gynecol* 160:646–647, 1989.

Van Hoesen KB, Camporesi EM, Moon RE, et al: Should hyperbaric oxygen be used to treat the pregnant patient for acute carbon monoxide poisoning? A case report and literature review. *JAMA* 261:1039–1043, 1989.

Wang PH, Yang MJ, Lee WL, et al: Acetaminophen poisoning in late pregnancy. *J Reprod Med* 42:367–371, 1997

Weaver LK, Hopkins RO, Chan KJ, et al: Hyperbaric oxygen for acute carbon monoxide poisoning. *N Engl J Med* 347: 1057–1067, 2002.

5

Human Milk and
Maternal Medications

Ruth A. Lawrence

HIGH-YIELD FACTS

- The benefits of breastfeeding and human milk are an important part of the equation when evaluating the risks of a particular maternal medication.

- Maternal medications are rarely a reason to interfere with breastfeeding.

- Drugs of abuse, including cocaine, phencyclidine, and heroin, are the only absolute contraindications to breastfeeding.

- Not only the maternal metabolism of a drug but the infant's ability to absorb, detoxify, and excrete a drug are part of the evaluation of a maternal drug.

- The impact of a given drug may be mitigated by changing dosing times, patterns, or temporarily pumping and discarding the milk when problem drugs are needed for a short time.

Breastfeeding is recommended for all infants under ordinary circumstances. According to the American Academy of Pediatrics (AAP), exclusive breastfeeding is recommended for the first 6 months of life, with continued breastfeeding while adding weaning food for the next 6 months, and then for as long thereafter that mother and child choose. Aggressive national and international efforts to encourage breastfeeding have led to a sustained increase in initiation and duration of breastfeeding, especially among high-risk populations. Meanwhile, accumulation of evidence confirms the tremendous value of

human milk to the infant and to the breastfeeding mother. These benefits play a significant role in determining the risk-benefit ratio of a specific drug in a breastfeeding infant.

The many benefits of breastfeeding to the infant are outlined in Table 5–1. The benefits of breastfeeding to the lactating women are outlined in Table 5–2. Unless a specific toxin or medication is clearly harmful for the infant, the benefits of continued breastfeeding will outweigh the risk of the agent in the breast milk.

Poison and Drug Information Centers are experiencing an increase in inquiries from professionals and the public regarding specific medications taken by lactating women. An understanding of the basic principles of drug transfer to breast milk will facilitate decision making about possible risks to the infant, and avoid unnecessary interference in breastfeeding. Lack of information does not justify the recommendation to just stop breastfeeding. In considering the question of risk of a given maternal medication to the suckling infant, both the mother's metabolism and clearance, as well as the infant's absorption and excretion of the compound must be considered.

PROPERTIES OF THE COMPOUND

Knowledge of the simple pharmacologic properties of a compound may quickly answer the question of whether the material will appear in the milk (Table 5–3). Solubility in water or in lipid will allow transport via the liquid or the fat fraction of the milk. Compounds of small molecular size will diffuse easily, but large molecules such as epinephrine, insulin, heparin, and even microheparins do not pass the membrane into milk. High protein binding also prevents the compound from passing into milk. Because breast milk is slightly acidic, compounds that

Table 5–1. Infant Benefits of Breastfeeding

- Species specificity—human milk is designed for the human infant
- Nutritional advantages—all the nutrients necessary in the right amount plus enzymes and ligands to facilitate digestion and absorption
- Infection protection—against otitis media, respiratory, gastrointestinal, sepsis, and genito-urinary infections
- Immunologic protection—reduced incidence of childhood cancer, celiac disease, diabetes mellitus, and other chronic disorders
- Allergy prophylaxis—reduced incidence of eczema, asthma, and other allergy symptoms
- Psychological and cognitive benefits

Table 5–3. Summary of Factors Affecting Drug Passage

  I. Drug
    A. Route of administration
      1. Oral (PO)
      2. Intravenous (IV)
      3. Intramuscular (IM)
      4. Transdermal drug delivery system (TDDS)
    B. Absorption rate
    C. Time to peak plasma concentration/half-life
    D. Dissociation constant
    E. Volume of distribution
  II. Size of molecule
 III. Degree of ionization
 IV. pH of substrate
    A. Plasma 7.4
    B. Milk 6.8
  V. Solubility
    A. In water
    B. In lipids
 VI. Protein binding more to plasma than to milk protein

are alkaline are attracted across the membranes, whereas acidic compounds are repelled. The rapidity with which the compound is metabolized has an impact on drug transport, but biological activity and persistence of its metabolites is more important. The half-life of the compound determines whether it clears quickly or accumulates over days of dosing, as with the selective serotonin-reuptake inhibitors (SSRIs). Occasional dosing, as with an acetaminophen tablet or two, is rarely a problem when compared to compounds that are taken daily until a steady state is reached.

MILK:PLASMA RATIO

Some drugs have actually been studied in relationship to their appearance in milk. The results are often reported as the milk:plasma (M:P) ratio, or the concentration measured in milk at the same time it is measured in maternal plasma. Such measurements are of limited value unless the time and dose of a drug are known. If the maternal plasma concentration is low, and the M:P ratio is 1, very little drug would reach the infant via the milk. This may be particularly true for a compound that has a large volume of distribution. For some substances, such

Table 5–2. Maternal Benefits of Breastfeeding

- More rapid postpartum recovery
- Reduced risk of long-term obesity
- Reduced risk of breast and ovarian cancers
- Reduced risk of long-term osteoporosis
- Psychological benefits—empowerment

as iodine, an M:P ratio that exceeds 1 would indicate a compound that is pumped into the milk.

INFANT EXPOSURE TO A DRUG

Calculations may be made regarding the fraction of the maternal dose that would be expected to reach the infant via the breast milk. If the concentration in the milk is known and the volume of milk that is consumed is also known, it is a simple calculation. It is unlikely that more than a small fraction of the maternal dose reaches the infant.

INFANT FACTORS THAT INFLUENCE DRUG EFFECTS

An essential factor in assessing potential toxicity is the bioavailability of the drug to the infant. If the gastrointestinal (GI) tract destroys or cannot absorb the compound, then the infant will not absorb it from the milk and it is of little risk. If the drug is poorly absorbed with food, it too will be poorly absorbed from breast milk, because the infant receives it with food.

In premature and newborn infants, age-specific dosing frequencies for caffeine and certain antibiotics demonstrate the fact that metabolic capabilities change with age

Table 5–4. Properties Affecting the Nursing Infant

1. Absorption from the gastrointestinal tract
2. Infant's ability to detoxify agent: maturity and age dependent
3. Infant's ability to excrete the agent: maturity and age dependent
4. The drug can be given directly to the infant

Table 5–5. Hale's Lactation Risk Categories

L1	Safest	Good studies showing safety
L2	Safer	Limited studies and/or demonstrated work
L3	Moderately safe	No controlled studies; risk is possible but remote
L4	Hazardous	Positive risk versus benefits of breastfeeding
L5	Contraindicated	Significant documented risk

Source: From Hale T: *Medications and Mother's Milk*. Amarillo, Tex: Pharmasoft Publishing; 2002.

and maturity. Other factors that influence the impact on the infant are listed in Table 5–4. The potential risk of a compound to a given infant cannot be estimated without knowing the infant's chronologic and corrected gestational age and the pattern of feedings. The fact that a compound may be given directly and safely to a neonate or child of the same age is helpful, suggesting the small amount received from the milk would be well tolerated.

SAFETY RATING SCALES FOR MEDICATIONS

In 1979, Lawrence published the first targeted description of the mechanisms of maternal drugs and the suckling infant, and the Swedish Drug Council prepared a rating scale in 1980. The AAP Committee on Drugs, which published its first statement on the transfer of drugs and chemicals into human milk in 1983, developed a rating scale of 1 to 8 that was the inverse of the Swedish scale. This position statement was updated in 1989, 1994, and 2001. Hale published a scale in 2002 that included definitions similar to those of the AAP scale, but used a scale (L1 to L5) in reverse order, from safe to contraindicated (Table 5–5).

DRUGS OF CONCERN

The AAP publication lists three categories of drugs of great concern (Table 5–6). Category 1 identifies cytotoxic drugs that may cause immune suppression and have as yet unknown effect on growth or association with carcinogenesis and possible neutropenia. The list includes cyclophosphamide, cyclosporine, oxorubicin, and methotrexate.

Category 2 includes drugs of abuse for which adverse effects on the infant during breastfeeding have been reported. The list includes amphetamine, cocaine, heroin,

marijuana, and phencyclidine. Some believe that occasional social marijuana smoking is acceptable, because little to none is absorbed from the infant's stomach when concentrations are low. Absorption of cannabis via inhalation represents a greater risk to infants exposed to second-hand marijuana smoke. The risk/benefit ratio is clearly in favor of the value of breastfeeding for the infant whose mother occasionally smokes marijuana.

Category 3 covers radioactive compounds that are used in single doses for diagnostic purposes. Clearance times in milk provide a guide for the mother to pump and discard her milk until radioactivity clears from her system (usually determined to be 5 times the half-life). Therapeutic doses of these radioactive compounds, however, require weaning if the total clearance time is weeks or months (e.g., iodine-131). These data on each com-

Table 5–6. The Transfer of Drugs and Other Chemicals Into Human Milk: AAP Classifications

1. Cytotoxic drugs that may interfere with cellular metabolism of the nursing infant
2. Drugs of abuse for which adverse effects on the infant during breastfeeding have been reported
3. Radioactive compounds that require temporary cessation of breastfeeding
4. Drugs for which the effect on nursing infants is unknown but may be of concern
5. Drugs that have been associated with significant effects on some nursing infants and should be given to nursing mothers with caution
6. Maternal medication usually compatible with breastfeeding
7. Food and environmental agents: effects on breastfeeding

pound are available so that unnecessary pumping and discarding may be avoided.

When specific information about the compound in breast milk is not available, the clinician should consider the pharmacology of the drug to estimate the risk that it enters the milk. Key features include oral bioavailability with food and first-pass metabolism.

Because is not possible for every clinician to maintain an adequate database of drugs in breast milk, such information may be accessed from the local poison center or the Breastfeeding and Human Lactation Study Center at the University of Rochester (1-585-275-0088), a dedicated line available from 9 AM to 5 PM (Eastern time), Monday through Friday, located in the Finger Lakes Poison and Drug Information Center.

There are very few instances where breastfeeding must be discontinued. The clinician should instruct the mother to avoid feeding when drug plasma concentrations peak to decrease exposure. Temporary pumping and discarding may become necessary after a brief exposure.

MEDICATION CATEGORIES OF PARTICULAR CONCERN

Psychotherapeutic Agents

A number of postpartum women diagnosed with depression require various psychotherapeutic agents that may present a problem during lactation. The most popular and frequently prescribed of this group are the SSRIs. The best known of these is fluoxetine (Prozac). The AAP rates fluoxetine as a drug whose effect on the nursing infant is unknown but may be of concern (Category 4). Studies of a small series of mothers taking fluoxetine have demonstrated its presence in breast milk, but the estimated concentration of the drug in milk is only about 7% of maternal plasma concentration. There is one case in the literature that suggests colic and fussiness in the breastfed infant of a mother taking fluoxetine, but these findings were never confirmed in subsequent literature. The long-term effects of limited exposure are as yet unknown, because few of these exposed infants have reached adulthood. One alternative to fluoxetine is sertraline (Zoloft), another SSRI whose metabolite is only marginally active. The concentrations found in breast milk in several studies have been reported to be very low (17 to 170 μg/L), and the concentrations in the plasma of nursing infants have been undetectable in most cases.

The infants in these studies had no reported clinical effects from this presumed exposure.

Another alternative is paroxetine (Paxil), a typical SSRI with inactive metabolites. Paroxetine is lipophilic and has a large volume of distribution, so plasma concentrations are low and breast milk concentrations are 7 to 8 μg/L. The estimated dose to the infant is only 0.34% of the mother's dose. In other studies, the drug was not detected in the plasma of seven of eight infants, and no adverse effects have been reported in any of the other nursing infants whose mothers have taken paroxetine. In the 2001 statement of the AAP Committee on Drugs, fluoxetine, paroxetine, and sertraline are all placed in Category 4. From the clinical standpoint, the clinician is left with the dilemma of treating the depressed mother while recognizing the risks or benefits of breastfeeding for both infant and mother. Untreated depression in mothers has a negative impact on infants, and treatment is important. The AAP Committee on Drugs commented that although the psychotropic drugs appear in low concentrations in milk, they have long half-lives and are dosed to produce a steady state in the mother. The Committee expressed concern about exposures of infants in the first few months of life when hepatic and renal function are immature, and when the central nervous system is developing. These drugs affect neurotransmitter function, and it is not possible to predict long-term neurodevelopmental impact.

The Committee also listed the anti-anxiety drugs diazepam, lorazepam, and prazepam in Category 4, which indicates an unknown but possible effect. Antipsychotic compounds clozapine, haloperidol, and mesoridazine are also in Category 4. A third compound, citalopram (Celexa), was not reviewed but has been detected in milk at low concentrations. It has been calculated that the infant would ingest about 4 μg/kg/d with a relative dose up to 6% of the maternal dose. There is a case report of an infant whose serum levels were 12.7 ng/mL and was reported to have "uneasy" sleep patterns that improved when the maternal dose was lowered from 40 mg/d.

Lithium is listed in Category 5 in the 2001 edition of the AAP drug list, signifying its potential for significant effects on the infant and advising that it should be given with caution. Several studies measured lithium in breast milk, whereas others reported symptomatic infants. It is very important to distinguish between infants exposed in utero and those exposed via breast milk. The M:P ratio is between 0.2 and 0.6. Once the maternal therapy has reached a steady state (after approximately 10 days), the infant should have serum lithium concentration measured. Close monitoring of the infant is advisable and relatively simple; most laboratories offer serum lithium concentrations.

HERBAL MEDICINES COMMONLY USED DURING LACTATION

Herbal medicine has become a popular alternative to traditional treatments. This is particularly true among patients who are pregnant or lactating because of the impression that compounds extracted from nature must be safe or the myth that they are benign (Table 5–7). There are no regulations or requirements for marketing herbs provided the container is labeled "not intended as a dietary supplement or a medication." The US Food and Drug Administration (FDA) has no control unless sufficient deaths have been reported, as in the case of comfrey (*Symphytum officinale*), which was very popular with midwives for use during labor, delivery, and lactation and contains hepatotoxic pyrrolizine alkaloids that have been associated with veno-occlusive disease and liver failure. Comfrey was eventually banned by the FDA. It had been banned in Canada and Europe for a decade.

Herbal products used during lactation to stimulate milk production are known as galactogogues, and include fenugreek, blessed thistle, and fennel. Fenugreek (*Trigonella foenum-graecum*) has been used as a digestive aid and for treatment of coughs and bronchitis. Lactation professionals recommend large doses (9 g) three times daily to enhance milk production. The odor of maple syrup becomes apparent in the urine, tears, and milk. In spite of thousands of years of tradition, herbal texts rarely mention any effect on lactation, and there are no placebo-controlled trials or scientific studies to confirm the lactogenic effect. An important caution is that fenugreek is in the same family as peanuts, which is the most common food allergy. Some infants whose mothers use fenugreek develop colic, stomach upset, and diarrhea, which clears when the herb is stopped.

Blessed thistle (*Silybum marianum*) is used as an anorexic, antidiarrheal, and antiseptic as well as a galactogogue. There are no known studies of its efficacy. There is no reported toxicity and it is considered quite benign.

Fennel (*Foeniculum vulgare*), a licorice-flavored herb, is centuries old and well known to fine chefs. It has a reputation for curing stomachache, colic, and gas. It is reputed to promote milk production, but there are no con-

Table 5–7. Herbal Products: Reminders for Clinicians

Ask patients about their use of herbal products.
Herbal products may interact with other traditional medications.
U.S. Food and Drug Administration has no regulatory control over safety, efficacy, quality, standardization, or sale of herbal products.
No placebo-controlled studies for most herbals in pregnancy and lactation.

trolled studies to support the claim. The seeds and fruit in small amounts are safe but the volatile oil is toxic, causing seizures and respiratory problems in doses as small as 1 to 5 mL.

The pharmacologically active ginkgo (*Ginkgo biloba*), ginseng (*Panax*), and kava are the best known of the herbs that allegedly enhance performance and build strength. Placebo-controlled blinded studies provide no evidence to support these claims. In fact, these herbs are capable of causing significant toxicity. The side effects of ginkgo include allergic skin reactions and GI symptoms. It is widely used in the elderly for dementia. The seeds contain ginkgotoxin and are too toxic for consumption.

Ginseng, the subject of thousands of books and papers, remains controversial. Although ginseng may be found in many vitamin products and health foods, the few placebo-controlled trials have not supported any therapeutic benefits. Because it is expensive, it is often laced with other roots. Ginseng may cause excitement, nervousness, hypertension, and hypoglycemia, as well as significant withdrawal when discontinued. It should not be used for more than 6 weeks consecutively.

Ephedra (ma huang) is the principal alkaloid of ephedrine. Known in China for over 500 years, it was employed as a therapy for asthma. Over 40 species differ in potency. Ma huang has become an herb of abuse and has been associated with the deaths of several celebrities who used it as a dietary supplement.

Kava (*Piper methysticum*) is prepared from roots cultivated in the South Pacific and is popular as a beverage. It has a strong taste that causes localized numbness associated with its complex chemistry of kavapyrones. Kava is thought to have muscle relaxant and anticonvulsant properties, and has been studied in the treatment of anxiety, tension, and agitation. The side effects of abuse may include yellow discoloration of the skin, hair, and nails;

allergic skin reactions; and sedation. Kava has not been associated with physical or psychological dependency, but is contraindicated in pregnancy, lactation, and depression.

Depression is a common postpartum symptom, and some patients self-diagnose and self-treat with St. John's Wort (*Hypericum perforatum*), credited for centuries with supernatural powers. The risks of self-medication are misdiagnosis and undertreatment; in addition, St. John's Wort is a member of the ragweed family and may cause cross-sensitization. This herb, which has activity similar to that of the SSRIs, is now openly marketed for depression although controlled drug trials that compare antidepressants show efficacy only in cases of mild depression. The main ingredient is hypericien, a photosensitizing substance that may cause sunburns in light-skinned individuals. There are 25 other chemicals in the concoction, which are under investigation and may be more antidepressant than hypericien.

MINIMIZING EFFECT OF MATERNAL MEDICATION ON NURSING THE INFANT

Although it is appropriate to avoid any unnecessary medication during lactation, it must be recognized that for the treatment of some diseases, medication is mandatory. In addition, the risk to the infant of an occasional acetaminophen, ibuprofen, or other over-the-counter medication is minimal if taken in one or two doses only. When a medication must be taken on a daily basis, the following should minimize the amount that passes into the breast milk:

1. Avoid long-acting preparations of the drug, because the infant may have difficulty excreting the agent, especially when hepatic detoxification is required. Accumulation of the compound may otherwise occur in the infant over time.

2. Schedule the doses so that the least amount possible is excreted into milk. If the dose is scheduled so that the peak plasma concentration does not occur during feeding, exposure should be minimized. Administration of the medication immediately after breastfeeding may be the safest time for many but not all drugs, because time to peak plasma concentration varies.

3. Observe the infant for any unusual signs or symptoms, such as change in feeding or sleeping patterns, fussiness, or rash that could be attributed to the medication.

4. When possible, choose the medication that produces the lowest concentration in milk.

SUGGESTED READINGS

Chambers C D, Anderson PO, Thomas RG, et al: Weight gain in infants breastfed by mothers who take fluoxetine. *Pediatrics* 104:e61, 1999.

Committee on Drugs of the American Academy of Pediatrics: The transfer of drugs and other chemicals into human breast milk. *Pediatrics* 72:375, 1983.

Committee on Drugs of the American Academy of Pediatrics: The transfer of drugs and other chemicals into human milk. *Pediatrics* 108:776, 2001.

Committee on Nutritional Status During Pregnancy and Lactation, Institute of Medicine: *Nutrition During Lactation.* Washington, DC: National Academy Press; 1991.

Foster S, Tyler VE: *Tyler's Honest Herbal.* 4th ed. New York, NY: Haworth Herbal Press; 1999.

Goldman AS: The immune system of human milk: Antimicrobials, anti-inflammatory and immune modulating properties. *Pediatr Infect Dis J* 12:664, 1993.

Hale T: *Medications and Mothers Milk.* Amarillo, Tex: Pharmasoft Publishing; 2002.

Howard CR, Lawrence RA: Drugs and breastfeeding (review). *Clin Perinatol* 26:447, 1999.

Koren G, Moretti M, Ito S: Continuing drug therapy while breastfeeding. Part 2. Common misconceptions of physicians. *Can Fam Physician* 45:1173–1175, 1999.

Lawrence RA: *Breastfeeding: A Guide for the Medical Profession.* St. Louis, Mo: Mosby; 1979.

Lawrence RA, Lawrence RM: *Breastfeeding: A Guide for the Medical Profession.* 5th ed. St. Louis, Mo: Mosby; 1999.

Llewellyn A, Stowe ZN, Strader JR: The use of lithium and management of women with bipolar disorder during pregnancy and lactation. *J Clin Psychiatry* 59(suppl):57–64, 1998.

Montgomery A: Use of lithium for treatment of bipolar disorder during pregnancy and lactation. *Acad Breastfeeding Med News Views* 3:4–5, 1997.

Mothers Survey. Ross Products Division, Abbott Laboratories, 2000.

Origliano MD: Herbal medicine. In: Hark L, Morrison G, eds: *Medical Nutrition & Disease.* 3rd ed. Malden, Mass: Blackwell; 2003:75–95.

Rotblatt M, Ziment I: *Evidence-based herbal medicine.* Philadelphia, Penn: Hanley & Belfus; 2002.

Sannerstedt R, Berglund F, Flodh H, et al: Medication during pregnancy and breastfeeding—A new Swedish system for classifying drugs. *Int J Clin Pharmacol Ther Toxicol* 18:45, 1980.

Stowe ZN, Cohen LS, Hostretter A, et al: Paroxetine in human milk and nursing infants. *Am J Psychiatry* 157:185–189, 2000.

Stowe ZN, Owens MJ, Landry JC, et al: Sertraline and des-methylsertraline in human breast milk and nursing infants. *Am J Psychiatry* 154:1255–1260, 1997.

Spigset O, Carleborg L, Ohman R, et al: Excretion of eltalo-pram in breastmilk. *Br J Clin Pharmacol* 44:295–298, 1997.

US Department of Health and Human Services: *Healthy People 2010* (Conference Edition, in Two Volumes). Stock no. 017-001-00537-1.Washington, DC: DHHS Printing Office; January 2000.

Work Group on Breastfeeding: Breastfeeding and the use of human milk. *Pediatrics* 100:1035, 1997.

6

Toxicity in the Premature Infant

Angela Anderson

HIGH-YIELD FACTS

- Skin–barrier function in infants less than 32 weeks' gestation is immature and may remain so until a chronological age of 8 weeks in severely premature infants. As a result, preterm infants may experience enhanced dermal absorption of potentially toxic drugs such as salicylates, phenol, povidone iodine, and hydrocortisone.

- Protein binding is reduced in premature infants, leading to increased amounts of free-active drug. Plasma drug concentrations may therefore underestimate pharmacologic effects.

- The volumes of distribution of hydrophilic drugs are relatively large in the fetus and preterm infant because the total body water content and extracellular fluid compartments are larger than those of older children and adults. In these infants, hydrophilic drugs are distributed over a larger volume, and therefore higher doses are required to achieve therapeutic plasma concentrations.

- Renal excretion is impaired in premature infants because of decreased glomerular filtration, decreased tubular secretion, and increased tubular reabsorption (of acidic drugs). Drugs that are excreted via glomerular filtration (e.g., gentamicin, indomethacin, and digoxin), or tubular secretion (e.g., penicillins, cephalosporins, and furosemide) require longer dosing intervals in premature infants.

- Many hepatic biotransformation pathways are less developed in preterm infants than in adults—other pathways are more active. Morphine clearance in infants 27 weeks' gestation is 25% that of term infants. In contrast, the enzyme methyltransferase allows prematures to clear theophylline via first-order kinetics and better tolerate concentrations that would be toxic in adults, who lack the enzyme.

Advances in technology have afforded medicine the ability to increase survival rates among premature infants. Babies born at an early gestational age often require pharmacologic intervention. However, there are still few studies evaluating the proper use of pharmacotherapy in these small, sick infants. An understanding of pharmacokinetics in premature infants is necessary to ensure proper drug administration and prevent potential toxicity.

PHARMACOKINETICS

Absorption

Dermal

Infants less than 32 weeks' gestation (Figure 6–1) have immature skin barrier function compared to full-term neonates. Their thin stratum corneum allows for increased fluid losses, and enhanced absorption of drugs

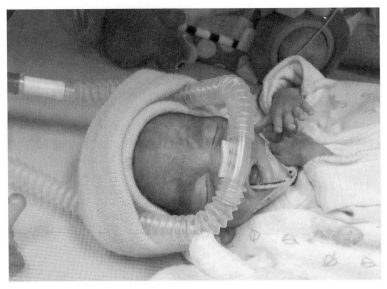

Fig. 6–1. Infants born at less than 32 weeks' gestation are considered premature and often require pharmacologic intervention.

and other potentially toxic substances. Mature skin barrier function is achieved approximately 2 to 4 weeks after birth, but may not occur until 8 weeks postpartum in severely premature infants. Dermal exposure to salicylates, ethanol, phenol, boric acid, hydrocortisone, aniline-containing disinfectant solutions, and hexachlorophene have caused toxicity in neonates.

At least one study suggests that the application of topical povidone-iodine antiseptic solutions to infants weighing less than 1500 g is associated with increased urinary iodine excretion and concomitant hypothyroidism. The observed hypothyroidism was transient: mean serum thyroxine concentrations increased back to normal at the time of discharge. Other studies have not supported this observation but admit potential confounding issues that may have precluded finding a similar association. A study of premature infants (≤33 weeks' gestation) who had transient hypothyroidism (blood thyroxine concentrations 2.6 standard deviations [SD] below the mean during the first week of life) found an associated increased risk of cerebral palsy and lower mental development scores at age 2 years. In premature newborns, therefore, chlorhexidine-containing antiseptics (e.g., Hibiclens and Betasept), which are not systemically absorbed, should be used in lieu of the potentially toxic povidone-iodine solutions.

Oral

A number of factors influence enteral drug absorption, including gastric pH, emptying time, and intestinal motility. Immature gastric mucosa decreases acid secretion in the premature neonate, in whom gastric pH is around 4.7. In the term infant, gastric pH ranges from 2.3 to 3.6, and after 3 years of age, adult gastric pH levels of 1.4 to 2.0 are usually achieved.

It is difficult to predict the net effect of relatively basic gastric pH. Non-ionic substances cross membranes more readily than ionic or charged substances. Consequently, acidic drugs are expected to be absorbed primarily in the acid environment of the stomach, whereas basic drugs are absorbed preferentially in the duodenum and small intestine. However, the thick mucosal layer of the mature stomach impedes gastric absorption, and the larger surface area of the duodenum and small intestine allow for greater absorption of both acidic and basic substances. Consequently—assuming the stomach mucosa is mature —most drug absorption occurs distal to the stomach regardless of drug pKa.

The relatively basic gastric pH of premature infants may be important when considering the absorption of drugs that are acid labile, such as penicillin. Increased gastric pH protects against the degradation of acid-labile substances; thus, the immature gastric mucosa of premature infants may allow greater absorption than that of adults. In fact, higher blood concentrations of penicillin have been reported in premature newborns.

Gastrointestinal motility is unpredictable and irregular in newborns. Although some preterm infants have adultlike duodenal activity, approximately 50% of preterm infants have immature function that diminishes the rate of duodenal contractions and delays gastric emptying following orogastric feedings. Delayed gastric emptying delays time to peak drug plasma concentrations in newborns. However, the *extent* of drug absorption in neonates may be similar to (e.g., digoxin and diazepam), greater than (penicillin G and ampicillin), or less than (phenobarbital and phenytoin) that in adults.

Rectal

Bioavailability following rectal drug administration may be variable, and depends partially on the site of absorption within the rectum. The height of insertion in the rectum may account for the differences seen in peak plasma drug concentrations achieved. The proximal rectum drains into the portal venous system via the inferior mesenteric vein, subjecting drugs to first-pass metabolism and thus decreased bioavailability. The anus and distal rectum drain directly into the systemic circulation via the inferior and middle hemorrhoidal veins.

A number of investigators have studied the pharmacokinetics of rectally administered acetaminophen in preterm neonates. Bioavailability following rectal administration decreases with increasing gestational age. Peak plasma acetaminophen concentrations following rectal acetaminophen administration are significantly higher in infants 28 to 32 weeks' gestation than in those 32 to 36 weeks' gestation. Bioavailability of rectally administered acetaminophen also depends on the preparation used: glycogelatin capsules have higher bioavailability than bullet-shaped triglyceride suppositories (Table 6–1).

Table 6–1. Bioavailability of Acetaminophen Suppositories Relative to Oral Elixir

	Gestational Age	
	28 Weeks	2 Years
Triglyceride suppository	0.86	0.50
Glycogelatin capsule suppository	0.92	0.86

Dosing of rectal capsules, therefore, is lower than that of triglyceride suppositories.

Overall, rectal preparations are less bioavailable than oral solutions; higher doses of acetaminophen are required rectally. One study of triglyceride suppositories revealed that the daily maintenance dose required to achieve a trough therapeutic acetaminophen concentration of 10 mg/L for newborns 30 weeks' gestation was 30 mg/kg/d. This dose increased with gestational age: for infants 34, 40, and 60 weeks' gestation, 60, 80, and 120 mg/kg/d are required, respectively. Although premature infants require lower doses of acetaminophen, drug clearance is significantly reduced (see hepatic elimination); consequently, dosage intervals for both rectal and oral preparations must be lengthened. To maintain a trough concentration of 10 mg/L, dosage intervals for infants 30, 34, 40, and 60 weeks' gestation are 12, 8, 6, and 4 hours, respectively.

Indomethacin has been administered rectally to premature infants to promote closure of a patent ductus arteriosus (PDA); success has been reported after a single rectal dose. Peak plasma concentrations were achieved in 1 to 3 hours.

Aminophylline suppositories have been used successfully in premature infants to treat apnea of prematurity. A loading dose of 10 mg/kg rectally led to therapeutic plasma concentrations within 2 hours, whereas a maintenance dose of 10 mg/kg/d achieved steady-state plasma levels and a reduction in apneic episodes within 24 hours.

Drug Distribution

A number of age-dependent factors influence drug distribution. Differences in protein binding, distribution of water in intracellular and extracellular body compartments, blood pH, and percent body fat all affect drug distribution. This may, in turn, influence pharmacologic responses to a given drug dose or plasma drug concentration. Protein binding is reduced in neonates. This decreased protein binding allows for an increase in the fraction of free drug, which potentially allows for heightened pharmacologic activity. Free drug is cleared more rapidly, however, and the increased activity is transient. The degree of protein binding of a drug depends on a number of factors, including the amount of binding proteins available, the affinity of various drugs for the available proteins, and the presence of substances that compete for protein binding sites.

Fetal albumin is present in the 4th week of gestation, and plasma concentrations rise with gestational age.

Although albumin concentrations approach adult levels by 40 weeks' gestation, the affinity of albumin to *acidic drugs* remains decreased until 10 to 12 months' post-gestational age.

Albumin is the most abundant plasma protein; however, it is not the only protein capable of binding drugs. Basic drugs and lipophilic cations bind to many plasma proteins, including alpha 1-acid glycoprotein (AAG). Although plasma albumin concentrations are close to adult levels (75% to 80%) at birth, AAG concentrations are only 50% of adult levels at birth. Consequently, during the newborn period, drugs that are bound primarily to albumin will parallel the pharmacologic activity and clearance seen in adults more closely than drugs bound primarily to AAG.

The binding affinity of albumin for *bilirubin* at birth is not related to gestational age, but is reduced relative to adult levels. After delivery, this affinity increases; the increase during the first week of life is related to gestational age. Adult levels are achieved at approximately 5 months of age. Increased neonatal susceptibility to kernicterus is postulated to be at least partially due to the lower affinity of albumin for bilirubin.

Free fatty acids are increased in the neonate as a consequence of increased lipolysis during the first week of life. Fatty acids and bilirubin both compete for drug binding sites on proteins, allowing increased free-drug concentrations in the blood. The relatively acidic (approximately 7.1 to 7.3) blood pH of neonates, as well as hypoxemia, contribute to reduced drug–protein binding. Whenever drugs have been displaced from binding proteins, total drug concentrations may underestimate potentially significant free-drug concentrations.

Changes in body water content also affect drug volume of distribution. As the fetus and infant mature, the proportion of adipose tissue increases while total body water and the size of the extracellular fluid compartment decrease. Alteration in fluid compartment size affects the dosage required to attain therapeutic plasma and tissue drug concentrations.

Body fat in fetuses less than 3 months' gestational age is less than 1%. The total body water content of these fetuses is 92% of body weight; extracellular and intracellular fluid compartments represent 65% and 25% of body weight, respectively. At term, total body water and the extracellular fluid compartment decrease in size to 75% and to 35% to 44% of body weight, respectively; the intracellular fluid compartment increases somewhat to 33% of body weight. These trends continue until puberty, when adolescent compartment sizes approximate those of adults.

As mentioned, the volume of distribution of a drug is related to the water compartments of the body: a comparatively large total body water compartment (as seen in the fetus and newborn infant) is associated with increased drug volume of distribution. Extrapolating this information to the equation

Steady-state drug concentration =
Dose/Volume of distribution

it is evident that premature infants and young children require higher per-kilogram doses of hydrophilic drugs to achieve comparable drug concentrations.

Elimination

Renal

Most drugs and many drug metabolites are eliminated from the body via the kidney. Renal function in preterm infants is dramatically reduced. Consequently, renally excreted drugs have a prolonged elimination half-life, and premature infants require longer dosing intervals of these drugs.

The components of renal excretion include glomerular filtration, tubular secretion, and tubular reabsorption, all of which are immature in the preterm neonate. Glomerular filtration, and therefore urine formation, begins around 10 weeks' gestation, and nephrogenesis is complete by 34 to 36 weeks' gestation. Infants less than 34 weeks' gestation have fewer glomeruli and significantly lower glomerular filtration rates (GFR) than neonates greater than 34 weeks' gestation. The GFR in the premature infant at birth ranges from 0.2 to 2 mL/min, whereas that of the term infant is between 1.5 and 4.0 mL/min. By comparison, the average adult GFR is 120 to 130 mL/min. Neonates at 30 and 40 weeks' gestation produce urine at rates of 10 and 27 mL/h, respectively.

Preterm infants who are also small for gestational age (SGA) have even lower glomerular filtration rates. One study compared the GFRs of SGA and appropriate for gestational age (AGA) premature infants: GFR (as measured by creatinine clearance) in the SGA infants on days 3, 7, and 14 days' postdelivery was 16, 21, and 37 mL/min/1.73 m^2, respectively. AGA infants, measured on the same time scale, had GFRs of 21, 36, and 58 mL/min/1.73 m^2, respectively. The difference between the SGA and AGA GFRs in preterm neonates continues until 2 weeks of life.

After delivery, increased cardiac output and decreased peripheral vascular resistance raise renal blood flow; increases occur in filtration surface area and membrane pore size. These factors contribute to a rise in GFR. The postnatal increase in GFR depends on postconceptual, not postnatal, age. The rise in GFR in term infants is substantial in the first 3 days of life. During this time, GFR of infants greater than 34 weeks' gestation increases to between 8 and 20 mL/min. Younger neonates, however, experience a rise in GFR to only 2 to 3 mL/min over the same period. GFRs for term infants reach adult values by age 2.5 to 5.0 months. GFR in very low birth weight infants does not reach the same levels as term infants until 9 months of age.

The importance of an immature GFR is evident when considering the administration of renally excreted drugs that are potentially toxic. Aminoglycosides are eliminated via glomerular filtration. Gentamicin is more effectively excreted with increasing postconceptual age. Blood elimination half-life between 26 and 34 weeks' gestation is approximately 8 hours, diminishing to 6.7 hours between 35 and 37 weeks', and to 4.9 hours in infants greater than 37 weeks' gestation. As a result, premature infants require longer dosing intervals than those born at term. Other examples of drugs eliminated via glomerular filtration include indomethacin and digoxin.

Tubular secretion in term infants is 20% to 30% of adult levels as a result of small tubular length and mass, reduced blood flow to the outer renal cortex, and immature energy-dependent processes, and does not mature fully until 6 to 10 months of age. Penicillins, sulfonamides, cephalosporins, and furosemide are among the medications excreted via tubular secretion.

Tubular immaturity may be even more pronounced in premature infants. Tubular secretion (as measured by the fractional excretion of sodium) was lower in one study of newborns younger than 36 weeks' gestation compared to term infants, but this finding did not achieve statistical significance. Studies that examine excretion of specific drugs concur that tubular secretion is dependent on gestational age. The elimination half-life ($t_{1/2}$) of penicillins

has been shown to decrease with increasing gestational and post-gestational age. The $t_{1/2}$ at birth for methicillin is 4.3 hours for newborns less than 33 weeks' gestation, but only 2.0 hours for term infants. Elimination half-lives of various antibiotics are noted in Table 6–2. Furosemide is both secreted and filtered in the kidney. Elimination $t_{1/2}$ following a single dose is 19.9 hours in premature infants, 7.7 hours in term infants, and 30 minutes in adults.

There is evidence that substrate stimulation of secretory pathways (i.e., the presence of a substance enhances the secretion of itself or another substance) occurs in infants as it does in adults. Administration of multiple doses of ampicillin induces a reduction in $t_{1/2}$ in both term and preterm neonates, compared to administration of a single dose. Gestational age and urine pH both affect tubular reabsorption of drugs. Newborn urinary pH values are relatively acidic; consequently, weak organic acids in this environment are expected to cross membranes more readily and have a high reabsorption rate. Higher reabsorption and lower tubular secretion rates, as well as low GFR, impair drug elimination, potentially prolonging the pharmacologic effects of renally excreted drugs.

Hepatic Drug Metabolism

Development of hepatic drug clearance mechanisms is quite important when considering drug administration to the premature newborn. Critically ill patients may have even lower enzyme activity, further compromising hepatic clearance. Intrauterine growth retardation also appears to adversely affect the development of hepatic function. Premature infants (28 to 36 weeks' gestation) who are small for gestational age (SGA; weighing 860 to 1850 g), are less able to perform biotransformation than appropriate for gestational age (AGA; weighing 980 to 2480 g) infants.

Table 6–2. Apparent Elimination Half-Lives ($t_{1/2}$), Hours

Drug	Premature Newborn	Full-Term Newborn	Adult
Amikacin	9.6–5.1 (1–4 weeks)	5.7 (2–8 days)	1.4–2.3
Ampicillin	6.2–1.7 (2–30 days)	3.5–1.7	0.6–1.6
Benzylpenicillin	4.9–2.1	1.2–1.3	0.95–1.20
Cefotaxime	2.4	1.5	1.2
Chloramphenicol	28 (2 days)		
	8 (13–23 days)		1.5–5.0
Kanamycin	18–20 (2–22 days)		2.1–2.4

Source: Adapted from Heimann (1981).

For hepatic metabolism of a drug to proceed, it must first interact with hepatic cells. The Y protein, known as ligandin or intracellular albumin, is housed in the cytoplasm of hepatic cells, and is one of the proteins responsible for facilitating transport of bilirubin and anionic substances, such as drugs, into the liver. The fetus and newborn have a relative deficiency of Y protein; adult concentrations are reached 5 to 10 days after birth.

Following hepatic uptake, drugs undergo phase I and phase II biotransformation reactions. Phase I reactions transform substances into polar (less lipid-soluble) compounds that undergo excretion via the kidney, biliary system, or lung. During this phase, drugs are hydroxylated, reduced, oxidized, or hydrolyzed.

The cytochrome P450 or CYP enzymes are the most widely studied phase I enzymes. They catalyze the metabolism of many endogenous substances, including steroids, fatty acids, fat-soluble vitamins, prostaglandins, leukotrienes, and thromboxanes. CYP enzymes also catalyze drug metabolism. High concentrations of endogenous substances (e.g., steroids found in premature infants) may compete for oxidative enzymes and therefore reduce oxidative metabolism of some drugs (e.g., theophylline).

Many phase I enzyme concentrations, or activities, are relatively deficient early in gestation and remain depressed at the time of birth. Although CYP oxidative enzyme activity is low at delivery, it undergoes rapid maturation after birth. As a result, drug clearance of hepatically metabolized drugs may be minimal at birth; however, clearance rates reach, and may even exceed, adult levels within the first several weeks to months of life. Six cytochromes are responsible for 90% of oxidative metabolism: CYP 1A2, 2C9, 2C19, 2D6, 2E1, and 3A4. The known ontogeny of these enzymes is listed in Table 6–3.

Phase II reactions are conjugation reactions in which drugs are combined with endogenous molecules, most commonly glucuronide, sulphate, glycine, acetate, and glutathione, a process that renders them even more water soluble and easier to eliminate. To be conjugated, a drug must have a functional group (e.g., carboxyl, sulfhydryl, hydroxyl, or amino group). Some drugs inherently contain one of these groups; others undergo a phase I reaction to acquire one.

Phase II enzymes are often transferases, and include glucuronosyltransferases (UGTs), sulfotransferases (STs), arylamine *N*-acetyltransferases (NAT1 and NAT2), and a variety of methyltransferases (MTs). Epoxide hydrolase is also a phase II enzyme. The ontogeny of phase II enzymes is not defined as well as that of phase I enzymes.

Glucuronic acid is plentiful and binds easily with all functional groups. As a result, glucuronidation is the most common conjugation pathway. Glucuronidation is also one of the best-studied phase II pathways in the pre-term infant, and UGT is responsible for catalyzing substrate conjugation with glucuronic acid. The fetal liver is capable of performing glucuronidation at 16 weeks' gestation. However, adult activity of most UGT enzymes is not achieved until 6 to 24 months postnatal age. Immature UGT activity is responsible for the causative association of neonatal chloramphenicol administration and cardiovascular collapse known as *gray baby syndrome*.

Bilirubin, morphine, and acetaminophen are also UGT substrates. Bilirubin conjugation depends on UGT 1A1 activity, which is absent in fetal liver but increases after birth; adult levels are reached by age 6 months. Neonatal jaundice is at least partially attributable to underdeveloped UGT 1A1 activity.

Morphine undergoes glucuronidation in the presence of UGT 2B7, which appears around 24 weeks' gestation; however, in vitro studies indicate that morphine glucuronidation in fetal liver is 10% to 20% of adult activity. Morphine clearance rates are low in premature infants and increase with gestational age. One study found that premature infants at gestational ages of 26.8, 29.8, 33.1, and 37.8 weeks have morphine clearance rates of 2.27, 3.21, 4.51, and 7.8 mL/kg/min, respectively; corresponding elimination half-lives were 13.5, 9.2, 7.0, and 7.7 hours. In essence, morphine clearance increases approximately fourfold between 26.8 weeks' postconception and term. Terminal elimination half-life in adults is 2 hours. Another study of infants born at 26 to 40 weeks' gestation revealed that morphine clearance increased at a rate of 0.9 mL/kg/min per week of gestation.

UGT 1A6 (and to a lesser extent UGT 1A9) promotes glucuronidation of acetaminophen, which is impaired in the neonate; in contrast, sulfation of acetaminophen is more active in neonates than in older children and adults (see below). Acetaminophen clearance is reduced at birth and increases with age until adult levels are achieved around 12 months of age. Clearance in premature infants at 28 weeks' gestation is impaired to an even greater extent at 0.74 L/h/70 kg. Clearance at 60 weeks postconception (5 months of age) is 10.9 L/h/70 kg, which is 86% of adult values.

Sulfotransferase activity during fetal life is variable and isoform specific. Maturation, in general, is more rapid than that of UGTs, and some ST isoforms exceed adult activity levels during infancy. Among the substrates for ST enzymes are acetaminophen and dopamine. Fetal livers, 19 to 22 weeks of age, are able to conjugate acetaminophen with sulfate. Acetaminophen ST does not appear to provide significant protection against hepatotoxic doses of acetaminophen in hamsters.

Table 6–3. Cytochrome P450

	CYP Presence/Activity in the Premature Infant and Neonate	Common Substrates	Notes
CYP 1A2	Low activity in premature infants and newborns. Activity reaches adult levels by 55 weeks postconceptual age or 4 months postnatal age. Activity exceeds adult levels between 1 and 2 years of age.	Theophylline, caffeine, acetaminophen, warfarin, estradiol.	Theophylline clearance, decreased at birth, increases linearly in 1st year of life. Clearance is approximately 10 mL/h/kg at 30 weeks' postconceptual age, rising to approximately 80 mL/h/kg at 100 weeks' postconceptual age. CYP 1A2 pathway metabolizes a small amount of APAP to NAPQI; CYP 2E1 generates most NAPQI.
CYP 2C9	Low activity in neonates; adult activity reached at approximately 6 months.	Phenytoin, ibuprofen, THC.	Apparent $t_{1/2}$ of DPH is approximately 75 h in premature infants, 20 h in term infants, and 8 h after 2 weeks.
CYP 2C19	No data found.	DPH, imipramine, citalopram.	Responsible for biotransformation of very few agents used in infants; involved in the metabolism of DPH to HPPH but contributes only 5% of HPPH production.
CYP 2D6	Fetal activity 1% of adult values; rises to 20% of adult by age 28 days.	Codeine, ondansetron, propranolol, oxycodone, captopril, diphenhydramine.	Bioactivates codeine to its active metabolite morphine.
CYP 3A7	Predominant fetal CYP, accounting for 30–50% of total; present in fetal liver by 50–60 days' gestation.	Dehydroepiandrosterone sulfate, ethinylestradiol, triazolam, 1,4-dihydropyridines	Activities decrease simultaneously with postnatal increases in CYP 3A4.
CYP 3A4	Very low concentrations in the fetus; expression activated within first few weeks of birth irrespective of gestational age. Activity is 30–40% of adult activity at 1 month of age, increasing 5-fold in the first 3 months of life.	Midazolam, diazepam, fentanyl, CBZ, amiodarone, lidocaine, digoxin, budesonide, acetaminophen, theophylline, EES.	Midazolam clearance impaired in young (<2 weeks of age), preterm (26–34 weeks) neonates, 2.3 mL/kg/min; infants 3 months, 3–9 mL/kg/min; children, 5–13 mL/kg/min; adults, 6–11 mL/kg/min.

Abbreviations: APAP, acetaminophen; CBZ, carbamazepine; DPH, diphenylhydantoin; EES, erythromycin; HPPH, 5-(para-hydroxyphenyl)-5-phenyhydantoin; NAPQI, *N*-acetyl-p-benzoquinoneimine; THC, tetrahydrocannabinol.

The major catecholamine-metabolizing ST in the fetal liver is SULT1A3. The activity of this dopamine ST is 75.6 pmol/min·mg at 16.2 weeks' gestation, but decreases rapidly to 6.7 pmol/min·mg at 48 weeks' gestation. The activity of this enzyme is absent in adults.

MT pathways are well developed in premature and term newborns, and are responsible for the biotransformation of theophylline into its *N*-methylated metabolite, caffeine. This pathway also appears to be absent in adults. Neonates biotransform theophylline via methylation, whereas adults metabolize theophylline via demethylation. Eighty percent of theophylline in adults is metabolized via CYP 1A2 to demethylated products: 1-methylxanthine and 3-methylxanthine. CYP 1A2 activity is deficient in the neonate, as described.

One study demonstrated that theophylline undergoes first-order kinetics in low birth weight (670 to 1800 g) premature (25 to 32 weeks' gestation) infants, even in the event of theophylline overdose and plasma concentrations as high as 10 times the therapeutic range. Older children and adults, in contrast, demonstrate saturable, zero-order theophylline kinetics. These findings suggest that premature infants may be better able to tolerate plasma theophylline concentrations that would be highly toxic to older children and adults.

NAT-2 activity is also immature in newborn infants. Infants remain slow acetylators of caffeine until 15 months of age. Premature infants metabolize caffeine to theophylline, primarily via N7-demethylation (a cytochrome P450 process).

EFFECTS OF A PATENT DUCTUS ARTERIOSUS ON DRUG DISPOSITION

In utero, the ductus arteriosus (DA) is responsible for carrying blood from the pulmonary artery to the fetal systemic circulation, thereby bypassing the lungs. After delivery, pulmonary vascular resistance decreases and allows flow to the newly functioning lungs. The DA is no longer required and, under normal circumstances, closes shortly after birth. Premature infants are at increased risk of maintaining a PDA. In these infants, a portion of the blood that would have traveled to the systemic circulation via the aorta now passes through the DA to the lungs. The final result is decreased organ perfusion, increased fluid reabsorption, fluid overload, and metabolic acidosis. Infants may have varying degrees of ductal patency; therefore, the pharmacokinetic effects of a PDA may have significant individual variation (Table 6–4).

Organ hypoperfusion influences drug absorption and clearance: decreases in intestinal blood flow may reduce enteral drug absorption and thereby impair bioavailability; reduced renal and hepatic blood flow may prolong drug elimination. Fluid overload increases the volume of distribution (V_d) of hydrophilic drugs. Drugs with larger V_d require higher initial doses to attain comparable plasma concentrations.

Metabolic acidosis from tissue hypoperfusion can decrease protein binding of some drugs, such as theophylline, leading to a larger V_d. Some drugs (e.g., phenobarbital: pKa 7.4) may become un-ionized in the presence of acidosis, leading to enhanced movement across cell membranes, elevated tissue concentrations, and further increases in V_d. A number of studies evaluating the pharmacokinetics of gentamicin have supported these theories,

with documented increases in V_d and $t_{1/2}$ in patients with a PDA compared to those with a closed DA. Other studies have documented that closure of the DA may lead to dramatic and abrupt decreases in drug V_d, which may cause elevations in plasma drug concentrations. Prolonged elimination half-lives may exacerbate this effect.

Indomethacin, which is administered to infants to promote closure of the DA, also decreases renal drug elimination and further confounds the picture. Accumulations of digoxin, gentamicin, amikacin, and vancomycin have been described in patients receiving indomethacin. Closure of the DA and indomethacin-related decreases in renal excretion are possible mechanisms.

SPECIFIC DRUG INFORMATION

Digoxin

Digoxin is used frequently to manage cardiac dysrhythmias in premature infants. Most studies evaluating the pharmacokinetics of digoxin in preterm neonates were carried out before the discovery that the fetus produces digoxin-like immunoreactive substances (DLIS). These DLIS, which cross-react with agents used to measure digoxin, cause false elevations in digoxin concentrations. The presence of DLIS has been described in patients who are pregnant or have renal failure, hypertension, or hypertrophic cardiomyopathy. Significant DLIS concentrations (≥0.5 ng/mL) have been documented in 64% of healthy neonates, 42% of premature infants, and 77% of full-term SGA babies.

Propylene Glycol

Propylene glycol (1,2 propanediol) is a solvent used in many drug preparations. Large quantities of propylene glycol have been known to cause seizures, cardiovascular collapse, cardiac dysrhythmias, hepatic damage, metabolic acidosis, hemolysis, and serum hyperosmolality. Medications that commonly contain propylene glycol include diazepam, phenobarbital, silver sulfadiazine, digoxin, phenytoin, and MVI-12 (an intravenous multivitamin, Armor Pharmaceuticals Co).

There are at least two studies documenting propylene glycol toxicity in premature infants. In one study of infants weighing less than 1500 g, administration of MVI-12 in a dose of 3 g/d led to an increased incidence of seizure activity, and in a report of a 27-week, 890-g infant, MVI-12 caused hyperosmolality.

The World Health Organization (WHO) recommends that the daily oral intake of propylene glycol be limited

Table 6–4. Pharmacokinetics of Various Drugs

Medication	Therapeutic Use	Oral Bioavailability	V_d (L/kg)	Protein Binding	$t_{1/2}$ (h)	Clearance	Ref.
Indomethacin 28–36 weeks' gestation (IV and PO)	Closure of DA	10–20%	0.33–0.40; no correlation with GA	99% (similar to adults)	17.2 in infants <32 w GA vs 12.5 in infants >32 w GA ($P < .05$)	25% of adult values	
Caffeine	Apnea of prematurity	100% peak concentrations reached in 0.5–2.0 h	0.78–0.92		65–103	8.5–8.9 mL/kg/h	Besunder
Theophylline (IV)	Apnea of prematurity		0.69	36.4%	24.7–36.5	17.6–39 mL/kg/h	Besunder; Lowry
Gentamicin					See renal excretion		
Midazolam (PO) 26–31 w GA	Sedation		1.4 (range 0.3–12.1)		7.6 (range 1.2–15.1)	2.7 mL/kg/min	
Midazolam (IV) 26–34 w GA	Sedation		1.1 (range 0.4–4.2)		6.3 (range 2.6–17.7)	1.8 mL/kg/min	
Morphine (IV)	Analgesia	72%	2.2–2.3	20%	See hepatic drug metabolism	See hepatic drug metabolism	
Digoxin (interpret with caution; see DLIS)	Myocardial rhythm disturbances	20%	LBW infants: 4.3–5.7; FT newborns: 7.5–9.7 (larger than LBW infants 2° to increased tissue binding)	20%	Preterm infants: 38–88 h (average 57 h) Term infants: 17–52 h (average 35 h)	26–29 w GA, 1.35 L/h/1.73 m²; 30–32 w GA, 1.77 L/h/1.73 m²; 3340 w GA, 3.54 L/h/1.73 m²	Besunder

Abbreviations: DA, ductus arteriosus; DLIS, digoxin-like immunoreactive substances; FT, full term; GA, gestational age; IV, intravenous; LBW, low birth weight; PO, orally; V_d, volume of distribution.

41

to less than 25 mg/kg. The typical loading dose of phenytoin for a 1-kg premature infant exceeds the WHO limit for propylene glycol by a factor of 7.

SUMMARY

Drug administration to the premature infant requires that special attention be paid to differences in drug absorption, distribution, and elimination. Changes in total body water, protein binding, renal structure, and hepatic and enzyme activity may affect drug activity and duration of action. One must keep in mind that these differences are not static, but a continuum. As the fetus and neonate mature, so do their body structures and metabolic processes. Until these processes reach adult levels, it is important to monitor drug levels when possible and to beware of potential toxicity.

SUGGESTED READINGS

Anderson BJ, van Lingen RA, et al: Acetaminophen developmental pharmacokinetics in premature neonates and infants: A pooled population analysis. *Anesthesiology* 96:1336–45, 2002.

Bertrand J, Langhendries J, et al: Digoxin-like immunoreactive substance in serum of preterm and full-term neonates. *Eur J Pediatr* 146:145–146, 1987.

Besunder JB, Reed MD, Blumer JL: Principles of drug biodisposition in the neonate. A critical evaluation of the pharmacokinetic-pharmacodynamic interface (Part I). *Clin Pharmacokinet* 14:189–216, 1988.

Chevalier RL: Developmental renal physiology of the low birth weight pre-term newborn. *J Urol* 156:714–719, 1996.

Gal P, Gilman J: Drug disposition in neonates with patent ductus arteriosus. *Ann Pharmacother* 27:1383–1388, 1993.

Glasgow A, Boeckx R, Miller MK, et al: Hyperosmolality in small infants due to propylene glycol. *Pediatrics* 72:353–355, 1983.

Heimann G: Drug disposition during the perinatal period. *Int J Biol Res Pregnancy* 2:1–14, 1981.

Kearns G: Meeting the needs of the modernization act: Challenges in developing pediatric therapies. Impact of developmental pharmacology on pediatric study design: Overcoming the challenges. *J Allergy Clin Immunol* 106:S128–138, 2000.

Leeder JS: Pediatric critical care: A new millennium. Pharmacogenetics and Pharmacogenomics. *Pediatr Clin North Am* 48:765–781, 2001.

Leeder JS, Kearns G: Pharmacogenetics in pediatrics. Implications for practice. *Pediatr Clin North Am* 44:55–77, 1997.

Lowry JA, Jarrett RV, Wasserman G, et al: Theophylline toxicokinetics in premature newborns. *Arch Pediatr Adolesc Med* 155:934–939, 2001.

MacDonald MG, Getson PR, Glasgow AM, et al: Propylene glycol: Increased incidence of seizures in low birth weight infants. *Pediatrics* 79:622–625, 1987.

McNamara PJ, Alcorn J: Protein binding predictions in infants. *AAPS PharmSci* 4:E4, 2002.

Reddy MD, Karan S, Reddy SV: Glomerular filtration rate in term and preterm infants in the first three weeks of life. *Indian Pediatr* 21:267–269, 1984.

Reuss ML, Paneth N, Pinto-Martin JA, et al: The relation of transient hypothyroxinemia in preterm infants to neurologic development at two years of age. *N Engl J Med* 334: 821–827, 1996.

Smerdely P, Lim A, Boyages SC, et al: Topical iodine-containing antiseptics and neonatal hypothyroidism in very-low-birth-weight infants. *Lancet* 2:661–664, 1989.

Touw DJ, Proost JH, Stevens R, et al: Gentamicin pharmacokinetics in preterm infants with a patent and a closed ductus arteriosus. *Pharm World Sci* 23:200–204, 2001.

Warner A: Drug use in the neonate: Interrelationships of pharmacokinetics, toxicity, and biochemical maturity. *Clin Chem* 32:721–727, 1986.

WHO: Joint Food and Agriculture Organization/WHO Expert Committee on Food Additives: Toxicological evaluation of some food additives. Geneva, Technical Report Series 539: 270–277, 1974.

7

Special Toxicologic Considerations in the Neonate

James F. Wiley II

High-Yield Facts

- The major modes of neonatal poisoning differ greatly from types seen in older children and adults.

- Understanding neonatal toxicology requires an appreciation of markedly different pharmacokinetics that place young infants at increased risk from toxins absorbed via the dermis, and from toxins requiring hepatic metabolism or renal excretion.

- Passive exposure to drugs of abuse, neonatal withdrawal, and child abuse by poisoning are prominent etiologies of neonatal toxin exposure.

- Certain toxin measurements, such as percent carboxyhemoglobin, percent methemoglobin, and cholinesterase activity, may be altered in the neonate in the absence of exogenous toxin exposure.

- Treatment of neonatal poisoning depends largely on stabilization measures and supportive care.

Neonates are arbitrarily defined as babies younger than 3 months of age (Figure 7–1). As a special population, they have patterns of poisoning quite different from those of older children and adults. Unintentional ingestions are the most common form of poisoning in children and adults, accounting for 76% of exposures in the United States in 2000. Unintentional ingestions occur rarely in the neonate. Secondary exposure, either in utero or via breast milk, and iatrogenic exposure are the major modes of poisoning in young infants.

An understanding of neonatal toxicology requires an appreciation of the unique physical vulnerabilities of this population. Because of their unique pharmacokinetics, neonates respond differently to toxins. This chapter focuses on the epidemiology, pharmacokinetics, common exposures, and treatment modalities in the full-term neonate.

EPIDEMIOLOGY

National poison control center data do not specifically report the number of neonatal exposures. Of the 2,168,248 human exposures reported to poison control centers in the United States in 2000, children younger than 12 months of age accounted for 6.5% of cases, and 0.5% of fatalities. Extrapolation from these data suggests that neonatal poisoning accounts for a small fraction of exposures.

Although toxic neonatal exposures are rare, the consequences can be severe. Classic examples of severe effects from iatrogenic neonatal exposures include the gasping syndrome, related to benzyl alcohol preservative in intravenous flush solutions, and the gray baby syndrome, associated with chloramphenicol (Table 7–1). In general, the neonate is predisposed to severe effects from dermal exposures, and from toxic agents requiring hepatic metabolism or renal excretion.

SPECIAL AGE CONSIDERATIONS

Understanding the pharmacologic basis for neonatal vulnerability to specific drugs begins with an appreciation of

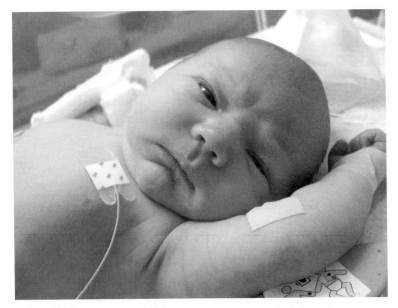

Fig. 7–1. Neonates are generally defined as babies younger than 3 months of age.

Table 7–1. Classic Iatrogenic Neonatal Exposures Resulting in Severe Effects

Agent	Mode of Exposure	Effect
Benzyl alcohol	IV fluids with 0.9% benzyl alcohol preservative	Respiratory depression with gasping, metabolic acidosis, hypotension, renal failure, CNS depression, death
Boric acid	Topical antiseptic, diaper rash treatment	Fever, vomiting, diarrhea, desquamation, coma, seizures, cardiovascular collapse, renal failure, death
Chloramphenicol	IV administration without monitoring of drug levels	Lethargy, metabolic acidosis, abdominal distension, hypotension, death
Hexachlorophene	Dermal absorption from contaminated talc powder	Coma, seizures, death, encephalopathy
Inorganic mercury	Oral (teething powder), mercurial diaper powders, mercurochrome cleansing of umbilical stump	*Acrodynia*: erythematous, swollen painful palms and soles with pink papular rash progressing to desquamation and ulceration *Associated findings*: tachycardia, diaphoresis, irritability, and tremors
Iodine	Dermal	Goiter, hypothyroidism
Isopropyl alcohol	Dermal	Hemorrhagic skin necrosis, hypotonia, coma, acetone odor
Methylmercury	Mercurial contamination of maternal food and in utero fetal and breast milk exposure	Delayed motor development, mental retardation, seizures, deafness
Pentachlorophenol	Dermal via diapers and linens	Fever, tachycardia, metabolic acidosis, diaphoresis, death

Abbreviations: CNS, central nervous system; IV, intravenous.

Table 7–2. Clinical Implications of Neonatal Pharmacokinetics on Therapeutic Drug Administration Compared with Adults

Pharmacokinetic Difference	Clinical Adjustment
Larger apparent volume of distribution	Increase single or loading dose of drug
Lower plasma protein binding (increased free-fraction drug activity)	Lower total plasma concentration for pharmacologic effect
Lower total drug clearance due to immature phase I and II metabolic pathways and diminished renal excretion	Lower weight-based daily doses when multiple doses of drug given
Rapid change in drug metabolism with increased age and large variation by gestational age	Rapidly alter dosing requirements based on close monitoring of drug effect and drug concentration (when feasible)

Source: Adapted from Rylance G: Pharmacological principles and kinetics, in Rylance G, Harvey D, Aranda JV (eds): *Neonatal Clinical Pharmacology and Therapeutics*. London: Butterworth-Heinemann Ltd.; 1991.

the differences in their pharmacokinetics relative to adults. These differences encompass the four basic processes of drug absorption, distribution, metabolism, and excretion. General clinical implications for these differences are summarized in Table 7–2.

Absorption

An elevated gastric pH and decreased gastric emptying relative to the adult alters gastric absorption of medications in the young infant. The elevated gastric pH retards the absorption of acidic drugs and enhances absorption of basic drugs in the neonate. Delayed gastric emptying delays drug absorption that occurs primarily in the duodenum. Typically, this delay results in a lower peak serum drug concentration, and prolonged time to peak concentration.

Dermal absorption occurs at a much higher rate in neonates than in adults. Term infants have mature skin but a greater surface area-to-mass ratio, resulting in approximately three times greater systemic availability of a percutaneous drug dose relative to an adult.

Premature infants (those born at less than 28 weeks' gestation) have a very immature epidermal layer that is only 1 to 2 cells thick, and a mostly absent stratum

corneum. In vitro studies on postmortem skin specimens have found skin absorption in 26-week-gestation premature infants to range from 3 to 50 times that of term infants for a variety of alcohols, and up to as much as 1000 times higher than term infants for salicylates. This marked dermal immaturity changes rapidly after birth, so that at a chronological age of about 3 weeks, the skin of a premature infant is similar to that of a term infant.

Distribution

Neonates display lower drug–protein binding and have higher total body and extracellular fluid spaces. Diminished protein binding results in increased free drug concentrations for a given dose relative to adults, and a potential for heightened pharmacologic effect. In addition, the apparent volume of distribution is increased and may prolong the half-life of the drug. On the other hand, the greater total body water and extracellular fluid space requires a higher dose of drug to reach the same concentration in these compartments in a neonate as opposed to an adult.

Metabolism

Elucidation of drug metabolism in the fetus and neonate has been derived from a complex array of information, much of which is extrapolated from murine models. The traditional view has suggested that drug metabolism and enzyme activity is essentially absent in the fetus, and severely limited in the neonate. However, recent evidence suggests that this belief does not adequately consider the variation in isoforms within the enzyme systems, such as cytochrome P450, the distribution and organ-specific patterns of expression of various enzymes, the potentiation of drug metabolism in individual fetuses exposed in utero, and the potential for alteration of enzyme expression created by chronic disease. Emerging information suggests that phase I fetal hepatic function (e.g., P450 system, alcohol dehydrogenase) is less than adult function, with variation from negligible activity to 50% that of adult levels. After birth, hepatic function develops at various rates depending on the system, individual exposure to xenobiotics, and organ site. Similarly, phase II metabolic pathways such as glucuronidation, sulfation, and acetylation are markedly depressed in the fetus and neonate, with development to adult levels occurring over months to years after birth.

Excretion

Renal excretion has direct impact on the elimination of drugs and their metabolites from the body, with very few exceptions. Glomerular filtration rate (GFR) and tubular secretion and reabsorption determine renal excretion. The GFR increases directly with age beyond 34 weeks' gestation, to the term infant value of 2 to 4 mL/min at birth. During the first 72 hours of life in the term infant, the GFR increases another 5- to 10-fold. The lower GFR relative to adults found in premature and term infants dictates reduced dose and increased intervals between doses of drugs that undergo primary renal excretion, such as aminoglycosides.

Tubular reabsorption is reasonably well developed in the neonate. However, tubular secretion is only 10% of adult values, and develops more slowly than GFR over the first 6 months of life. Diminished tubular secretion leads to prolonged elimination half-life for drugs such as penicillins and furosemide that rely on active tubular secretion in the kidney.

MOST COMMON TOXINS

Passive Fetal Exposure

The categories of human in utero exposure consist of maternal drugs of abuse, maternal environmental exposure, and maternal prescription drug use. Major fetal exposures from maternal drug abuse associated with specific postnatal abnormalities occur most commonly from ethanol, opiates, and cocaine. Maternal and perinatal factors (Table 7–3) dictate monitoring for perinatal exposure to drugs of abuse. Toxicologic screening of the mother includes urine testing for drugs of abuse and plasma alcohol after obtaining informed consent, and screening of neonatal meconium. The specimen must be the size of a quarter and obtained before the passage of transitional stool to provide valid neonatal exposure results.

Fetal Alcohol Syndrome

Fetal alcohol syndrome occurs in the children of 0.5% to 4.0% of alcoholic women. Signs in each of the three following categories define this syndrome: (1) pre- or postnatal growth retardation, (2) neurologic abnormalities including jitteriness, developmental delay, and hyperactivity, and (3) at least two of the following: microcephaly, short palpebral fissures, poorly developed philtrum, thin upper lip, or flattened maxilla. Other neurodevelopmental abnormalities associated with maternal alcohol use include motor dysfunction, tremors, decreased visual perceptual ability, and poor hand–eye coordination. As little as one drink per day has been associated with abnormalities in fine and gross motor

Table 7–3. Maternal and Infant Factors Associated With Maternal Substance Use

Maternal Factors	Infant Factors
Positive history of maternal substance use within 1 year of infant conception	Prematurity without cause
	IUGR without cause
	Vascular accidents in a term baby (stroke, CNS hemorrhage)
Poor prenatal care	Jittery or lethargic infant beyond 6 h of life with no hypoglycemia
Precipitous delivery	
Unplanned delivery out of the hospital or in the emergency department	Neonatal seizures
Placental abruption without previa	
Sexually transmitted disease in the mother	
Violence/incarceration within the past year	
Maternal altered mental status	
Maternal intoxication or withdrawal	
Track marks	
Loss of custody of other children	

Abbreviations: CNS, central nervous system; IUGR, intrauterine growth retardation.

tasks 4 years after birth. This effect is linear, with no clear threshold below which alcohol ingestion is safe.

Neonatal Abstinence Syndrome

An estimated 70,000 neonates annually are exposed to opioids during gestation and at risk for neonatal abstinence syndrome (NAS) after birth. NAS occurs in up to 50% of heroin-exposed infants, and 70% of methadone-exposed infants. Symptoms include abnormal arousal, difficulty maintaining a stable mental status, hyperresponsiveness, jitteriness, irritability, feeding difficulty, vomiting, diarrhea, diaphoresis, and constant movement that result in abrasions on the elbows and knees. Typically, a heroin-exposed infant will begin to withdraw 24 hours after birth, and will complete withdrawal in 7 to 10 days. A methadone-exposed infant usually begins withdrawal 2 to 7 days after birth, and ends withdrawal 3 to 8 weeks later. A variety of neonatal withdrawal scores exist to determine which infants will benefit from pharmacologic intervention. Finnegan has provided a

Table 7–4. NAS Scoring Systems

Score	Assessment	Evaluator
Neonatal Abstinence Scale	33 numerically weighted items	Nurse
Neonatal Narcotic Withdrawal Index	15 numerically weighted items	Physician
Moro Scale Score	5 specific Moro observations, 3 specific tremor observations	Physician
Kahn et al.	Subjective: mild, moderate, or severe	Nurse or physician
Ostrea et al.	Subjective: grades I–III	Nurse or physician

Abbreviation: NAS, neonatal abstinence syndrome.
Source: Adapted from Ananand KJS, Arnold JH: Opioid tolerance and dependence in infants and children. *Crit Care Med* 22:334–342, 1994.

system to grade degree of NAS according to nursing assessment of 21 symptoms (Neonatal Abstinence Scale; Table 7–4). A score of 8 on three successive screenings suggests the need for therapy, with dosing adjustments and eventual cessation based on subsequent scores. Several therapeutic agents may be used for NAS, but

tincture of opium has gained favor because of its low ethanol content, lack of neurologic stimulation, and lower risk of displacing bilirubin (Table 7–5). Recent research suggests that a combination of phenobarbital and diluted tincture of opium may provide optimal results.

Opioid-exposed neonates may also experience life-threatening respiratory depression at birth. Treatment consists of naloxone 100 µg/kg, to a maximum dose of 400 µg given intramuscularly, intravenously, or endotracheally. Care must be taken not to exceed the maximum dose, or potentially lethal withdrawal seizures may occur.

Cocaine Exposure

Intrauterine growth retardation, abruptio placenta with neonatal asphyxiation, seizures, and stroke are prominent prenatal effects of cocaine. After birth, cocaine-exposed neonates may display jitteriness, sleep disturbance, general lability, and poor sucking. Passive cocaine exposure through breast milk or crack-cocaine smoke inhalation may cause acute toxicity with seizures, tachycardia, hypertension, and irritability. Longitudinal evaluation of cocaine-exposed infants over several years has found no neurodevelopmental effects of cocaine independent of any postnatal deprivation or poor upbringing.

Heavy Metals

Passive environmental exposure to toxins such as heavy metals or polychlorinated compounds may have a major

Table 7–5. Therapeutic Agents Used for NAS

Agent	Dose	Side Effects/Limitations
Tincture of opium (10% opium tincture)	Dilute 1:25 with sterile water (morphine equivalent 0.4 mg/mL), 0.1–0.2 mL/kg with feeds q4h, increase 0.05 mL/dose every 12 h until symptoms controlled	Lethargy, constipation, respiratory depression, hypotension (0.75% ethanol content)
Paregoric (0.4% camphorated tincture of opium)	Morphine equivalent 0.4 mg/mL 0.1–0.2 mL/kg with feeds q4h, increase 0.05 mL/dose every 12 h until symptoms controlled	Lethargy, constipation, respiratory depression, hypotension, seizures (camphor), hyperbilirubinemia (benzoic acid) (45% ethanol content)
Phenobarbital	2–4 mg/kg q8–12h	Greater sedation than from opiates, decreased sucking behavior, respiratory depression; does not control diarrhea or vomiting, long half-life, induces hepatic enzymes, rapid tolerance
Chlorpromazine	0.30–0.75 mg/kg q6h	Cardiac dysrhythmias, tachycardia, hypotension, dystonia, (?endocrine)
Clonidine	3–4 µg/kg	No controlled clinical trials

impact on the developing nervous system and other organs. Heavy metal poisoning with lead or mercury occurs primarily via prenatal placental transfer (see Chapters 69 and 70). Women exposed to organochlorine insecticides and polychlorinated biphenyls concentrate these lipophilic substances in their breast milk, with significant toxic potential (see Chapter 4). Environmental exposure to ubiquitous toxins, such as lead and nitrates, also has specific toxic potential shortly after birth (see Chapters 69 and 74).

Up to 33% of women require drug therapy during pregnancy. A significant subset of this group requires chronic treatment for underlying diseases such as diabetes mellitus, seizures, and rheumatologic disorders. A lack of human data for most new drugs hampers the identification of drugs that are safe during pregnancy. Therefore, the list of drugs approved for pregnancy is limited. Table 7–6 lists drugs for which strong scientific evidence allows recommendation for various medical conditions during pregnancy. Table 7–7 lists drugs that are contraindicated in pregnancy.

Maternal Poisoning

Estimates suggest that up to 12% of women who attempt or commit suicide are pregnant. Maternal overdose raises many concerns regarding the appropriate treatment that will ensure the best outcome for both mother and child. In general, what is best for the mother in terms of supportive care, decontamination, and definitive treatment is also best for the fetus. Acetaminophen and carbon monoxide (CO) poisoning in pregnancy pose two specific instances that may require adjustments in therapeutic approach.

Fetal toxicity from maternal acetaminophen overdose requires transplacental transfer of acetaminophen and development of sufficient cytochrome oxidase in the fetal liver to produce the toxic metabolite, *N*-amino-*p*-benzoquinoneimine. Animal and human data show that both do occur, with significant potential for fetal demise. *N*-acetylcysteine (NAC) also crosses the placenta and may prevent fetal toxicity. It has no known teratogenic effect. Fetal loss is correlated with delay in NAC therapy. Therefore, any pregnant woman who has ingested a toxic amount of acetaminophen should receive an initial loading dose of NAC as soon as possible after ingestion. Therapy should not be delayed while awaiting maternal plasma acetaminophen determination. No evidence supports an optimal route of administration, although excessive vomiting associated with oral NAC administration may be deleterious in the pregnant patient if not adequately controlled.

Table 7–6. Drugs Safe for Use During Pregnancy

Condition	Drug
Acne (topical agents)	Benzoyl peroxide
	Clindamycin
	Erythromycin
	Tretinoin
Constipation	Docusate sodium
	Glycerin
	Sorbitol
	Lactulose
	Mineral oil
Cough	Diphenhydramine
	Dextromethorphan
	Codeine
Depression	Cyclic antidepressants
	Fluoxetine
	Lithium[a]
Diabetes	Insulin
Gastritis, esophagitis	Oral antacids
	Ranitidine
	Sucralfate
Hypertension	Labetalol, other β-blockers
	Methyldopa
	Hydralazine
	Prazosin
Hyperthyroidism	Propylthiouracil
	Methimazole
	β-blockers
Mania	Lithium[a]
	Chlorpromazine
	Haloperidol
Migraine headache	Acetaminophen
	Codeine
	Dimenhydrinate
	Prophylaxis
	β-blockers
	Cyclic antidepressants
Pain	Acetaminophen
	Codeine
Pruritus	Calamine lotion
	Topical glucocorticoids
	Hydroxyzine
	Diphenhydramine
Thrombophlebitis	Heparin

[a]If lithium is given in first trimester, fetal echocardiogram and ultrasound are indicated.
Source: Adapted from Koren G, Pastuszak A, Shinya I: Drug therapy: Drugs in pregnancy. *N Engl J Med* 338:1128–1137, 1998.

Table 7–7. Prescription Drugs That Are Known Human Teratogens[a]

Drug	Fetal/Neonatal Effect
ACE inhibitors	Renal failure, renal tubular dysgenesis, impairment of skull ossification
Carbamazepine	Neural tube defects
Cyclophosphamide	CNS malformations
Danazol	Masculinization of females
Hypoglycemic drugs	Neonatal hypoglycemia
Isotretinoin	Retinoic acid embryopathy: CNS (hydrocephalus, microcephaly, major cerebellar abnormalities), cardiovascular (conotruncal malformations, e.g., transposition of the great vessels, tetralogy of Fallot, truncus arteriosus, hypoplastic left heart), craniofacial (microtia, anotia, hypertelorism, flat depressed nasal bridge)
Lithium	Ebstein anomaly and other cardiac defects when given in first trimester
Misoprostol	Moebius sequence (bilateral cranial nerve palsy, typically VI and VII)
NSAIDs	Closing of ductus arteriosus in third trimester, necrotizing enterocolitis
Phenytoin	Fetal hydantoin syndrome: mental retardation, craniofacial anomalies (hypertelorism, broad nose with depressed ridge, cleft lip and palate), hypoplasia of phalanges and nails, digitalized thumbs
Tetracycline	Staining of teeth, enamel hypoplasia, inhibition of bone growth when taken in second and third trimesters
Thalidomide	Limb hypoplasia, phocomelia, amelia, microtia, anotia, renal anomalies, cryptorchidism
Valproic acid	Neural tube defects, cardiovascular (coarctation of the aorta, hypoplastic left heart, atrial septal defect, pulmonary atresia), craniofacial anomalies (long philtrim, small mouth, epicanthal folds, broad nasal bridge)
Warfarin	Mental retardation, seizures, Dandy–Walker syndrome, skeletal stippling of uncalcified epiphyses, craniofacial anomalies (depressed nasal bridge, nasal groove between alae nasi and tip)

[a]Partial list of known teratogens.
Source: Adapted from Koren G, Pastuszak A, Shinya I: Drug therapy: Drugs in pregnancy. *N Engl J Med* 338:1128–1137, 1998.
Abbreviations: ACE, angiotensin-converting enzyme; CNS, central nervous system; NSAIDs, nonsteroidal anti-inflammatory drugs.

Several physiologic factors in the fetus accentuate the toxicity of maternal CO exposure: (1) low ambient P_{O_2} (20 to 25 mmHg); (2) elevated hemoglobin F concentration that decreases O_2 delivery to fetal tissues; (3) immature free-radical scavenger enzyme systems to counteract CO effect at the cellular level; and (4) slower CO elimination. Because of slower CO absorption and elimination in the fetus, maternal carboxyhemoglobin levels do not correlate well with fetal levels. As a result, the fetus is at high risk following maternal exposure. Major fetal effects and death may occur despite minimal symptoms in the mother. For this reason, aggressive therapy should follow any maternal CO exposure. Hyperbaric oxygen (HBO) therapy has produced good fetal outcomes despite severe maternal CO poisoning. Maternal symptoms, evidence of fetal distress, and a maternal carboxyhemoglobin level $\geq 15\%$ are all potential indications for HBO therapy. In addition, HBO may be beneficial to the fetus beyond the typical 6-hour window of maximal potential benefit. If HBO is not available, then the mother should receive 100% oxygen for a period of time that is 5 times longer than required to ameliorate maternal symptoms and to reduce the maternal carboxyhemoglobin level below 5%.

Adverse Fetal Effects of Perinatal Drug Administration

Perinatal drug administration has improved outcomes for the neonate in several specific instances, such as prenatal antibiotics for prolonged rupture of membranes or maternal fever, digoxin for fetal supraventricular tachycardia, corticosteroids to enhance fetal lung maturation when premature delivery is imminent, and magnesium sulfate for maternal preeclampsia. Tocolysis for premature labor and analgesia for labor and delivery provide significant benefit to both mother and newborn, but pose risks for the latter.

Table 7–8. Maternal Tocolytic Therapy and Adverse Neonatal Effects

Tocolytic Medication	Neonatal Effects
Magnesium sulfate	Hypotonia, lethargy, respiratory depression
β-Adrenergic agonists (terbutaline, ritodrine)	Tachycardia, neonatal hypoglycemia
NSAIDs (indomethacin, ibuprofen, sulindac)	Renal insufficiency, prenatal PDA constriction with postnatal pulmonary hypertension, ileal perforation, meconium peritonitis, necrotizing enterocolitis, intraventricular hemorrhage
Calcium-channel blockers	None

Abbreviations: NSAIDs, nonsteroidal anti-inflammatory drugs; PDA, patent ductus arteriosus.

Eleven percent of deliveries in the United States are preterm. Tocolytic therapy allows time to optimize lung maturation of the infant with corticosteroid therapy, to transport the mother to a center prepared to manage a preterm infant, and to allow treatment of the underlying cause of preterm labor. Table 7–8 summarizes the tocolytics currently in common use and their potential toxic effects on the neonate. Intravenous magnesium sulfate remains the most commonly used tocolytic in the United States. It crosses the placenta easily and causes neuromuscular depression in the neonate proportionate to that seen in the mother. The resultant hypotonia can complicate respiratory disease in the newborn, who may require respiratory support and/or endotracheal intubation in the delivery room or nursery.

Maternal pain management during labor and delivery poses the specific challenge of providing comfort safely while avoiding adverse effects of drug administration on both the mother and newborn. Each class of analgesics and each mode of delivery has potential direct or indirect toxicity for the newborn (Table 7–9). Preterm infants are

Table 7–9. Maternal Sedation and Analgesia During Labor and Adverse Neonatal Effects

Agent	Mode	Neonatal Effect
Diazepam	IV	*Small doses*: minimal effect *Large doses*: prolonged CNS depression
Meperidine	IV	Minimal if delivery <1 h after maternal administration; respiratory/CNS depression maximum 2–3 h after maternal administration
Local anesthestics (lidocaine, bupivacaine, chloroprocaine)	Epidural, subarachnoid	None, if maternal hypotension and accidental maternal vascular injection with seizures avoided
Opiates	Epidural, subarachnoid	None, if maternal hypotension and respiratory depression avoided
Local anesthetics	Paracervical block	Bradycardia, metabolic acidosis, hypotonia especially if delivery <30 min after injection
General anesthesia (nitrous oxide, isoflurane, desflurane)	Inhaled	CNS depression, hypotonia, apnea, bradycardia; coordination with delivery avoids these effects
General anesthesia (thiopental)	IV	Minimal effect if maternal dose <4 mg/kg
General anesthesia (propofol)	IV	Respiratory depression, lethargy

Abbreviations: CNS, central nervous system; IV, intravenous.

more likely to experience problems than term infants. Judicious selection of agent and coordination of analgesia administration with delivery should minimize the impact on the newborn.

Intentional Poisoning by a Caretaker

Intentional poisoning, although a relatively rare manifestation of physical abuse, is a potential form of poisoning among neonates. Social factors, such as teenage pregnancy and maternal drug abuse, raise the risk of prematurity in subsequent offspring. These same factors elevate the risk of parental abuse of the neonate. Furthermore, in predisposed parents, the intense exposure to a highly technical hospital environment with a high level of attention given to the parent of the ill child can facilitate the emergence of Munchausen syndrome by proxy (MSP). The withdrawal of attention when the child is discharged from the nursery sets the stage for intentional administration of harmful doses of drugs prescribed for the child. This behavior results in readmission and renewal of the parents' secondary gain during the victim's rehospitalization. The discovery of any unprescribed ingestion in the neonatal age group must raise high suspicion for MSP by the caretaker. Once identified, abuse by poisoning dictates that the child be taken into protective custody and that child welfare and police be notified.

Patterns of neonatal abuse by poisoning fall into the categories of drugs given to quiet or sedate an infant, passive exposure to drugs of abuse, and malicious administration. A caretaker may intentionally administer an opioid or benzodiazepine to quiet an infant, who subsequently may present to medical attention with the chief complaint of lethargy, hypotonia, apnea, or cyanosis. Antipsychotic medications, especially phenothiazine derivatives, may cause coma with increased muscle tone. The author has cared for an infant who was given cocaine for teething and presented with seizures. Reports detail caretaker administration of injected heroin to stop crying that resulted in two infant deaths, and maternal administration of methadone to treat an infant's withdrawal symptoms. Urine enzyme-mediated immunoassay (EMIT) for drugs of abuse readily detects opioids, cocaine, barbiturates, amphetamines, and phencyclidine; certain benzodiazepines that lack an oxazepam intermediate when metabolized may go undetected. Urine EMIT also identifies passive exposure to drugs of abuse. Screening should occur in neonates with altered mental status or seizures and no clear underlying etiology.

Malicious poisoning by the parent challenges the health provider because the manifestations may mimic a variety of disease states (Table 7–10). Mortality frequently occurs in these cases. A high index of suspicion and a willingness to entertain the possibility of child abuse by poisoning and to do the appropriate tests is essential to good outcomes for the infant.

THERAPY

Treatment

The management principles for the poisoned neonate are the same as for any other age group: stabilization, decontamination, toxin identification, elimination enhancement, and antidote administration. Neonates are fragile and prone to apnea, respiratory distress, and hemodynamic instability when faced with a toxin exposure. Aggressive resuscitation with timely airway, breathing, and circulatory interventions are essential in the seriously poisoned infant.

Decontamination

Decontamination commences after appropriate supportive care has been initiated. Dermal exposures require bathing and irrigation. An overhead warmer prevents the potential for cold stress during this care. There are age-related limitations on gastric decontamination. Syrup of ipecac is contraindicated in the young infant. Large-bore gastric lavage is not possible. However, nasogastric lavage of a liquid medication, if attempted soon after ingestion, is possible using small aliquots of normal saline. Activated charcoal must be dosed properly (1 g/kg), and used without cathartic to avoid serious morbidity from fluid/electrolyte shifts. Furthermore, very young infants may be at risk for necrotizing enterocolitis. Therefore, the risk and benefit of activated charcoal use in the poisoned neonate should be weighed individually, based on the gestational age of the infant, the seriousness of the exposure, and the availability of other therapeutic modalities.

Laboratory

Neonates have important differences in the normal range for certain toxicology laboratory measurements that may falsely indicate poisoning has occurred. This may cause significant difficulties when attempting to identify specific toxins. Carboxyhemoglobin levels in neonates typically range from 2% to 5%, because CO is a byproduct of protoporphyrin metabolism. In the absence of exposure to exogenous toxins, neonates may develop severe

Table 7–10. Presenting Signs and Symptoms by Etiologic Agent in Neonates Abused by Poisoning

Signs and Symptoms	Etiologic Agent	Detection Methods
Vomiting, dehydration, hypotonia, metabolic alkalosis, metabolic acidosis, failure to thrive, cardiomyopathy	Syrup of ipecac	Emetine/cephaline screening of urine, vomitus or ingested substance (thin layer chromotography)
Diarrhea, metabolic alkalosis, hypokalemia, dehydration, failure to thrive	Laxatives	Phenophthalein screening of stool (alkalinization with pink color), elevated stool magnesium, sulfate or anthracine melanosis coli on colonoscopy (chronic anthracene administration)
Nonketotic hypoglycemia, lethargy, coma, seizures	Exogenous insulin	Low serum C-peptide insulin level and high total insulin levels
Jaundice, direct hyperbilirubinemia	Acetaminophen	Toxic serum acetaminophen level (may not be present if remote exposure), centrilobular necrosis on liver biopsy
Lethargy, severe metabolic acidosis with elevated anion gap, renal failure	Ethylene glycol	Serum ethylene glycol level, urinary dipartite calcium oxalate crystals, elevated urinary glyoxylic acid and oxalic acid
Hyponatremia, seizures, low urine specific gravity	Water	Measurement of formula concentration (overdiluted formula possibly related to abject poverty), association with trading of formula for drugs

methemoglobinemia and metabolic acidosis from gastroenteritis. Neonates also have a lower baseline cholinesterase activity that may interfere with the interpretation of plasma pseudocholinesterase and red blood cell cholinesterase levels. Finally, the abnormal metabolic products present in the disease methylmalonic acidemia may be mistaken for ethylene glycol. Those investigating poisoning in the neonate must be aware of these important age-related differences in laboratory measurements.

Enhanced Elimination

Small patient size, propensity to fluid and electrolyte abnormalities, and challenging circulatory access impede enhancement of toxin elimination in the neonate. Hemodialysis, charcoal hemoperfusion, continuous arteriovenous or venovenous hemofiltration are technically difficult modalities in the neonate, and are performed only in specialized pediatric centers. Single-volume exchange transfusion has alleviated symptoms of theophylline and salicylate toxicity in neonates. Exchange transfusion offers an alternative to potentially harmful antidotal therapy in the setting of neonates with severe methemoglobinemia or CO exposure.

Multiple-dose activated charcoal has treated severe theophylline poisoning successfully. However, misuse of sorbitol as a cathartic during this therapy has also caused severe hypernatremia in young infants. Any decision to utilize elimination enhancement techniques in neonates must involve careful consideration of major morbidities associated with these therapies. In many instances, watchful waiting is most beneficial.

Antidotes

Limited data exist regarding antidote administration to neonates. In certain settings, antidote doses need to be reduced. For example, no more than 0.4 mg of naloxone should be given to heroin- or methadone-exposed infants to avoid withdrawal seizures in the first few days of life. Also, methylene blue administration for neonatal methemoglobinemia should be closely monitored to avoid Heinz body hemolytic anemia. In other instances, such as digoxin overdose and organophosphate poisoning, the same criteria for antidote administration apply. As for any other poisoned patient, the majority of neonatal poisonings do not have a readily available antidote, and the best outcome occurs with diligent supportive care.

ACKNOWLEDGMENTS

Special thanks to Dr Victor Herson for his review of this chapter.

SUGGESTED READINGS

Abel EL: An update on incidence of Fetal Alcohol Syndrome (FAS): FAS is not an equal opportunity birth defect. *Neurotoxicol Teratol* 17:437–443, 1995.

Amin-Zaki L, Ethassani SB, Majeed MA : Studies of infants postnatally exposed to methyl mercury. *J Pediatr* 85:81–84, 1974.

Anand KJS, Arnold JH: Opioid tolerance and dependence in infants and children. *Crit Care Med* 22:334–342, 1994.

Armstrong RW, Eichner ER, Klein DE, et al: Pentachlorophenol poisoning in a nursery for newborn infants. II. Epidemiologic and toxicologic studies. *J Pediatr* 75:317, 1969.

Avner JR, Henretig FM, McAneney CM: Acquired methemoglobinemia: The relationship of cause to course of illness. *Am J Dis Child* 144:1229–1230, 1990.

Banzaw TM: Mercury poisoning in Argentine babies linked to diapers. *Pediatrics* 67:637, 1981.

Barker N, Hadgraft J, Rutter N: Skin permeability in the newborn. *J Invest Derm* 88:409–411, 1987.

Bauman WA, Yalow RS: Child abuse: Parenteral insulin administration. *J Pediatr* 99:588, 1981.

Bays J: Child abuse by poisoning. In: Reece RR, Ludwig S, eds: *Child Abuse: Medical Diagnosis and Management.* 2nd ed. Lippincott, Williams and Wilkins; 2001:405–442.

Berkner P, Kaster T, Skolnick L: Chronic ipecac poisoning in infancy: A case report. *Pediatrics* 82:384–386, 1988.

Biggs BS, Bronstein AC, Kulig K, et al: Acute acetaminophen overdose during pregnancy. *Obstet Gynecol* 74:247, 1989.

Blumer JL, Reed MD: Principles of neonatal pharmacology, In: Yaffe SJ, Aranda JV, eds: *Pediatric Pharmacology: Therapeutic Principles in Practice.* 2nd ed. Philadelphia, Penn: Saunders; 1992:164–177.

Chabrolle JP, Rossier A: Goiter and hypothyroidism in the newborn after cutaneous absorption of iodine. *Arch Dis Child* 53:495–498, 1978.

Clarren SK, Smith DW: The fetal alcohol syndrome. *N Engl J Med* 298:1063, 1978.

Coles CD: Impact of prenatal alcohol exposure on the newborn and the child. *Clin Obstet Gynecol* 36:255–256, 1993.

Ducey J, Brooke D: Transcutaneous absorption of boric acid. *Pediatrics* 43:644–651, 1953.

Coyle MG, Ferguson A, Lagasse L,et al: Diluted tincture of opium (DTO) and phenobarbital versus DTO alone for neonatal opiate withdrawal in term infants. *J Pediatr* 140:561–564, 2002.

Farley TA: Severe hypernatremic dehydration after use of an activated charcoal-sorbitol suspension. *J Pediatr* 109:719–722, 1986.

Fine JS: Reproductive and perinatal principles. In: Goldfrank LR, Flomenbaum NE, Lewin NA, et al, eds: *Goldfrank's Toxicologic Emergencies.* 6th ed. Stamford, Conn: Appleton & Lange; 1998:1672–1675.

Friesen RH: Anesthesia and analgesia: Issues for the fetus and newborn. In: Taeusch HW, Ballard RA, eds: *Avery's Diseases of the Newborn.* 7th ed. Philadelphia, Penn: Saunders; 1998:167–168.

Gershanik JJ, Boecher B, Ensley H, et al: The gasping syndrome and benzyl alcohol poisoning. *N Engl J Med* 307:1364, 1982.

Goebel J, Gremse DA, Artman M: Cardiomyopathy from ipecac administration in Munchausen syndrome by proxy. *Pediatrics* 92:601–603, 1993.

Griffith DR, Azuma SD, Chasnoff IJ: Three-year outcome of children exposed prenatally to drugs. *J Am Acad Child Adolesc Psychiatry* 33:20–27, 1994.

Hoder EL, Leckman JF, Ehrenkranz R, et al: Clonidine in neonatal narcotic-abstinence syndrome. *N Engl J Med* 305:1284, 1981.

Horowitz RS, Dart RC, Jarvie DR, et al: Placental transfer of *N*-acetylcysteine following human maternal acetaminophen toxicity. *Clin Toxicol* 35:447, 1997.

Kandall SR: Managing neonatal withdrawal. *Drug Therapy* 6:47–59, 1976.

Karlsen RL, Sterri S, Lyngaas S, et al: Reference values for erythrocyte acetylcholinesterase and plasma activities in children: Implications for organophosphate intoxications. *Scand J Clin Lab Invest* 4:301–302, 1981.

Katz VL, Farmer RM: Controversies in tocolytic therapy. *Clin Obstet Gynecol* 42:802, 1999.

Koren G, Pastuszak A, Shinya I: Drug therapy: Drugs in pregnancy. *N Engl J Med* 338:1128–1137, 1998.

Koren G, Sharav T, Pastuszak A, et al: A multicenter, prospective study of fetal outcome following accidental carbon monoxide poisoning in pregnancy. *Reprod Toxicol* 5:397–403, 1991.

Langkamp DL, Nutt A, Raasch R: Child abuse by poisoning: Why is alprazolam difficult to detect. *Clin Pediatr* 32:250–251, 1993.

Leeder JS, Kearns GL: Pharmacogenetics in pediatrics: Implications for practice. *Pediatr Clin North Am* 44:55–77, 1997.

Linakis JG: Toxic emergencies in the neonate. In: Haddad LM, Shannon MW, Winchester JF, eds: *Clinical Management of Poisoning and Drug Overdose.* 3rd ed. Philadelphia, Penn: Saunders; 1998:277–287.

Litovitz TL, Klein-Schwartz W, White S, et al: 2000 Annual report of the American association of poison control centers toxic exposure surveillance system. *Am J Emerg Med* 19:337–395, 2001.

Longo LD, Hill EP: Carbon monoxide uptake and elimination in fetal and maternal sheep. *Am J Physiol* 232:H324–H330, 1977.

Mack RB: Boric acid—Bad news for cockroaches and other little beings. *Contemp Pediatr* June:83–89, 1987.

Manikan A, Stone S, Hamilton R: Exchange transfusion as an alternative to hemodialysis in severe infant salicylism. *J Toxicol Clin Toxicol* 34:585, 1996 (abstract).

Martin-Boyer G, Lebreton R, Toga M, et al: Outbreak of accidental hexachlorophene poisoning in France. *Lancet* 1:91, 1982.

McClung H, Murray R, Braden N, et al: Intentional ipecac poisoning in children. *Am J Dis Child* 142:637–639, 1988.

McElhatton PR, Sullivan FM, Volans GN, et al: Paracetamol poisoning in pregnancy: An analysis of the outcomes of cases referred to the teratology information service of the national poisons information service. *Hum Exp Toxicol* 9:147, 1990.

National Institute on Drug Abuse: National pregnancy and health survey. Rockville, Md: National Institutes of Health; 1996.

Osborn HH, Henry G, Wax P, et al: Theophylline toxicity in a premature neonate—Elimination kinetics of exchange transfusion. *J Toxicol Clin Toxicol* 31:639–644, 1993.

Paech M: Newer techniques of labor analgesia. *Anesthesiol Clin North Am* 21:1–17, 2003.

Petrie RH: Tocolysis using magnesium sulfate. *Semin Perinatol* 5:266, 1981.

Plessinger MA, Woods JR: Maternal, placental, and fetal pathophysiology of cocaine exposure during pregnancy. *Clin Obstet Gynecol* 36:267–278, 1993.

Powell PP: Minamata disease: A story of mercury's malevolence. *South Med J* 84:1352–1358, 1991.

Rubin P: Fortnightly review: Drug treatment during pregnancy. *BMJ* 317:1503–1506, 1998.

Rutter N: Percutaneous drug absorption in the newborn: Hazards and uses. *Clin Perinatol* 14:911, 1987

Rutter N: Absorption of drugs through the skin. In: Rylance G, Harvey D, Aranda JV, eds: *Neonatal Clinical Pharmacology and Therapeutics*. London: Butterworth-Heinemann; 1991: 233–249.

Rylance G: Pharmacological principles and kinetics. In: Rylance G, Harvey D, Aranda JV, eds: *Neonatal Clinical Pharmacology and Therapeutics*. London: Butterworth-Heinemann; 1991:1–25.

Saladino R, Shannon M: Accidental and intentional poisonings with ethylene glycol in infancy: Diagnostic clues and management. *Pediatr Emerg Care* 7:93–96, 1991.

Shannon M, Amitai Y, Lovejoy FH: Multiple dose activated charcoal for theophylline poisoning in young infants. *Pediatrics* 80:368–370, 1987.

Shoemaker JD, Lynch RE, Hoffman JW, et al: Misidentification of proprionic acid as ethylene glycol in a patient with methylmalonic acidemia. *J Pediatr* 120:417–421, 1992.

Sills MR, Zinkham WH: Methylene blue-induced Heinz body hemolytic anemia. *Arch Pediatr Adolesc Med* 148:306, 1994.

Sutherland JM: Fatal cardiovascular collapse in infants receiving large amounts of chloramphenicol. *Am J Dis Child* 97: 761, 1959.

Tomaszewski C: Carbon monoxide. In: Ford MD, Delaney KA, Ling LJ, et al, eds: *Clinical Toxicology*. Philadelphia, Penn: Saunders; 2001:664.

Vivier PM, Lewander WJ, Martin HF, et al: Isopropyl alcohol intoxication in a neonate through chronic dermal exposure: A complication of a culturally-based umbilical care practice. *Pediatr Emerg Care* 10:91, 1994.

Walker M, Hull A: Preterm labor and birth. In: Taeusch HW, Ballard RA, eds: *Avery's Diseases of the Newborn*. 7th ed. Philadelphia, Penn: Saunders; 1998:144–153.

Wang LH, Rudolpgh AM, Benet LZ: Pharmacokinetic studies of the disposition of acetaminophen in the sheep maternal-placental-fetal unit. *J Pharmacol Exp Ther* 238:198, 1986.

Warkany J, Hubbard DM: Adverse mercurial reactions in the form of acrodynia and related conditions. *Am J Dis Child* 81:335–373, 1951.

Webster RC, Noonan PK, Cole MP, et al: Percutaneous absorption of testosterone in the newborn rhesus monkey: Comparison to the adult. *Pediatr Res* 11:737–739, 1979.

Woolf A, Wenger T, Smith TW, et al: The use of digoxin-specific Fab fragments for severe digitalis intoxication in children. *N Engl J Med* 326:1739–1744, 1992.

Wright GR, Shephard RJ: Physiological effects of carbon monoxide. *Int Rev Physiol* 20:311–368, 1979.

Yeh, TF, Pildes RS, Firor HV, et al: Mercury poisoning from mercurochrome therapy of infected omphalocele. *Lancet* 1:210, 1978.

Zwiener RJ, Ginsburg CM: Organophosphate and carbamate poisoning in infants and children. *Pediatrics* 81:121–126, 1988.

8

Special Toxicologic Considerations in the Toddler

Holly Perry

A child learns by doing. He gains experience by investigating the world around him.

Toddlers frequently ingest potentially hazardous substances. In 2002, poison control centers participating in the American Association of Poison Control Centers Toxic Exposure Surveillance System (AAPCC-TESS) reported 2.3 million inquires, more than half of which involved children younger than 6 years of age, with 1- and 2-year-olds exposed most frequently (Figure 8–1). There are many reasons why toddlers account for a disproportionate number of potentially toxic exposures (Figure 8–2).

Toddlers are curious about the world around them and learn by exploring, frequently with their mouths. The pincer grasp develops between 6 months and 1 year of age, and children are delighted to be able to pick up small objects such as pills or tablets. A toddler's abilities are continually evolving and he may have capabilities today, such as opening the garage door and unscrewing the cap of an antifreeze-containing bottle, that he did not have yesterday. A disruption of household routine may be an important factor in poisoning if it transforms a previously safe environment into an unsafe one. For example, visitors without toddlers may not be as attuned to locking cabinets and keeping all medications out of the child's reach. Other disruptions include moving, birth of a baby, and preparation for a holiday. In addition, toddlers often mimic behavior of older siblings and caretakers resulting in a greater rise of toxic exposures (Figure 8–3).

EPIDEMIOLOGY

Data from two large national databases, AAPCC-TESS and the National Electronic Injury Surveillance System (NEISS), demonstrate that most unintentional poisonings in toddlers are inconsequential. According to the NEISS, a database that captures all injury-related visits to representative emergency departments, only 80,313 children younger than 6 years of age were evaluated for toxic exposure in an emergency department in 2002. Nearly 90% of these children were treated and released. The AAPCC-TESS database, which records inquiries to poison control centers, adds further evidence of the benign nature of these unintentional poisonings. In 2002, poison control centers received more than 1.2 million inquiries about children under 6 years of age. The vast majority of exposures caused either a minor and transient

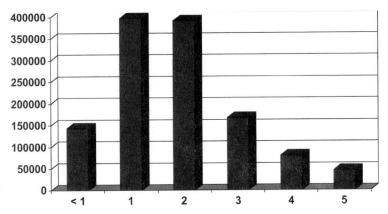

Fig. 8–1. Age distribution (years) of poison exposures reported to poison control centers. (Source: Watson WA, Litovitz TL, Rodgers GC, et al: 2002 Annual report of the American Association of Poison Control Centers Toxic Exposure Surveillance System. *Am J Emerg Med* 21:353–421, 2003).

effect, such as mouth irritation, or no effect at all. Fewer than 1% resulted in symptoms that may have required some form of treatment but were not life threatening, and left no residual disfigurement or disability. Only 0.1% (739 children) of all exposures caused symptoms that were either life threatening or left the child with some

disability or disfigurement. AAPCC-TESS reported 23 deaths in this age group for 2002.

There are two important reasons why most potentially hazardous exposures in the toddler age group are nontoxic. First, a large proportion of ingestions involve household products or plants, which typically have a low order of toxicity. For example, in 2002 nearly 20% of all exposures in this age group were to cosmetics, personal care products, or plants. The most commonly ingested substances reported to poison control centers are listed in Table 8–1. Not surprisingly, these are products and medications kept in most homes and therefore readily available to children.

The second reason that the majority of exposures are nontoxic is the small amount ingested. Frequently, a toddler ingests only one or two pills or sips (equivalent to 2 to 4 mL) of a liquid product. The one-pill rule—"one pill of anything won't hurt anybody"—generally holds

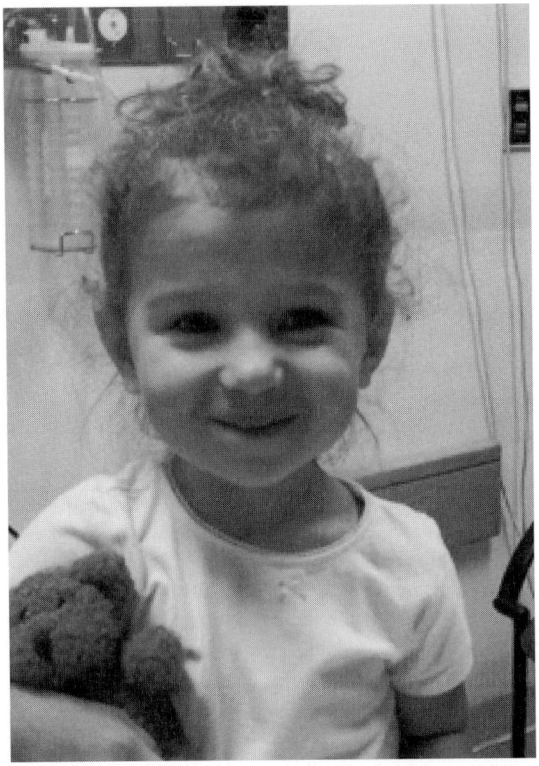

Fig. 8–2. Toddlers are more prone to accidental poisonings.

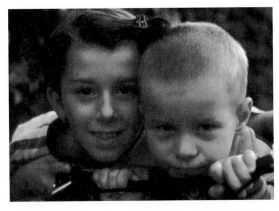

Fig. 8–3. Toddlers often mimic behavior of older siblings.

Table 8–1. Substances Most Frequently Involved in Exposures Among Children ≤5 Years Old 1995–2001

Cosmetics and personal care products	0.75 million
Cleaning substances	0.63 million
Analgesics	0.44 million
Plants	0.40 million
Foreign bodies	0.36 million
Cough and cold preparations	0.33 million
Topicals	0.32 million

Total number of exposures, 5.7 million.
Source: From Litovitz et al. (1996).

Table 8–2. Primary Agents Involved in Fatal Poisonings Among Children 5 Years and Younger Between 1995 and 2000

Category (Number of deaths reported)	Specific Agents
Analgesic drugs (17)	Acetaminophen, ibuprofen, methadone, morphine, oxycodone, salicylates
Cleaning products (8)	Corrosives, fluoride-based solutions
Electrolytes and minerals (8)	Elemental iron, lead
Hydrocarbons (10)	Gasoline, lamp oil, paint thinner, pine oil, kerosene, lighter fluid
Antidepressant drugs (5)	Amitryptiline, imipramine, desipramine
Insecticides and pesticides (7)	Propoxur, organophosphates, aluminum phosphate, paraquat
Cosmetics and personal care products (4)	Ethanol, baby oil, hair oil
Anticonvulsant drugs (3)	Carbamezapine, valproate sodium
Stimulants and illicit drugs (3)	Cocaine, heroin
Plants (2)	Cayenne pepper, pennyroyal tea
Foreign bodies (3)	Activated charcoal, kitty litter
Sedatives and hypnotic drugs (2)	Promethazine, chloral hydrate
Cardiovascular drugs (3)	Nifedipine, clonidine
Tobacco (1)	Cigarette butts
Cough and cold preparations (3)	Phenylpropanolamine, codeine, hydrocodone
Hormones and hormone antagonists (1)	Glipizide
Chemicals (1)	Diethylene glycol
Alcohols (2)	Ethanol, methanol
Gastrointestinal preparations (2)	Lomotil, bismuth salicylate
Essential oils (1)	Citronella

Source: From Litovitz et al. (1996).

true, although there are a few important exceptions. Medications that can harm a toddler who ingests only a single pill include theophylline, tricyclic antidepressants, thio-ridizine, chlorpromazine, and antimalarials. A few other drugs may be associated with significant toxicity, including include sulfonylureas, clonidine, and Lomotil (diphenoxylate/atropine). Liquid medications that cause significant toxicity after only a sip or two include topical preparations, such as imidazoles in eye drops, benzocaine in teething ointments, and concentrated solutions of camphor used as a rubeficiant. Even small sips of non-pharmaceuticals like caustics, pesticides, and hydrocarbons are hazardous. Many of these are required to be stored in child-resistant packaging.

Agents involved in fatal poisonings reported to AAPCC-TESS over a 5-year period are listed in Table 8–2. *Hazard analysis,* in which the number of major toxic effects or death is divided by the total number of reported cases of exposure to the substance, then normalized to the rate of major toxic effects or death in that age group, is a way to determine which agents are particularly dangerous to children. On the basis of this type of analysis, agents found to be particularly dangerous to children include tricyclic antidepressants, antimalarials, anticonvulsants (carbamazepine), cocaine, gun-bluing compounds, and cleaning agents such as alkalis and acids.

Mortality from poisoning in children has declined dramatically over the past 60 years. In the 1940s, there were over 500 pediatric deaths annually from poisoning, compared to 26 in 2001. The AAPCC-TESS has demonstrated a steady downward trend since 1983, the year data collection began; young children accounted for 10.5% of all deaths from poisonings. In contrast, by 2001, pediatric cases accounted for only 2.4% of all poisoning deaths. The causes of this dramatic decline are multifactorial and include creation of poison information centers, heightened parental awareness of poisons in the home, development of lower-toxicity drugs to replace those of greater toxicity, and federally mandated use of child-resistant packaging for certain products.

The efficacy of child-resistant packaging in reducing the incidence of childhood poisonings was shown in two studies conducted in the late 1960s. In part because of these data, Congress passed the Poison Prevention Packaging Act (PPPA) in 1970. This act grants authority to the Consumer Product Safety Commission (CPSC) to require "special packaging" of household products and drugs to protect children from serious illness or injury. *Special packaging* is defined as a container that fewer than 20% of children can open within 5 minutes, but is not difficult for adults aged 50 to 70 to use. Under this act, all prescription drugs must be placed in child-resistant packaging unless the recipient specifically requests otherwise. Additionally, a number of nonprescription medications must be placed in child-resistant packaging if they exceed predetermined amounts. Examples of nonprescription medications thus regulated include acetaminophen and iron. A large number of nonpharmaceutical substances are also regulated, including mouthwash with a high ethanol concentration and concentrated liquid turpentine. The scope of the PPPA is broad, and the CPSC may add new products to the list of regulated substances. Typically this occurs only after significant poisoning has been reported. In 1998, for example, following reports of deaths in children exposed to ammonium bifluoride in wheel cleaner, products containing more than 50 mg of elemental fluoride (the minimal toxic dose for a 10-kg child) required child-resistant packaging. The PPPA has been credited with reducing childhood mortality from prescription drug poisoning by 45%, which translates into approximately 24 fewer deaths per year.

Intentional Poisonings

Most poisonings in young children are unintentional and a consequence of exploratory behavior. However, intentional poisoning of young children does occur, and should be considered when a child presents with symptoms and signs not consistent with the clinical history. Suspicion should be aroused when the child's medical problems do not respond as expected to therapy, the medical course is highly unusual, family history elicits numerous medical problems that are implausible, or when other children have unexplained illness while under the supervision of the caregiver. Many of these intentional poisonings are a result of feelings of hatred or violence toward the child, and are purely malicious. However, some may be classified as Munchausen syndrome by proxy (MSBP). In this

syndrome, the motivation is the attention gained through the perpetrator's involvement with the child's illness. The harm to the child that the perpetrator causes is a means to an end, not the end itself. Although the definition of MSBP is evolving, the currently accepted set of diagnostic criteria includes the following: (1) parent or someone *in loco parentis* fabricates the child's illness; (2) the child is brought, usually persistently, to medical attention and may undergo multiple medical procedures; (3) the perpetrator denies the etiology of the child's illness; and (4) acute symptoms and signs of the illness cease when the child and perpetrator are separated. Hettler (2002) describes MSBP as "a form of child maltreatment in which the caretaker-perpetrators exaggerate, feign, or induce symptoms and/or illness in children and are motivated by the need to assume the sick role by proxy or to gain another form of attention."

MSBP is an uncommon form of child abuse. In a prospective study conducted in the United Kingdom and the Republic of Ireland between 1992 and 1994, the annual reported incidence was only 0.3 per 100,000 for children younger than 16 years. The majority of cases were in children younger than 5 years, with the peak incidence occurring in the first year of life. The reported age range is 19 days to 16 years, with median age of 20 to 24 months. The victim usually has a prolonged hospitalization and extensive investigations before the diagnosis is made. Boys and girls are affected equally, and the mother is the sole perpetrator in 94% to 99% of the cases described. The mothers, who are described as friendly and socially adept, frequently have some training in a medical field and may be overly helpful with the child's care in the hospital. In contrast, parents who maliciously poison their child are likely to spend little time in the hospital with their child, and to be antagonistic toward the medical professionals who are caring for the child.

Any toxic substance may be used to poison a child. Poisons that have been used are diverse and include prescription medications, over-the-counter medications, household products, and gases such as carbon monoxide. Victims of poisoning may have other forms of abuse inflicted upon them, such as suffocation. MSBP is an important diagnosis to make; mortality is estimated to be between 9% and 15%. Siblings are also at risk: up to 40% of MSBP children in whom MSBP involved poisoning had siblings who were also victims.

Treatment

The initial decision of whether to observe the child at home or to evaluate them at a health care facility is made after information regarding substance ingested, quantity ingested, and symptoms since ingestion is obtained. If the ingestion is deemed to be nontoxic or to have limited toxicity, a responsible caregiver may observe the toddler at home. More than 60% of toxic exposures reported to AAPCC-TESS fall into this category. The method of gastrointestinal decontamination best suited for a poisoned toddler in the home or hospital setting is detailed in Chapter 16.

REFERENCES

Bamshad MJ, Wasserman GS: Pediatric clonidine intoxications. *Vet Hum Toxicol* 32:220–223, 1990.

Consumer Product Safety Commission: Accessed July 16, 2003. Available from URL: http://www.cpsc.gov/CPSCPUB/PUBS/384.pdf

Consumer Product Safety Commission: 16 CFR Part 1700. Accessed July 16, 2003.Available from URL: http://www.cpsc.gov/businfo/frnotices/fr98/fluoride.html

Davis P, McClure RJ, Rolfe K, et al: Procedures, placement, and risks of further abuse after Munchausen syndrome by proxy, non-accidental poisoning, and non-accidental suffocation. *Arch Dis Child* 78:2172–2121, 1998.

Dine MS, McGovern ME: Intentional poisoning of children—An overlooked category of child abuse: Report of seven cases and review of the literature. *Pediatrics* 70:32–35,1982.

Hettler J: Munchausen syndrome by proxy. *Pediatr Emerg Care* 18:371–374, 2002.

Knapp JF, Kennedy C, Wasserman GS, et al: Case 01-1994: A toddler with a caustic ingestion. *Pediatr Emerg Care* 10:54–58, 1994.

Koren G: Medications which can kill a toddler with one tablet or teaspoonful. *J Toxicol Clin Toxicol* 31:407–413, 1993.

Liebelt EL, DeAngelis CD: Evolving trends and treatment advances in pediatric poisoning. *JAMA* 282:1113–1115, 1999.

Liebelt EL, Shannon MW: Small doses, big problems: A selected review of highly toxic common medications. *Pediatr Emerg Care* 9:292–297, 1993.

Litovitz TL, Felberg L, White S, et al: 1995 annual report of the American Association of Poison Control Centers Toxic Exposure Surveillance System. *Am J Emerg Med* 14:486–537, 1996.

Litovitz TL, Smilkstein M, Felberg L, et al: 1996 annual report of the American Association of Poison Control Centers Toxic Exposure Surveillance System. *Am J Emerg Med* 15:447–500, 1997.

Litovitz TL, Klein-Schwartz W, Dyer KS, et al: 1997 annual report of the American Association of Poison Control Centers Toxic Exposure Surveillance System. *Am J Emerg Med* 16:443–497, 1998.

Litovitz TL, Klein-Schwartz W, Caravati EM, et al: 1998 annual report of the American Association of Poison Control Centers Toxic Exposure Surveillance System. *Am J Emerg Med* 17:435–487, 1999.

Litovitz TL, Klein-Schwartz W, White S, et al: 1999 annual report of the American Association of Poison Control Centers Toxic Exposure Surveillance System. *Am J Emerg Med* 18:517–574, 2000.

Litovitz TL, Klein-Schwartz W, White S, et al: 2000 annual report of the American Association of Poison Control Centers Toxic Exposure Surveillance System. *Am J Emerg Med* 19:337–395, 2001.

Litovitz TL, Klein-Schwartz W, Rodgers GC, et al: 2001 annual report of the American Association of Poison Control Centers Toxic Exposure Surveillance System. *Am J Emerg Med* 20:391–401, 2002.

Litovitz T, Manoguerra A: Comparison of pediatric poisoning hazards: an analysis of 3.8 million exposure incidents. *Pediatrics* 89:999–1006, 1992.

McCarron MG, Challoner KR, Thompson GA: Diphenoxylate-atropine (Lomotil®) overdose in children: An update (report of 8 cases and review of the literature). *Pediatrics* 87:694–700, 1991.

McClure RJ, Davis PM, Meadows SR, et al: Epidemiology of Munchausen syndrome by proxy, non-accidental poisoning, and non-accidental suffocation. *Arch Dis Child* 75:57–61, 1996.

Meadow R: What is, and what is not, "Munchausen syndrome by proxy"? *Arch Dis Child* 72:534–538, 1995.

National Electronic Injury Surveillance System. Accessed July 16, 2003. Available from URL: http://www.cpsc.gov/library/neiss.html

Quadrani DA, Spiller HA, Widder P: Five year retrospective evaluation of sulfonylurea ingestion in children. *J Toxicol Clin Toxicol* 34:267–270, 1996.

Rodgers GB: The safety effects of child-resistant packaging for oral prescription drugs: Two decades of experience. *JAMA* 275:1661–1665, 1996.

Rosenberg DA: Web of deceit: A literature review of Munchausen syndrome by proxy. *Child Abuse Negl* 11:547–563, 1987.

Scharman EJ, Cloonan HA, Durback-Morris LF: Home administration of charcoal: Can mothers administer a therapeutic dose? *J Emerg Med* 21:357–361, 2001.

Shannon M: Ingestion of toxic substances by children. *N Engl J Med* 342:186–191, 2000.

Tenenbein M: Poisoning pearls regarding the very young. *Clinical Pediatric Emergency Medicine* 1:176–179, 2000.

Watson WA, Litovitz TL, Rodgers GC, et al: 2002 annual report of the American Association of Poison Control Centers Toxic Exposure Surveillance System. *Am J Emerg Med* 21:353–421, 2003.

9

Special Toxicologic Considerations in the Adolescent

Alan Woolf

HIGH-YIELD FACTS

- By their senior year in high school, 80% of teenagers have experimented with alcohol, 61% with cigarettes, and 58% with illicit drugs (including inhalants).

- As a cohort, U.S. adolescents who start cigarette smoking today will suffer 5.5 million premature deaths and will account for over $200 billion in future health care costs.

- Suicide is the third most common cause of death among children 10 to 19 years old. Poisoning by drug overdose is a common mechanism of self-harm.

- Adolescents who suffered childhood plumbism have a 5.8-fold higher risk of a reading disability and a 7.4-fold higher risk of dropping out of high school.

- As many as 3% to 5% of adolescent girls develop an eating disorder, either anorexia nervosa (prevalence 0.5% to 1.0%) or bulimia nervosa (prevalence 3%). Intentional abuse of ipecac, laxatives, and/or diuretics and suicide attempts by poisoning often play a role in the pathology of the disorder.

Adolescents are confronted with risks of poisoning related to a variety of circumstances in the course of their physical, sexual, cognitive, and psychosocial growth and development. They suddenly find themselves in new or newly stressful situations: the workplace, social gatherings and parties, dating, and intense competition on the sports field and in the classroom. The struggles for peer approval, independence from family, and personal and sexual identity often present adolescents with difficult decisions about alcohol, cigarette, and substance abuse. For some, estrangement from family, friends, and community supports may lead to inner turmoil and feelings of hopelessness associated with self-destructive acts of poisoning, either through the abuse of drugs and alcohol or suicide attempts.

EPIDEMIOLOGY

Adolescents 13 to 19 years of age constitute a secondary peak (after the preschool-aged child) in the incidence of poisonings, accounting for 7% of all exposures reported to poison control centers. Unlike poisonings involving young children, adolescent poisonings are more likely to be intentional incidents and have serious medical implications. Whereas only about 10% of early childhood poisonings are referred to health care facilities, almost 50% of those involving teens are serious enough to require emergency department management. Illicit drugs account for the majority of adolescent deaths owing to intentional poisoning, whereas alcohol and carbon monoxide poisoning are important causes of adolescent deaths owing to unintentional poisoning.

SPECIAL AGE CONSIDERATIONS

Adolescents undergo a variety of developmental changes, including physical and sexual maturation, cognitive growth, and behavioral and psychosocial changes. Such considerations leave them especially vulnerable as a group to certain poisonings. Athletic prowess and the mastery of a sport are valued for contributing to an adolescent's self-image and competence. However, such pressures may also lead to experimentation with amphetamine-based stimulants, anabolic steroids, or ephedra- or caffeine-containing herbs and dietary supplements to improve physical performance. Dietary supplements, often containing caffeine or ephedrine, may cause toxic side effects, including anxiety, gastrointestinal disturbance, hypertension, or, with ephedrine use, seizures and stroke. Adolescents may also abuse anabolic steroids or weight loss products to improve their physical appearance and self-image. In doing so, they risk the many side effects of chronic anabolic steroid use, such as acne, hirsutism, loss of libido, testicular atrophy, behavioral changes, and even psychosis (see Chapter 55).

Adolescents may also experience toxic exposures in the workplace. For example, many adolescents are recruited into lower-tier, entry-level jobs that involve cooking, cleaning, painting, construction, or landscaping, often with little preparatory training or instruction in the use of protective equipment. As such, they constitute a group likely to experience a toxic exposure. In one study of 8779 U.S. teenagers aged 12 to 17 years who experienced toxic exposures while at work, alkaline corrosive agents, gases and fumes, bleach, and cleaners accounted for over 43% of the substances implicated.

EATING DISORDERS

Adolescents and young adults represent the age groups most prone to eating disorders. *Anorexia nervosa* is described as insufficient caloric intake to maintain weight, accompanied by a delusion of being fat and an obsession with being thin. More than 90% of patients with anorexia nervosa are white females; the prevalence rate for the illness is 0.5% to 1.0% among adolescent women. *Bulimia,* defined as binge eating and then purging to prevent weight gain, is usually first manifested in adolescence, and has a lifetime prevalence in the United States of 3%. Eating disorders are associated with a notable risk of intentional poisoning, either to assist in purging and weight loss, or in a suicide attempt. A clustering of other unhealthy behaviors, including drug and alcohol abuse, suicidality, delinquency, and sexual promiscuity often accompanies eating disorders.

Physicians may encounter such patients because they present with physical symptoms related to starvation, weight loss, or repeated emesis. These symptoms can be associated with ipecac, diuretic, and/or laxative abuse; and the acute or chronic toxic effects of diet pill use. In one survey of 39 adolescents with eating disorders, 64% used weight-loss aides and 34% used diuretics regularly. Table 9–1 lists a number of weight-loss product ingredients and their side effects.

Drugs used in the therapy of eating disorders, such as cisapride, selective serotonin reuptake inhibitors, cyclic antidepressants, and other psychopharmaceuticals (such as sedatives, phenothiazines, MAO inhibitors, venlafaxine, bupropion, and atypical antipsychotics) have their own toxicities and side effects. Adolescents may abuse these same therapeutic agents to attempt suicide, another consideration in the assessment of symptomatic patients with underlying eating disorders. In one study of 23 cases of poisoning among adolescents with anorexia nervosa, psychotherapeutic drugs, cathartics, and/or analgesics were the most common agents employed. Delays seeking medical care, as well as unusual fluid and electrolyte abnormalities, complicated case management.

Cardiovascular features of eating disorders include resting bradycardia, hypotension, exaggerated orthostasis, and hypovolemia. Electrocardiographic (ECG) changes such as low voltage, prolonged QT_C interval, and nonspecific T-wave changes have also been described. These cardiotoxic signs may indicate poisoning from ipecac, antihypertensives, or other cardiotropic agents, to which adolescents may have access. Ipecac abuse is associated with repeated vomiting of acidic contents, dental-enamel erosions, metabolic alkalosis, and hypokalemia. Emetine, a component of ipecac that is toxic when used chronically and excessively, produces ECG and echocardiogram changes consistent with reversible cardiomyopathy, as well as elevated muscle enzymes and electromyographic changes associated with skeletal myopathy. Chronic ipecac abuse may lead eventually to irreversible cardiomyopathy and death.

Laboratory abnormalities, including hypokalemia, hypochloremia, other electrolyte disturbances, metabolic alkalosis, hypoglycemia, and elevated liver function tests are features of chronic, pathologic purging and weight loss. Table 9–2 differentiates the serum and urine electrolyte and acid–base disturbances seen with different types of purging behaviors.

Up to 15% of patients with bulimia report laxative abuse and purging behaviors. Laxatives of the stimulant category, which include phenolphthalein, senna, bisacodyl, and castor oil, are commonly used. Table 9–3 lists some of the symptoms and signs of laxative abuse, which may include such severe complications as atonic colon and protein-losing enteropathy.

OTHER PSYCHIATRIC DISORDERS

Clinical depression, other mood disorders, and chronic anxiety states in adolescence may manifest themselves

Table 9–1. Toxicity of Selective Ingredients in Weight Loss Products

Ingredient	Adverse Effects
Ashwagandha	CNS depression
Bladder wrack kelp	Hyperthyroidism, exacerbated acne
Bromelain	Gastric upset, diarrhea
Caffeine	Insomnia, restlessness, agitation, irritability
Calcium salts	Anorexia, vomiting, headache, dizziness, kidney stones, milk-alkali syndrome
Cascara sagrada	Vomiting, electrolyte abnormalities, hypokalemia
Cayenne	Hypothermia, diarrhea, gallstones
Chitosan	Allergies?
Choline	Anorexia, nausea, diarrhea, vomiting, abdominal pain, sedation, fishy body odor
Chromium picolinate	Hypoglycemia, nephrotoxicity, rhabdomyolysis, pustulosis, personality disturbances
Creatine pyruvate	Nausea, diarrhea, cramps, dizziness, renal dysfunction
DHEA	Androgenic effects (acne, hirsutism, voice change)
Echinacea	Allergies, asthma, anaphylaxis
Ephedrine	MI, hemorrhagic and ischemic stroke, tremor, palpitations, tachycardia, anxiety, headache, hypertension, nervousness, insomnia
Fenugreek	Hypoglycemia
Gingko biloba	Headache, GI upset, allergic skin reactions, cerebral hemorrhage, abnormal platelet function
Ginseng, Panax	Nervousness, insomnia, nausea, headache
Guarana	*See* caffeine
Horse chestnut	Pruritus, nausea, GI complaints
Inositol	Flatulence, loose bowels, behavioral effects
Kola nut	*See* caffeine
Lactobacillus acidophilus	Flatulence, constipation
Licorice	Pseudoaldosteronism, hypokalemia, hypertension
Phenylpropanolamine	Headache, hypertension, hemorrhagic or ischemic stroke, seizures, dystonia, MI, psychosis
Psyllium	Bloating
Senna	Hepatitis, nausea, hypokalemia, hypocalcemia, melanosis coli, atonic bowel
St. John's wort	Photosensitivity, restlessness, allergic reaction, drug interactions
Tinnevelly senna	*See* senna
Tryptophan	Eosinophilia-myalgia syndrome
Vanadium	Nausea, vomiting, diarrhea, cramps, green tongue
Vitamin B_{12}	Itching, diarrhea
Vitamin B_6	Nausea, vomiting, peripheral neuropathy
Yohimbe	Tachycardia, hypertension, tremor, anxiety

Abbreviation: MI, myocardial infarction.
Source: Modified with permission from Table 1 in Roerig et al: *Int J Eat Disord* 33:446–468, 2003.

through suicidal ideation. Comorbidities of suicidal adolescents include cigarette or alcohol use, access to firearms, witnessed violence, previous attempts, and psychiatric problems. As many as 12% of girls and 6% of boys in high school report making at least one suicide attempt. Young women are 3 to 4 times as likely as young men to take an overdose in a suicide attempt. Adolescents who attempt suicide by poisoning often do so as an impulsive act, and frequently choose medications that are convenient and close at hand. Not unexpectedly, analgesics such as acetaminophen and psychotherapeutic agents are often involved in such suicide attempts.

Table 9–2. Electrolyte Abnormalities Often Associated With Purging

	Serum					Urine		
	Na	**K**	**Cl**	**HCO$_3$**	**pH**	**Na**	**K**	**Cl**
Vomiting	↑–↓	↓	↓	↑	↑	↓	↓	↓
Laxatives	↑–	↓	↑↓	↑↓	↑↓	↓	↓	↓–
Diuretics	↓–	↓	↓	↑	↑	↑	↑	↑

↑ increased; – normal; ↓ decreased.
Source: Reproduced, with permission, from Mehler PS: Bulimia nervosa. *N Engl J Med* 349:875–880, 2003.

CHRONIC DISEASES

Adolescents with chronic illnesses are particularly vulnerable to the risks of experimentation with substances of abuse. In some cases, such as those with sickle cell disease who use tobacco or cocaine, injury from the toxic agent directly compounds the injury from the underlying illness.

Adolescents with a chronic illness such as cystic fibrosis also may self-medicate with herbs and dietary supplements. Some remedies, such as those containing vitamins and trace elements, may be innocuous or even have nutritional benefits; others such as gingko, ginger, feverfew, or garlic have the potential to interfere with platelet aggregation or other functions and to exacerbate pulmonary bleeding. Herbs and dietary supplements may also interact with other drugs in the therapeutic regimen to complicate an illness. For example, adolescents who are organ transplant recipients may not realize that self-therapy with St. John's wort for dysthymia may induce cytochrome P450-metabolizing enzymes that reduce plasma levels of a critical antirejection drug such as cyclosporine.

LEARNING AND COGNITION

Throughout this age period, adolescents develop the higher-order cognitive skills and executive function needed for the advanced learning demands of high school, college, and job training. Studies by Needleman and colleagues have suggested that chronic exposures to the heavy metal lead, experienced in early childhood, may result in higher rates of reading disability and higher drop-out rates later in high school. Young adults suffering from chronic inhalant abuse and associated early solvent encephalopathy may experience school failure. Those with chronic addictions to hallucinogens, amphetamines, cocaine, opiates, and/or marijuana may suffer memory problems, amotivational syndromes, cognitive weaknesses, and behavioral problems associated with school failure.

Table 9–3. Physical and Laboratory Signs of Chronic Laxative Abuse

Physical
  Abdominal pain
  Diarrhea
  Protein-losing enteropathy
  Rectal bleeding
  Dehydration
  Hypovolemic hypotension
  Cathartic colon
  Smooth muscle atrophy
  Melanosis coli
Laboratory
  Hypokalemia
  Hypocalcemia
  Cardiac arrhythmias
  Rhabdomyolysis
  Renal failure
  Osteomalacia

PREGNANCY

Although the rate of adolescent pregnancy has declined in recent years, it still remains an important public health issue. Among pregnant women who suffered lead poisoning earlier in childhood, the fetus may sustain lead-induced neurologic injuries during fetal maturation. Pregnant adolescents are vulnerable to the same pressures of substance abuse and other risk-taking behaviors as other teens. However, injurious effects to the fetus are inevitable consequences of such behaviors. Cigarette smoking in pregnancy is associated with a higher incidence of low birthweight and health problems during infancy and childhood. Ethanol use, even in small amounts, may cause fetal alcohol syndrome, with neurologic damage and long-term learning disabilities. Use of illegal drugs, such as cocaine, during pregnancy is associated with increased rates of fetal wastage and neurologic problems later in childhood (see Chapter 4).

MOST COMMON TOXINS

Besides traditional substances of abuse, such as tobacco, alcohol, marijuana, cocaine, opiates, and sedative-hypnotics, recent trends have pointed to the popularity among teens of newer chemicals such as methylene dioxymethamphetamine (MDMA), other amphetamine congeners (so-called designer drugs), dextromethorphan, gamma hydroxybutyrate (GHB) and its congeners, ketamine, and khat. The Internet serves as a vehicle for dissemination of information about substances of abuse; many newer, as yet unregulated abusable chemicals may be ordered directly from Internet sources. The emergence of prescription drugs—baclofen, clonazepam, methylphenidate, hydrocodone, and oxycontin—as targets for misuse is a new and worrisome development. When adolescent poisoning is suspected, a toxicologic screen of the blood and urine is indicated. However, some substances such as ketamine or GHB are not assayed in conventional screens. Some amphetamine assays can detect MDMA, but with reduced sensitivity (see Chapter 20). Determination of blood ethanol concentration is also indicated.

Table 9–4 presents recent results of the Monitoring the Future nationally weighted survey of high school seniors and their lifetime prevalence of substance abuse. The trends in adolescents' views of substance abuse are revealing. Whereas an overwhelming number of 12th graders continue to disapprove of heroin (93.1%) and crack cocaine (87%) use even once or twice, only 49% disapprove of marijuana use, a moderating view toward the drug that has trended downward for over a decade.

MOST DANGEROUS TOXINS

Cigarettes, alcohol, inhalants, cocaine, narcotics, and other substances of abuse also represent the most dangerous toxins to teenagers. Some adolescents suffer short-term complications of drug use. These include adverse effects directly related to drugs such as coma, seizures, and cardiac dysrhythmias. Indirect injuries such as those resulting from poor judgment leading to motor vehicle

Table 9–4. National Prevalence, 2001: Lifetime Substance Abuse Among High School Students

Drug or Chemical	8th Graders (N = 16,200) (%)	10th Graders (N = 14,000) (%)	12th Graders (N = 12,800) (%)
Any illicit drug (+inhalants)	34.5	48.8	58.0
Alcohol	50.5	70.1	79.7
Cigarettes	36.6	52.8	61.0
Marijuana/hashish	20.4	40.1	59.0
Inhalants	17.1	15.2	13.0
Amphetamines	10.2	16.0	16.2
MDMA (ecstasy)	5.2	8.0	11.7
Hallucinogens	4.0	7.8	12.8
LSD	3.4	6.3	10.9
Tranquilizers	4.7	8.1	9.2
Cocaine	4.3	5.7	8.2
Crack cocaine	3.0	3.1	3.7
Steroids	2.8	3.5	3.7
Heroin	1.7	1.7	1.8

Source: Summarized from Table 1, Monitoring the Future National Results on Adolescent Substance Abuse, Overview of Key Findings, 2001. University of Michigan Institute for Social Research under contract with NIDA, DHHS, Bethesda, MD, 2002.

Table 9–5. A Brief Screening Test for Adolescent Substance Abuse: The CRAFFT Questions*

C	Have you ever ridden in a CAR driven by someone (including yourself) who was high or had been using alcohol or drugs?
R	Do you ever use alcohol or drugs to RELAX, feel better about yourself, or fit in?
A	Do you ever use alcohol or drugs while you are by yourself, ALONE?
F	Do you ever FORGET things you did while using alcohol or drugs?
F	Do your family or FRIENDS ever tell you that you should cut down on your drinking or drug use?
T	Have you ever gotten into TROUBLE while you were using alcohol or drugs?

*Two or more answers suggest a significant problem, abuse, or dependence.
Source: Knight et al.: *Arch Pediatr Adolesc Med* 156:607–614, 2002.

collisions or other incidental trauma are also common. Clinicians should query adolescents who present with unexplained trauma or change in consciousness for possible substance abuse or an undeclared suicide attempt. Confronted with the medical consequences of their substance abuse, adolescents may be evasive and give an unreliable history. Friends or family can be alternative sources of information.

Adolescents may experience toxic injuries to organ systems from their chronic use of harmful substances. The Centers for Disease Control and Prevention estimated that more than 16.6 million American youth, aged 17 and under in 1995, would become smokers. This cohort alone will suffer a national toll of 5.5 million premature deaths and will account for $200 billion in future health care costs. In one prospective study of younger adolescents who initiated smoking, changes in lung maturation and airway flow were documented by the time they reached older adolescence.

Long-term neurologic damage, some of which is readily apparent in adolescence, results from chronic abuse of some drugs and chemicals. Adolescents using hallucinogens such as D-lysergic acid diethylamide (LSD) may experience flashbacks. Amphetamines and cocaine use may induce personality change and psychosis. Chronic inhalant abuse is known to cause slow cognition and memory defects associated with a syndrome of solvent

encephalopathy. Animal and clinical studies have found that MDMA-induced injury to serotonergic pathways leads to long-term changes in serotonin fiber architecture, with drop out of neurons populating specific regions of the brain. Clinical correlates of such studies on MDMA are unknown, but there seems an important potential for long-term injury.

Table 9–5 presents the CRAFFT questions, a validated brief questionnaire that ascertains whether or not an adolescent has a significant substance abuse addiction problem. Such tools can help clinicians decide which adolescents need a more intensive approach to the management of substance abuse problems.

PREVENTION

Adolescent poisoning is preventable. Measures as simple as training and the use of protective barriers when handling caustics or cleaning agents may prevent workplace-associated toxic exposures. School-based health care professionals, primary care providers, mental health centers, church support groups for teens and their families, and other community group-based counseling are some of the resources available for adolescents in trouble.

Adolescents are good candidates for interdiction of substance abuse. Consistent and frequent anti–drug abuse messages from parents should begin early in childhood. Parents should not engage in substance abuse themselves to serve as role models. Restricted access, educational campaigns designed to forestall initiation and experimentation, peer-initiated guidance, and an emphasis on parental awareness and involvement are all powerful yet underutilized strategies. Many adolescents recognize the dangers of such experimentation and want to avoid its risks. Those who already suffer from addiction may be ready for help with strategies to quit. Expansion of inpatient detoxification programs and outpatient cognitive-behavioral therapy options can help those with established substance abuse addiction.

SUGGESTED READINGS

Boyer EW, Woolf A: What's new on the street? *Clin Pediatr Emerg Med* 1:180–185, 2000.
Centers for Disease Control and Prevention: Projected smoking-related deaths among youth: United States. *Morb Mortal Wkly Rep* 45:971–974, 1996.
Colton P, Woodside DB, Kaplan AS: Laxative withdrawal in eating disorders: Treatment protocol and 3- to 20-month follow-up. *Int J Eat Disord* 25:311–317, 1999.

Gold DR, Wang X, Wypij D, et al: Effects of cigarette smoking on lung function in adolescent boys and girls. *N Engl J Med* 335: 931–937, 1996.

Ho PC, Dweik R, Cohen MC: Rapidly reversible cardiomyopathy associated with chronic ipecac ingestion. *Clin Cardiol* 21:780–783, 1998.

Johnston LD, O'Malley PM, Bachman JG: *Monitoring the Future—National Results on Adolescent Drug Use: Overview of Key Findings, 2001.* University of Michigan Institute for Social Research. Bethesda, MD: National Institute on Drug Abuse, U.S. DHHS, 2002. Available from URL: http://www.monitoringthefuture.org.

Kann L, Warren CW, Harris WA, et al: Youth risk behavior surveillance—United States, 1993. *MMWR CDC Surveillance,* Summary 44:1–56, 1995.

Knight JR, Sherritt L, Shrier LA, et al: Validity of the CRAFFT substance abuse screening test among adolescent clinic patients. *Arch Pediatr Adolesc Med* 156:607–614, 2002.

Kreipe RE, Birndorf SA: Eating disorders in adolescents and young adults. *Med Clinic North Am* 84:1027–1049, 2000.

Lewinsohn PM, Striegel-Moore RH, Seeley JR: Epidemiology and natural course of eating disorders in young women from adolescence to young adulthood. *J Am Acad Child Adolesc Psychiatr* 39:1284–1292, 2000.

Litovitz TL, Klein-Schwartz W, Rodgers GC, et al: 2001 annual report of the American Association of Poison Control Centers—Toxic Exposure Surveillance System. *Am J Emerg Med* 20:391–452, 2002.

MacDorman MF, Minino AM, Strobino DM, et al: Annual summary of vital statistics—2001. *Pediatrics* 110:1037–1052, 2002.

Mehler PS: Bulimia nervosa. *N Engl J Med* 349:875–880, 2003.

Needleman HL, Schell A, Bellinger D, et al: The long-term effects of exposure to low doses of lead in childhood—An 11-year follow-up report. *N Engl J Med* 322:83–88, 1990.

Reneman L, Booij J, de Bruin K et al: Effects of dose, sex, and long-term abstention from use on toxic effects of MDMA (ecstasy) on brain serotonin neurons. *Lancet* 258:1864–1869, 2001.

Ricaurte GA, Forno LS, Wilson MA et al: (+) 3,4-Methylenedioxy methamphetamine selectively damages central serotonergic neurons in nonhuman primates. *JAMA* 260:51–55, 1988.

Roerig JL, Mitchell JE, de Zwaan M, et al: The eating disorders medicine cabinet revisited: A clinician's guide to appetite suppressants and diuretics. *Int J Eat Disord* 33:443–457, 2003.

Shepherd G, Klein-Schwartz W: Accidental and suicidal adolescent poisoning deaths in the United States, 1979–1994. *Arch Pediatr Adolesc Med* 152:1181–1185, 1998.

Woolf AD, Gren JM: Acute poisonings among adolescents and young adults with anorexia nervosa. *Am J Dis Child* 144: 785–788, 1990.

Woolf AD: Smoking and nicotine addiction: A pediatric epidemic with sequelae in adulthood. *Curr Opin Pediatr* 9:470–947, 1997.

Woolf AD, Garg A, Alpert H, et al: Adolescent workplace toxic exposures: A national study. *Arch Pediatr Adolesc Med* 155: 704–7, 2001.

10

Pediatric Toxicokinetics and Pharmacology

Frank P. Paloucek

HIGH-YIELD FACTS

- Pharmacokinetic principles such as drug absorption, distribution, elimination, and metabolism are important parameters to consider in the poisoned pediatric patient.

- Serum drug concentrations in the poisoned child are frequently determined, and more difficult to interpret, than in the patient undergoing routine therapeutic drug monitoring.

- Understanding the basic fundamentals of clinical toxicokinetics is essential for the optimal selection of a therapeutic intervention and proper disposition of an intoxicated patient.

Pharmacokinetics is the science of drug movement through the body and can be described in terms of absorption, distribution, and elimination. Toxicokinetics is used to describe these three principles in the setting of drug toxicity. Poisoned pediatric patients frequently manifest wide changes in physiologic and pharmacokinetic parameters. This may be further compounded by various iatrogenic or therapeutic interventions. These patients frequently require aggressive therapy, including recognition of the dynamic changes in an individual's pharmacokinetic parameters in the overdose setting. Serum drug concentrations are frequently obtained, and are more difficult to interpret than in the patient undergoing routine therapeutic drug monitoring. Understanding

the basic fundamentals of clinical toxicokinetics is crucial to the optimal selection of a therapeutic intervention and proper disposition of the patient.

This chapter discusses the relationships of physiologic alterations and pharmacokinetic parameters describing drug disposition in poisoned pediatric patients. The basic pharmacokinetic and toxicokinetic principles and equations that can be used as a basis for evaluating serum drug concentrations are discussed. The concepts of physiologic clearance and applied pharmacokinetics are important clinical tools to optimize treatment and improve outcome.

ABSORPTION

The absorption or administration rate is clinically important because it influences or determines the time required to achieve desired serum concentrations. In most ill patients, this should occur as quickly as possible, which explains the strong preference for intravenous (IV) administration. Drug absorption from the gastrointestinal (GI) tract and intramuscular (IM) or subcutaneous (SC) administration is frequently unreliable or inconsistent.

Blood supply to the GI tract or capillary flow within the muscle may be altered by acute pathology affecting drug absorption. In slow cardiac output or poor perfusion states, inadequate and delayed absorption is possible. Time to, and magnitude of, peak drug concentrations can be delayed and reduced. In high cardiac output states, the reverse may be seen, with earlier time to peak and higher peak concentrations. In poor perfusion states as with a hypodynamic overdosed patient, the rapid provision of

IV fluids can improve blood flow sufficiently to allow oral, IM, or SC medications to be better absorbed. Similar processes have been described with the provision of enteral fluids in patients with oral overdoses where significantly delayed and large increases in drug concentrations were observed owing to the presumed enhancement of tablet dissolution in the GI tract. Effects are also seen with therapeutic interventions such as multiple-dose oral activated charcoal for elimination enhancement in a drug overdose. It has been shown in in vitro animal models that the effectiveness of charcoal is directly related to mesenteric blood flow.

Orally administered drug must first undergo dissolution to be absorbed. Dissolution depends on the chemical properties of the drug, the formulation, and physiologic factors such as GI pH and concomitant fluids or medications. A drug with a slow dissolution rate, or administered as a sustained-release product, in a patient with increased GI motility or a short bowel may not dissolve completely. Hence, bioavailability will be decreased and less drug will be absorbed. Many drugs are primarily absorbed via passive diffusion in the small bowel. Thus, gastric emptying time can be a rate-limiting step following dissolution. Many drugs can slow or hasten gastric emptying. Most acute illnesses decrease gastric motility, reducing drug absorption. As patients improve, drug absorption, and hence serum drug concentrations, may increase. In these patients, follow-up monitoring of serum concentrations or dosage adjustments may be necessary to prevent toxicity.

Another consideration for the absorption process is bioavailability (F). *Bioavailability* is calculated by dividing the area under the serum drug concentration versus time curve (AUC) resulting from the oral dose compared with that of the intravascular dose, assuming that 100% of the latter is absorbed. Changes (decreases) in F are typically assumed to be due to the first-pass effect. This is for most drugs, assumed to be due to hepatic metabolism. It ignores incomplete dissolution or absorption from GI lumen, or any metabolism that occurs in the GI wall during absorption. The first-pass effect is taken into account when calculating the normal dosage for a drug, and explains the relatively large differences in doses for highly metabolized drugs such as propranolol or verapamil when comparing oral and parenteral doses. Increased bioavailability for drugs with a large first-pass effect following oral administration is seen in liver dysfunction. This may be due to diminished enzymatic capacity or shunting of blood flow. Finally, absorption from the GI tract depends on the integrity of the GI lumen and luminal contents.

With IM or SC administration, the extent of absorption usually approaches 100%; however, the rate of absorption varies greatly, depending on the formulation and chemical properties of the drug, and factors such as tissue composition, temperature, blood pH, and perfusion at the site of administration. All the physiologic factors can be altered in the poisoned patient. If the patient experiences an adverse reaction, the effect may be more prolonged, although often of lower magnitude, than generally observed after IV administration.

After IV administration, the dose, rate of administration, and length of infusion influence resultant serum concentrations. If the dose remains the same, the serum concentration-time curve differs, but the AUC is similar for most drugs. Common drugs that do not follow this linear pharmacokinetic principle include alcohols, phenytoin, and salicylates.

Common methods of IV drug administration for patients in the pediatric intensive care unit (PICU) are IV bolus, intermittent infusion, and continuous administration. Retrograde infusions are also frequently used. These methods of IV administration produce different serum concentration time profiles and can therefore result in different dose–response effects. Recognition of the variances may allow selection of a specific method to optimize drug therapy and avoid toxicity.

A *bolus infusion* is an IV dose administered directly into the vascular compartment via a vein or artery, or by injecting into the distal end of the IV catheter. The method allows for rapid delivery of drug to the systemic circulation. This is advantageous, especially for the cardiovascular agents, but can be problematic for drugs with rapid neurologic or direct respiratory depressant effects, such as sedative-hypnotics.

Intermittent IV infusion is administration at a fixed rate at a specific frequency. It is important to emphasize that considerable mixing can occur in the line. The patient thus receives an infusion with a smaller peak concentration than if infused directly into a vein alone. This even occurs with the use of infusion pumps on the same IV catheter where a Y-site connection is being used. Variations in compatibilities of the agents administered to a patient and the number of IV lines can result in intrapatient variations for the same dose of an intermittent infusion. Using faster rates of drug administration, smaller-bore catheter lines, catheter sets with less dead space, and solutions with similar osmolarity can decrease in-line mixing of drug.

A drug administered as a *continuous infusion* is infused at a constant rate over a prolonged period. This delays attaining therapeutic values, which may be a disadvantage, especially with drugs with slower elimination half-lives. Serum concentrations are assumed to have reached steady-state values following continuous or intermittent infusion after three to five elimination half-lives of the drug. Therapeutic serum concentrations can be achieved more quickly with the use of a bolus injection or a more rapid rate of infusion when initiating therapy, after which a continuous infusion would be started. Lidocaine and phenytoin are drugs commonly administered in this matter.

DISTRIBUTION

Once in the systemic circulation, drug is available for transport into peripheral tissue compartments. The apparent volume of distribution (V_d) is an abstract constant that relates the total dose or amount of drug in the body to the resulting serum drug concentrations. This volume is termed *apparent* because it is generally not a true physiologic or anatomic volume. A simplified mathematical version of V_d is

$$V_d = \text{Dose}/C_p$$

Here, the serum drug concentration (C_p) is the result of a single instantaneously administered dose. This assumes that the initial serum drug concentration is 0; 100% of the drug is administered instantaneously; distribution is uniform and instantaneous; and there is no elimination from the body. In simpler terms, the dose in the body is equal to the dose administered. As calculated above, the lower the C_p drug concentration relative to a dose, the larger the volume of distribution. Factors that can increase the volume of distribution are high lipid solubility, high tissue binding, or low serum protein binding. The predominant factor that results in a very low volume of distribution is plasma protein binding. It is critical to note that a drug's V_d is independent of its clearance.

The V_d is not a true physiologic entity, but rather an indicator of where the drug distributes in relative concentrations throughout the body. V_d generally correlates well with body weight, and is often expressed in liters per kilogram. A volume of distribution of 0.25 L/kg of total body weight is associated with distribution primarily in extracellular fluid. A volume of distribution of 0.65 L/kg with a drug that is highly water soluble suggests distribution to total body water. A large volume of distribution (>1.00 L/kg) suggests extensive tissue distribution and peripheral concentrations, commonly found with lipophilic drugs.

The assumption that there is instantaneous and uniform drug distribution is consistent with a one-compartment model. In reality, the distribution of most drugs occurs over a measurable time period and in a non-homogenous pattern. In a two-compartment model, the drug distributes initially into a central compartment consisting of blood and the highly perfused tissues whose properties are most compatible with the drug's physicochemical characteristics. Subsequent distribution occurs to the less well-perfused or less compatible sites (peripheral compartment). Distribution between the central and peripheral compartments is described by the rate constants K_{12} and K_{21}. A serum drug concentration obtained immediately after administration of an initial IV bolus dose reflects the volume of the central compartment (V_{dc}).

$$V_{dc} = \text{Dose}/C_{p0}$$

Here, C_{p0} is the drug concentration immediately after an instantaneous dose. As distribution takes place, the serum drug concentration rapidly decreases. The rate of decline reflects the processes of both distribution and elimination. Drug distribution is usually a first-order process and is associated with the distribution rate constant α. Using this constant, distribution half-life can be calculated as follows:

$$t_{1/2}\alpha = 0.693/\alpha$$

Here, $t_{1/2}\alpha$ is the time required for distribution to be 50% complete. Most drugs have a $t_{1/2}\alpha$ value between 5 and 30 minutes. Notable exceptions are digoxin and lithium. When distribution is complete, the slope of the decline decreases, remaining linear, reflecting the elimination process alone. Similarly, when elimination is a first-order process, the elimination phase is associated with an elimination rate constant (K_e) or β. K_e and β are common abbreviations, and are used interchangeably in this text. Using this constant, the elimination half-life can be calculated as follows:

$$t_{1/2} = 0.693/K_e$$

Here, $t_{1/2}$ (also referred to as *elimination $t_{1/2}$*) is the time required for the serum drug concentration to decline by 50%. There is continued distribution occurring during the elimination phase, but the rate between compartments is in equilibrium (*steady state*) with the elimination rate. A serum concentration drawn at the time of beginning of the elimination phase is what is commonly considered the *peak* concentration for a drug, because it is believed to reflect the maximum concentration that would occur following a dose in any given tissue site. Recommended sampling times for most drugs are specific to waiting a specified time period following the dose administration to account for this effect. In addition, most reported V_d represent the value determined by dividing the dose by the serum concentration found at the end of distribution. Otherwise, all drugs would share the essentially same volume of distribution for the central compartment.

Recommended total loading doses of drugs are usually calculated using the apparent volume of distribution and desired serum concentration. When the dose is administered much more rapidly than the distribution half-life, the initial (peridistribution) serum drug concentrations are high. This can lead to a misdiagnosis of drug intoxication. The actual clinical importance of this high serum drug concentration is determined by the drug's pharmacodynamics. The peridistribution concentration value becomes important and determines the safe maximal rate of administration if a drug's toxicologic affects are seen in the central compartment. A slower rate of administration decreases the magnitude of the peak concentration in the central compartment and minimizes adverse effects. If the response is correlated only with postdistribution serum drug concentrations, the initial level is irrelevant. For example, with lidocaine, seizures are associated with high initial concentrations and may be avoided by splitting the total loading dose into several smaller bolus doses to reduce predistribution serum drug concentrations. Conversely, the pharmacologic effects of digoxin or lithium are correlated with postdistribution serum drug concentration; initial predistribution concentrations are usually irrelevant.

Other impacts of distribution on therapeutic interventions are less well studied or understood. Examples include elimination enhancement procedures, such as hemodialysis. In controlled settings or at maintenance hemodialysis sessions, all of a patient's medications are withheld prior to the session to avoid excessive removal. Conversely, it is commonly recommended that only drugs with low volumes of distribution (<1 L/kg) and other favorable physicochemical properties can undergo hemodialysis in the management of toxicity or overdose. This is based on a mathematical modeling that assumes initiation of the extracorporeal procedure only after distribution had occurred. This ignores the potential benefits in drugs with prolonged distribution rates. It also ignores the impact that prolonged absorption (e.g., sustained-release dosage forms) or delayed elimination has on extending the distribution phase, thus extending the period where higher concentrations are available for removal from the central compartment. In summary, the various V_d can influence the rate of administration of a dose (central compartment) or the dose necessary to obtain desired serum drug concentrations.

An important determinant of distribution is protein binding. Many drugs bind, usually competitively, to plasma proteins, predominantly albumin and α_1-acid glycoprotein, which results in very small volumes of distribution. This is usually readily reversible, and an equilibrium between bound and free drug is established such that the free fraction remains relatively constant for any given protein concentration. Only the free drug is pharmacologically active. In most cases, protein-binding capacity is much larger than necessary and the fraction of free drug is independent of the total serum drug concentrations. A few drugs of exception are valproic acid and salicylates, for which binding sites can be saturated with therapeutic or supratherapeutic doses. If saturation occurs, the total serum drug concentrations can be within the normal range, but the free fraction, and hence the pharmacologic effect, can be increased. In overdose, saturation of protein binding sites becomes clinically more important. Also, the acute administration of a competitive binding drug can result in transient increases of the free drug concentration of the drug with lower affinity, and result in toxic effects. Endogenous ligands can also displace of drugs from their binding sites. In uremic patients, free drug concentrations of both diazepam and phenytoin are greatly increased. This causes an increased free fraction of drug, which can be confirmed by determining the free and total serum drug concentrations simultaneously.

Anionic drugs and weak acids, such as phenytoin, warfarin, and salicylates, usually bind to albumin. Malnutrition, burns, sepsis, renal disease, and liver disease are associated with significant decreases in plasma albumin concentrations in children. If the albumin concentration is decreased, binding sites are proportionally decreased and the percentage of free drug increases. If the free fraction (f) is greater than 0.5, less than one-half of the drug is bound, and changes in albumin concentrations usually have an insignificant effect on free serum drug concentrations. For example, for a drug with f of 0.5, decreasing albumin concentration by 25% increases the free drug concentration from 50.0% to 62.5% of the total drug. In contrast, if f is 0.1, a 25.0% decrease in albumin concentration increases free serum drug concentration from 10% to 33% of the total drug, more than a threefold increase. A drug for which clinical significance of this issue is well known is phenytoin, whose normal therapeutic total drug concentration is 10 to 20 mg/L. Because f is 0.1 for this drug, the equivalent free drug therapeutic range is 1 to 2 mg/L.

It is important to note that drug–drug interactions affecting distribution processes, such as the inhibition or induction of p-glycoprotein, result in no observable change in the free fraction of the affected drug, yet still result in pharmacodynamic changes owing to the change in distribution ratio between compartments. Similarly, it has been noted in severe overdoses that significant differences exist between simultaneously obtained venous and arterial samples for drug concentration determinations, which may be due to a back diffusion process. This may have relevance for comparing published pharmacokinetic studies in critically ill patients or in comparing results within a specific patient, and possibly when comparing samples obtained in the emergency department versus those obtained in the PICU.

ELIMINATION AND METABOLISM

Consistent with the absorption and distribution processes, elimination of drugs from the body depends on the physicochemical properties of the drug and the patient's physiologic status. In humans, the primary routes of elimination are the liver, kidneys, GI tract, and lungs.

Lipophilic drugs usually must undergo metabolism to more polar compounds to be eliminated. *Phase I metabolism* transforms lipophilic drugs into relatively polar substances. Oxidation reactions generally occur in the hepatic microsomal enzyme system. Hydrolysis often takes place in the plasma, and reduction often occurs in the GI tract. *Phase II metabolism* combines relatively polar compounds with other lipophilic substances, rendering the latter hydrophilic. Common conjugation reactions are *glucuronidation* and *sulfonation,* which generally take place in the hepatic microsomal enzyme system.

Metabolites formed in the liver can be excreted into the intestinal tract via bile, and then eliminated in the feces or reabsorbed into the blood via enterohepatic recirculation. Multidose oral activated charcoal can enhance the elimination of such drugs by providing a concentration sink in the GI tract. This effect of multiple dose oral activated charcoal, often called *gastrointestinal dialysis,* is also seen with drugs that do not undergo enterohepatic recirculation, particularly those that are easily hemodialyzed. The kidneys often excrete hydrophilic substances. Volatile anesthetics are the only major pharmacologic agents that undergo primarily pulmonary excretion.

Clearance refers to the abstract volume of blood, plasma, or serum from which a drug is completely removed per unit time. Clearance is expressed in units of volume per time (L/h or mL/min). This volume is theoretical; no single liter of blood necessarily has all contained drug removed during one pass through the clearance organ. Instead, a fraction of drug is removed from each of the many liters perfusing the organ(s) of elimination. This fraction is expressed as though it were derived by completely clearing a smaller volume of blood of total drug.

Clearance usually involves more than one organ. Total body clearance (Cl) is the sum of all the individual organ clearances, as shown in the equation:

$$Cl = Cl_H + Cl_R + Cl_{other}$$

Here, Cl_H is hepatic clearance, Cl_R is renal clearance, and Cl_{other} represents the sum of all other routes of drug elimination. Typically, an organ is felt to contribute to clearance when the concentration in vessels leading into the organ significantly exceeds the concentration found in outflow from the organ. Thus, clearance by any single organ is usually extremely dependent on blood flow to the organ.

Table 10–1. Clinical Implications of Neonatal Pharmacokinetics on Therapeutic Drug Administration Compared with Adults

Pharmacokinetic Difference	Clinical Adjustment
Larger apparent volume of distribution	Increase single or loading dose of drug
Lower plasma protein binding (increased free fraction drug activity)	Lower total plasma concentration for pharmacologic effect
Lower total drug clearance due to immature phase I and II metabolic pathways and diminished renal excretion	Lower weight-based daily doses when multiple doses of drug given
Rapid change in drug metabolism with increased age and large variation by gestational age	Rapidly alter dosing requirements based on close monitoring of drug effect and drug concentration (when feasible)

Source: Adapted from Rylance G: Pharmacological principles and kinetics. In: Rylance G, Harvey D, Aranda JV eds: *Neonatal Clinical Pharmacology and Therapeutics.* London: Butterworth-Heinemann; 1991:1–25.

Table 10–2. Considerations for Unexpectedly High Serum Drug Concentrations in a Pediatric Patient

Pharmacokinetic Process

Absorption
    Inaccurate history of time of administration
    Inaccurate history of dose administered
    Inaccurate history of dosage form
    Improved perfusion at the absorption site (late peaks with GI or SC absorption sites)
    Increased dissolution of oral dosage forms (dose-dumping of oral dosage forms with food or physical destruction
        of SR dosage forms)
    Increased gastric motility (also hastens time to peak)
    Increased parenteral delivery mechanics (failure of infusion control devices)
Distribution
    Inaccurate assessment of patient's V_d
        Volume loss (especially for hydrophilic drugs or extensive serum protein binding)
        Obesity (especially for lipophilic drugs)
        Altered morphology (amputations/limb loss—inaccurate body size determination)
    Inappropriate timing of sample
        Sampling time too early (distribution incomplete, can result in very fast elimination rate calculations)
        Sampling time too late (redistribution in post mortem samples)
Elimination/Metabolism
    Inaccurate assessment of patient's elimination or metabolic capacity
        Renal clearance
            Calculated renal clearance (using SCr) too high
            Impaired renal blood flow
            Inhibition of interactions inhibiting renal tubular secretion
            Elimination of tubular reabsorption
    Hepatic clearance
        Impaired hepatic blood flow (especially for flow-limited or flow/capacity sensitive)
        Decreased metabolic capacity
            Hypometabolic states (shock, sepsis, severe toxicity)
        Drug interactions affecting relevant metabolic processes
            Presence of inhibiting effects—this could also be seen late in the co-administration of interacting drugs
                if the process is noncompetitive and requires the normal physiology aging of active enzymes, e.g.
                CYP3A4 inhibition with diltiazem
            Removal of inducing effects
    Impaired enterohepatic elimination

Nonpharmacokinetic Considerations

Laboratory considerations
    Assay interference with endogenous compounds
    False positives
    Sampling considerations
        Sample collection from, or near, the site of administration
        Prolonged or inappropriate sample storage
            Drug generation by serum or tissue contents (e.g., ethanol post mortem)
Pharmacy/nursing considerations
    Medication errors
        Inappropriate admixture or filling process (especially in neonatology—10-fold dosing errors)
    Manufacturing errors

The only organ for which approximation of true clearance can be readily made is the kidney. When a drug is freely filtered and neither secreted nor reabsorbed, renal clearance is equivalent to *glomerular filtration rate* (GFR). Thus:

$$Cl_R = C_{pfree} \times GFR$$

After filtration, many drugs undergo either tubular secretion or reabsorption. Drugs that undergo significant tubular secretion have renal clearance values greater than the GFR. Drugs that are filtered and then reabsorbed have renal clearance values less than the GFR. Neither process can be easily assessed by clinical parameters. Thus, for renally eliminated drugs, dosage adjustments are based on estimates of the fractional reduction in GFR. Clinical estimations of GFR take advantage of the close correlation of GFR with creatinine clearance (Cl_{Cr}). When otherwise stable physiologically, a patient's Cl_{Cr} and their S_{Cr} (serum creatinine) are highly correlated; thus, S_{Cr} is often used to estimate Cl_{Cr} and thus glomerular filtration rate. The most common estimation is as follows:

$$Cl_{Cr} \text{ (mL/min)} = (140 - \text{Age}) \times$$
$$\text{Lean body weight}/72 \times S_{Cr}$$

Hepatic clearance depends on blood flow to the liver, the intrinsic activity of hepatic enzymes, and the fraction of drug that is unbound and free to interact with these enzymes. Changes in blood flow to the liver affect the drug delivery rate and alter hepatic clearance and elimination. This commonly occurs in the PICU patient with shock or heart failure, leading to increased serum drug concentrations of the affected medication. The reverse occurs with therapeutic recovery phases of low-flow states or with drugs that increase hepatic blood flow, such as dopamine, glucagon, and isoproterenol drugs.

USING PHARMACOKINETIC PRINCIPLES TO INTERPRET ELEVATED DRUG CONCENTRATIONS

Recommended doses for any specific drug are based on preapproval pharmacokinetic studies, and the accumulation of further data following marketing. These doses are intended to result in concentrations that fall within the *normal range,* in which therapeutic benefits are far more likely to result than drug toxicity. To summarize some of the principles described for the processes of absorption, distribution, and elimination/metabolism and their relation to the daily interpretation of serum drug concentrations in pediatric patients, Table 10–1 lists clinical impli-

cations of neonatal pharmacokinetics on therapeutic drug administration compared with adults. Table 10–2 lists reasons for drug concentrations being markedly higher than expected in the pediatric patient.

SUGGESTED READINGS

Bauer L: Interference of oral phenytoin absorption by continuous nasogastric feedings. *Neurology* 32:570, 1982.

Bauer LA: *Applied Clinical Pharmacokinetics.* New York: McGraw-Hill, 2001.

Baumann T, Staddon J, Horst H, et al: Minimum urine collection periods for accurate determination of creatinine clearance in critically ill patients. *Clin Pharm* 6:393, 1987.

Bickley SK: Drug dosing during continuous arteriovenous hemofiltration. *Clin Pharm* 7:198–206, 1988.

Bjornsson TD: The method of relative drug accumulation: A simple method for illustrating the effects of different drug dosing regimens and variability in drug elimination on time courses of drug concentrations. *Clin Pharmacol Ther* 51: 266–270, 1992.

Chyka PA: Multiple-dose activated charcoal and enhancement of systemic drug clearance: Summary of studies in animals and human volunteers. *J Toxicol Clin Toxicol* 33:399–405, 1995.

Chiou WL: The phenomenon and rationale of marked dependence of drug concentration on blood sampling site. *Clin Pharmacokinet* 17:175–199, 1989.

Cockroft D, Gault M: Prediction of creatinine clearance from serum creatinine. *Nephron* 16:31, 1976.

Ekstrand R, Alvan G, Borga O: Concentration dependent plasma protein binding of salicylate in rheumatoid patients. *Clin Pharmacokinet* 4:137, 1979.

Evans W, Schentag J, Jusko W, eds: *Applied Pharmacokinetics: Principles of Therapeutic Drug Monitoring.* 3rd ed. Vancouver, WA: Applied Therapeutics; 1992.

Gubbins P, Bertch K: Drug absorption in gastrointestinal disease and surgery. *Pharmacotherapy* 9:285, 1989.

Jones J, Burnett P: Creatinine metabolism in humans with decreased renal function: Creatinine deficit. *Clin Chem* 20: 1204, 1974.

Kellum JA, Angus DC, Johnson JP, et al: Continuous versus intermittent renal replacement therapy: A meta analysis. *Intensive Care Med* 28:29–37, 2002.

Leissing N, Story K, Zaske D: Inline fluid dynamics in piggyback and manifold drug delivery systems. *Am J Hosp Pharm* 46:89, 1989.

Nimmo W: Drugs, diseases and altered gastric emptying. *Clin Pharmacother* 1:189, 1976.

Nimmo W, Heading R, Wilson J, et al: Inhibition of gastric emptying and drug absorption by narcotic analgesics. *Br J Clin Pharmacol* 2:509, 1975.

Reetze-Bonorden P, Bohler J, Keller E: Drug dosage in patients during continuous renal replacement therapy. *Clin Pharmacokinet* 24:362–379, 1993.

Rowland M, Tozer TA: *Clinical Pharmacokinetics: Concepts and Applications.* 3rd ed. Hagerstown, Md: Lippincott, Williams & Wilkins; 1995.

Rylance G: Pharmacological principles and kinetics. In: Rylance G, Harvey D, Aranda JV, eds: *Neonatal Clinical Pharmacology and Therapeutics.* London: Butterworth-Heinemann; 1991:1–25.

Tillement J, Lhoste F, Giudicelli J: Diseases and drug protein binding. *Clin Pharmacokinet* 3:144, 1978.

Tiula E, Neuvonen P: Effect of total drug concentration on the free fraction in uremic sera. *Ther Drug Monit* 8:27, 1986.

Uchebbu IF, Florence AT: Adverse drug events related to dosage forms and delivery systems. *Drug Safety* 14:39–67, 1996.

Venho V, Aukee S, Jussila J, et al: Effect of gastric surgery on the gastrointestinal drug absorption in man. *Scand J Gastroenterol* 10:43, 1975.

Welling P: Interactions affecting drug absorption. *Clin Pharmacokinet* 9:404, 1984.

Winter ME: *Applied Clinical Pharmacokinetics.* 3rd ed. Vancouver, WA: Applied Therapeutics; 1994.

Yu H: Clinical implications of serum protein binding in epileptic children during sodium valproate maintenance therapy. *Ther Drug Monit* 6:414, 1984.

11

Pediatric Toxic Syndromes (Toxidromes)

Asim F. Tarabar
Robert S. Hoffman

Recognition or exclusion of classic toxic syndromes (toxidromes) is important when evaluating the poisoned pediatric patient. Toxidromes are specific signs and symptoms associated with a particular class of toxins. A great deal of emphasis is placed on mental status assessment and vital signs, noting that normal vital signs vary significantly with age. Not only can vital signs provide important clues to help differentiate toxidromes from each other, they can also be indicative of the patient's progress after interventions are made. The physical examination should also include an assessment of the pupils, skin and mucous membranes, pulmonary status, as well as bowel and bladder activity. In addition, knowing the nature and progression of symptoms that are associated with a particular toxidrome can be a useful prognostic tool.

There are several toxidromes with distinct clinical findings. However, it is important to recognize that exposures involving multiple substances may not develop as a classic toxidrome. Also, patients may not present with all of the findings associated with a single toxidrome. Understanding the basic toxidromes can help the clinician determine if the patient was exposed to a toxin from the one of the following classes: sympathomimetic, anticholinergic, cholinergic, opioids, or sedative-hypnotic. While presenting typical features of each syndrome, we also list the prototypical agent for each toxidrome. For detailed information regarding a particular substance or agent, please refer to the individual chapters presented later in this book.

SYMPATHOMIMETIC TOXIC SYNDROME

HIGH-YIELD FACTS

- The sympathomimetic toxidrome results from activation of sympathetic system, manifesting as hypertension, tachycardia, hyperthermia, agitation, diaphoretic skin, and dilated pupils.

- The sympathomimetic toxidrome resembles the anticholinergic toxidrome. Diaphoresis is characteristic of sympathomimetic agents, whereas dry skin, urinary retention, and diminished bowel sounds are characteristic of anticholinergic agents.

- The sympathomimetic toxidrome and ethanol or sedative-hypnotic withdrawal can present with similar clinical manifestations.

- The majority of sympathomimetic exposures require no specific treatment apart from supportive measures and possible benzodiazepine administration.

Introduction and Epidemiology

Sympathomimetic agents are available as prescription drugs, most of which are used to treat asthma and attention deficit hyperactivity disorder (ADAD). Other sympathomimetic drugs include over-the-counter diet and cold preparations, and illicit drugs such as cocaine and 3,4-methylenedioxy methamphetamine (MDMA or ecstasy). According to the 2002 National Survey on Drug Use and Health, there are 1.2 million Americans abusing stimulants. Another 676,000 are current ecstasy users (defined as use within the past month). Among those aged 12 to 17 years, lifetime prevalence of illicit amphetamine use increased from 0.7% to 4.3% between 1990 and 2002. Users of ecstasy and other stimulants total over 1.8 million, approaching the prevalence of cocaine use.

Pharmacology and Pathophysiology

All physiologic and toxic effects caused by sympathomimetic agents occur through α- and β-adrenergic receptors. Which symptoms predominate clinically depends on which group or subgroup of receptors are activated (Table 11–1). Activation of the receptors can occur through different mechanisms:

1. Direct stimulation of the α- and β-adrenergic receptors
2. Indirect release of catecholamine from the presynaptic neuron
3. Prevention of presynaptic uptake of catecholamines
4. Prevention of catecholamines metabolism (e.g., monoamine oxidase [MAO] inhibitors)

Regardless of the mechanism of the toxicity, signs and symptoms are almost identical.

Table 11–1. Symptoms Associated with Common Sympathomimetics

Agent	Specific Clinical Features
Asthma medications	
Albuterol	
Terbutaline	
Theophylline	Wide pulse pressure (β-2 agonist); $\downarrow K^+$, $\uparrow$glucose; GI symptoms, seizures
Decongestants (pseudoephedrine)	
Dieting agents (ephedrine, caffeine)	
Metabolife 356	
Ripped Fuel	
Xenadrine RFA-1	
Illicit drugs	
Amphetamines	
Cocaine	
MDMA/ecstasy	Hyponatremia (altered mental status, seizures), hyperthermia
MAO inhibitors	
Isocarboxazide	Delayed presentation (up to 24 h)
Phenelzine	Severe toxicity
Selegiline	$\uparrow\uparrow\uparrow$ NE, DA, serotonin followed by catecholamine depletion
Tranylcypromine	Ping-pong gaze
Stimulants (dextroamphetamine, methylphenidate)	
Adderal	
Concerta	
Dexedrine	
Ritalin	
Thyroid hormones (T_3, T_4)	
Liothyronine (T_3)	Majority of exposures are benign
Synthroid (T_4)	T_3: symptoms within 24 h; T_4: symptoms within 1 w

Abbreviations: $\downarrow$, depressed; $\uparrow$, elevated; DA, dopamine; GI, gastrointestinal; MDMA, 3,4-methylenedioxy methamphetamine; NE, norphephrine; T_3, triiodothyronine; T_4, thyroxine.

Table 11–2. Clinical Findings Associated With the Sympathomimetic Syndrome

Vital Signs	Neurologic	Pupils	Skin	End-Organ Effects
Hypertension Hyperthermia Tachycardia Tachypnea	Agitation Psychosis (can progress to seizures and coma)	Mydriasis	Diaphoresis	CVA, MI, rhabdomyolysis, DIC

Abbreviations: CVA, cerebrovascular accident; DIC, disseminated intravascular coagulation; MI, myocardial infarction.

Clinical Presentation

The majority of patients develop symptoms within 2 hours of exposure (Table 11–2). Most of the life-threatening complications occur within first 6 hours. This does not apply to exposures to MAO inhibitors, which can have a late presentation and severe toxicity, or thyroid hormones, which can have a delayed presentation but rarely cause severe toxicity. The patient may become hyperthermic owing to increased muscle activity. Severe toxicity can be complicated by cardiovascular and neurologic manifestations. Extreme and prolonged elevation of blood pressure can produce headache, hypertensive encephalopathy, seizures, and intracranial bleeding. End-organ complications are somewhat dose related, and are rare in young children with small unintentional exposures. Adolescents, on the other hand, may be involved in high-risk exposures such as cocaine or MDMA.

Laboratory Studies

Sympathomimetics can cause leukocytosis and hyperglycemia. Rhabdomyolysis may occur due to severe agitation, with subsequent development of hyperkalemia, hyperphosphatemia, hypocalcemia, ventricular dysrhythmias, and acute renal failure.

Treatment

The majority of sympathomimetic exposures require no specific treatment other than supportive measures, including hydration and active cooling for hyperthermia. Agitation, tachycardia, and hypertension generally respond well to benzodiazepine administration.

Special Considerations

Amphetamines

MDMA is an amphetamine derivative with rather atypical complications. Its use can result in severe hypona-

tremia, associated with altered mental status and seizures. This occurs due to increased release of antidiuretic hormone, and excessive hydration, often during rave parties (see Chapter 54).

Cocaine Body Packing

Clinicians should also be aware that children and adolescents might be used as mules for smuggling of the cocaine. Rupture of a package in the intestines can cause local ischemia with perforation, as well as life-threatening systemic toxicity (See Chapter 57).

ANTICHOLINERGIC TOXIC SYNDROME

HIGH-YIELD FACTS

- The anticholinergic toxidrome presents with tachycardia, hyperthermia, dry/warm skin, hallucinations, urinary retention, and dilated pupils resulting in blurred vision.
- Neurologic manifestations range from sedation to irritability, agitation, seizures, and coma.
- Skin should be thoroughly examined, looking especially for scopolamine patches.
- An electrocardiograph (ECG) is necessary to look for the signs of cyclic antidepressant poisoning.
- Antihistamines are often sold as combination drugs with acetaminophen.
- Doxylamine can cause idiosyncratic rhabdomyolysis and a serum creatinine kinase (CPK) should be checked in suspected exposures.

• Physostigmine is relatively safe drug but should be used selectively for children with severe neurologic effects of anticholinergic poisoning and no signs of cyclic antidepressant poisoning.

Introduction and Epidemiology

The anticholinergic syndrome can result after exposure to a wide variety of prescription and over-the-counter medications, as well after abuse of hallucinogenic plants such as *Datura stramonium* or jimson weed. Antihistamines are a common cause of anticholinergic toxicity owing to their wide spread availability. Tricyclic antidepressants (TCAs) are another class of drugs with anticholinergic properties. However, these agents are potentially more dangerous due to their toxic effects on the myocardium.

Pharmacokinetics and Pathophysiology

Both anticholinergic and cholinergic toxidromes are mediated through acetylcholine, one of the major transmitters of the peripheral (PNS) and central nervous systems (CNS) (Table 11–3). Acetylcholine exerts its effects through both nicotinic and muscarinic receptors. Nicotinic receptors are located on postganglionic autonomic neurons (sympathetic and parasympathetic), at the neuromuscular junction, and in the CNS (mainly spinal cord). Muscarinic receptors reside at postganglionic parasympathetic nerve endings and postganglionic sympathetic nerves (sweat glands), and also in the CNS (brain).

The anticholinergic toxidrome, which can be referred to as the antimuscarinic toxidrome, is caused by agents that oppose or block the action of acetylcholine and cholinergic neurotransmission at muscarinic receptor sites. The majority of effects are on the heart, salivary and sweat glands, the gastrointestinal (GI) tract, and the genitourinary tract. Antagonism of the central cortical/subcortical muscarinic receptors cause CNS manifestations.

Clinical Presentation

The anticholinergic toxidrome is similar to the sympathomimetic toxidrome in its presentation. Agitation, hypertension, tachycardia, hyperthermia, and mydriasis are prominent findings. However, dry, flushed skin, urinary retention, and decreased bowel sounds are distinguishing

Table 11–3. Common Anticholinergics

Typical Agents Class	Representative
True anticholinergics	Atropine, glycopyrrolate, benzotropine, scopolamine (available in patches)
Antihistamines	Doxylamine, diphenhydramine
Antipsychotics	Chlorpromazine, thioridazine
Antispasmodics	Dicyclomine, hyoscyamine
Cyclic antidepressants	Amitriptyline, doxepine, imipramine
Incapacitating agents	3-Quinuclidinyl benzilate (BZ)
Mydriatics	Cyclopentolate, tropicamide
Plants	*Atropa belladonna, Datura stramonium*

features of anticholinergic poisoning, as opposed to the diaphoresis and increased bowel sounds that occur in sympathomimetic poisonings. The mnemonic listed in Table 11–4 helps clinicians to recognize some of the antimuscarinic effects. It is also important to include the following in the differential diagnosis of anticholinergic poisoning:

1. sympathomimetic drugs (skin is usually moist, rather than flushed, and hot)

2. alcohol withdrawal (more likely in tolerant adolescents with chronic abuse)

3. CNS infection (fever, stiff neck, septic appearance, focal CNS deficit)

4. hallucinogenic drugs (D-lysergic acid diethylamide [LSD], amphetamines, phencyclidine [PCP], and ketamine)

Laboratory Studies

A serum CPK should be checked in agitated, febrile children, as well as those with suspected doxylamine exposure owing to its intrinsic ability to cause rhabdomyolysis. Every patient with an unknown cause of anticholinergic poisoning should have an ECG to exclude TCA toxicity and to screen for possible cardiac dysrhythmias. It is important to note that young children normally have a right axis deviation. Thus, a screening ECG may not ade-

Table 11–4. Clinical Findings Associated With Anticholinergic Toxidrome

Vital Signs	Neurologic	Pupils	Skin/Mucous Membranes	GI	GU
Mnemonic: *"Red as a beet, dry as a bone, blind as a bat, mad as a hatter, and hot as a hare."*					
Hyperthermia, tachycardia, tachypnea	Agitation or sedation; can result in coma and seizures	Mydriasis	Dry, flushed skin; dry mucous membranes	Decreased bowel sounds	Urinary retention

Abbreviations: GI, gastrointestinal; GU, genitourinary.

quately exclude early TCA toxicity. Because many over-the-counter preparations containing antihistamines also contain acetaminophen, serum acetaminophen measurement is recommended.

Treatment

Physostigmine

Physostigmine is an antidote for pure anticholinergic toxicity. It is a carbamate that can reversibly inhibit cholinesterases. This process, which occurs in both PNS and CNS, inhibits metabolism of acetylcholine, and allow its accumulation, thereby overcoming antimuscarinic effects. Indications for use include the following:

1. Evidence of severe CNS and peripheral anticholinergic toxicity.
2. Normal QRS interval (<0.08 msec).
3. No history of seizure disorder.
4. Severe agitation, coma, or cardiovascular instability unresponsive to other treatments, such as benzodiazepine administration.
5. No history of cyclic antidepressant ingestion.

The dose of physostigmine for children is 0.02 mg/kg, infused slowly over 5 minutes, with maximum of 0.5 mg total. In older adolescents, depending on their size, the adult dose should be used at 1 mg IV slowly over 5 minutes. Lack of cholinergic symptoms or improvement of delirium and anticholinergic symptoms may reassure clinician in the diagnosis of anticholinergic poisoning. Additional doses may be required if clinical symptoms reoccur. The usual duration of action for physostigmine is 60 to 70 minutes (see Chapter 29).

CHOLINERGIC TOXIC SYNDROME

HIGH-YIELD FACTS

- Excess of acetylcholine results in the cholinergic toxidrome.
- The major causes of cholinergic syndrome in children are pesticides and insecticides.
- The typical presentation includes increased secretions from salivary, lacrimal and sweat glands, as well from the GI and respiratory tracts.
- Carbamates reversibly bind to acetylcholinesterase, whereas organophosphorous compounds bind irreversibly. Clinically, it is difficult to distinguish between the two entities.

Introduction and Epidemiology

The most common source of cholinergic exposure in children is ingestion or dermal exposure to pesticides. Other agents are listed in Table 11–5.

Pathophysiology

Acetylcholine is a major neurotransmitter that acts on nicotinic and muscarinic receptors. The nicotinic receptors are located predominantly in preganglionic autonomic nerve endings and at the neuromuscular junction. The muscarinic receptors are located at all parasympathetic and some sympathetic postganglionic nerve endings. In addition to peripheral locations, acetylcholine

Table 11–5. Common Cholinergic Agents

Acetylcholinesterase inhibitors
    Carbamate insecticides
    Neostigmine
    Organophosphorous compounds
        Warfare agents: sarin, soman, tabun, Vx
        Pesticides (e.g., malathion)
    Physostigmine
    Pyridostigmine
Nicotine alkaloids
    Coniine
    Lobeline
    Nicotine
Cholinomimetics
    Arechnol
    Bethanechol
    Carbachol
    Cevimeline
    Choline
    Metacholine
    Muscarine-containing mushrooms (*Boletus spp,*
        Clitocybe spp, Inocybe spp)

receptors can be found at some CNS synapses. The cholinergic toxidrome results from excessive stimulation of muscarinic acetylcholine receptors. It can occur either from increased production or decreased degradation of acetylcholine (e.g., inhibition of acetylcholinesterase).

Clinical Presentation

Depending on the severity of the exposure, patients present with altered mental status, diffuse muscle weakness, and excessive secretory activity (Table 11–6). The actual symptoms that predominate depend on whether muscarinic, nicotinic, or CNS receptors are stimulated. If muscarinic receptors are predominantly activated, the patient manifests increased parasympathetic activity, including bradycardia, diaphoresis, excessive lacrimation, increased bronchial secretions, and vomiting. Additional signs of muscarinic hyperactivity include urinary and fecal incontinence. Patients may also experience dimmed vision owing to pinpoint pupils.

The activation of nicotinic receptors manifests with the signs of increased sympathetic activity, including tachycardia, hypertension, and dilated pupils. Fasciculations and neuromuscular paralysis may result from overstimulation at the neuromuscular junction. The CNS effects can range from agitation, psychosis, and confusion to coma and seizures.

Laboratory Studies

Decreased activity of serum and erythrocyte acetylcholinesterase is diagnostic, but of no value in acute management. Levels should be sent prior administration of pralidoxime. Owing to increased secretions and possible metabolic abnormalities, exposed patients should have electrolytes, renal function, and serum glucose concentrations measured. It is important to assess the respiratory status of the patient and their ability to ventilate and oxygenate, with continuous pulse oximetry, arterial blood gases (if hypoxic), and a chest radiograph.

Treatment

Atropine

Atropine is the drug of choice, and should be given as soon as diagnosis is established. Its effect is on the muscarinic receptors, where it is a competitive antagonist, and is useful in the control of secretions. Sometimes the total dose re-

Table 11–6. Clinical Findings Associated With Cholinergic Toxidrome

Vital Signs	Neurologic	Pupils	Skin/Mucous Membranes	Lungs	GI Tract	GU Tract
Mnemonic: Sialorrhea, Lacrimation, Urination, Defecation, Gastrointestinal effects (emesis, diarrhea), Emesis (SLUDGE)						
Hypertension, hyperthermia, bradycardia, *or* tachycardia, tachypnea	Altered mental status (can progress to seizures)	Miosis	Diaphoresis, lacrimation, sialorrhea	Bronchorrhea, bronchospasm	Emesis, defecation	Polyuria

Abbreviations: GI, gastrointestinal; GU, genitourinary.

quired for control of secretion could be as high as 100 mg. Clinicians may be hesitant to administer large doses of atropine because of concerns of causing worsening tachycardia. In reality, as secretions are better controlled, and hypoxia improves, the heart rate frequently decreases.

Pralidoxime

Pralidoxime should be initiated in severe pesticide poisoning, together with atropine. It is a quaternary ammonium oxime that is capable or reactivating cholinesterase if applied early in the course of disease (see Chapter 51).

OPIOID TOXIC SYNDROME

HIGH-YIELD FACTS

- The typical opioid toxidrome includes decreased mental status, respiratory depression, and miosis.
- Patients who overdose on meperidine, pentazocine, and propoxyphene can have dilated pupils.
- Some opioids, such as meperidine and propoxyphene, can cause seizures.
- Removal of fentanyl patches is an important means of dermal decontamination.
- Naloxone can be given rapidly to the opioid-naïve child; caution should be exercised in opioid-dependent patients, in whom gradual administration of naloxone is recommended.

Introduction and Epidemiology

Opioids are commonly used analgesics and drugs of abuse. Because of their availability, young children are at risk for unintentional exposure. Some medicinal preparations such as fentanyl come in the form of a patch; a child may mistake it for a Band-Aid and apply it to the skin. Parents or caretakers who suffer from chronic pain syndromes may be taking very potent and long-acting opioids, including methadone and Oxycontin, to which children can be exposed.

Unfortunately, there is also evidence of a resurgence of heroin abuse among adolescents, as well as reports of young adolescents being used as body-packers for smuggling of large quantities of heroin across international borders (see Chapter 60).

Clinical Presentation

Classic opioid toxicity presents with the clinical triad of respiratory depression, depressed mental status, and miosis. The onset of the symptoms may range from minutes after intravenous (IV) exposure, to up to 2 to 4 hours after dermal application.

Special Considerations

Some heroin users combine heroin with cocaine a combination commonly referred to as *speedball*. Their clinical presentation may initially be dominated by the sympathomimetic effects of cocaine. Heroin can also be adulterated with scopolamine, because of its hallucinogenic properties. These patients may present with an anticholinergic toxidrome.

Miosis

Miosis is one of the key features of the opioid toxidrome. It is important to remember, however, that certain opioids—including meperidine, pentazocine, dephenoxylate/atropine, and propoxyphene—can be associated with normal or dilated pupils. The pupils may be also dilated in the patient who had prolonged respiratory depression and suffered from a CNS hypoxic insult.

Skin

It is important to perform a thorough skin examination in every patient, looking for transdermal fentanyl patches and for signs of IV or subcutaneous administration of heroin. A patch, if found, should be removed. The skin should then be cleaned with soap and water to reduce absorption.

Laboratory Studies

Toxicology screens are not helpful in the initial management of the opioid overdosed child. Serum assays may only detect opioid compounds for up to 6 hours. Urinary qualitative screens may be useful in ruling out an opioid exposure in a child presenting with altered mental status. These are typically positive for up to 48 to 72 hours postingestion. Most urinary screens lack sensitivity, and may not detect many of the synthetic opioids including methadone, hydrocodone, and propoxyphene. In addition, routine screens may not detect potent opioids such as fentanyl. Along with other routine baseline laboratory tests, serum acetaminophen and salicylate levels should be measured, because many opioid compounds like hydrocodone and codeine also contain these common analgesics.

Treatment

Naloxone

Naloxone is a competitive opioid antagonist capable of reversing opioid toxicity. It acts on μ, κ, and δ receptors, and should be administered IV to achieve adequate ventilation and restoration of protective airway reflexes. It is important to remember the children typically overdose on adult doses of opioids, and may require adult doses of naloxone. More cautious dosing is required when treating young patients with heroin/methadone dependence, or a child who was receiving opioids for a prolonged period owing to chronic pain. Such patients may experience withdrawal symptoms following naloxone administration, usually consisting of agitation and vomiting.

Naloxone has the greatest affinity toward μ receptors, and the treatment of opioids with greater affinity toward κ and δ receptors (e.g., pentazocine, propoxyphene) may require administration of higher-than-usual doses of naloxone. If 10 mg of naloxone is administered without response, it is unlikely that the patient's respiratory and CNS depression is due to the effect of an opioid.

SEDATIVE-HYPNOTIC TOXIC SYNDROME

HIGH-YIELD FACTS

- The sedative-hypnotic toxidrome usually presents as obtundation or coma, with normal vital signs
- The majority of patients with severe sedative-hypnotic overdose respond to supportive treatment alone.
- γ-Hydroxy butyrate (GHB) toxicity is characterized by respiratory failure and CNS depression that resolves rapidly (2 to 3 hours after exposure).
- Flumazenil is a competitive benzodiazepine antagonist. It is indicated only in benzodiazepine-naïve persons presenting with a pure benzodiazepine overdose, whether accidental, intentional, or iatrogenic.

Introduction and Epidemiology

Sedative-hypnotics are readily available, both as pharmaceutical and nonpharmaceutical agents (Table 11–7). Benzodiazepines and barbiturates are commonly used during diagnostic procedures and conscious sedation. Alcohol is one of the most commonly used nonpharmaceutical sedative-hypnotics, and naïve children respond with significant CNS depression to very low level exposures. GHB and its precursor γ-butyrolactone (GBL) are increasingly used by teenagers at rave parties, and unfortunately as chemical submission (date rape) drugs.

Pharmacology and Pathophysiology

All sedative-hypnotics cause CNS depression, and the majority of them act by increasing the effect of the major inhibitory transmitter, δ-amino butyric acid (GABA). The majority of sedative-hypnotics are rapidly absorbed from the GI tract. These highly lipophilic agents rapidly penetrate the blood–brain barrier and cause prompt CNS and respiratory depression. Some agents, including diazepam, are metabolized to an active intermediate that can prolong their duration of effect.

Clinical Presentation

Because of their wide availability, exposures to sedative-hypnotics are common. There are predominantly three at-risk populations in pediatric patients. The first is the young child with an unintentional exposure. The second is composed of children undergoing a diagnostic or interventional procedures in the hospital setting, and the third consists of adolescents with either accidental or intentional exposure.

Typically, a patient presents with a depressed mental status and relatively normal vital signs. Mild bradycardia, hypoventilation, hypotension, and hypothermia can occur

Table 11–7. Common Sedative Hypnotics Agents

Pharmaceutical	Nonpharmaceutical
Benzodiazepines	Ethanol
Barbiturates	γ-Hydroxy butyrate (GHB)
Carisoprodol	γ-Butyrolactone (GBL)
Chloral hydrate	
Etomidate	
Propofol	
Zolpidem	
Zaleplon	

owing to suppressed CNS stimulation. Chloral hydrate may be associated with nausea, vomiting, abdominal pain, and cardiac dysrhythmias. Some agents, such as GHB, typically produce significant respiratory depression, whereas in benzodiazepines respiratory effort is preserved.

Exposure to multiple agents is more lethal than exposure to the single agents, because of their synergistic effect on GABA receptors. This is especially true when ethanol is used in combination with sedatives. The majority of deaths and complications occur from respiratory depression.

Laboratory and Diagnostic Testing

Many benzodiazepines are not detected in the standard urinary tests, and serum drug levels have not been valuable during the acute treatment phase. However, a positive urine test may have significant medicolegal implications, especially if child neglect or sexual assault is suspected. A standard urine test will not be able to detect flunitrazepam or GHB, so urine should be collected, stored, and sent to a specialized laboratory with the appropriate chain of custody. Chloral hydrate is radiopaque and abdominal radiographs may be helpful if obtained in the acute setting after a recent ingestion.

Treatment

Flumazenil

Flumazenil is a competitive benzodiazepine antagonist. It is indicated only in benzodiazepine naïve persons presenting with a pure benzodiazepine overdose, whether accidental, intentional, or iatrogenic. Flumazenil should not be used in patients with mixed overdose, because seizures and cardiac dysrhythmias may occur. Flumazenil can also be dangerous in patients who are chronically using benzodiazepines, because they can experience severe withdrawal symptoms, including seizures (see Chapter 39).

SUMMARY

The recognition of toxic syndromes is a useful tool for the diagnosis and treatment of poisoned patients. Clinicians should be familiar with these typical signs and symptoms, as well as with some variability as that might be associated with specific toxins. It is important to be aware that children do not always respond in the same manner as adults, and that pediatric toxidromes may not always present with classic clinical features.

SUGGESTED READINGS

Abbruzzi G, Stork C: Pediatric toxicologic concerns. *Emerg Med Clin North Am* 20:223–247, 2002.

Ajaelo I, Koenig K, Snoey E: Severe hyponatremia and inappropriate antidiuretic hormone secretion following ecstasy use. *Acad Emerg Med* 5:839–840, 1998.

American Academy of Pediatrics Committee on Drugs and Committee on Environmental Health: Use of chloral hydrate for sedation in children. *Pediatrics* 92:471–473, 1993.

Amitai Y, Degani Y: Treatment of phenobarbital poisoning with multiple dose activated charcoal in an infant. *J Emerg Med* 8:449–450, 1990.

Anon: *Overview of Findings From the 2002 National Survey on Drug Use and Health* (DHHS Publication No. SMA 03-3774). Rockville, MD: SAMHSA Office of Applied Studies, 2003.

Ashbourne J, Olson K, Khayam-Bashi H: Value of rapid screening for acetaminophen in all patients with intentional drug overdose. *Ann Emerg Med* 18:1035–1038, 1996.

Bamshad M, Wasserman: Pediatric clonidine intoxications. *Vet Hum Toxicol* 32:220–223, 1990.

Berkovitch M, Matsui D, Fogelman R, et al: Assessment of the terminal 40-millisecond QRS vector in children with a history of tricyclic antidepressant ingestion. Pediatr Emerg Care 11:75–77, 1995.

Erich J, Shih R, O'Connor R: Ping-pong gaze in severe monoamine oxidase inhibitor toxicity. *J Emerg Med* 13;653–635, 1995.

Hoffman RJ, Nelson L: Rational use of toxicology testing in children. *Curr Opin Pediatr* 13;183–188, 2001.

Litovitz TL, Klein-Schwartz W, Rodgers GC, et al: 2001 Annual Report of poison control centers toxic exposure surveillance system. *Am J Emerg Med* 20:391–452, 2002.

Malis DJ, Burton DM: Safe pediatric outpatient sedation: The chloral hydrate debate revisited. *Otolaryngol Head Neck Surg* 116: 535–537, 1997.

Schexnayder S, James L, Kearns G, et al: The pharmacokinetics of continuous infusion pralidoxime in children with organophosphate poisoning. *J Toxicol Clin Toxicol* 36:549–555, 1998.

Shannon M, Amitai Y, Lovejoy FH Jr: Muliple-dose activated charcoal for theophylline poisoning in young infants. *Pediatrics* 80:368–370, 1987.

Stegmayr BG: On-line hemodialysis and hemoperfusion in a girl intoxicated by theophylline. *Acta Med Scand* 223:565–567, 1988.

Suner S, Szlatenyi, Wang R: Pediatric gamma hydroxybutyrate intoxication. *Acad Emerg Med* 4:1041–1045, 1997.

Wiley J, Wiley C, Torrey , et al: Clonidine poisoning in young children. *J Pediatr* 116:654–658, 1990.

Wolfe L, Cavavati E, Rollins D, et al: Terminal 40-ms frontal plane QRS axis as a marker for tricyclic antidepressants overdose. *Ann Emerg Med* 18:348–351, 1989.

12

Airway Management

Rebekah Mannix
Michele Burns Ewald

Airway management is among the most crucial issues confronting those caring for pediatric patients suffering from acute toxicologic exposures. Although many fundamentals of airway management are no different than those for any other patient requiring endotracheal intubation, the poisoned patient may present unique clinical situations. The poison exposure may cause increased secretions, physical distortion of the airway, or rapid loss of airway reflexes, all of which must be considered in assessing the best approach to management. The pediatric airway warrants even further special consideration in the case of toxic exposures.

EPIDEMIOLOGY

In 2002, children under 20 years of age accounted for 66% of all poison exposure cases reported to the American Association of Poison Control Centers, but only 9.1% of fatalities. Oral ingestions were responsible for most of these fatalities; inhalational agents accounted for the next largest number of deaths. Four common toxins that lead to respiratory failure in the pediatric age group are carbon monoxide, hydrocarbons, opioids, and caustics.

DEVELOPMENTAL CONSIDERATIONS: THE PEDIATRIC AIRWAY

Pediatric upper airways are of small diameter and easily obstructed by a foreign body or edema. The tongue occupies a large proportion of the upper airway, an anatomic feature that necessitates proper airway positioning. Whereas children who are awake and alert should be permitted to remain in a position of comfort, unconscious children should be positioned using a head tilt or jaw thrust. Infants in particular are obligate nose breathers, and any nasal obstruction may seriously impair effective respirations. The narrowest part of the pediatric airway is subglottic.

Compared to adults, children are at higher risk for aspiration because the larynx is more cephalad and anterior. Toxins such as hydrocarbons can cause significant alveolar toxicity in the pediatric population owing to this propensity for aspiration.

The chest wall of the infant and child is much more compliant than that of the adult. Accessory chest muscles are underdeveloped, and the diaphragm is the primary muscle of respiration. Until about 3 years of age, alveolar space is very limited, and the predominant response to respiratory insult is tachypnea. Limited metabolic reserve renders infants and young children relatively vulnerable to muscle fatigue and, therefore, respiratory failure. The thin, soft, and compliant chest wall of the child facilitates the auscultation of breath sounds. Children may not demonstrate the classic metabolic changes seen in adults. For example, children who have ingested salicylates may lack the initial hyperpnea and resultant respiratory alkalosis typically observed in adults, and metabolic acidosis is characteristically observed earlier in the clinical course. Children have metabolic rates greater than those of adults, and have lesser respiratory reserves. These differences in part explain the increased relative dose that children receive of inhaled toxins (e.g., carbon monoxide), and leave them more susceptible to hypoxia and respiratory failure.

Some of the most important anatomic differences between the pediatric airway and the adult airway are summarized in Table 12–1.

AIRWAY MANAGEMENT

The initial evaluation of any ill child includes an assessment of the airway, breathing, and circulation. The poi-

soned child who is at risk for loss of airway patency or protective reflexes requires immediate assistance, and may require basic airway interventions such as suction, 100% oxygen, cardiorespiratory monitoring, with pulse oximetry, airway positioning, oral/nasal airway placement, and gastric decompression via orogastric or nasogastric tube. If these interventions do not improve the situation rapidly, more advanced techniques, including bag-mask ventilation and endotracheal intubation, should be considered. Personnel skilled in pediatric airway management, preferably those trained in pediatric emergency medicine or anesthesiology, should be present or available on-call to ensure a successful outcome.

Proper bag-mask ventilation should include the basic interventions described, as well as a mask fitted to form a tight seal around the child's nose and mouth. If bag-mask ventilation is unsuccessful and oxygen saturation does not improve, rapid-sequence intubation (RSI) of the trachea should be considered. This technique is summarized in Table 12–2. RSI may be contraindicated in the child who has ingested caustics that damage the airway.

Several caveats should be noted with regard to the paralytic agents. The depolarizing agent succinylcholine is not advisable in a patient in the midst of status epilepticus in whom excess potassium release is a risk. It is contraindicated in patients with hyperkalemia, muscular dystrophy, massive trauma, and eye injury. In children,

Table 12–1. The Pediatric Airway

Anatomic Structure	Comparison to Adult Structure	Implication
Adenoidal tissue	Larger	Nasopharyngeal airways may be more difficult to pass in infants <1 y
Tongue	Relatively larger	Tongue is most common cause of airway obstruction in children → necessitates better head positioning or judicious use of airway adjuncts
Epiglottis	Softer, more flexible, U-shaped	Straight laryngoscope blade may facilitate endotracheal procedures
Larynx	Position more cephalad and anterior	More difficult to visualize vocal cords
Cricoid ring	Narrowest portion of the airway	Allows use of uncuffed tubes up to internal diameter of 6 mm (for children up to about 8 y)
Trachea	Narrower diameter; shorter distance between tracheal rings; shorter length	Tracheostomy difficult Right mainstem intubation common
Airways	Narrower diameters	Greater airway resistance (R proportional to $1/r^4$) R = airway resistance r = airway diameter

Table 12–2. Rapid-Sequence Intubation

Step	Notes
Preparation	Suction
	Oxygen
	IV access
	Monitors
	Appropriate personnel available
Premedication (vagolytic)	Atropine (0.02 mg/kg, minimum 0.1 mg; maximum 1.0 mg)
Cricoid pressure	
Sedation (choose one)	Midazolam (0.05–0.10 mg/kg)
	Thiopental (4–6 mg/kg)
	Ketamine (1–2 mg/kg)
	Etomidate (0.3 mg/kg)
Paralysis (choose one; see cautions in text)	Succinylcholine (1 mg/kg IV; 2 mg/kg IM; consider premedication with midazolam)
	Rocuronium (0.6–1.2 mg/kg)
	Vecuronium or pancuronium (0.1–0.2 mg/kg)
Intubation	ETT internal diameter (mm) = (age + 16)/4
	Full-term infant: approximately 3.5 mm
	Use uncuffed tube if <6 mm (subglottic narrowing)
	Depth of insertion (cm) = 3× inner diameter (mm)
Check ETT placement	Auscultation
	In-line CO_2 detection
Release cricoid pressure	
Confirm ETT position	Chest radiograph

Abbreviations: ETT, endotracheal tube; IM, intramuscular; IV, intravenous.

succinylcholine can induce excessive vagal tone. In addition, succinylcholine may cause prolonged neuromuscular blockade in patients whose cholinesterase concentrations are decreased because of genetic variants or exposure to cocaine or organophosphates. The sedative-hypnotics such as midazolam and thiopental should be used with caution in the patient who is hypotensive and at risk for cardiovascular collapse.

The choice of ventilator settings for the intubated patient may vary according to physiologic disturbances associated with the toxin in question.

THE MOST COMMON AND DANGEROUS AIRWAY TOXINS

The relatively large tongue of the child may obstruct the pharynx under certain circumstances. For example, in-gestion of angiotensin-converting enzyme inhibitors or angiotensin II–receptor antagonists may cause angio-edema of the tongue and glottis. Plants that contain insoluble calcium oxalate crystals (*Dieffenbachia, Philodendron*) can also produce acute swelling of mucous membranes to obstruct airways.

Caustic and thermal injuries to the upper airway, which may lead to complete airway obstruction, must be managed aggressively to prevent the need for emergency endotracheal intubation. Warning signs that respiratory compromise is imminent include (1) patient sitting up, leaning forward with the mandible protruded; (2) an inability to swallow; (3) stridor; and (4) hot potato voice. Patients with a known caustic injury and any of the above signs should undergo endotracheal intubation using direct visualization, because perforation is associated with blind intubation attempts. Chemical paralysis to facilitate intubation in these situations should be ap-

Table 12–3. Respiratory Toxins

Mechanism of Respiratory Compromise	Examples
Airway obstruction	Caustics, plants, angiotensin-converting enzyme inhibitors (angioedema)
Increased secretions/bronchorrhea	Acetylcholinesterase inhibitors (organophosphates, nerve gases), Alzheimer medications (rivastigmine, galantamine)
Loss of protective airway reflexes	CNS depression (benzodiazepines, barbiturates, ethanol), cerebrovascular accident (sympathomimetics) seizures (INH, theophylline)
Frank respiratory failure	Pneumonitis (hydrocarbons, inhalationals)
	Paralysis (botulism, tetanus)
Noncardiogenic pulmonary edema or acute lung injury	Opioids, aspirin

Abbreviations: CNS, central nervous system; INH, isoniazid.

proached cautiously, and only if a high degree of certainty exists that the procedure will be successful.

In contrast to caustic ingestions, there are some situations for which paralysis may ameliorate symptomatology. Paralysis and intubation may be considered a useful adjuvant in the patient with seizures refractory to pharmacologic management, such as with isoniazid or theophylline toxicity. Another acceptable scenario would be a patient whose condition and hemodynamic stability are rapidly deteriorating after a severe cyclic antidepressant overdose.

Special considerations may arise in the patient who is paralyzed, intubated, and ventilated. The salicylate-poisoned patient, for example, must be allowed a respiratory rate adequate to compensate for metabolic acidosis and to maintain an optimal serum pH. Toxins that may cause hyperkalemia (see succinylcholine, above) include cardiac glycosides, such as digoxin, and sympathomimetic agents such as phencyclidine, cocaine, and amphetamines secondary to hyperthermia, rhabdomyolysis, and myoglobinuria. The mechanisms of respiratory toxicity of some of the most common and most dangerous poisonings are highlighted in Table 12–3.

CONCLUSION

Although the basic principles of airway management apply to the pediatric population, effective management of toxic exposures in this population requires special knowledge of the epidemiologic, anatomic, and physiologic differences between children and adults.

SUGGESTED READINGS

Abbruzzi G, Stork CM: Pediatric toxicologic concerns. *Emerg Med Clin North Am* 20:223–247, 2002.

Bryant S, Singer J: Management of toxic exposure in children. *Emerg Med Clin North Am* 21:101–119, 2003.

Cerf C, Mesguish M, Gabriel I, et al: Screening patients with prolonged neuromuscular blockade after succinylcholine and mivacurium. *Anesth Analg* 94:421–426, 2002.

Krauss BS, Shannon M, Damian FJ, et al: *Guidelines for Pediatric Sedation.* Dallas: American College of Emergency Medicine; 1995.

Leikin JB, Paloucek FP, eds: *Poisoning & Toxicology Handbook.* 3d ed. Hudson, OH: Lexi-Comp; 2002.

Murphy MF, Schneider R: Airway management in the poisoned patient. In: Ford MD, Delaney KA, Ling L, et al eds: *Clinical Toxicology.* Philadelphia: Saunders; 2001:5–11.

Gunn VL, Nechyba C, eds: *The Harriet Lane Handbook.* 16th ed. St. Louis: Mosby; 2002.

Olson KR, Anderson IB, Benowitz NL, et al, eds: *Poisoning & Drug Overdose.* 4th ed. New York: Lange Medical Books/McGraw-Hill; 1999.

Watson WA, Litovitz TL, Rodgers GC, et al: 2002 annual report of the American Association of Poison Control Centers Toxic Exposure Surveillance System. *Am J Emerg Med* 21:353–421, 2003.

13

Advanced Pediatric Life Support

Gary R. Strange

HIGH-YIELD FACTS

- Pediatric cardiac arrest is usually the result of deterioration of an underlying medical condition rather than from a primary cardiac event, as is the case in adults. This is one factor that leads to poorer prognosis in pediatric cardiac arrest.

- The etiology of cardiac arrest in children is more diverse than in adults. In infants and young children, the most common cause of cardiac arrest is respiratory failure, which may be a result of many common medical conditions encountered in the pediatric population.

- Sudden infant death syndrome is the most common cause of cardiac arrest in infants under the age of 12 months, with a peak incidence at 5 months.

- Additional causes of respiratory failure leading to cardiac arrest are bronchiolitis, asthma and upper airway obstruction.

- In children over the age of 1 year, trauma continues to be the most common cause of cardiopulmonary arrest and death.

- Toxic ingestion and drug overdose are less common causes, but become more prevalent among adolescents.

- After establishing airway control, a route for administering fluids and medications is essential for advanced life support. A peripheral intravenous line is preferred but

may be difficult to establish in an infant or child in circulatory collapse. If necessary, most medications can be administered via an endotracheal tube or interosseous route.

- Whenever ventricular fibrillation or pulseless ventricular tachycardia is diagnosed, immediate defibrillation is indicated and may be life saving.

- Cardiotoxins in the pediatric arrest patient include carbon monoxide, cyanide, cocaine, cyclic antidepressants, calcium channel antagonists, β-blockers, theophylline, and digitalis.

- Case reports have documented pediatric survival after prolonged periods of resuscitation when the cardiac or respiratory arrest was secondary to a drug overdose, particularly when the child had no serious underlying chronic disease state.

Cardiopulmonary resuscitation is a technique for providing artificial support of ventilation and circulation during periods when spontaneous cardiopulmonary function is interrupted. The goal is restoration of spontaneous cardiac activity and respirations with the preservation of intact neurologic function. In addition to cardiopulmonary resuscitation, advanced pediatric life support includes advanced airway techniques, pharmacologic, and electrical interventions.

Pediatric cardiac arrest is usually the result of deterioration of an underlying medical condition rather than from a primary cardiac event, as is the case in adults.

This is one factor that leads to poorer prognosis in pediatric cardiac arrest.

EPIDEMIOLOGY

Approximately 16,000 children die unexpectedly in the United States each year. The annual incidence of cardiopulmonary arrest is reported to be 20 in 100,000. About 60% of these arrests occur in the home. Approximately half of pediatric arrests occur in infants under 1 year of age.

The etiology of cardiac arrest in children is more diverse than in adults. In infants and young children, the most common cause of cardiac arrest is respiratory failure, which may be a result of many common medical conditions encountered in the pediatric population. Sudden infant death syndrome is the most common cause of cardiac arrest in infants under the age of 12 months, with a peak incidence at 5 months. Additional causes of respiratory failure leading to cardiac arrest are bronchiolitis, asthma, and upper airway obstruction. In children over the age of 1 year, trauma continues to be the most common cause of cardiopulmonary arrest and death. Toxic ingestion and drug overdose are less common causes, but become more prevalent among adolescents. Other common causes are submersion injury, cardiac disease, and sepsis.

PROGNOSIS

Survival rates for cardiopulmonary arrest in children are much lower than in adults. The overall survival-to-discharge rate for pediatric cardiopulmonary arrest is reported to be 13%. For arrests occurring outside hospitals, the rate is lower (8%). For the subgroup who are pulseless on arrival in the ED, the survival rate is only about 2% and severe neurologic sequelae are virtually universal. For patients with respiratory arrest only, the survival rate is much higher, at approximately 75%, and these patients almost all survive without significant neurologic impairment.

Survival rate appears to be poorer for infants younger than 1 year. Submersion injuries have significantly better prognosis than cardiopulmonary arrest owing to other causes, with reported survival-to-discharge rate of 26%. Bradyasystolic arrest is associated with poor survival rate, approximately 5%. Whereas only about 10% of pediatric arrests are associated with ventricular fibrillation or ventricular tachycardia, these have a much better prognosis, with survival rates of about 30%.

As with adults, bystander cardiopulmonary resuscitation appears to be associated with significant improvement in outcomes (20% survival). Successful prehospital endotracheal intubation also appears to be correlated with increased return of spontaneous circulation, but data are insufficient to confirm correlation with improved survival-to-discharge rate.

BASIC LIFE SUPPORT

The initial approach to an unresponsive child is to open the airway and begin ventilatory support. Simply opening the airway may allow for resumption of spontaneous breathing. The head-tilt, chin-lift maneuver (Figure 13–1A) is used unless there is concern for the possibility of cervical spine injury. In that case, the jaw-thrust maneuver (Figure 13–1B) is used.

If no spontaneous respirations are noted after opening the airway, ventilatory support is initiated. This may be accomplished by mouth-to-mouth breathing in the older child and by mouth-to-nose or mouth–to–nose-and-mouth breathing in an infant. If available, a mouth-to-mask technique may be used. When using the mouth-to-mouth technique, the nose is sealed by pinching it between the thumb and forefinger. Two slow breaths are provided with enough volume to cause the chest to rise. If there is no obstruction to air flow, ventilations are continued at a rate of 20 per minute. If there is obstruction to airflow af-

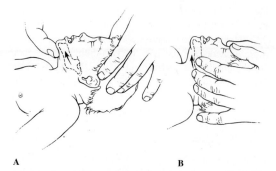

A **B**

Fig. 13–1. A. The head-tilt chin-lift maneuver. To open the airway, place one hand on the patient's forehead and tilt the head back into a neutral or slightly extended position. Use the index finger of the other hand to lift the patient's mandible upward and outward. **B.** The jaw-thrust maneuver. To open the airway wile maintaining cervical spine stabilization, place two or three fingers under each side of the lower jaw angle and lift the jaw upward and outward. Maintain the neck in a neutral position manually to prevent craniocervical motion.

ter repeated attempts to open the airway, a foreign body should be suspected (see below). For rescue units and in health care settings, ventilation is usually provided by the bag-valve-mask (BVM) technique. BVM ventilatory support is an effective method of ventilation, when performed correctly, and recent evidence indicates that, at least in systems with short transport times, BVM may be superior to endotracheal intubation for field airway management. The proper technique should be emphasized in basic life support training for health care providers. Regardless of the technique used, high-flow oxygen should be used to increase the partial pressure of oxygen in the inspired air whenever it is available.

After opening the airway and establishing ventilation, assess for the presence of a pulse. In infants the best location for palpating a pulse is over the brachial or femoral arteries. In children, a carotid pulse is usually palpable if there is spontaneous circulation. If no pulse is detected, initiate chest compressions at a rate of 100 per minute regardless of age. After every fifth compression, pause for a ventilation before continuing. After 20 cycles, pause and reassess for spontaneous pulses and respirations. If none, continue chest compressions and ventilations, checking for spontaneous pulses and respirations every few minutes.

Chest compressions are provided by placing the infant or child on a firm surface in the supine position and providing compression to the lower half of the sternum with enough pressure to compress the chest one-third to one-half of the anterior-posterior diameter of the chest or about 0.5 to 1.0 inch in the infant and 1.0 to 1.5 inches in the child. In infants, two fingers may be used, placed one finger width below the intermammary line (Figure 13–2A). However, for health care providers when two or more rescuers are present, the two-thumb, chest encircling technique is preferred (Fig. 13–2B). For children ages 1 to 8 years, the heel of the hand is placed two finger widths above the xiphoid process (Fig. 13–2C). Avoid compressing the xiphoid process because this may result in laceration to the liver, spleen, or stomach.

A major difference in the provision of basic life support for the child versus the adult is the timing for calling emergency medical services. In the child, this notification is delayed until rescue breathing is initiated. This variation is used because of the high rate of respiratory problems causing arrest in children and the high rate of survival with respiratory support alone in such cases.

A major advance in the area of basic life support over the past several years has been the use of automatic external defibrillators (AEDs). These devices have conclusively been shown to be safe and effective in the resuscitation

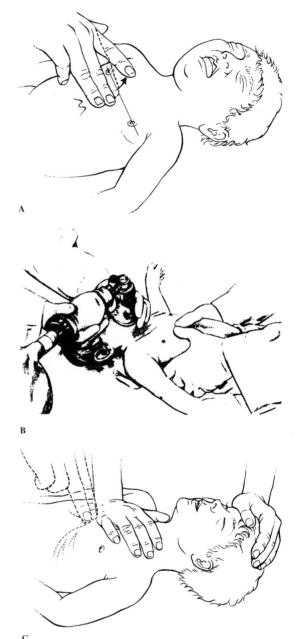

A

B

C

Fig. 13–2. A. Proper finger position for chest compressions in infants less than 1 year of age: use two fingers to perform compression one finger width below the intermammary line. **B.** Proper technique for two-thumb encircling hands technique over lower third of sternum. **C.** Proper finger position for chest compression in children from 1 to 8 years of age: use the heel of one hand to perform compressions two finger widths above xiphoid.

of adults, even when used by the lay public with minimal training. Although ventricular fibrillation and ventricular tachycardia are less common among children than adults, they do occur in about 10% of arrests. Standard AEDs can be used in children over 8 years of age or those weighing more than 55 pounds. There have been concerns about the ability of the devices to differentiate shockable from nonshockable rhythms in children and about the electrical energy delivered relative to the small body weight of the child. A pediatric AED that delivers approximately 50 J, compared to 150 to 360 J for the standard AED, has been developed but as yet had not been endorsed by the American Heart Association for use in children under the age of 8.

FOREIGN BODY ASPIRATION

When an infant or child cannot be ventilated after proper use of airway opening techniques, obstruction owing to infection of the upper airway or aspiration of a foreign body is usually the cause. Infants and small children are likely to put all sorts of objects in their mouths, including medications, and are therefore prone to aspiration. Sudden onset of dyspnea in a previously well child, associated with coughing, gagging, or stridor, is highly suggestive of a foreign body partially occluding the airway. As long as the child is coughing or able to vocalize, intervention is contraindicated for fear of converting a partial obstruction into a complete one. However, if the cough becomes weak, there is severe respiratory distress, or the child begins to lose consciousness, immediate intervention is essential.

For those less than 1 year of age, place the infant face down over the forearm of the rescuer (which can be rested on the ipsilateral thigh) with the infant's head lower than the trunk. Deliver five back blows between the scapulae with the heel of the hand. If unsuccessful, turn the infant and deliver five chest thrusts over the midsternum. Remove the foreign body if it can be visualized, but do not use blind finger sweeps. Ventilation is again attempted and if still not effective, the sequence is repeated.

For those over 1 year of age who are still conscious, the Heimlich maneuver is used. Five subdiaphragmatic thrusts are used, with the rescuer positioned behind the victim, arms encircling with one fist in the subxiphoid area and the other hand over the closed fist. If the child in unconscious, she or he is place in the supine position on a flat surface. The rescuer positions him- or herself a-straddle the child and uses the heel of one hand positioned above the umbilicus and below the xiphoid process, with the other hand overlaid, to provide five quick upward thrusts. If ineffective, the sequence is repeated.

Once advanced airway equipment is available, the airway can be visualized with a laryngoscope and the foreign body may be removed with the aid of Magill forceps. Bronchoscopy may be required for removal of subglottic foreign bodies.

ADVANCED AIRWAY TECHNIQUES

Endotracheal intubation is used to secure the airway and provide ventilation in the vast majority of infants and children requiring cardiopulmonary resuscitation. This procedure and adjuncts related to its use are discussed in Chapter 12.

VASCULAR ACCESS

A route for administering fluids and medications is essential for advanced life support. A peripheral intravenous (IV) line is preferred, but may be difficult to establish in an infant or child in circulatory collapse. Fortunately, most medications can be delivered via the endotracheal tube while other access is being established. If a peripheral line cannot be established immediately, alternative access should be established either by inserting a central line or an intraosseous (IO) catheter.

If central venous catheterization is chosen, the preferred site in infants and small children is the femoral vein because it is large, has a predictable anatomic location, and can be accessed without interfering with other resuscitative efforts. The tip of the femoral venous catheter should be advanced to a point above the diaphragm to provide rapid delivery of resuscitative medications. In the setting of trauma, where fluid resuscitation is needed, a short femoral catheter is preferred, because the long catheter produces significant resistance to fluid infusion.

Intraosseous catheters are relatively easy to place and provide a reliable route for delivery of resuscitative medications and fluid when a peripheral line is not available. It is now recognized that IO catheters can be inserted and used in children of any age. The preferred site of insertion is the proximal tibia.

FLUID RESUSCITATION

A common cause of arrest in children is hypovolemic shock, which may be due either to severe dehydration or to acute blood loss. In either case, administration of isotonic crystalloid solutions, such as Ringer's lactate or normal saline, is an essential part of the initial resuscitative effort. A fluid bolus of 10 to 20 mL/kg may be used as a part of the resuscitation of any arrest, even when the etiology is unknown, in an effort to ensure adequate circulating volume.

PHARMACOLOGIC THERAPY

Epinephrine

Epinephrine, with both β- and α-adrenergic effects, is a primary resuscitative drug in all cases of pediatric cardiac arrest, regardless of the underlying cardiac rhythm (Figure 13–3). The principle effect that makes epinephrine useful in the arrest situation is the production of vasoconstriction, which elevates the blood pressure and coronary perfusion pressure. For bradyasystolic arrests, which constitute the majority of pediatric arrests, epinephrine is the first intervention after attention to airway and breathing.

The recommended dose is 0.01 mg/kg (0.1 mL/kg of the 1:10,000 solution) IV or IO. If used by the endotracheal tube, the recommended dose is 0.1 mg/kg (0.1 mL/kg of the 1:1000 solution). The endotracheal dose should be delivered beyond the tip of the endotracheal tube through a suction catheter and followed by a 3 to 5 mL saline flush. In an arrest situation, these doses are repeated every 3 to 5 minutes.

The use of higher doses of epinephrine has been proposed to provide improved survival, but the evidence is inconclusive. Subsequent IV or IO doses of epinephrine may be increased to 0.1 mg/kg (0.1 mL/kg of the 1:1000 solution). Note that the volume of the epinephrine dose is the same regardless of whether standard or high doses are being used; the difference is the concentration of the solution.

An epinephrine infusion at a rate of 0.1 to 1.0 μg/kg/min may be used in the presence of a perfusing rhythm but inadequate blood pressure.

Atropine

Atropine is a parasympatholytic agent that accelerates supraventricular pacemakers and enhances atrioventricular (AV) nodal conduction. It is a second-line drug for the treatment of persistent bradycardia unresponsive to ventilation, oxygenation, and epinephrine therapy. It is most frequently used to prevent or treat vagally mediated bradycardia associated with intubation. It may also be ef-

fective for some AV blocks, but defects of the conduction system are rare in children.

The recommended dose of atropine is 0.02 mg/kg IV or IO. The minimum dose is 0.1 mg; smaller doses may produce paradoxical bradycardia. The dose can be repeated at 5-minute intervals until a maximum dose of 1 mg in a child and 2 mg in an adolescent is reached. For endotracheal administration, the dose should be increased by 2 to 3 times and followed by 3 to 5 mL of saline. In cases of organophosphate or nerve agent poisoning, much higher doses of atropine may be required to counteract the acute cholinergic effects of these agents.

Lidocaine

Lidocaine suppresses ventricular dysrhythmias primarily by decreasing automaticity. It is indicated for persistent ventricular tachycardia and ventricular fibrillation unresponsive to defibrillation and epinephrine therapy. These rhythms are found in only about 10% of pediatric cardiac arrests. They are usually secondary to metabolic abnormalities, drug intoxications, myocarditis, or congenital heart disease. Lidocaine is also indicated for ventricular tachycardia with a pulse. The dose of lidocaine is 1 mg/kg IV or IO, followed by an infusion of 20 to 50 μg/kg/min.

Amiodarone

Amiodarone may be considered an alternative to lidocaine for the treatment of persistent ventricular fibrillation or pulseless ventricular tachycardia. It may also used for supraventricular tachycardias. The dose is 5 mg/kg IV or IO by rapid push in the arrest situation and over 20 to 60 minutes in the non-arrest situation.

Magnesium

Magnesium is another alternative to lidocaine in the management of persistent ventricular fibrillation or pulseless ventricular tachycardia. It is the drug of choice for polymorphic ventricular tachycardia (torsades de pointes). The dose is 25 to 50 mg/kg IV or IO.

Glucose

Severe hypoglycemia can be a cause of cardiac arrest or may result from the stress of the event. Therefore, blood glucose should be checked at the outset of resuscitation and monitored carefully during all arrest situations. Infants and young children have limited glycogen stores and are prone to develop hypoglycemia when stressed

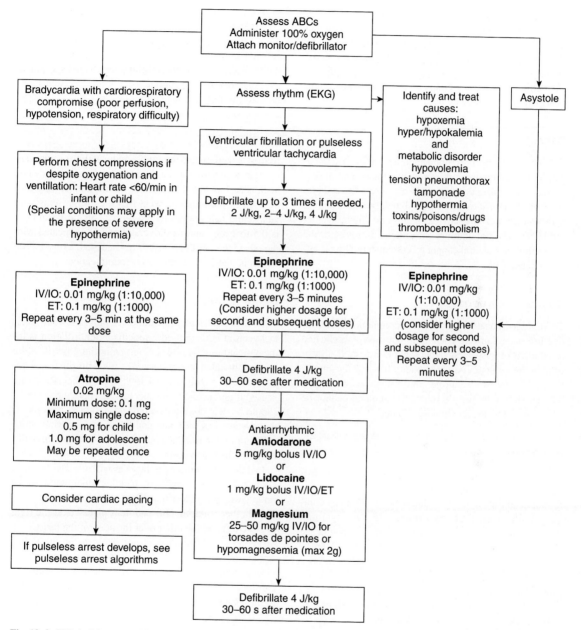

Fig. 13–3. CPR decision tree. *Abbreviations:* ABCs, airway, breathing, circulation; ET; endotracheal; IO, intraosseous; IV, intravenous.

from any cause. If hypoglycemia is found, glucose is administered at 0.5 to 1.0 g/kg (2 to 4 mL/kg of 25% solution). Common toxins associated with pediatric hypoglycemic reactions include ethanol, salicylates, oral hypoglycemic agents, and insulin.

Naloxone

Naloxone is a pure narcotic antagonist that can be used to reverse the effects of narcotic poisoning, including respiratory depression, sedation, hypotension, and hypoperfusion. When the cause for an arrest is unknown and toxic injection or ingestion is considered possible, it is prudent to administer naloxone presumptively, because it may be effective and is an extremely safe drug. The dose is 0.1 mg/kg for infants and children under the age of 5. For older children or those weighing more than 20 kg, a standard dose of 2 mg may be used.

Calcium

Calcium is no longer recommended for routine use in pediatric resuscitation, but it is indicated for known or suspected hyperkalemic arrest. It is also used for calcium channel antagonist overdose, ethylene glycol poisoning, hydrofluoric acid burns, hypocalcemia, and hypermagnesemia. The dose of calcium chloride is 20 mg/kg of the 10% solution. Calcium cannot be administered by the endotracheal route.

Sodium Bicarbonate

Sodium bicarbonate is no longer recommended for routine use in pediatric resuscitation, but it too is indicated for known or suspected hyperkalemic arrest. It is also used in the setting of cardiac toxicity from cyclic antidepressant overdose. It can be administered as 1 mEq/kg infused slowly by the IV route. Bicarbonate cannot be administered by the endotracheal route.

Adenosine

Adenosine is an endogenous nucleoside that has the ability to interrupt reentrant circuits. Its primary indication is for supraventricular tachycardia, which is the most common dysrhythmia in children (Figure 13–4). Vagal maneuvers, such as carotid massage or placing a bag of ice on the face, may also be effective for this dysrhythmia. The dose of adenosine is 0.1 to 0.2 mg/kg IV. It has a very short half-life and must be administered at a site not more distal than the antecubital veins. It is injected rapidly and followed immediately by a saline flush of 2 to 5 mL. If ineffective, the dose is doubled.

ELECTRICAL THERAPY

Transcutaneous Pacing

Although there are limited data specific to pediatric patients, transcutaneous pacing may be used in the setting of bradycardia unresponsive to ventilation, oxygenation, epinephrine, and atropine. Adhesive-backed electrodes are used, placing the negative electrode over the heart and the positive electrode behind the heart on the patient's back. For infants weighing less than 15 kg, pediatric electrodes are recommended. Adult electrodes may be used for children weighing more than 15 kg.

Cardioversion

Synchronized cardioversion is indicated for supraventricular tachycardia when the patient is unstable or when adenosine has failed to convert the rhythm. It may also be used in the unlikely event that a child presents with ventricular tachycardia with a pulse. The electrical dose is 0.5 to 1 J/kg and cardioversion may be repeated with the dose increased to 1 to 2 J/kg if needed. Consultation with a pediatric cardiologist is recommended.

Defibrillation

Whenever ventricular fibrillation or pulseless ventricular tachycardia is diagnosed, immediate defibrillation is indicated and may be life saving. An initial dose of 2 J/kg is recommended and, if unsuccessful, defibrillation is repeated immediately using 4 J/kg. A third shock at 4 J/kg is used if the second is not successful. These three shocks should be delivered in as rapid succession as possible. If the rhythm has still not converted, epinephrine, lidocaine, or amiodarone are administered with repeat defibrillation after each dose.

Paddle size should be as large as will allow good chest contact. In general, pediatric paddles should be used for infants who weigh less that 10 kg. Adult paddles are used for all other children. One paddle is placed over the right upper chest and the other over the apex of the heart.

Ventricular fibrillation is not likely to be an agonal rhythm in children and is usually due to underlying cardiac pathology such as myocarditis, cardiac contusion, cardiomyopathy, or electrical shock. It may also be due to intoxication with digitalis.

TOXINS COMMONLY ASSOCIATED WITH CARDIAC ARREST

Carbon Monoxide

Carbon monoxide (CO) is the most common cause of death due to poisoning. CO is a colorless, odorless, tasteless, and nonirritating gas that is formed as a byproduct of incomplete combustion of organic fuels. It binds to hemoglobin with 240 times the affinity of oxygen and competitively displaces oxygen. The ultimate result is tissue hypoxia. The most oxygen-sensitive organs, the brain and heart, are most affected. Symptoms are non-specific and a high index of suspicion must be maintained to make the diagnosis. If more than one person from the same environment presents with nonspecific symptoms, including cardiac arrest, especially during the winter months, CO intoxication must be considered. The diagnosis is confirmed by specifically measuring the carboxyhemoglobin level. When CO poisoning is suspected, the most important initial treatment is high-flow oxygen, followed by hyperbaric oxygen therapy for patients with cardiac or central nervous system involvement (see Chapter 72).

Cyanide

Cyanide is increasingly recognized as a toxin in victims of fires. Toxic hydrogen cyanide gas is a product of combustion from many common household materials. Cyanide toxicity may also result from ingestion of silver polishes and sculptured nail removers, as well as fruit pits. Cyanide is now also feared as a possible agent for use by terrorists. It produces severe tissue hypoxia by binding to the ferric ion in cytochrome oxidase. Again, the central nervous system and heart are the most vulnerable to its effects. With inhalation, loss of consciousness can occur within seconds. In addition to supportive care, the treatment is with specific antidotal therapy. The Taylor Cyanide Antidote Kit contains amyl nitrite perles, sodium nitrite solution, and sodium thiosulfate solution. All three should be used if cyanide intoxication is suspected. The amyl nitrite perles are crushed for the patient to inhale. Sodium nitrite is then administered IV, followed by sodium thiocyanate (see Chapter 73).

Cocaine

The toxic effects of cocaine result from stimulation of the cardiovascular and central nervous systems. Cardiovascular effects include tachycardia, hypertension, cardiac ischemia and infarction, and ventricular dysrhythmias. Cocaine should be suspected whenever an adolescent or young adult patient with no history of cardiac disease presents with any of these findings. Benzodiazepines are effective for mild to moderate manifestations. Nitro-

prusside or labetalol in combination with an α-blocker, (such as phentolamine) is recommended for severe hypertension. Pure β-blockers are contraindicated because they may lead to unopposed α-stimulation and even worse hypertension (see Chapter 57).

Cyclic Antidepressants

The major toxicities of the cyclic antidepressants result from their effects on the cardiovascular and central nervous systems. Tachycardia is the most common cardiovascular manifestation. Patients with cyclic antidepressant overdoses may arrive in the ED looking stable and then deteriorate suddenly. Cardiac monitoring is essential. Persistent tachycardia and QRS prolongation (>100 msec) are associated with increased risk of seizures and dysrhythmias. When the QRS interval is >100 msec, alkalinization and sodium administration are indicated. This can be accomplished with sodium bicarbonate, 1 to 2 mEq/kg IV bolus, followed by a bicarbonate infusion. Hyperventilation may also be used to assist in bringing the pH to the goal level, which is between 7.45 and 7.50. Ventricular dysrhythmias unresponsive to sodium bicarbonate therapy may be treated with lidocaine or cardioversion. Benzodiazepines are recommended for neurotoxicity and seizure activity (see Chapter 43).

Calcium Channel Antagonists

Calcium channel antagonists decrease contraction of vascular smooth muscle and myocardium by inhibiting the influx of calcium into the cell. In overdose situations, they may cause significant bradycardia, heart blocks, and asystole. Decreased cardiac contractility can be severe enough to result in cardiogenic shock. Vasodilatation may lead to hypotension. The primary antidote is calcium, which is indicated for patients with hypotension, bradycardia, or heart blocks. The recommended pediatric dose is 10 to 20 mg/kg of 10% calcium chloride slow IV push. The dose may be repeated in 10 to 15 minutes. Atropine may also be administered for bradycardia. Glucagon may also counter some of the effects of the calcium channel blockers, but its use should be reserved for toxicity unresponsive to the measures above. In the setting of persistent hypotension, pressors may be required and amrinone has been reported to be effective.

Recent literature has suggested that IV insulin/glucose rescue therapy may be effective in managing severe calcium channel antagonist toxicity (see Chapter 35).

β-Adrenergic Blockers

The β-blockers suppress cardiovascular activity and may result in hypotension, bradycardia, heart block, and congestive heart failure. For patients with symptomatic bradycardia and hypotension, glucagon has been shown to reverse the toxic effects via its interaction with cyclic adenosine monophosphate. For patients unresponsive to glucagon, fluids and epinephrine are recommended. Epinephrine infusion is started at a rate of 1 μg/kg/min and titrated to perfusion parameters (see Chapter 35).

Theophylline

Acute theophylline toxicity can result in tachydysrhythmias, hypotension, and cardiac arrest. Supraventricular tachycardias are the most common, with multifocal atrial tachycardia frequently seen. Ventricular ectopy is common; significant ventricular dysrhythmias are rarely seen. The dysrhythmias are treated with β-blockers or calcium channel blockers. Short-acting agents such as esmolol are preferred. Verapamil may inhibit theophylline metabolism and is avoided. Gastrointestinal decontamination with repetitive dosing of activated charcoal has also proven efficacious in management of theophylline poisoning. Other treatment considerations in theophylline toxicity such as extracorporeal methods of elimination are discussed in Chapter 38.

Digitalis

Digoxin is a positive inotrope and the presentation of toxicity is highly varied. Cardiovascular toxicity is the most important factor in determining morbidity and mortality. Multiple dysrhythmias can occur, with premature ventricular contractions being the most common. Other common disturbances include junctional escape beats, accelerated junctional rhythm, paroxysmal supraventricular tachycardia with AV block, and various AV blocks. Antidotal therapy is with digoxin immune Fab fragments (Digibind). In addition, standard treatment of dysrhythmias and heart blocks is indicated. In addition to standard treatments, phenytoin and magnesium have been shown to be effective for digoxin-induced tachydysrhythmias. With digoxin toxicity, cardioversion is used only as a last resort for life-threatening dysrhythmias. Calcium, sotalol, and quinidine are avoided (see Chapter 37).

DISCONTINUING LIFE SUPPORT

In the emergency department, the decision to terminate resuscitative efforts is based primarily on the failure to respond to standard resuscitative efforts. Although there are no strict guidelines, there is general consensus that failure to respond to two standard doses of epinephrine, along with all the appropriate accompanying resuscitative efforts, is highly correlated with death. Each physician must decide based on the facts of each individual case how far to go and when to cease resuscitative efforts. Prolonged resuscitative efforts run the risk of getting a return of spontaneous circulation in a patient who has undergone such severe cerebral anoxia that severe permanent neurologic impairment is inevitable.

However, case reports and anecdotal experience have documented pediatric survival after prolonged periods of resuscitation when the cardiac or respiratory arrest was secondary to a drug overdose, particularly when the child had no serious underlying chronic disease state.

SUGGESTED READINGS

AAP Committee on Child Abuse and Neglect: Investigation and review of unexpected infant and child deaths. *Pediatrics* 104:1158–1160, 1999.

American Heart Association: Guidelines 2000 for cardiopulmonary resuscitation and emergency cardiovascular care. *Curr Emerg Cardiovasc Care* 11:3, 2000.

American Heart Association: Pediatric basic life support. *Circulation* 102(suppl I):I-253, 2000.

American Heart Association: Pediatric advanced life support. *Circulation* 102(suppl I):I-291, 2000.

Atkins DL, Hartley LL, York DK: Accurate recognition and effective treatment of ventricular fibrillation by automated external defibrillators in adolescents. *Pediatrics* 101:393–397, 1998.

Brown K, Bocock J: Update in pediatric resuscitation. *Pediatr Clin North Am* 20:1–26, 2002.

Dembofsky DA, Gibson E, Nadkarni V, et al: Assessment of infant cardiopulmonary resuscitation rescue breathing technique: Relationship of infant and caregiver facial measurements. *Pediatrics* 103:17, 1999.

Derlet RW, Horowitz BZ: Cardiotoxic drugs. *Pediatr Clin North Am* 13:771–791, 1995.

Gausche M, Lewis RJ, Stratton SJ, et al: A prospective randomized study of the effect of out-of-hospital pediatric endotracheal intubation on survival and neurologic outcome. *JAMA* 283:783–790, 2000.

Hickey RW, Zuckerbraun NS: Pediatric cardiopulmonary arrest: Current concepts and future directions. *Pediatr Emerg Med Rep* 8:1–12, 2003.

Nadkarni V, ed: *Pediatric Advanced Life Support*. Dallas: American Heart Association; 1997:4–8.

Primm PA, Reamy RR: Cardiopulmonary resuscitation. In: Strange G, Ahrens WR, Lelyveld S, et al, eds: *Pediatric*

Emergency Medicine: A Comprehensive Study Guide. 2nd ed. New York: McGraw-Hill; 2002:18–27.

Sirbaugh PE, Pepe PE, Shook JE, et al: A prospective, population-based study of the demographics, epidemiology, management and outcome of out-of-hospital pediatric cardiopulmonary arrest. *Ann Emerg Med* 33:174, 1999.

Whitelaw CC, Slywka B, Goldsmith LJ: Comparison of a two-finger vs two-thumb model. *Resuscitation* 43:213–216, 2000.

Young KD, Seidel JS: Pediatric cardiopulmonary resuscitation: A collective review. *Ann Emerg Med* 33:195–205, 1999.

14

Pediatric Hazardous Materials Exposure

Suzanne R. White
Frank G. Walter

HIGH-YIELD FACTS

- Physiologic differences make children more susceptible to chemical exposures than adults.

- Most chemically exposed patients are not decontaminated prior to arrival at the hospital.

- Children are prone to hypothermia during decontamination.

- Key toxidromes to recognize are irritant gas, asphyxiant, caustic, cholinergic, and hydrocarbon/solvent.

- *Toxic time bombs* can be associated with delayed onset of symptoms.

INTRODUCTION AND EPIDEMIOLOGY

A *hazardous material* can be defined as any substance (chemical, radiologic, nuclear, or biological) that poses a risk to health, safety, property, or the environment. It is estimated that 600 new chemicals are introduced yearly in the United States, some finding their way into homes and schools, where they can potentially poison children. In fact, 10% of the 24,359 chemical incidents registered in the Hazardous Substances Emergency Events Surveillance database between 1993 and 1997 occurred in schools or hospitals. The presentation of victims of hazardous materials incidents includes traumatic injury, respiratory compromise, burns, eye irritation, nausea, vomiting, dizziness, headache, and neurologic effects. Most injuries and deaths are associated with exposure to chlorine, ammonia, nitrogen fertilizer, or hydrochloric acid. Other commonly involved chemicals include petroleum products, pesticides, corrosives, metals, and volatile organics. It is important to note that more than 40% of hazardous materials victims are decontaminated at hospital emergency departments (ED), not at the scene.

DEVELOPMENTAL ISSUES

Unique physiologic variables can increase pediatric patients' susceptibility to hazardous materials versus adults. Higher minute ventilation and short stature can enhance the pulmonary absorption of aerosols and gases. The thin pediatric stratum corneum promotes dermal absorption of some chemicals. Other unique susceptibilities include (1) a predisposition to methemoglobinemia after exposure to oxidant stresses owing to low NADH methemoglobin reductase activity; (2) lower oxygen-carrying capacity due to a lower baseline hematocrit; (3) greater susceptibility due to bronchospasm from inhaled toxicants; and (4) smaller fluid reserves predisposing to dehydration and shock in the setting of vomiting, diarrhea, or burns. A larger relative body surface area (approximately 2.5 times that of adults on a pound-per-pound basis) facilitates heat loss during decontamination. Thus, a high-volume, low-pressure, heated water system, and control of ambient temperature, are necessary to prevent hypothermia. Finally, developmental and psychological immaturity (or loss of a caregiver) can prevent appropriate actions that limit further exposure. These factors can also predispose to posttraumatic stress disorder.

MANAGEMENT OF VICTIMS DURING A HAZARDOUS MATERIALS INCIDENT

Appropriate management of the chemically contaminated child hinges on pre-identification of potential community hazards, timely recognition of a contaminated victim, and rapid identification of the involved material, as well as its toxicity and secondary contamination potential. Hospital personnel and other patients must be protected from injury, and the facility protected from contamination and loss of serviceability. The victim must be decontaminated, stabilized, and treated for injuries. Finally the community must be protected from secondary contamination. One excellent planning resource is the Agency for Toxic Substance and Disease Registry's *Managing Hazardous Materials Incidents,* available at: www.atsdr.cdc.gov/mhmi.html.

Identification of the Chemical

Details about the incident are important to the overall response. Information is obtained regarding the reason for the incident, the presence and status of other victims, the routes of exposure, whether it occurred in a confined space, and the duration of the exposure. Exact chemical identification can be facilitated by Regional Poison Control Centers that provide 24-hour service nationwide through 1-800-222-1222. Additionally, the Material Safety Data Sheet (MSDS) provides limited health and safety information for any product containing hazardous materials. The MSDS can be obtained from on-scene supervisors, some poison centers, Chemtrec, National Response Center, or the Internet. Other resources are listed in Table 14–1.

Preparation for Receipt of the Patient

Patient decontamination ideally occurs outside the hospital or in a predesignated indoor decontamination area by staff garbed in appropriate personal protective equipment (PPE). Hot, warm, and cold zones are established. The *hot zone* is the area of the spill or chemical release, or the hospital area where arriving patients with no prior decontamination are held. Only the most immediate life threats are addressed in the hot zone. The *warm zone* is an area where thorough decontamination and some medical stabilization occurs. The *cold zone* is the area to which fully decontaminated patients are transferred and where definitive medical care can be rendered. There is no personnel flow between hot, warm, and cold areas

without proper decontamination. Consideration should be given to a special pediatric triage, decontamination, and secured observation area that allows for decontamination of parent–child pairs, is staffed by those familiar with pediatric medical and behavioral issues, and provides the highest security for children unaccompanied by an adult.

Personal Protective Equipment

Levels of PPE are categorized as follows:

- *Level A*—fully encapsulating chemical-resistant suit and self-contained breathing apparatus (SCBA) for the highest level of eye, mucous membrane, skin, and respiratory protection.

- *Level B*—skin splash protection chemical-resistant suit and an SCBA.

- *Level C*—skin splash protection chemical-resistant suit and a full-face, air-purifying canister-equipped respirator.

- *Level D*—a standard work uniform.

There is currently no consensus regarding the level of PPE needed for health care workers decontaminating ambulatory patients at hospitals, although many hospitals are opting for Level C. Factors that have complicated this decision include physical limitations while providing patient care in PPE, deconditioned ED staff, heat stress, limited oxygen tank supply, specialized training requirements, fit testing, and the potential for a false sense of security while in PPE.

Receipt of the Contaminated Patient

ED triage must be efficient, and should ideally occur outdoors. *First and foremost, the contaminated patient should not be allowed to enter the ED.* The incoming ambulance or ambulatory patients should be met by a triage officer, wearing an appropriate level of PPE, who determines whether decontamination has been adequately performed. It is prudent to err on the side of decontamination before treatment. Examples of substances with little or no risk of secondary contamination include gases and vapors. Patients exposed only to gases or vapors who have no symptoms other than respiratory irritation and who have no signs of condensation of vapor generally do not require decontamination, other than considering clothing removal.

Table 14–1. Aids in Chemical Identification and Hazard Determination

Department of Transportation (DOT) Placards (used with DOT ERG*) are diamond-shaped placards on tank
trucks or rail cars, etc.
United Nations Classification numbering system on vehicles is at the bottom of placards or on shipping papers, and
defines hazard.
Bill of lading (cargo manifest in cab of truck)
Waybill (with train conductor)
Shipping papers
National Fire Protection Association (NFPA) 704 marking system labels on containers at fixed facilities
Material Safety Data Sheet (MSDS) from company records or company safety officer
CAS number (unique number assigned to specific chemical or mixture) http://chemfinder.cambridgesoft.com/
On-scene chemical analysis (by fire department or HazMat Team)
Regional Poison Control Center: 1-800-222-1222
Chemtrec
    24-hour assistance to emergency responders for chemicals spills: 1-800-424-9300 or
        www.chemtrec.org/Chemtrec/chemtrec.nsf/NavERFS
REAC/TS
    24-hour emergency consultative assistance for radiation accidents: 423-576-3131
        (after business hours): 423-481-1000
Motherisk Program
    teratology information service, 416-813-6780;
        after business hours, 416-813-5900
ATSDR Emergency Response 24-hour Hotline: 404-639-0615
EPA Environmental Response Hotline: 201-321-6660
National Response Center (NRC): 800-424-8802
Local Emergency Planning Committee (LEPC)
Local FBI (suspected terrorist incident)
Local Health Department
U.S. Army Medical Research Institute of Infectious Diseases, (USAMRIID), Fort Detrick, Maryland: 888-872-7443
Centers for Disease Control (CDC): 404-639-3311
National Pesticide Telecommunication Network: 800-858-7378
ATSDR Managing Hazardous Materials Incidents: 404-639-6360 or online at www.atsdr.cdc.gov/mhmi.html
*DOT Emergency Response Guidebook 2000: (obtain by calling 1-800-327-6868 or online at www.tc.gc.ca/canutec/
erg_gmu/erg2000_menu.htm
Advanced HazMat Life Support (AHLS) Manuals and Course Materials: (obtain by calling 520-626-1982, online at
www.ahls.org or via e-mail at ahlsinfo@aemrc.arizona.edu)

Patient Decontamination Techniques

The goals of decontamination are to decrease the absorbed dose for the victim and to prevent secondary contamination of health care providers. Ocular exposures and are treated immediately with irrigation, ideally starting in the prehospital setting. Eye irrigation in children is difficult, and can be facilitated by utilizing a topical ocular anesthetic and by irrigating the bridge of the nose. The use of pH paper, with a range of 1 to 14, can help to guide the duration of irrigation, until a pH of 7 is re-

corded. Wounds are irrigated, debrided of gross contaminants, and then covered with a water-occlusive dressing to prevent recontamination during subsequent showering. Clothing should be removed quickly because this step alone can accomplish significant decontamination. Particulate or radioactive matter should be removed by a careful roll-down of clothing or carefully cutting off clothing in a rostral to caudal direction. Any remaining particulate matter should be brushed away prior to showering, because interaction of some dry chemicals with water can produce heat. All clothing and personal possessions are double bagged and tracked. Whole-body decontamination should begin with the hands, face, and head, which are generally the most heavily contaminated areas. Most chemicals are readily removed with copious amounts of tepid water; special decontamination solutions are rarely necessary. In fact, attempting to locate or prepare such decontamination solutions can delay decontamination. A mild liquid soap, shampoo, or detergent is necessary for nonpolar, water-insoluble substances. In children, the focus should be on using a high-volume, low-pressure warm water delivery system that allows decontamination of parent–child pairs to facilitate both supervision and thermoregulation. Typically, 3 to 5 minutes of showering is recommended, although 15 minutes or longer can be required for concentrated, strongly alkaline materials or oily, adherent substances. The use of abrasives, such as corn meal or scrub brushes, is not advised, because abrading the skin can increase toxicant absorption.

Certain metals such as elemental sodium, lithium, and potassium react violently with water, releasing heat, hydroxide ion, and hydrogen gas to produce chemical and thermal burns. Treatment of alkali metal burns involves clothing removal, covering the affected area with mineral or cooking oil, followed by removal of any remaining metal with dry forceps. Wounds can then be copiously irrigated with water. Burning fragments should be extinguished by smothering or with a class D fire extinguisher.

Some adherent toxicants are extremely difficult to remove from the skin. Epoxy resins and cyanoacrylates (glues) can be removed by swabbing with acetone. Use of vegetable or mineral oil or saline-soaked gauze pads for the eyes and mucous membranes is safe. Hot tar typically inflicts burns to the face and upper extremities, and should be allowed to cool prior to removal. Effective tar removal has then been reported using Neosporin cream, Tween 80, plain Vaseline, Shur Clens, Desolv-It, or may-

Table 14–2. Common Hazardous Material Toxidromes

Irritant gas
> *Symptoms*: Mucous membrane irritation, coughing, dyspnea, bronchospasm, and pulmonary edema
> *Substances*: Ammonia, chlorine, hydrogen chloride, acrolein, isocyanates, sulfur dioxide, and formaldehyde
> *Therapy*: Humidified oxygen, and β-2 agonist bronchodilators

Asphyxiant (simple or systemic)
> *Symptoms*: *Early:* nausea, vomiting, headache, dizziness; *Late:* syncope, coma, seizures, dysrhythmias, cardiac arrest
> *Substances*: *Simple:* carbon dioxide, methane, propane, butane; *Systemic:* nitrites, hydrogen cyanide, hydrogen sulfide, azides
> *Antidotes*: *All asphyxiants:* 100% oxygen; *cyanide:* cyanide antidote kit (see Chapter 73); nitrites/methemoglobinemia (methylene blue) (see Chapter 74)

Caustic
> *Symptoms*: Irritation or burning of skin or mucous membranes
> *Substances*: Acids or alkalis
> *Therapy*: Copious irrigation to a pH of 7.0 and burn care

Cholinergic
> *Symptoms*: Pinpoint pupils, eye pain, dyspnea, bronchospasm, pulmonary edema, muscle fasciculations/weakness, coma, seizures, tachycardia or bradycardia, diaphoresis, salivation, lacrimation, vomiting, diarrhea, and abdominal cramps
> *Substances*: Organophosphates, carbamates, nerve agents
> *Antidotes*: Atropine 1–2 mg IV bolus; titrate to drying of pulmonary secretions (pediatric dose = 0.05–0.10 mg/kg); *Pralidoxime*: 1–2 g slow IV infusion over 10 min, then 500 mg/h infusion (pediatric dose = 25–50 mg/kg slow IV infusion over 10 min then 10–20 mg/kg/h infusion)

Hydrocarbons and solvents
> *Symptoms*: Mucous membrane irritation, headache, lightheadedness, dizziness, nausea, chest tightness, dyspnea, dysrhythmias, lethargy, confusion, coma
> *Substances*: Chloroform, gasoline, toluene, etc.
> *Therapy*: 100% oxygen and β-blockers for myocardial irritability

onnaise. No attempt should be made to remove tar by mechanical means, because this can increase tissue destruction and result in hair follicle loss.

Nausea and vomiting are common following chemical exposures. These symptoms may reflect ingested toxicants causing gastrointestinal irritation or, more commonly, systemic toxicant effect or psychogenic emesis. Regardless of the cause, secondary contamination by toxic vomitus can occur, and the need for its containment should be anticipated. Furthermore, some materials react with stomach acid to produce toxic gas. For instance, sodium azide is converted to hydrazoic acid; cyanide salts, to hydrogen cyanide gas. Suction with outdoor venting should be available to prevent secondary poisoning of personnel. If a chemical has been ingested, decisions regarding gastrointestinal tract decontamination can be guided by the regional poison control center. Placing decontaminated patients into body bags hooded Tyvek suits prior to transport to the support zone is not recommended. This technique is not effective in minimizing the transfer of toxicants to hospital staff, and poses the risk of increased toxicant absorption by the patient. The patient simply should be wrapped in clean blankets or sheets prior to transfer to the cold zone.

Complete medical assessment and specific medical treatment can be carried out in the support cold zone. ED personnel in this area should utilize universal precautions, with blood- and bodily fluid-resistant gowns, latex or nitrile gloves, and eye protection.

Toxidrome Recognition and Medical Management

Following decontamination and the primary survey, a secondary survey is carried out with attention to the identification of common hazardous materials toxidromes. Key toxidromes involve exposure to irritant gases, asphyxiants, caustics, cholinergics, hydrocarbons, and solvents (Table 14–2).

POSTINCIDENT RESPONSE

Prolonged observation is necessary following significant exposures to agents listed in Table 14–3 that are associ-

Table 14–3. Toxicants with Delayed Onset of Symptoms, Requiring Prolonged Monitoring

Toxicant	Toxicity
Aniline	Methemoglobinemia
Arsine	Hemolysis
Benzene	Bone marrow suppression and leukemia
Cadmium	Pulmonary toxicity
Chlorine	Airway and pulmonary edema
Ethylene oxide	Pulmonary edema and neurotoxicity
Halogenated solvents	Hepatorenal toxicity, etc
Hydrofluoric acid	Pulmonary edema, dermal burns
	Electrolyte changes (hyperkalemia, hypocalcemia, hypomagnesemia)
Hydrogen sulfide	Pulmonary edema
Metals	Hepatorenal, neurotoxicity
Methanol	Neurologic, acid–base disturbance
Methyl bromide	Pulmonary edema
Methylene chloride	Carbon monoxide toxicity, dysrhythmias
Nitriles acetonitrile, acrylonitrile	Cyanide toxicity
Nitrogen oxides	Pulmonary edema, methemoglobinemia
Organophosphates	Cholinergic toxicity
Ozone	Pulmonary edema (rare)
Paraquat	Pulmonary edema/fibrosis
Phosgene	Pulmonary edema
Phosphine	Pulmonary edema
Zinc phosphide	Pulmonary edema

ated with delayed onset of toxicity. Certain patients require special medical follow-up, depending on the nature of the contaminant. Counseling may be needed following pediatric exposure to carcinogens and reproductive or developmental toxicants.

Psychological factors affect health after toxicologic disasters. Victims of a hazardous materials incident may experience posttraumatic stress disorder consisting of anxiety, depression, insomnia, amplification of symptoms, and somatization. This is estimated to occur in 25% of victims, as evidenced by abnormal psychological test scores. Early psychological debriefing and interviews with patients and personnel may help prevent postexposure stress syndrome.

SUGGESTED READINGS

Advanced Hazmat Life Support Provider Manual. 3rd ed. Tucson: Walter FG and Arizona Board of Regents; 2003.

Agency for Toxic Substance and Disease Registry: *Managing Hazardous Materials Incidents.* Accessed September 30, 2003. Available from URL: www.atsdr.cdc.gov/mhmi.html

Burgess JL: Hospital preparedness of hazardous materials incidents and treatment of contaminated patients. *West J Med* 167:387, 1997.

Burgess JL, Kirk M, Borron SW, et al: Emergency department hazardous materials protocol for contaminated patients. *Ann Emerg Med* 34:205, 1999.

Burgess JL, Kovalchick DF, Lymp JF, et al: Risk factors for adverse health effects following hazardous materials incidents. *J Occup Environ Med* 43:558–566, 2001.

Greenberg MI, Cone DC, Roberts JR: Material Safety Data Sheet: A useful resource for the emergency physician. *Ann Emerg Med* 27:347, 1996.

Hall HI, Dhara VR, Price-Green PA, et al: Surveillance for emergency events involving hazardous substances: United States, 1990–1992. *MMWR, CDC Surveillance Summaries* 43:1, 1994.

Hazardous Substances Emergency Events Surveillance (HSEES): *Five-Year Cumulative Report 1993–1997.* Atlanta: Department of Health and Human Services, Agency for Toxic Substances and Disease Registry; 2001.

Kales SN, Polyhronpoulos GN, Castro MJ, et al: Injuries caused by hazardous materials accidents. *Ann Emerg Med* 30:598, 1997.

Phelps AM, Morris P, Giguere M: Emergency events involving hazardous substances in North Carolina, 1993–1994. *N Carolina Med J* 59:120, 1998.

Rotenberg JS, Burklow TR, Selanikio JS: Weapons of mass destruction: The decontamination of children. *Pediatr Ann* 32:261, 2003.

Saari KM, Leinonen J, Aine E: Management of chemical eye injuries with prolonged irrigation. *Acta Ophthalmol Suppl* 161:52, 1984.

15

Weapons of Mass Destruction

Suzanne R. White
Frank G. Walter

HIGH-YIELD FACTS

- Children are more likely than adults to have severe illness following a chemical, biological, or nuclear attack.

- Biological terrorism will likely involve nontraditional first responders, such as hospital, primary care, and public health providers.

- Antibiotics that are infrequently used in children, such as tetracyclines and fluoroquinolones, may be the drugs of choice in the setting of bioterrorism.

- Infection control practices should be employed because secondary transmission is likely with biologic agents such as plague, smallpox, and hemorrhagic fevers.

- Secondary contamination with liquid and solid chemical agents is likely unless personal protection equipment and proper decontamination techniques are utilized.

Planning for a medical response to terrorism has primarily focused around the needs of healthy military recruits or the population as a whole. There has been little discussion pertaining to vulnerable populations such as children. Unfortunately, entire communities are now at risk for terrorism. Furthermore, there is no reason to believe that terrorists would avoid children when carrying out an attack, and they may even target locations such as daycare centers, schools, or hospitals to maximally terrorize a population. If this were to occur, affected pediatric victims would pose diagnostic and therapeutic challenges, and would be at higher risk for developing complications than adults.

DEVELOPMENTAL CONSIDERATIONS

The general physiologic and developmental concepts relating to hazardous materials exposures outlined in Chapter 14 also apply to weapons of mass destruction incidents. Specific to bioterrorism, more fulminant infectious diseases are possible in children because of immunologic immaturity and a more permeable blood–brain barrier. Furthermore, many drugs used to treat illness from bioagents were historically avoided during childhood because of potential developmental toxicity. Finally, it is anticipated that specific vulnerabilities such as lack of pediatric expertise, equipment, or facilities within disaster planning and emergency medical services systems might be exacerbated by a terrorist attack involving children.

BIOLOGICAL AGENTS

In contrast to a chemical attack, a covert biological attack will simulate a natural outbreak with an incubation period, rather than producing immediate mass casualties. The Centers for Disease Control and Prevention (CDC) has developed a list of critical agents for health preparedness that encompasses organisms with the most potentially devastating consequences that would require the most critical medical responses if released by a bioterrorist. According to this classification scheme, the highest overall public health impact and requirement for intensive preparedness and intervention would stem from an aerosolized release of the Variola virus (smallpox), *Bacillus anthracis* (anthrax), *Yersinia pestis* (plague), *Clostridia botulinum* (botulism), *Francisella tularensis* (tularemia), or the filoviridae/arenaviridae, such as Ebola, Marburg, and Lassa fever viruses that produce hemorrhagic fevers.

Anthrax

Anthrax occurs in nature following contact with infected animals or animal products. *B. anthracis* spores are highly stable and highly infectious upon inhalation and have been manufactured for use in biological warfare. Illness resulting from an aerosolized release of anthrax spores would likely be associated with an incubation period of 1 to 60 days, followed by fever, myalgias, cough, and chest pain. Transient improvement might occur, but would be followed by the abrupt onset of sepsis, hypotension, and death within 24 to 36 hours. Hemorrhagic meningitis would be expected in 50% of cases, as would a very high overall case fatality rate. Hallmarks of the illness include gram-positive bacilli on tissue biopsy, blood smear, or spinal fluid microscopy, and chest X-ray findings of mediastinal widening from lymphadenitis. Pulmonary infiltrates or effusions may also be seen. All forms of anthrax may occur in children, although cutaneous infection is said to account for 90% of natural pediatric cases. The cutaneous form of illness is associated with a relatively painless papule that progresses to a vesicle, a necrotic ulcer, and then a depressed black painless eschar with marked surrounding edema. Several gastrointestinal anthrax cases have been reported following the ingestion of contaminated meat in Asia and Africa. In addition, a unique case was reported in a 2-day-old baby with fever and erythema surrounding the umbilicus that had been tied with a wool thread from an infected hide. The infant had positive blood, urine, and umbilical cultures for *B. anthracis*. During the United States 2001 mail-borne anthrax outbreak, the one pediatric victim was a 7-month-old thought to have suffered a brown recluse spider bite, who was initially treated for cellulitis.

Historically, a severe course of illness, including hemolysis, thrombocytopenia, and renal insufficiency, as well as meningitis with the cutaneous form anthrax in children, raises concerns of enhanced pediatric susceptibility to *B. anthracis*. There are no clinical trials assessing the treatment of inhalational anthrax in humans, let alone in children. Early antibiotic administration is likely to be the most important determinant of outcome in the setting of anthrax infection. Those patients potentially exposed to anthrax spores should receive antibiotic prophylaxis for 60 days. Treatment and prophylaxis recommendations are summarized in Table 15–1. Secondary transmission of inhalational anthrax does not occur, although it has been described with cutaneous anthrax. Standard blood and bodily fluid precautions are indicated.

Plague

Yersinia pestis, the bacteria that causes plague, classically spreads in nature from infected fleas to humans. An aerosol-mediated bioterrorist attack would be associated with pneumonic plague, with nonspecific respiratory signs and symptoms beginning 1 to 6 days after exposure, and progressing to death in those not treated with antibiotics within 24 hours of symptom onset. Hemoptysis is a characteristic finding. Most natural cases of plague in children are of the bubonic type. Complicating sepsis and meningitis can occur, but undifferentiated septicemic plague is less common than among adults. When it does occur, primary plague sepsis in children has a much higher fatality rate than the bubonic form, 71% versus 3% in one pediatric series. Gastrointestinal signs and symptoms can be very prominent, and at times mimic an acute abdomen. Petechiae, purpura, and an overwhelming picture of disseminated intravascular coagulation may occur. A clue to the diagnosis of *Y. pestis* is bipolar, safety pin-staining bacilli on Gram staining of the sputum or lymph node aspirate. Secondary transmission of pneumonic plague occurs. As such, standard blood and bodily fluid, as well as droplet precautions are necessary, as is postexposure prophylaxis for those exposed to pneumonic plague victims. Treatment and prophylaxis recommendations are summarized in Table 15–1.

Smallpox

Declared eradicated in 1980 by the World Health Organization, smallpox was caused by a member of the Orthopoxvirus group. The illness was known for its highly contagious nature and relatively high mortality rate. The possibility of the reemergence of smallpox as the result of a deliberate release is a concern. Smallpox has an incubation period of 7 to 17 days. Clinical illness is characterized by a severe prodrome of high fever, rigors, vomiting, headache, and backache. The classic exanthem begins 2 to

Table 15–1. Initial Antibiotic Therapy for Selected Bacterial Agents of Bioterrorism in Children[a]

Agent	Antibiotics	Dose and Route
Inhalational anthrax[a]	Ciprofloxacin *or*	10–15 mg/kg IV q12h (max 400 mg/dose)
	Doxycycline *and*	2.2 mg/kg IV (max 100 mg) q12h
	Clindamycin *and*	10–15 mg/kg IV q8h
	Penicillin G	400–600K μ/kg/d IV divided q4h
Cutaneous anthrax[a]	Ciprofloxacin *or*	10–15 mg/kg PO q12h (max 1 g/d)
	Doxycycline	2.2 mg/kg PO (max 100 mg) q12h
Plague	Streptomycin *or*	15 mg/kg IM q12h (max 2 g/d)
	Gentamicin *or*	2.5 mg/kg IM or IV q8h (q12h in neonates <1week old)
	Doxycycline	2.2 mg/kg IV q12h (max 200 mg/d) (ciprofloxacin 15 mg/kg IV q12h or chloramphenicol 25 mg/kg IV q6h (max 4 g/d) might also be considered; especially chloramphenicol for plague meningitis)
Tularemia	Streptomycin *or*	15 mg/kg IM q12h (max 2 g/d)
	Gentamicin *or*	2.5 mg/kg IM or IV q8h (q12h in neonates <1 week old)
	Doxycycline	2.2 mg/kg IV q12h (max 200 mg/d) (chloramphenicol or ciprofloxacin may also be considered)
Mass Casualty Setting or Prophylaxis		
Inhalational anthrax[a]	Ciprofloxacin *or*	10–15 mg/kg PO q12h (max 1 g/d) × 60d
	Doxycycline	2.2 mg/kg (max 100 mg) PO q12h × 60d
Plague	Doxycycline *or*	2.2 mg/kg PO q12h (max 200 mg/d)
	Ciprofloxacin	20 mg/kg PO q12h (max 1 g/d)
Tularemia	Doxycycline *or*	2.2 mg/kg PO q12h (max 200 mg/d)
	Ciprofloxacin	15 mg/kg PO q12h (max 1 g/d)

[a]Amoxicillin could be substituted after 14 days of ciprofloxacin or doxycycline if strain susceptible at 40 to 80 mg/kg/d divided q8h to complete a 60-day course of therapy.
Abbreviations: IM, intramuscular; IV, intravenous; max, maximum; PO, orally.

4 days later, on the face and distal portions of the extremities, with macules progressing to papules, umbilicated pustules, and then scabs. The centrifugal onset and synchronous nature of the rash helps to distinguish it from chickenpox. Death has been reported in 30% of infected patients from toxemia and shock. Historically, children younger than 5 years of age had the highest mortality.

Currently in the United States, virtually all children and adults under the age of 32 years are unvaccinated and have no immunity to smallpox. Thus, their potential susceptibility to fulminant disease might actually be greater than in Americans who were immunized before 1972.

There are few reports that distinguish between pediatric and adult presentations. During the prodromal phase, in addition to high fever, head and muscle aches, chills and prostration, a child may develop delirium, coma, and seizures. Also, viral osteomyelitis has been described, involving multiple bones and joints. This could be accompanied by radiographic evidence of bony destruction, and might lead to serious sequelae including deformed bones, stunted growth, and ankylosis. The diagnosis of smallpox is made clinically, with laboratory confirmation through the CDC.

Vaccination with the smallpox vaccine within 4 days of exposure may prevent disease. Historically, the vaccine was given to children. Currently, it is not being offered to children for pre-event prophylaxis and it is not recommended for postexposure use in children younger than 1 year. The smallpox vaccine may be associated with a high rate of serious complications from the vaccinia virus in certain patients. Such complications are likely to disproportionately affect children who are primary vaccinees.

Secondary transmission of smallpox is likely. Airborne, droplet, and standard blood and bodily fluid precautions are indicated when caring for victims until all their scabs separate. Universal fluid precautions are also recommended for close contacts of victims until 17 days from their last exposure.

Botulism

Clinical manifestations of botulism are very similar in adults and children. Even the infant botulism syndrome is now described in adults as classification undetermined or intestinal botulism (botulism is discussed fully in Chapter 77). The trivalent botulinum antitoxin available through the CDC may be used to treat children of any age with subtypes A, B, or E. The United States Army hepatavalent antitoxin is currently an Investigational New Drug status drug. Botulism immune globulin is used to treat infant botulism.

Tularemia

Tularemia is a zoonotic illness that most commonly manifests in an ulceroglandular form after exposure to diseased animal fluids or bites from infected deerflies, mosquitoes, or ticks. Although not highly fatal, its extremely high infectivity and its ability to escape laboratory detection make it an agent of potential use in bioterrorism. An aerosolized release would likely result in clinical findings similar to a community-acquired pneumonia. Specifically, following a 2- to 10-day incubation period, fever, prostration, dry cough, abdominal pain, and chest pain develop.

Patchy infiltrates and hilar adenopathy might be seen on chest radiograph. Person-to-person transmission does not occur, and respiratory isolation is not required. Treatment is outlined in Table 15–1.

Viral Hemorrhagic Fevers

Certain RNA viruses can cause fulminant illnesses with fever, hypotension, and diffuse bleeding. Filoviruses cause Ebola and Marburg hemorrhagic fevers and an arenavirus causes Lassa fever. Supportive care and blood product replacement are the mainstays of therapy with ribavirin possibly efficacious in arenaviral illness. Secondary transmission is likely, necessitating airborne isolation with standard blood and bodily fluid precautions.

BIOLOGICAL AGENT TREATMENT

Recent consensus recommendations for the antibiotic treatment and prophylaxis of anthrax, plague, and tularemia in children are based on clinical and evidence-based criteria and do not necessarily correspond to the Federal and Drug Administration (FDA) approved indications or labeling of these drugs. Foremost, as detailed in Table 15–1, many of the highest threat bioterrorist agents are appropriately treated in adults with ciprofloxacin or doxycycline. The fluoroquinolone and tetracycline classes of antibiotics have each been considered as relatively contraindicated in young children. The fluoroquinolone concern has primarily stemmed from arthropathy and growth abnormality noted in animal studies. The tetracyclines are known to stain children's teeth, particularly in children younger than 8 years old taking prolonged or repeated courses.

The past decade has seen a great deal of clinical use of ciprofloxacin in young children with cancer, cystic fibrosis, shigellosis, typhoid fever, and neonatal sepsis. There is no evidence of arthropathy or slower rates of bone growth in these children. In fact, in 2001, the FDA approved ciprofloxacin for use in bioterrorist-related anthrax exposures for children, as well as for adults. Among the tetracyclines, doxycycline is least likely to cause dental staining. It is now recognized as the drug of choice for treatment in children with life-threatening rickettsial infections, such as Rocky Mountain spotted fever and erlichiosis. In this setting, has been used without evidence of dental staining. This reevaluation has mitigated much of the previous concern regarding fluoroquinalone and doxycycline use in children.

Chemical Agents

Nerve Agents

Nerve agents are highly toxic organophosphates developed circa World War II, that were placed in munitions and yet never employed in battle. Liquid compounds currently recognized as nerve agents are tabun, sarin, soman, and VX. Properties of these liquids vary in terms of vapor pressure, persistence in the environment, and potency. Sarin is the most volatile. VX is the most potent and persistent, with a potentially fatal exposure involving a skin area of only 2 to 3 mm in diameter in adults and proportionately much less in children. Animal studies suggest that infants and juveniles succumb to 10% to 33% of the lethal adult dose on an equivalent mg/kg basis. The nerve agents are minimally irritating to the eyes, mucous membranes, and respiratory tract. Their odors are described as fruity (tabun), odorless (sarin, VX), or fruity/camphorous (soman). The nerve agents are powerful inhibitors of acetylcholinesterase (AChE) located in nerves, skeletal muscles, glands, and other tissues innervated by cholinergic neurons. The ability of nerve agents to interfere with normal acetylcholine hydrolysis at cholinergic synapses causes acetylcholine accumulation and abnormal neurotransmission. Excess acetylcholine at brain synapses, for example, results in seizures, coma, respiratory depression, and apnea. Acetylcholine accumulation at the motor endplate causes initial fasciculations that progress to weakness and paralysis. Overstimulation of sympathetic and parasympathetic ganglia of the peripheral nervous system results in tachycardia, hypertension, diaphoresis, miosis, lacrimation, salivation, bronchorrhea, bronchospasm, bradycardia, vomiting, diarrhea, and urination. Miosis and peripheral muscarinic effects are less common in children, who are more likely to present with central nervous system (CNS) depression, hypotonia, and weakness. Children may have a greater tendency toward seizures because of their more permeable blood–brain barrier and relatively lower paroxonase (detoxifying enzyme) activity.

The onset and type of symptoms are determined by both the concentration and route of exposure to nerve agents. For example, sarin vapor inhalation or massive VX dermal exposure may cause death within minutes, whereas mild VX dermal exposure may be associated with delayed symptom onset up to 18 hours later. Vital sign abnormalities may result from stimulation of both the sympathetic and parasympathetic ganglia. Although bradycardia is expected from stimulation of the parasympathetic nervous system, 90% of patients exposed to nerve agents in Tokyo in 1995 had either normal heart rates or were tachycardic.

Vapor exposure typically creates a triad of ocular, nasal, and respiratory symptoms. The eyes and nose are most sensitive, with miosis, conjunctival injection, pain, and rhinorrhea developing at low doses. At higher concentrations, respiratory effects such as chest tightness, dyspnea, and copious secretions occur. Neurologic findings associated with severe exposures include giddiness, collapse, convulsions, fasciculations, and flaccid paralysis. The predominant cause of death is respiratory depression and apnea.

In contrast to vapor exposure, dermal exposure results in a unique pattern of symptom onset and progression. Miosis may not be evident initially, but localized sweating and fasciculations can be noted near the exposed area. Nausea, vomiting, diarrhea, and fatigue develop with increasing doses. As with vapor exposures, the presence of respiratory and neurologic symptoms indicates severe toxicity. There is little information that allows distinction to be made between expected pediatric and adult presentations after nerve agent exposures, but two case series involving cholinesterase pesticides suggest a disproportionate degree of depressed sensorium and muscle weakness in children.

Once a nerve agent release has been recognized, self-protection and patient decontamination take precedence over other medical treatment. There is an extremely high risk of secondary contamination of medical personnel caring for patients exposed to liquid or aerosolized nerve agents. Appropriate skin and respiratory protection should be donned by hospital staff because these agents are readily absorbed by the skin, mucous membranes, and respiratory tract. Neither surgical nor HEPA masks render protection from these agents. Even double latex gloves are ineffective in preventing dermal exposure; butyl rubber gloves should be worn. Although a 0.5% sodium hypochlorite solution (9:1 dilution of household bleach in water) effectively inactivates nerve agents, its use on children is not advisable. Copious amounts of tepid/warm water washing with a mild soap should be adequate for skin decontamination. However, a considerable amount of VX may remain on the skin even after initial decontamination, necessitating several washings and awareness of the potential for secondary contamination.

Following decontamination, restoring ventilation and oxygenation is the critical step in medical management, because most deaths are respiratory in nature. Succinylcholine, if used to facilitate intubation, may have a prolonged effect because plasma cholinesterase is inhibited.

Cardiac monitoring for dysrhythmias should be instituted, as torsades de pointes has been described.

Specific antidotes are atropine and pralidoxime (2-PAM). Atropine blocks muscarinic receptors and reverses the parasympathetic findings of lacrimation, bronchorrhea, bronchoconstriction, bradycardia, salivation, and gastrointestinal dysfunction, along with CNS manifestations. Atropine does not affect the motor endplate fasciculations and weakness. The atropine dose is 0.05 to 0.10 mg/kg IV or IM (minimum 0.1 mg, maximum 5 mg), to be repeated every 2 to 5 minutes as needed for marked secretions. In contrast to organophosphate pesticide poisoning, high-dose or continuous atropine therapy generally may not be necessary beyond 2 to 3 hours following nerve agent exposure. The endpoint of dosing for atropine is drying of pulmonary secretions. Miosis is not a useful therapeutic endpoint, and sinus tachycardia is not a contraindication for use of atropine.

Oximes, like 2-PAM, are effective nerve agent antidotes via their ability to reactivate AChE. They carry out a nucleophilic attack on the nerve-agent–phosphorylated-AChE complex. Subsequent liberation of the enzyme occurs along with detoxification of the nerve agent. Whereas atropine is not effective in treating neuromuscular findings such as weakness or fasciculations, oximes reverse the nicotinic, muscarinic, and CNS effects of the nerve agent. One caveat when using oximes is the need for administration prior to aging of the nerve-agent–AchE complex. *Aging* is the process whereby permanent inhibition of AChE activity occurs because of the nerve agent's alkyl group hydrolysis, resulting in irreversible covalent binding. Aging half-life time, which occurs within 2 minutes of soman exposure and within 5 hours of sarin exposure, provides a rationale for early 2-PAM therapy. 2-PAM is given at 25 to 50 mg/kg IV or IM (maximum 1g IV or IM) and may be repeated within 30 to 60 minutes. While repeat doses for adults are recommended every 1 to 2 hours for persistent weakness or in the setting of high atropine requirements, the threefold longer half-life of 2-PAM in children may obviate the need for such frequent dosing. In contrast to organophosphate pesticide exposures, long-term or continuous infusions of 2-PAM have not been required in the management of adult victims with nerve agent poisoning.

Seizures generally are not persistent once ventilatory support, atropine, and 2-PAM therapy are instituted. However, severe exposures, even in the absence of obvious seizures, should be treated aggressively with benzodiazepines, which may be neuroprotective. The dose is diazepam 0.05 to 0.30 mg/kg (max 10 mg) IV, or lo-razepam 0.1 mg/kg IV or IM (max 4 mg), or midazolam 0.1 to 0.2 mg/kg (max 10 mg) IV or IM.

Military Mark I autoinjector kits contain 2 mg of atropine and 600 mg of 2-PAM for immediate IM administration in the field. The emergency physician should be familiar with this form of these antidotes, because these kits may be stockpiled for civilian first responder use. Although not approved for use in children, adult autoinjectors may be considered as initial treatment in circumstances for children with severe, life-threatening nerve agent toxicity for whom IV treatment is not possible or available, or when more precise IM mg/kg dosing would not be logistically possible. Adult autoinjectors discharged into emptied, sterile 10-mL vials may provide a readily available source of concentrated atropine and 2-PAM for IM use in children. Symptomatic patients or those with dermal exposures should be kept under close observation for at least 24 hours.

Blister Agents (Vesicants)

Terrorist use of vesicants, or agents that produce blisters, would result in severe dermal manifestations in children. The three primary vesicants are sulfur mustard, lewisite, and phosgene oxime. Sulfur mustard is the most viable threat among the three; more than a dozen countries have sulfur mustard in their arsenals, and it is the easiest of the chemical agents to synthesize. During World War I, sulfur mustard caused more casualties than all other chemical agents combined. In the 1980s, 45,000 casualties occurred with their use during the Iran–Iraq war.

Sulfur mustard (H and HD) is an alkylating agent that is highly reactive and electrophilic. It induces toxicity through rapid adduct formation with peptides, proteins, RNA, DNA, and cell membranes and disappears from extracellular fluids within a few minutes. Sulfur mustard is an oily liquid with an odor of garlic, horseradish, or mustard. The LD_{50} is approximately 1.5 teaspoons, which can result in a 25% body surface area burn in adults. Clinical effects are somewhat dose dependent. At low doses, vessication occurs, whereas at higher doses, vessication and systemic toxicity are seen. Characteristically, symptoms are delayed for 4 to 8 hours. Skin, eyes, and airways are relatively equally affected. Skin findings include initial erythema that progresses to blister formation over 24 hours. Warm, moist areas are predominantly affected. Ocular findings are similarly delayed and include edema of the lids, conjunctival injection, and with severe exposures, corneal ulceration. Respiratory involvement manifests as a dry, barking cough and hoarseness beginning 4 to 6 hours postexposure. Early tachypnea or dyspnea indicates exposure to a potentially lethal amount of sulfur mustard. In such cases, bronchospasm, bronchiolar obstruction by sloughed pseudomembranous bronchial epithelium, and hemorrhagic pulmonary edema may ensue over 1 to 2 days. Systemic absorption is seen with greater exposures, and results in hematopoietic, gastrointestinal tract, and CNS involvement. Overall, the expected mortality is approximately 3% for those reaching medical facilities. In children, more rapid onset and more severe dermal lesions have been noted and are attributed to their more delicate skin. In addition, Iranian children had a higher frequency of eye, facial, and pulmonary injury that was attributed to a higher vapor concentration closer to the ground, and the children's shorter stature relative to adults.

Lewisite (L) is an oily colorless liquid with the odor of geraniums. It has a potency similar to that of sulfur mustard. It was released by Japan during wartime, and known stockpiles of a Lewisite–mustard mixture are possessed by Russia. Lewisite's active ingredient, trivalent arsenic, inhibits various enzymes throughout the body and interferes with glycolysis; the mechanism for vesication is unclear. In contrast to sulfur mustard exposure, skin irritation and pain are characteristically present within 15 to 30 minutes of Lewisite exposure. Blister formation also occurs more quickly than with sulfur mustard exposure, usually within 2 hours. Lewisite lesions have less surrounding erythema and result in more tissue destruction than those caused by sulfur mustard. Ocular pain and irritation also occur within minutes; however, in most cases, reflex blepharospasm seems to prevent the severe ocular injury seen with mustard exposure. Pulmonary involvement is characterized by immediate upper airway irritation and central airway inflammation. Parenchymal involvement is rare and progression to pulmonary edema occurs only in the most severe cases. Hypotension and hemolytic anemia are rarely seen and result from systemic arsenic toxicity.

Phosgene oxime (CX), an agent that causes extensive tissue damage, is discussed here even though it is not a true vesicant. It is actually a corrosive urticaric with an unknown mechanism of action. Following exposure, instantaneous pain and irritation of the skin, eyes, and airways occur. The affected skin then blanches, turns grayish, and becomes urticarial, erythematous, and edematous. True vesicle formation does not occur. Necrosis of the area may penetrate to the muscle layers and result in eschar formation. Ocular findings are similar to those described for Lewisite exposure. Pulmonary edema is common and bronchiolitis has been described.

The diagnosis of vesicant toxicity is a clinical diagnosis. Urinary thiodiglycol metabolites will confirm exposure to sulfur mustards, but this test is not widely available. Treatment begins with immediate skin and eye decontamination, ideally within 1 to 2 minutes of exposure. This is the only effective way of preventing tissue damage. Late decontamination is recommended to prevent spread to uninvolved areas of the skin and to rescue or medical personnel. Copious detergent and water decontamination is appropriate for the skin. A dilute hypochlorite solution has been recommended in adults for skin decontamination of the relatively water-insoluble mustards and Lewisite; however, this is not recommended in children. Water alone is the preferred decontamination solution for phosgene oxime.

There are no antidotes for sulfur mustard poisoning, although mustard scavengers, antioxidants, nicotinamide-adenine dinucleotide precursors, polymerase inhibitor, corticosteroids, and granulocyte colony stimulating factor are under investigation. As with thermal burns, aggressive airway, fluid, electrolyte, and pain management coupled with prevention of secondary infection with topical antibiotics and sterile dressing changes are the mainstays of therapy. In contrast to thermal burns, mustard burns do not trigger the same magnitude of fluid loss. All burns resulting from caustic chemical agents are classified as major by the American Burn Association and require referral to a burn surgeon. Death most frequently occurs 5 to 10 days after exposure, usually from pulmonary insufficiency and infection. Long-term hospitalization is expected.

British anti-Lewisite (BAL or dimercaprol) is an arsenic chelator that prevents or greatly decreases the severity of skin and eye lesions if applied topically within minutes of Lewisite exposure; however, the topical form is not widely available. Given intramuscularly, BAL reduces the mortality from systemic effects of Lewisite.

Irritant Gases

Phosgene (CG, carbonyl chloride, D-Stoff, or green cross) is a gas with a density four times that of air. Beyond its military application, it is found in the plastics, pharmaceutical, and textile industries. Upon release, it forms a white cloud with a characteristic odor of newly mown hay. It is relatively water insoluble. Only mild initial eye, nose, throat, and upper airway irritation are expected and these may be entirely absent. The major toxicity involves an acid burn to lower airways as phosgene reaches the alveoli and slowly hydrolyzes to carbon dioxide and hydrochloric acid. Acylation of alveolar capillary membranes results in diffuse capillary leak and noncardiogenic pulmonary edema, whose appearance is characteristically delayed for up to 24 hours. This clinically latent period is followed by dyspnea and chest tightness, heralding the onset of pulmonary edema. If the exposure is massive, immediate dyspnea and mucous membrane and eye irritation can occur. The onset of dyspnea or pulmonary edema within 4 hours of exposure suggests a very poor prognosis. Those victims who become symptomatic after 6 hours of exposure generally survive, if intensive medical care is available. Recovery occurs in 3 to 4 days with respiratory supportive care and management of noncardiogenic pulmonary edema. Because exertion is known to increase pulmonary edema from phosgene, rest is mandatory for those exposed. Furthermore, a 24-hour observation period with frequent reassessments is indicated even for asymptomatic patients.

Chlorine is also widely available in the industrial sector, in the setting of laboratories, paper manufacture, swimming pool chemical distribution, and municipal water treatment. When dispersed, this dense green-yellow gas has an acrid, pungent odor. It is of intermediate water solubility, which is consistent with the observation that moderately exposed soldiers in World War I exhibited both central airway damage and pulmonary edema. Early inflammatory injury results from the formation of acids and oxidants upon contact with moist membranes. Immediate ocular and upper airway irritation along with nausea and vomiting are common following mild exposures. More significant exposure results in coughing, hoarseness, and pulmonary edema, usually within 12 to 24 hours. Permanent reactive airways disease has been described following significant chlorine gas inhalation. Care is primarily supportive with the use of humidified oxygen and bronchodilators as needed. The role of nebulized sodium bicarbonate as a neutralizing therapy is controversial. Chlorine may cause dermal injury at high concentration and skin decontamination may be required.

Nitrogen oxides are encountered in the form of silo gas (silo filler's disease), as products of fire combustion, in industrial processes, or as components of military blast weapons, smokes, and obscurants. These oxides have limited water solubility and generally result in mainly lower airway toxicity. Slow conversion of nitrogen oxide to nitric acid in the alveoli results in delayed alveolar injury and pulmonary edema. A triphasic illness typically is seen with initial dyspnea and flulike symptoms, transient improvement, and then worsening dyspnea, heralding the onset of pulmonary edema 24 to 72 hours after exposure. Methemoglobinemia also can occur. Bronchiolitis obliterans, a potential late complication, may be prevented by the use of steroids.

Ammonia, widely available as a fertilizer and industrial chemical, is a highly water soluble, colorless, alkaline corrosive gas. It has good warning properties and rapidly reacts with water to form ammonium hydroxide. The presence of ammonia is usually obvious based on its characteristic pungent odor and immediate induction of symptoms of eye, mucous membrane, and throat irritation. Lower airway involvement resulting in bronchospasm, pulmonary edema, and residual reactive airways disease have all been described following massive exposures, especially in those who have been trapped in confined spaces. Treatment is supportive with humidified oxygen and bronchodilators. Anhydrous ammonia is extremely hazardous to the eyes and can penetrate the anterior chamber within 1 minute of exposure. Therefore, following ocular irrigation in symptomatic patients, evaluation for corneal burns should be considered and a careful ophthalmologic examination is warranted.

Overall treatment for irritant gases is supportive and involves removal from the source of exposure, application of humidified oxygen, and enforced rest. Flushing of the eyes and skin may be necessary. Copious airway secretions, hypoxia, bronchospasm, and pulmonary edema should be anticipated. Antibiotics are reserved for those with positive sputum gram stains or cultures. No human studies have shown benefit from the use of steroids. Their use may be considered in those with underlying reactive airway disease or nitrogen oxide exposure (see above).

Cyanides

Cyanides (AC, hydrocyanic acid; CK, cyanogen chloride) are discussed in detail in Chapter 73.

Riot Control Agents

Riot control agents are a group of compounds that cause transient but intensely noxious effects on exposure. They include CS, CN or mace, and OC or capsaicin or pepper spray. Although generally considered to be only briefly incapacitating, fatalities from pulmonary edema have occurred following large exposures in confined spaces. Typically, symptoms include immediate irritation of the eyes and respiratory tract, blepharospasm, lacrimation, coughing, sneezing, and rhinorrhea, followed by a burning sensation of exposed skin and mucous membranes. Nausea, vomiting, headache, and photophobia may be seen. These symptoms usually disappear within a few hours after cessation of the exposure. Burns and sensitization of the skin have been described, especially if contact with the agent is prolonged. Long-term corneal damage is more likely to occur with CN than CS. Management includes removal of the patient from the area, copious irrigation of the eyes with normal saline, and skin decontamination with detergent and water. Contact with water can briefly exacerbate skin symptoms from CN. The use of bleach solutions to decontaminate the skin is not recommended because this may increase irritation or trigger blister formation from some agents. Patients with preexisting lung disease should be observed carefully for bronchospasm.

Incapacitating Agents

Military incapacitating agents produce physiologic or mental effects that render the exposed victim unable to perform assigned duties. These agents are generally not lethal, but recovery may take several hours to days. The anticholinergic deliriant, 3-quinuclidinyl benzilate (QNB, BZ) is of military interest. BZ's clinical profile most closely represents that of atropine, with a slower onset and longer duration of action. Recognition of an anticholinergic toxidrome is key to diagnosing BZ toxicity. Expected signs and symptoms are delirium, hallucinations, mydriasis, tachycardia, ileus, dry mucous membranes, absent axillary sweat, urinary retention, and hyperthermia. Treatment involves supportive care and sedation with benzodiazepines to prevent hyperthermia and rhabdomyolysis. In the past, physostigmine was used to reverse the action of BZ, and was associated with untoward side effects. Its use should be reserved for patients with refractory seizures or profound tachycardia. Incapacitation can be produced by a variety of other chemical agents including stimulants, potent opioids, such as carfentanyl, hallucinogens, or nausea-producing drugs. Their battlefield use is problematic, but covert or terrorist use is possible. As a recent example of non-battlefield use, the Russian military ended a hostage crisis in Moscow by deploying a potent gas. Over 100 fatalities and more than 400 hospitalizations resulted. Definitive identification of the chemical is pending at this time, but based on clinical features that included a response to naloxone, an opioid derivative is suspected.

RADIOLOGIC AND NUCLEAR AGENTS

Children may be exposed to radiation through the detonation of a nuclear weapon, an accident at a nuclear power plant, dispersal of radionuclides by conventional explosives, or the crash of a transport vehicle. The short- and long-term consequences of a radiation disaster are significantly greater in children. Acutely, this is based on increased incorporation of radionuclides due to a relatively higher minute ventilation. Long-term, children, with their longer life expectancy, have a greater risk of developing cancer or other radiation effects, even when exposed in utero.

Potassium iodide (KI) is of proven value for thyroid protection, but must be given before or within several hours of exposure, suggesting its placement in homes, schools, and child care centers. Radioactive dispersal devices (dirty bombs) generally would not contain radioiodines, so administering KI after detonation is currently not recommended. Graded dosing scales for KI exist (www.fda.gov/cder/guidance/index.htm). These should be adhered to whenever possible, but if impractical, the overall benefits for small children receiving standard adult doses of KI (130 mg) instead of lower doses far exceed the small risks of overdosing.

Children exposed only to radiation energy do not require decontamination. Those who have surface contamination with radioactive particulate matter or have internal contamination from inhaled or ingested particles are a potential hazard. Decontamination is outlined in Chapter 14. This process is guided by health physicists with appropriate radioactivity detection equipment and swabs of the nares and skin surfaces, along with surveying all urine and stool.

REPORTING

Recognition of a large number of patients presenting with similar or unexpected signs and symptoms, a similar exposure histories, at an unexpected time of the year, should trigger the suspicion of an outbreak. Any suspected outbreak or bioterrorism incident should be reported immediately to the local health department. Local and federal law enforcement agencies should also be notified of suspected terrorism. The risk of civilian uses of personal protective equipment, such as gas masks for children, is believed to currently outweigh any potential benefit. The misuse of such devices has led to fatalities from suffocation.

SUGGESTED READINGS

Advanced Hazmat Life Support (AHLS) for Toxic Terrorism. 1st ed. Tuscon: Walter FG and Arizona Board of Regents; 2003. Available from URL: aemrc.Arizona.edu.

American Academy of Pediatrics Policy Statement: Radiation disasters and children. *Pediatrics* 1111455, 2003.

American Academy of Pediatrics: Chemical-biological terrorism and its impact on children: A subject review. *Pediatrics* 105:662, 2000.

Bradley BJ, Gresham LS, Sidelinger DE, et al: Pediatric health professionals and public health response. *Pediatr Ann* 32:87, 2003.

Burklow TR, Yu CE, Madsen JM: Industrial chemicals: Terrorist weapons of opportunity. *Pediatr Ann* 32:230, 2003.

Henretig FM, Ciesklak TJ, Eitzen EM: Biological and chemical terrorism. *J Pediatr* 141:311, 2002.

Lifschitz M, Shahak E, Lafer S: Carbamate and organophosphate poisoning in young children. *Pediatr Emerg Care* 15:102–103, 1999.

Markenson D, Redlener I: *Pediatric preparedness for disasters and terrorism: A national consensus conference executive summary.* Available from URL: www.bt.cdc.gov/children/pdf/working/execsumm03.pdf

Patt HA, Feigin RD: Diagnosis and management of suspected cases of bioterrorism: A pediatric perspective. *Pediatrics* 109: 685, 2002.

Rotenberg JS, Burklow TR, Selanikio JS: Weapons of mass destruction: The decontamination of children. *Pediatr Ann* 32:261, 2003.

Rotenberg JS: Diagnosis and management of nerve agent exposure. *Pediatr Ann* 32:242, 2003.

Waecker NJ, Hale BR: Smallpox vaccination: What the pediatrician needs to know. *Pediatr Ann* 32:178, 2003.

Wax PM, Becker CE, Curry SC: Unexpected "gas" casualties in Moscow: A medical toxicology perspective. *Ann Emerg Med* 41:700–705, 2003.

Yu CE: Vesicant agents and children. *Pediatr Ann* 32:254, 2003

Yu CE: Medical response to radiation-related terrorism. *Pediatr Ann* 32:169, 2003.

Zweiner RJ, Ginsberg CM: Organophosphate and carbamate poisoning in infants and children. *Pediatrics* 81:121–126, 1988.

16

Gastrointestinal Decontamination

Timothy B. Erickson
Ken Kulig

HIGH-YIELD FACTS

- In asymptomatic children presenting with nontoxic ingestions, observation alone is adequate without any gastrointestinal decontamination.

- Ipecac is rarely useful in pediatric ingestions in either the home or the emergency setting and is no longer recommended by the American Academy of Pediatrics.

- Activated charcoal is the safest mode of gastrointestinal decontamination method, has the fewest side effects, and should be used in the majority of toxic ingestions.

- Cathartic agents are not necessary in the pediatric patient and multiple doses may result in significant dehydration and electrolyte disturbances

- Whole bowel irrigation with an osmotically neutral and electrolyte safe polyethyleneglycol solution may be indicated in a limited number pediatric toxic ingestions.

CASE PRESENTATION

A normally healthy 3-year-old child presents after ingesting several over-the-counter (OTC) medications from the family bathroom medicine cabinet 2 hours prior to presentation in the emergency department (ED). The child is crying, but alert with stable vital signs. The parents are frantic and demanding their child's stomach be pumped. What is the best management approach in regards to gastric decontamination in this child?

GASTROINTESTINAL DECONTAMINATION

Gastrointestinal (GI) decontamination is one of the more controversial topics in toxicology. Whether patients are managed with syrup of ipecac, gastric lavage, cathartics, or activated charcoal alone depends on the toxicity of the particular drug, the quantity and time of ingestion, and patients' conditions. If children ingest a nontoxic agent or a very small amount of a poison unlikely to cause toxicity, no gastric decontamination measures are necessary. However, if the ingestion is recent and the child is symptomatic, or the toxin ingested may cause delayed toxicity, gastric evacuation is recommended. Several clinical trials have been conducted to determine which of the gastric decontamination modalities are most efficacious. However, the investigations either involve adult volunteers who ingested subtoxic amounts of an agent and received decontamination at a set postingestion time or involve mild-to-moderately poisoned patients, and exclude patients with significant overdoses. Few children have been included in these trials. Therefore, these studies must be critically interpreted prior to their definitive application in the clinical setting, especially in the pediatric patient. Most treatment modalities have focused on stomach evacuation; however, the ultimate goal should be to decontaminate the entire GI tract. According to the

2001 American Poison control database, of the approximately 250,000 adult and pediatric patients who received some form of gastric evacuation, 59% received activated charcoal, 22% a cathartic agent, 12% gastric lavage, 6% syrup of ipecac, and 1% whole bowel irrigation.

Induction of Emesis

Syrup of ipecac is the most commonly used emetic agent (Figure 16–1). It is a mixture of alkaloids consisting of emetine and cephaeline, which are strong emetic agents that stimulate the gastric mucosa as well as the brain's chemoreceptor trigger zone. Ipecac gained popularity for home use in pediatric poisonings in the 1960s. However, its use has largely fallen out of favor in the ED and prehospital settings and is no longer advocated in the heath care setting for treatment of the acutely poisoned patient. In 1985, it was administered in 15% of all oral exposures reported to poison control centers. In 2001, it was administered in only 0.7% of cases.

Ipecac can be expected to induce vomiting within 20 to 60 minutes. The recovery of ingested material in the vomitus is approximately 30% if ipecac is administered within 5 minutes of ingestion, and far less if delayed beyond 1 hour. Unfortunately, most children experience three episodes of vomiting, which often delays the administration of activated charcoal. In human volunteer studies, ipecac was not able to significantly decrease absorption of drugs after 30 to 60 minutes, and was inferior when compared to activated charcoal alone.

Ipecac is contraindicated in children under 6 months of age, in patients with evidence of a diminished gag reflex and potential for coma or seizures, and in the ingestion of most hydrocarbons, acids, alkalis, and sharp

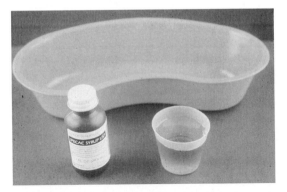

Fig. 16–1. Routine induction of emesis with syrup of ipecac is no longer recommended.

objects. Complications following ipecac use that have been reported in the literature include aspiration pneumonia, dehydration owing to protracted vomiting, diaphragmatic rupture and death, Mallory-Weiss tears of the esophagus, and gastric rupture.

Currently, the use of ipecac is not recommended by the American Academy of Pediatrics or the American Association of Poison Centers. However, there are selected toxicologists who continue to believe that ipecac may have a very limited role in specific pediatric ingestions in the prehospital setting. The use of ipecac syrup may be an acceptable benefit-to-risk ratio in *rare* situations in which:

- There is no contraindication to the use of ipecac syrup and there is substantial risk of serious toxicity to the victim with no alternative therapy available or effective means to decrease GI absorption (e.g., activated charcoal).

- There will be a delay of greater than 1 hour before the patient will arrive at an emergency medical facility and ipecac syrup can be administered within 60 minutes of the ingestion.

- Ipecac administration will not adversely affect more definitive treatment that might be provided at a hospital.

Owing to the ethical considerations involving clinical trials with pediatric patients, the use of ipecac in the prehospital setting will remain an area of controversy for the foreseeable future.

Gastric Lavage

Ideally, gastric lavage mechanically removes toxins from the stomach through a large-bore orogastric tube. In pediatric patients, the size of the lavage tube ranges from 16 to 32 Fr, depending on the age of the patient. In fact, gastric lavage removes, at best, up to 40% of the ingested toxin. In some cases, the holes at the end of the evacuation tube are too small to allow pill fragments to be suctioned into the lavage tube lumen (Figure 16–2). It is important to note that gastric lavage does not remove toxic agents from the intestinal tract, where the majority of drug absorption occurs. It is also important to realize that there have been no clinical trials evaluating the efficacy of gastric lavage in neonates, infants, and toddlers.

Gastric lavage should not be routinely performed in overdosed pediatric patients. This mode of gastric decontamination is reserved for intoxicated children who present within 1 hour after ingesting a potentially life-

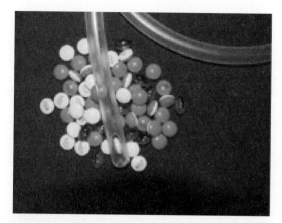

Fig. 16–2. Even large bore gastric lavage tubes may not have sufficient size to aspirate pills and medication fragments.

threatening amount of a drug. Airway protection by endotracheal intubation prior to lavage is indicated in children with a depressed level of consciousness to avoid aspiration pneumonitis. In these cases, the risk of intubation must be weighed against the potential benefits of gastric lavage. After verifying proper orogastric tube placement, the stomach contents are aspirated, then irrigated with 50- to 100-mL aliquots of normal saline until the returned lavage fluid is clear; in adolescents, 250-mL aliquots are recommended.

In patients in whom lavage may be indicated, it is theoretically attractive to give charcoal down the tube immediately upon insertion, followed by lavage, followed by charcoal. This obviously would not apply to drugs not bound to charcoal, but it does address the concern that process of lavage moves drugs from the stomach into the small intestine, thereby enhancing absorption. Theoretically, the charcoal administered prior to lavage binds to drug that would be forced through the pylorus by the lavage fluid, limiting the drug's absorption.

If the child has recently ingested an elixir or liquid, a simple nasogastric tube is adequate to avoid orogastric injury from traumatic insertion of a large-bore tube. Theoretically, there may be some efficacy for lavage beyond 1 hour when the agent ingested slows gut motility, such as with anticholinergics or opioids, or when the toxin forms concretions, such as with iron and salicylates. However, this has never been substantiated in the toxicology literature.

Gastric lavage is contraindicated in ingestions of most hydrocarbons, acids, alkalis, and sharp objects. Although relatively safe when performed properly, complications including aspiration, esophageal perforation, bleeding,

electrolyte imbalance, and hypothermia have been described. Therefore, the clinician must have adequate rationale to perform lavage.

Activated Charcoal

The majority of poisoned children who are not critically ill can be managed safely and effectively in the ED setting with charcoal alone. Activated charcoal is an odorless, tasteless, fine black powder that is effective in adsorbing many toxins. Recent charcoal products have been superactivated, resulting in large surface areas of up to 3000 m^2/g, allowing for maximum absorptive power. It has now become the most frequently used and most effective GI decontamination agent. Activated charcoal can be administered rapidly and is most beneficial when administered within 1 hour after the ingestion. Activated charcoal's absorptive properties are effective beyond the gastric mucosa; it absorbs drugs throughout the small intestine.

Most younger children will refuse to drink charcoal due to its gritty texture and threatening appearance (Figure 16–3). Children can be distracted by administrating the charcoal in an opaque Styrofoam cup with a lid and straw, or by adding flavoring to enhance its palatability. Additionally, medical personnel may allow reliable parents to administer the charcoal to the child. Occasionally a patient may be unable to or may refuse to drink charcoal. In these scenarios, when charcoal is clearly

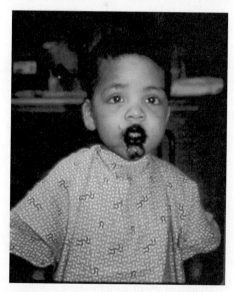

Fig. 16–3. Although safe and effective, activated charcoal administration may a challenge in younger pediatric patients.

indicated, a small nasogastric tube may need to be inserted to facilitate its administration.

The recommended initial dose of activated charcoal is summarized in Table 16–1. Although most sources recommend an activated charcoal dose of 1 mg/kg, if the amount of drug ingested is known, an accurate dose of activated charcoal can be calculated as a 10:1 ratio of charcoal to the ingested agent. However, even this 10:1 ratio, although adequate in most scenarios, has never been shown to be as efficacious or superior to higher ratios. Most patients, however, will not tolerate larger doses.

For some drugs, such as theophylline, phenobarbital, and carbamazepine, multiple dosing of activated charcoal may enhance elimination due primarily to enteroenteric circulation of the drug. Repeated use of charcoal preparations premixed with cathartics such as sorbitol is to be avoided, because dehydration and electrolyte imbalance may result.

Activated charcoal is probably the safest method of decontamination. It is the preferred mode of GI decontamination when the history of the overdose or time of ingestion is unclear, because delayed administration may be beneficial with minimal adverse side effects. Rare cases of vomiting, constipation, obstruction, and aspiration have been reported, but the incidence, particularly in pediatric cases, is extremely low. The administration of activated charcoal in the home or prehospital setting is gaining popularity as a superior substitute for syrup of ipecac. Activated charcoal is neither effective nor indicated in heavy metal poisonings, such as with iron, lithium, or borates, ingestions of ethanol-containing products, or following ingestion of acids or alkalis where gastric visualization or endoscopy may be required.

Cathartics

Cathartics are osmotically active agents that eliminate toxins from the GI tract by inducing diarrhea. The most common agents are sorbitol, magnesium citrate, and magnesium sulfate (Figure 16–4). It is often recommended that one dose of a cathartic be administered with the first dose of charcoal, but studies have not shown a benefit of cathartic plus charcoal versus charcoal alone. No studies have been conducted to evaluate cathartics as the sole decontamination modality in the overdose setting. Studies investigating the use of sorbitol in combination with activated charcoal have found that it enhances charcoal's palatability. As a result, younger children may be more accepting of its oral administration. In the pediatric population, cathartic agents have been reported to result in hypermagnesemia, severe dehydration, and electrolyte imbalances if used excessively or in repeated doses. In children less than 12 months of age, it is generally recommended that activated charcoal be administered with water only, without any cathartic agent.

Whole Bowel Irrigation

Originally used as a preoperative bowel preparation, whole bowel irrigation is now used in the overdose setting to flush the toxin through the GI tract and prevent further absorption. In theory, it may also produce a concentration gradient that allows previously absorbed toxins to diffuse back into the gastrointestinal tract. The solution used is nonabsorbable, isotonic polyethylene glycol electrolyte solution that, unlike cathartic agents, does not appear to create fluid or electrolyte disturbances (Figure 16–5). The dose is 25 mL/kg/h for small children and 1 to 2 L/h for adolescents. The irrigation process is continued until the rectal effluent is clear, which is usually in 2 to 6 hours.

Although much of the evidence for whole bowel irrigation is anecdotal, this modality has been used in the pediatric population with minimal to no side effects. In case reports, it has been effective in ingestions not well absorbed by activated charcoal such as lead paint chips, iron tablets, and button batteries. With these cases, an ab-

Table 16–1. Doses for Gastric Decontamination

Syrup of ipecac
    6–12 months of age: 5–10 mL with 15 mL/kg
      clear fluids
    12 months–12 years: 15 mL ipecac plus 8 oz
      clear fluids
    >12 years: 30 mL ipecac plus 16 oz water
Activated charcoal
    1–2 g/kg prepared as a slurry in water or sorbitol
      to achieve a 25% concentration
    For repetitive dosing: 1 g/kg every 2–3 h without
      sorbitol or cathartic
Cathartics
    Sorbitol (35% solution): 4 mL/kg of commercial
      solution diluted
    1:1 Magnesuim citrate (10% solution): 4 mL/kg
    Magnesium sulfate: (10% solution): 1–2 mL/kg
Whole bowel irrigation
    High-molecular-weight polyethylene glycol
      solution @ 25 mL/kg/h for small children
    1–2 L/h for adolescent

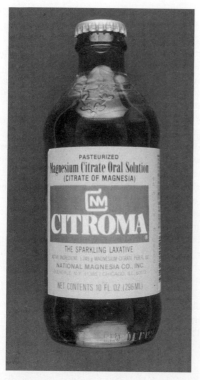

Fig. 16–4. Cathartic agents can cause severe electrolyte and fluid disturbances in young children and should be used cautiously.

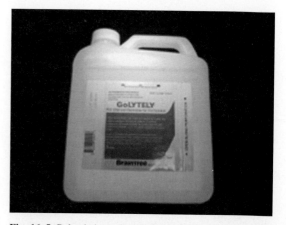

Fig. 16–5. Polyethylene glycol solution is an osmotically safe solution used for whole bowel irrigation

dominal radiograph demonstrating radio-opacities can be followed serially to document the effectiveness of whole bowel irrigation. In addition, its use has been documented with cocaine and opiate packet ingestions as well as sustained-release products such as calcium channel antagonists. For agents well absorbed by charcoal, whole bowel irrigation is discouraged because it may actually decrease the efficacy of activated charcoal.

CASE OUTCOME

The 3-year-old child continues to demonstrate stable vital signs. One dose of activated charcoal is administered orally, and the child tolerates it well. The parents return to the ED with an OTC decongestant containing diphenhydramine, children's chewable acetaminophen, mouthwash, and vitamin pills without iron. The child's labs including serum glucose are within normal limits. Serum acetaminophen, salicylate, and iron levels are determined to be nontoxic. The ethanol level is 10 mg/dL. The

child is admitted for overnight observation and recovers uneventfully.

SUGGESTED READINGS

American Academy of Pediatrics: Committee on Injury, Violence, and Poison Prevention: Poison treatment in the home. *Pediatrics* 112:1182–1185, 2003.

Arnold FJ, Hodges JB, Barta PA, et al: Evacuation of the efficacy of lavage and emesis in the treatment of salicylate poisoning. *Pediatrics* 23:286, 1959.

Barceloux D, McGuigan M, Hartigan-Go K: Position statement: Cathartics. American Academy of Clinical Toxicology; European Association of Poisons Centres and Clinical Toxicologists. *J Toxicol Clin Toxicol* 35:742–752, 1997.

Bond GR: Home syrup of ipecac use does not reduce emergency department use or improve outcome. *Pediatrics* Nov 112: 1061–1064, 2003.

Buckley N, Dawson AH, Howarth D, et al: Slow-release verapamil poisoning: Use of polyethylene glycol whole bowel irrigation lavage and high dose calcium. *Med J Aust* 158:202–204, 1993.

Burton BT, Bayer MJ, Barron L, et al: Comparison of activated charcoal and gastric lavage in the prevention of aspirin absorption. *J Emerg Med* 1:411, 1984.

Chyka PA, Seger D: Position statement: Single-dose activated charcoal. American Academy of Clinical Toxicology; European Association of Poisons Centres and Clinical Toxicologists. *J Toxicol Clin Toxicol* 35:721–741, 1997.

Corby DC, Decker W: Clinical comparison of pharmacologic emetics in children. *Pediatrics* 42:361, 1968.

Corby DC, Lisiandro RC, Lehman RH, et al: The efficacy of methods used to evacuate the stomach after acute ingestions. *Pediatrics* 40:871, 1967.

Erickson T: Toxicology: Ingestions and smoke inhalation. In: Gausche-Hill M, Fuchs S, Yamamoto L, eds: *APLS: The Pediatric Emergency Medicine Resource*. 4th ed. Boston: AAP and ACEP; 2004:234–267.

Everson GW, Bertaccini EJ, O'Leary J: Use of whole bowel irrigation in an infant following iron overdose. *Am J Emerg Med* 9:366, 1991.

Henretig FM: Special considerations in the poisoned pediatric patient. *Emerg Med Clin North Am* 12:549–567, 1994.

Holt LE, Holz PH: The black bottle. *Pediatrics* 63:306, 1963.

Kaczorowski JM, Wax PM: Five days of whole bowel irrigation in a case of pediatric iron ingestion. *Ann Emerg Med* 27:258, 1996.

Koren G: Medications which can kill a toddler with one tablet or teaspoonful. *Clin Toxicol* 31:407–414, 1993.

Kornberg AE, Dolgin J: Pediatric ingestions: Charcoal alone versus ipecac and charcoal. *Ann Emerg Med* 20:648, 1991.

Kulig K: Initial management of toxic substances. *N Engl J Med* 326:1677–1681, 1992.

Kulig K: Gastrointestinal decontamination. In: Ford M, DeLaney K, Ling Let al, eds: *Clinical Toxicology*. Philadelphia: Saunders; 2001:34–41.

Liebelt EL, Shannon MW: Small doses, big problems: A selected review of highly toxic common medications. *Pediatr Emerg Care* 9:292–297, 1993.

Litovitz TL, Schwartz-Klein W, Rogers, GC, et al: 2001 Annual Report of the AAPCC Toxic Exposure/Surveillance System. *Am J Emerg Med* 20:391–452, 2002.

Roberge RJ, Martin TG: Whole bowel irrigation in acute oral lead intoxication. *Ann Emerg Med* 10:577, 1992.

Rosenberg PJ, Livingstone DJ, McLellan BA: Effect of whole-bowel irrigation on the antidotal efficacy of oral activate charcoal. *Ann Emerg Med* 17:681, 1988.

Shannon M: The demise of ipecac? *Pediatrics* 112:1180–1181, 2003.

Smith SW, Ling LJ, Halstenson CE: Whole-bowel irrigation as a treatment for acute lithium overdose. *Ann Emerg Med* 20:536, 1991.

Tenenbein M: Whole bowel irrigation for toxic ingestions. *Clin Toxicol* 23:177, 1985.

Tenenbein M: Whole bowel irrigation in iron poisoning. *Pediatrics* 111:142, 1987.

Tennenbein M: Position statement: Whole bowel irrigation. American Academy of Clinical Toxicology; European Association of Poisons Centres and Clinical Toxicologists. *J Toxicol Clin Toxicol* 35:753–762, 1997.

Vale JA: Position statement: gastric lavage. American Academy of Clinical Toxicology; European Association of Poisons Centres and Clinical Toxicologists. *J Toxicol Clin Toxicol* 35:711–719, 1997.

17

Antidotes

Suzan Mazor
Steven E. Aks

HIGH-YIELD FACTS

- Antidotes should not be used indiscriminately, particularly in the pediatric patient with an unknown ingestion or overdose, because overuse often complicates the clinical situation.

- It is important for practitioners involved in the care of poisoned patients to be aware of their hospital's antidote supply.

- A critical action when administering any antidote is to routinely double check the dose and concentration of the drug.

An *antidote* is a remedy or other agent used to neutralize or counteract the effects of a poison. Experimentally, an antidote can also be described as an agent that can raise the LD_{50} (lethal dose for 50% of subjects) of a toxin. There are a limited number of pharmaceutical antidotes that are clinically efficacious, and it is important for clinicians to know the specific indications for their administration. Antidotes should not be used indiscriminately, particularly in the pediatric patient with an unknown ingestion or overdose, because overuse often complicates the clinical situation. In weighing the benefits and risks of giving a particular antidote, consider the patient's clinical status, laboratory values, expected pharmaceutical action of the toxin, and possible adverse reactions associated with the antidote.

It is important for practitioners involved in the care of poisoned patients to be aware of their hospital's antidote supply. Several studies have demonstrated inadequate stocking of common antidotes. A list of minimum recommended stocking amounts for common antidotes is listed in Table 3–2.

Finally, a critical action when administering any antidote is to routinely double check the dose and concentration of the drug. A pediatric patient can be easily poisoned because of an iatrogenic 10-fold dosing error. Some dosing errors, such as with naloxone, can be relatively inconsequential, whereas a 10-fold dosing error of sodium nitrite can have a significant clinical consequence. In addition to Table 17–1, a regional poison control center, clinical toxicologist, or neonatologist can be excellent sources for dosing confirmation, particularly in small children weighing less than 10 kg.

Table 17–1. Common Antidotes

Antidote	Indications	Dose	Comments
n-Acetyl cysteine (NAC)	Acetaminophen overdose, possibly useful for carbon tetrachloride, chloroform, pennyroyal.	PO/NGT: 140 mg/kg then 70 mg/kg q4h × 17 doses; if started late after ingestion, continue dosing until resolution of hepatic dysfunction. IV: (consult poison center) 140 mg/kg then 70 mg/kg q4h × 11 doses; if started late after ingestion, continue dosing until resolution of hepatic dysfunction.	Most effective if given in first 8 hours postingestion. *Caution:* Unpleasant odor, nausea, vomiting with oral dosing; anaphylactoid reaction with IV dosing; IV dosing may be useful for patients with hepatic failure, pregnancy or inability to tolerate PO dosing. In young pediatric patients such as infants, IV preparation and dosing may cause fluid overload if not monitored carefully.
Antivenin, Black widow spider (*Lactrodectus mactans*)	Severe hypertension, muscle spasms not alleviated by analgesics and muscle relaxants. Indicated for patients at the extremes of age.	1–2 vials IV slowly over 15–30 min.	*Caution:* Equine serum derived—immediate hypersensitivity, serum sickness 10–14 days. Premedicate for anaphylaxis if known equine serum hypersensitivity. Most symptoms of *Lactrodectus* envenomation are alleviated by supportive care; consider antivenin in extremes of age (<5 or >65 y), pregnant women with threatened abortion.
Antivenin, Crotaline	Significant envenomation by Crotaline species: rattlesnake, cottonmouth, copperhead snakes	*Equine-derived (Wyeth-Ayerst polyvalent):* Mild: 5 vials slow IV Moderate: 10 vials slow IV Severe: 15 vials slow IV *Ovine-derived (CroFab):* 4–6 vials IV slowly, may repeat dose of 4–6 vials if control of envenomation not achieved, then 2 vials IV q6h × 3	*Caution:* Equine- or ovine-derived products: immediate hypersensitivity; serum sickness 10–14 days. Premedicate for anaphylaxis if known equine/ovine serum hypersensitivity. Close monitoring in ICU setting during infusion. Dosage not weight based; children may require as much as adults.
Antivenin, Elapid (*Micrurus fulvius*)	Eastern or Texas coral snake.	4–10 vials IV over 15–30 min.	Equine serum derived—immediate hypersensitivity; serum sickness 10–14 days. Premedicate for anaphylaxis if known equine serum hypersensitivity.

Atropine	Bradycardia due to cardiotoxic drugs. Cholinergic poisoning due to organophosphate/ carbamate insecticides, nerve gas agents.	*Cardiotoxic drugs:* Pediatric: 0.02 mg/kg (min 0.1 mg) IV Adult: 0.5–1.0 mg IV *Organophosphates/carbamates:* Pediatric: Test dose 0.05 mg/kg IV, double the dose q5–10 min until clearing of tracheo bronchial secretions. Adult: Test dose 1–2 mg IV, double the dose q5–10 min until clearing of tracheobronchial secretions.	*Caution:* Myasthenia gravis, narrow-angle glaucoma, hypertension, coronary ischemia, and urinary obstruction. Large repeated doses needed in organophosphate poisoning.
Benzodiazepine	Agitation, seizures, stimulant overdose (cocaine/ amphetamines) chloroquine or aminoquinolone overdose.	*Midazolam* Pediatric: 0.1 mg/kg IV/IM Adult: 1 mg IV/IM q2–3 min PRN *Diazepam* Pediatric: 0.1 mg/kg IV/IM Adult: 2–5 mg IV/IM, repeat in 10–15 min. *Lorazepam* Pediatric: 0.04 mg/kg IV/IM Adult: 1–2 mg IV/IM	*Caution:* Respiratory/CNS depression
Bicarbonate, sodium	Cyclic antidepressants, salicylate, phenobarbital poisoning, metabolic acidosis, wide-complex tachydysrhythmias, urinary alkalinization.	*Serum alkalinization:* 1 mEq/kg IVP, repeat PRN, goal is serum pH 7.50–7.55 *Urine alkalinization:* 150 mEq in 1L D_5W at twice maintenance IV, goal is urine pH 7–8.	*Caution:* May cause CHF, excessive alkalosis, hypokalemia. Monitor potassium, must have adequate potassium, or it will be difficult to alkalinize the urine.
Botulin antitoxin trivalent A,B,E	Clinical botulism, prior to onset of paralysis.	1–2 vials IV slowly q2–4h for 4–5 doses.	*Caution:* Distributed by the CDC. Not for infant botulism. Only binds free toxins. Equine serum derived—immediate hypersensitivity, serum sickness 10–14 days. Premedicate for anaphylaxis if know equine serum hypersensitivity.

(Continues)

Table 17–1. Common Antidotes (*continued*)

Antidote	Indications	Dose	Comments
Calcium	Calcium channel blocker overdose, hypocalcemia due to ethylene glycol, hydrofluoric acid toxicity. Hypermagnesemia. Hyperkalemia with cardiac toxicity. Hydrofluoric acid burn.	*Pediatric:* 0.1–0.2 mL/kg 10% Ca chloride, or 0.2–0.3 mL/kg 10% Ca gluconate. *Adult:* 5–10 mL 10% Ca chloride, or 10–20 mL of 10% Ca gluconate *Cutaneous hydrofluoric acid burns:* Topical Ca gluconate gel: Mix 25 mL 10% Ca gluconate with 5 oz KY jelly Subcutaneous injection: 10% Ca gluconate	*Caution:* Avoid in digoxin toxicity, can cause asystole, CaCl corrosive to skin, SC tissue. Incompatible with certain IV solutions.
Charcoal, activated	Toxins well adsorbed by activated charcoal.	*Pediatric:* 1 g/kg *Adults:* 50–100 g	*Contraindications:* Unprotected airway, hydrocarbon ingestion, caustic ingestion, absence of anatomically intact GI tract. *Caution:* Some preparations of activated charcoal are premixed with a cathartic agent (sorbitol). Repeat doses of sorbitol have been associated with an increased likelihood of emesis and hypernatremic dehydration. Repeat doses of charcoal with sorbitol should never be used.
Cyanide antidote kit (Taylor cyanide antidote kit)	Cyanide poisoning	*Nitrites:* Amyl nitrite: 1–2 amp crushed, inhaled *or* Sodium nitrite (preferred): *Pediatric:* 0.15–0.30 mL/kg of 3% solution IV (10 cc maximum) (slow, over at least 5 min) *Adult:* 300 mg (10 mL of 3% solution) IV over 5 min	*Caution:* Nitrites may cause hypotension, anemic patients at risk for excessive methemoglobinemia. Sodium thiosulfate may cause hypernatremia, sulfa allergic reaction. *Note:* Dosing of sodium nitrite can be based on weight and hemoglobin if known. See cyanide kit for table.

		Sodium thiosulfate: Pediatric: 1.65 mL/kg of 25% solution IV, may repeat in 1 hour. Adult: 12.5 g (50 mL of 25% solution) IV, may repeat in 1 hour.	
Dantrolene	Muscle rigidity due to malignant hyperthermia, neuroleptic malignant syndrome, possibly miscellaneous causes of drug-induced muscular hyperactivity/hyperthermia.	1–2 mg/kg IV bolus, repeat q5–10 min PRN, max 10 mg/kg.	*Caution:* Muscle weakness, respiratory depression, hepatitis, venous irritation, thrombophlebitis.
Deferoxamine (Desferal)	Iron toxicity	10–15 mg/kg/h IV, may increase to 35 mg/kg/h in severe poisonings, continue until metabolic acidosis has resolved.	*Caution:* Hypotension if >15 mg/kg/h, flushing, urticaria. Prolonged (>24 h) infusion associated with ARDS, *Yersinia* sepsis, transient blindness (rare).
Digoxin-specific antibody fragments (Digibind, Digifab)	Digoxin, digitoxin, cardiac glycoside toxicity.	1 vial (38 mg) binds 0.5 mg digoxin. If digoxin level is known: # vials = digoxin level (ng/mL) × wt (kg)/100. Empiric dosing: Acute overdose in child or adult: 10–20 vials, chronic overdose in child: 1–2 vials, adult 3–6 vials.	*Caution:* Falsely elevated digoxin levels after use; exacerbation of heart failure, atrial fibrillation in patients requiring digoxin.
Dimercaprol (BAL)	Use in conjunction with EDTA for lead-induced encephalopathy and severe lead toxicity. Chelation of inorganic mercury and arsenic.	*For lead encephalopathy and severe lead toxicity:* 75 mg/m² IM q4h for 5 days (25 mg/kg/d in 6 divided doses IM). First dose should precede the first EDTA dose by 4 hours.	*Caution:* Renal toxicity, fever, nausea, vomiting, urticaria, cholinergic symptoms. Contraindicated in peanut allergy (uses peanut oil vehicle).

(Continues)

Table 17–1. Common Antidotes (*continued*)

Antidote	Indications	Dose	Comments
		For severe arsenic poisoning: 3 mg/kg IM q4h × 2 days, then q12h × 7–10 days. *For inorganic mercury poisoning:* 5 mg/kg IM once, then 2.5 mg/kg q8–12h for 1 day, then 2.5 mg/kg q12–24h until clinical improvement is evident.	*Caution:* Nausea, vomiting, chills, nephrotoxicity, hypercalcemia.
EDTA (calcium disodium EDTA, CaNa$_2$-EDTA)	Use in conjunction with dimercaprol in the management of symptomatic lead poisoning and lead encephalopathy.	*For lead encephalopathy:* 50 mg/kg^2/d continuous IV infusion over 24 h (1500 mg/m^2/d), start infusion 4 h after dimercaprol dose. *For symptomatic children without encephalopathy:* 20–30 mg/kg/d continuous IV infusion (1000 mg/m^2/d), start infusion 4 hours after dimercaprol dose.	
Ethanol	Methanol or ethylene glycol poisoning when fomepizole is not available.	IV: 10 mL/kg load as 10% solution, maintenance 1–2 mL/kg/h. PO: 2.5 mL/kg load as 40% (80 proof) dose, maintenance 0.3–0.5 mL/kg/h. Goal: level of 100 mg/dL.	*Caution:* Hypoglycemia in pediatric population disulfiram reaction, inebriation, CNS and respiratory depression. Double infusion rate during hemodialysis.
Flumazenil (Romazicon)	Known, pure benzodiazepine overdose in a benzodiazepine-naïve patient.	*Pediatric:* 0.01–0.05 mg/kg IV over 30 min–1 hour. *Adult:* 0.2 mg IV slow, repeat q2–3min to 1 mg max.	*Caution:* Contraindicated in TCA overdose, unknown overdose, patients with chronic benzodiazepine use. Lowers seizure threshold; avoid in patients with seizure disorder. Induces benzodiazepine withdrawal.
Folic acid Leucovorin (Folinic acid)	Methanol poisoning, methotrexate poisoning.	*Methanol:* Folic acid or leucovorin: 1 mg/kg IV q4h for 1–2 doses or until tolerating PO, then 1 mg/kg PO q4h, max 50 mg/dose.	*Caution:* Do not substitute folic acid for leucovorin in methotrexate poisoning. Slow IV infusion recommended for leucovorin owing to high calcium content. Avoid benzyl alcohol–containing solution in neonates receiving leucovorin.

Methotrexate:		Leucovorin: If dose of methotrexate is known, administer and equal amount of leucovorin. Empiric dose: 10 mg/m²/dose IV/PO q6h for 72 hours.	
Fomepizole (4-MP, Antizol)	Methanol or ethylene glycol poisoning	15 mg/kg IV load, then 10 mg/kg q12h × 4, then 15 mg/kg q12h.	*Caution:* Nausea, dizziness, headache Increase frequency of dosing to q4h during dialysis.
Glucagon	β-blocker or calcium channel blocker overdose with bradycardia/ hypotension.	*Pediatric:* 0.05–0.10 mg/kg rapid IVP, if effective, follow by continuous infusion: 0.07 mg/kg/h IV. *Adult:* 3–5 mg rapid IVP may repeat to max 10 mg, if effective, follow by continuous infusion: dose which caused improvement/hour.	*Caution:* Nausea, vomiting, hyperglycemia, hypokalemia.
Hyperinsulinemia/ euglycemia therapy	Calcium channel blocker overdose with severe hypotension/symptomatic bradycardia refractory to other therapies.	*Bolus:* 0.5–1.0 IU/kg regular insulin, followed by 25 g glucose (1 amp D50). *Maintenance:* Insulin: 0.5 IU regular insulin/ kg/h, titrate to 1.0 IU regular insulin/kg/h. Glucose: D10 start at 100 cc/h (10 g/h) and titrate to keep glucose ≥ 100 mg/dL.	*Caution:* Experimental therapy: consult a poison center/medical toxicologist. Follow serum glucose q15min for 1 hour after the first bolus or after any increase in dose, then q1h.
Methylene blue	Methemoglobinemia with symptoms of hypoxia, concurrent medical illness, or >30%.	1–2 mg/kg (0.1–0.2 mL/kg) slow IV as 1% solution, repeat in 1 hour.	*Caution:* Ineffective in reversing methemoglobinemia in patients with G-6-PD deficiency; hemolysis may occur with G-6-PD deficiency, high doses (>15 mg/kg).
Naloxone (Narcan)	Opiate, α-2 agonist (e.g., clonidine), imidazoline poisoning, empiric treatment of coma.	*Pediatric:* 0.1 mg/kg IV or IM, max 2 mg. Higher doses may be required for certain agents (e.g., methadone, fantanyl, lomotil). *Adult:* 0.4–2.0 mg IV or IM, repeat to 10 mg.	*Caution:* Acute opiate withdrawal may be precipitated in opiate-habituated patients. Duration of action short (<30 min), repeat doses may be necessary.

(Continues)

127

Table 17–1. Common Antidotes (*continued*)

Antidote	Indications	Dose	Comments
Octreotide	Hypoglycemia due to oral hypoglycemic overdose, quinine, if IV dextrose fails to maintain euglycemia.	*Pediatric:* 1 μg/kg SC/IV q6h max 50 μg *Adult:* 50–100 μg SC/IV q6–12h.	*Caution:* Nausea, abdominal pain, diarrhea.
Oxygen, hyperbaric	CO poisoning. Can be considered for managing cyanide, hydrogen sulfide, carbon tetrachloride poisoning.	100% oxygen at 2–3 ATM.	*Caution:* TM perforation, seizures due to oxygen toxicity; contraindicated if unvented pneumothorax is present. Difficulty monitoring critically ill patient in monoplace chambers.

Penicillamine	Second-line agent for chelation of lead, arsenic, mercury, copper.	*Lead:* (use only when succimer, EDTA not tolerated)
		 10 mg/kg/d PO for 1 week, increase to 10 mg/kg BID for 1 week, then TID.
		 Arsenic: (use only if BAL/succimer are unavailable)
		 25 mg/kg/dose PO q6h (maximum: 1 g/d).
		 Mercury: (use only if succimer is unavailable)
		    Pediatric: 20–30 mg/kg/day PO in 4 divided doses
		    Adult: 250 mg PO QID.
		 Copper:
		    Pediatric: 20–30 mg/kg/d PO QID
		    Adult: 1–2 g/d PO QID.
			Caution: Contraindicated in penicillin allergy, pregnancy, renal insufficiency. Hematologic toxicity, GI upset, rash, proteinuria, hematuria.

Phentolamine	Hypertensive crisis due to stimulants, sympathomimetics, MAO-tyramine reaction. Extravasated vasoconstrictive agents.	*Hypertension:*
		    Pediatric: 0.02–0.10 mg/kg bolus, repeat q5–10 min PRN.
		    Adult: 1–5 mg IV bolus, repeat q5–10 min PRN.
			Caution: Hypotension, tachycardia, dysrhythmias.

Drug	Indication	Dose	Caution
		Extravasation: Pediatric: 0.1 mg/kg, max 10 mg diluted in 10–15 mL saline SC. Adult: 5–10 mg diluted in 10–15 mL saline SC.	
Physostigmine (Antilirium)	Severe *pure* anticholinergic poisoning; diphenhydramine, jimsonweed, atropine.	*Pediatric:* 0.02 mg/kg IV, infuse over at least 5 min, max 0.5 mg, repeat in 10 min PRN. *Adult:* 1–2 mg IV, repeat in 10 min PRN.	*Caution:* Contraindicated in TCA overdose; may exacerbate cardiotoxicity. Check ECG prior to administration. If QRS is prolonged, do not use. *Relative contraindications:* bronchospasm, peripheral vascular disease, intestinal/bladder obstruction, interventricular conduction defects, AV block. Can cause allergic reaction in patients with salicylate allergy.
Polyethylene glycol (whole bowel irrigation, Golytely)	Lead paint chips, iron tablets, cocaine, and opioid drug packet ingestions.	*Pediatric:* 25 mL/kg/h PO or NG tube. *Adult:* 1–2 L/h.	*Contraindications:* Bowel obstruction, bowel perforation, recent abdominal surgery. In young children, monitor electrolytes, glucose, and fluid status.
Pralidoxime (2-PAM, Protopam)	Organophosphate, insecticide, chemical nerve agent toxicity with cholinergic toxidrome. Use in conjunction with atropine.	*Pediatric:* 25–50 mg/kg IV over 30 min, repeat in 1 hour PRN, repeat in 6 hours if symptoms return. *Adult:* 1–2 g in 100 mL NaCl IV over 15–30 min, repeat in 1 hour PRN, repeat in 6 hours if symptoms return.	*Caution:* Rapid IV infusion can lead to respiratory and cardiac arrest. Long-term dosing may be necessary depending on patient's clinical condition.
Protamine sulfate	Heparin overdose with prolonged PTT and persistent bleeding.	1 mg for each 100 IU heparin, 1/2 dose if 30–60 min and 1/4 dose if 2 hours after heparin bolus.	*Caution:* Hypotension, anaphylaxis have been reported. Hypersensitivity in patients with fish allergy. Avoid benzyl alcohol diluent in neonates.

(Continues)

Table 17–1. Common Antidotes (*continued*)

Antidote	Indications	Dose	Comments
Pyridoxine (vitamin B$_6$)	Isoniazid-induced seizures, *Gyromitra* mushroom, monomethylhydrazine; ethylene glycol.	*INH induced seizures:* Dose (mg) = amount INH ingested (mg). Unknown ingested amounts: 1 g for pediatrics or 5 g for adult slow IV infusion.	*Caution:* Ataxia, sensory neuropathy following massive/chronic dosing.
Succimer (DMSA, Chemet)	Pediatric lead poisoning with blood lead level ≥ 20 µg/dL. Chelation of organic and inorganic mercury, and arsenic.	10 mg/kg (350 mg/m^2) PO q8h × 5 days, then q12h × 14 days, then reassess blood metal levels.	*Caution:* Nausea, vomiting diarrhea, rarely, fever, chills, urticaria, eosinophilia, elevated liver transaminases. If lead encephalopathy is present, treat with BAL and EDTA first. Must remove child from the source of exposure.
Thiamine (vitamin B$_1$)	Ethylene glycol poisoning, chronic alcohol use, malnutrition.	*Pediatric:* 50 mg IM or IV q6h. *Adult:* 100 mg IM or IV q6h.	*Caution:* Rare reports of anaphylaxis following rapid IV injection
Vitamin K$_1$ (Phytonadione, Aqua Mephyton)	Treatment of prolonged PT due to ingestion of drugs/toxins interfering with vitamin K$_1$ metabolism (coumadin, brodifacoum).	*Pediatric:* 1–5 mg/dose PO: dose q6–8h SC/IV: dose q6–8h. *Adult:* PO: 25–50 mg q6–8h SC: 10–25 mg q6–8h IV: 10–25 mg slow push q6h	*Caution:* Anaphylaxis from IV administration, IV route reserved for life-threatening coagulopathy; PO/SC route preferred.

Abbreviations: ARDS, acute respiratory distress syndrome; ATM, atmosphere; AV, atrioventricular; BID, twice a day; Ca, calcium; CDC, Centers for Disease Control and Prevention; CHF, congestive heart failure; CNS, central nervous system; CO, carbon monoxide; ECG, electrocardiograph; EDTA, ethylenediaminetetraacetic acid; G-6-PD, glucose-6-phosphate dehydrogenase; GI, gastrointestinal; IM, intramuscular; INH, isoniazid; IV, intravenous; max, maximum; MAO, monoamine oxidase; NGT, nasogastric tube; PO, orally; PRN, as needed; PT, prothrombin time; PTT, partial thromboplastin time; QID, four times a day; SC, subcutaneous; TCA, tricyclic antidepressants; TID, three times a day; TM, tympanic membrane.

SUGGESTED READINGS

Burda AM: Poison antidotes: Issues of inadequate stocking with review of uses of 24 common antidotal agents. *J Pharm Pract* 10:235–248, 1997.

Dart RC, Goldfrank LR, Chyka PA, et al: Combined evidence-based literature analysis and consensus guidelines for stocking of emergency antidotes in the United States. *Ann Emerg Med* 36:126–132, 2000.

Dart RC, Stark Y, Fulton B, et al: Insufficient stocking of poisoning antidotes in hospital pharmacies. *JAMA* 276:1508–1510, 1996.

Woolf AD, Chrisanthus K: On-site availability of selected antidotes: Results of a survey of Massachusetts hospitals. *Am J Emerg Med* 15:62–66, 1997.

18

Extracorporeal Removal of Toxins

Janis M. Orlowski
Susan Hou
Jerrold B. Leikin

HIGH-YIELD FACTS

- Fewer than 0.05% of all toxic exposures require extracorporeal therapy.

- Toxins most commonly removed by extracorporeal therapy include lithium, barbiturates, salicylates, and toxic alcohols.

- Common complications from use of extracorporeal therapy include hypotension, bleeding, and problems from obtaining proper vascular access.

- Correction of metabolic complications including metabolic acidosis is a common indication for hemodialysis.

- Phenobarbital and theophylline are most effectively removed via charcoal hemoperfusion.

Although very few toxic exposures require or are effectively treated by extracorporeal techniques, these are essential modalities that may be life saving in the treatment of selected poisoned patients. The medical literature does report successful treatments of pediatric patients with extracorporeal techniques. The extracorporeal techniques most commonly employed for the removal of toxins are hemodialysis and charcoal hemoperfusion, although plasmapheresis, exchange transfusion, and continuous ultrafiltration techniques may also be used. In 2002, the American Association of Poison Control Centers (AAPCC) reported a total of 1.2 million poisonings of children younger than 6, of which 132,055 required treatment in a medical facility. According to the AAPCC

data, extracorporeal procedures were utilized in fewer than 0.05% of cases, with hemodialysis accounting for approximately 90% of these interventions. Implementation of these invasive techniques requires the 24-hour availability of nephrologists and other critical care specialists, dialysis equipment, technicians, and reference laboratory personnel who monitor the efficacy of treatment.

According to Pond, employing extracorporeal techniques to remove toxins should be considered if the total body elimination of the toxin can be potentially increased by 30% or more. Specific criteria related to physical characteristics of the toxin, the efficacy of alternative therapies, the presence of renal failure, and the severity of poisoning guide decisions regarding the utilization of these techniques (Table 18–1). Certain agents that predictably cause severe toxicity are routinely dialyzed, based on an assessment of blood levels and clinical manifestations of toxicity. These include lithium, ethylene glycol, methanol, and salicylates (Table 18–2). Rarely, theophylline toxicity requires hemodialysis. Extracorporeal techniques may also be beneficial in the treatment of severe poisoning with other agents (Tables 18–3 and 18–4). Physical characteristics that predict the successful removal of an agent by dialysis or charcoal hemoperfusion include low volume of distribution (<1 L/kg), the presence of the toxin in the central compartment, and low endogenous clearance (<4 mL/min/kg). For hemodialysis, a low molecular weight (<500 daltons), low protein binding, and water solubility of the toxin are necessary. For some drugs, hemodialysis results in not only removal of the drug but also correction of the metabolic consequences of the poisoning. An example is the metabolic acidosis associated with salicylates, ethylene glycol, methanol, or metformin. Although the great majority

Table 18–1. Indications for Extracorporeal Removal of Drugs and Toxins

Intoxication with a drug or poison whose removal is enhanced 30 percent or more by extracorporeal techniques along with one or more of the following:

> Blood level or ingested quantity that is generally associated with severe or lethal toxicity
> Natural removal mechanism impaired
> Clinical condition deteriorating with supportive care
> Clinical evidence exists of severe toxicity, including hypotension, coma, metabolic acidosis, respiratory depression, dysrhythmias, or cardiac decomposition
> Ingestion of a toxin with serious delayed effects

of patients poisoned with barbiturates and sedative-hypnotic agents, such as phenobarbital, chloral hydrate, ethanol, or isopropyl alcohol, do well with supportive care, extracorporeal removal may be indicated for unstable patients. Patients with renal or cardiac insufficiency may not tolerate the alkaline load required for treating salicylism, and may benefit from the earlier institution of dialysis. In addition to removal of a toxin, the treatment of renal failure and the correction of the metabolic abnormalities associated with poisoning, hemodialysis increases the temperature of the blood in poisonings complicated by hypothermia.

EXTRACORPOREAL THERAPY

Hemodialysis

Hemodialysis is accomplished by actively pumping blood past a semipermeable membrane, most commonly configured as a bundle of hollow fibers that has a nonsterile solution on the outer membrane. The diffusion of dialyzable substances across the membrane as well as flux caused by circulation removes toxins from an area of high concentration to an area of low concentration. Solutes dissolved in fluid are also removed by convection, which has a more prominent role in some of the continuous forms of dialysis therapy.

Most of the hemodialysis systems currently in use are single-pass systems; that is, the dialysate comes in contact with the blood only one time. Single-pass systems use 30 to 40 L/h of nonsterile treated water, which dilutes a concentrated solution of electrolytes. The maximum gradient between the serum and the dialysate is maintained throughout the treatment.

In the acute setting, the REDY sorbent system, which regenerates dialysate and requires only 6 L of water per treatment, is rarely used today in place of a single-pass system. Dialysate is regenerated by passage through a five-layered sorbent cartridge that uses urease to convert urea to ammonium carbonate and binds other toxins at other levels of the cartridge. A disadvantage of this system is that the toxin may be incompletely bound by the cartridge, so that over time the concentration of the toxin in the dialysate increases, thereby decreasing the gradient

Table 18–2. Toxins for Which Extracorporeal Removal May Be Efficacious

Toxin	Serum Level	Molecular Weight (Daltons)	Volume of Distribution (L/kg)	Protein Binding	Modality
Ethylene glycol	>50 mg/dL	62	0.6–0.7	Negligible	HD
Lithium	Clinical	74	0.8	Negligible	HD
Methanol	>50 mg/dL	32	0.6–0.7	Negligible	HD
Phenobarbital	Clinical	232	0.50–0.88	50%	HP/HD
Salicylates	Acute >100 mg/dL	138	0.15–>0.30 (increases with increasing levels)	50–90% (binding decreases with increasing levels)	HD
Theophylline	*Acute:* 90 mg/L *Chronic:* 40 mg/L and poorly responsive to therapy				

Abbreviations: HD, hemodialysis; HP, hemoperfusion.

Table 18–3. Toxins and Drugs Removed by
Hemodialysis or Hemoperfusion

Common	Uncommon[a]
Barbiturates	Aminoglycosides
Ethylene glycol	Atenolol
Lithium	Boric acid
Methanol	Bromide
Salicylates	Carbamazepine
Theophylline	Chloral hydrate (trichlorethanol)
Monobutyl ether	Diethylene glycol
(Z-butoxyethinal)	Ethanol
	Ethylene glycol
	Isopropanol
	Magnesium
	Metformin
	Methotrexate (high flux)
	Paraquat (very early)
	Phenytoin (albumin dialysis)
	Procainamide/
	N-acetylprocainamide
	Sotalol
	Thallium
	Valproic acid

[a]Not usually utilized or performed.

Table 18–4. Pharmaceutical Agents Removed by
Hemodialysis or Hemoperfusion

Aminoglycosides
β-Adrenergic receptor antagonists
    (atenolol, sotalol)
Carbamazepine
Gluethimide
Isoniazid
Methaqualone
Methyldopa
Metronidazole
Penicillins
Procainamide
Pyrazinamide
Quinidine
Sulfonamides
Thyroid hormone
Valproic acid
Vidarabine

of toxin from blood to dialysate and markedly decreasing
the efficiency of toxin removal. This system is less efficient for poison removal, and should be used only if
standard hemodialysis is not available.

Toxin Removal and the Dialysis Membrane

Many characteristics of the dialysis system influence the
efficacy of dialysis, including membrane surface area,
pore size, rate of blood flow through the dialyzer, and
rate of dialysate flow through the artificial kidney. The
ability of a substance to cross the membrane depends on
membrane thickness, on pore size, and pore shape. There
is significant variation in the characteristics of dialysis
membranes. They are divided into three basic categories
based on permeability to solutes and ease of ultrafiltration of fluid: standard, high efficiency, and high flux.
High-flux membranes can be used only with specialized
dialysis machines that continuously adjust ultrafiltration
based on computerized measurements. Dialysis machines
require recalibration to switch from standard to high-flux
membranes. For the treatment of acute poisoning, time
constraints and availability of personnel usually make
it necessary to use the more readily available standard
hemodialysis systems. There is little advantage to a more
efficient dialyzer for small molecules such as lithium,
which are almost completely removed by the passage of
blood through any dialyzer. Larger molecules, such as
methotrexate, are poorly removed by standard dialyzers,
but may be removed by high-flux dialyzers and highly
permeable filters used for continuous therapies. The permeability of the membrane is usually expressed in terms
of the clearance of urea. Most manufacturers also spec-
ify the clearance of vitamin B_{12} as a representative of
molecules of middle molecular weight. A knowledge of
the permeability characteristics of the dialyzers available in a specific setting allows the nephrologist to better predict the efficacy of dialysis for the removal of a
given substance.

Toxin Characteristics and Dialysis Effectiveness

There are several characteristics of toxins that determine
the efficacy of dialysis in the treatment of poisoning or
overdose.

Size and Charge

The rate at which molecules travel down a concentration
gradient and across the dialysis membrane is inversely

proportional to molecular weight. Simply put, large molecules move more slowly than small molecules. For example, a molecule of vitamin B_{12} (molecular weight = 1355 daltons) would be dialyzed more slowly than molecule of urea (molecular weight = 60 daltons).

Protein Binding

The dialysis membrane is designed to prevent the movement of large quantities of plasma proteins into the dialysate. For this reason, only drugs that are not protein bound are removed by dialysis. Protein binding may vary with the concentration of a drug. Although both salicylates and valproic acid are highly protein bound at therapeutic levels, the fraction of protein binding is decreased at toxic levels, allowing for their removal by hemodialysis.

Volume of Distribution

The volume of distribution is the theoretical space over which a substance is distributed. Substances that are widely distributed in tissues have a higher calculated volume of distribution than substances that are confined to the intravascular space. For example, the administration of a given amount of toxin that is confined to the intravascular space results in a higher serum concentration and a lower volume of distribution than the same amount of a substance that is distributed into the intravascular space plus fat and muscle. Hemodialysis removes only the toxins that are in the intravascular space. Substances that can be effectively removed by dialysis have a volume of distribution that is less than 1 L/kg (Table 18–5). Although widely distributed substances may be efficiently extracted from the blood by hemodialysis or hemoperfusion, they are still not effectively removed

because only a small percentage of the toxin is in the intravascular space. An example is cyclic antidepressants, which have a volume of distribution of more than 10 L/kg. Although easily removed from the intravascular space by dialysis, they are so widely distributed in tissue that their removal has little impact on total body burden and toxicity. For some of these substances, there is a critical time period between ingestion of the toxin and its concentration in tissues.

Water Solubility

To be removed by hemodialysis, a substance must be soluble in the aqueous phase of plasma. Lipid-soluble drugs are poorly removed. Lipid-soluble drugs also frequently have a large volume of distribution.

Transfer Rates From Tissues

As a substance is removed from the intravascular space, a portion of the drug distributed in tissue (including red blood cells) and an interstitial water diffuses into the serum. This movement accounts for the postdialysis rebound in the blood level of some drugs that occurs independent of continued gastrointestinal absorption. The rate of transfer during the treatment affects the efficiency of removal. This rebound effect is prominent following the removal of lithium by hemodialysis.

Hemoperfusion

Hemoperfusion is similar to hemodialysis, except that blood passes through a cartridge containing either charcoal or a resin that adsorbs the toxin directly, rather than passing through a hollow fiber. Hemoperfusion efficiently removes toxins that adsorb to activated charcoal or resin, including substances that are lipid soluble or have a higher molecular weight than those able to pass through a hollow-fiber hemodialyzer. It is also more effective in removing substances that are protein bound. Hemoperfusion is very efficient in removing toxin located within the intravascular space, including the lipid portion of plasma and red blood cells. It does not overcome the problem of removing a toxin that has a large volume of distribution.

Although the machine used for hemodialysis can be used for hemoperfusion, hemoperfusion is not as readily available as hemodialysis. Cartridges are not available in many hospitals, and familiarity with hemoperfusion, even among nephrologists, is limited. Certain complications occur frequently, including hypotension, thrombo-

Table 18–5. Pharmacokinetic Parameters of Toxins for Optimal Removal by Extracorporeal Therapy

	Hemodialysis	Hemoperfusion
Distribution time	Short	Short
Low endogenous clearance (mL/min/kg)	<4	<4
Volume of distribution (L/kg)	<1	<1
Protein binding	Low	Low or high
Solubility	Water	Water or lipid
Molecular weight (D)	<500	<40,000

cytopenia, leukopenia, and electrolyte disturbances. The causes of hypotension are multifactorial. It may be caused by the toxin itself, the blood volume used to prime the filter, or a pyrogen reaction to the filter itself. Leukopenia and thrombocytopenia are frequently seen, although with newer hemoperfusion cartridges, thrombocytopenia is usually limited to approximately a 30% drop in platelet count. Nonselective binding of important molecules, such as calcium, phosphate, and glucose, to the charcoal or the resin in the hemofiltration cartridge can cause hypocalcemia, hypophosphatemia, and hypoglycemia. Systemic anticoagulation, which is necessary to prevent clotting of the filter, may lead to bleeding problems. Charcoal embolization has been reported, but is uncommon with the newer hemofiltration cartridges.

The efficiency of hemoperfusion may be increased by using a standard hemodialyzer and hemoperfusion cartridges in series. The removal of small molecules, such as urea, by hemodialysis decreases their concentration in the blood reaching the hemoperfusion cartridge, thus decreasing their binding to the charcoal or resin. This leaves a greater portion of the cartridge surface area available for binding the targeted toxin, increasing the time before the cartridge is saturated and must be replaced. As with any extracorporeal system for toxin removal, repeated treatments may be necessary because plasma levels of the toxin rebound. *Rebound* occurs when toxins are removed from the blood space. After extracorporeal treatments is discontinued, there may be a reequilibration of the toxin from extravascular stores (tissue) resulting in an increase in the toxins serum level. Thus, toxin serum levels should be repeated several times after a treatment. Although hemoperfusion has been used in the treatment of numerous poisonings, there are few studies comparing the long-term outcomes of patients treated with hemoperfusion versus those treated with conservative therapy.

Continuous Extracorporeal Methods

Continuous renal replacement therapies, introduced for the treatment of acute renal failure in hemodynamically unstable patients, allow ongoing removal of small volumes of fluid and toxins at low blood flow rates. Blood is pumped continuously through a very permeable hollow-fiber membrane or flat filter membrane either from an artery to a vein, relying on the patient's own blood pressure, or by a blood pump from a large vein with a double-lumen catheter. The permeable membrane allows for an ultrafiltration rate as high as 1 to 1.5 L/h. When continuous arteriovenous hemofiltration (CAVH) is performed

without the use of a blood pump, the ultrafiltration rate is determined by the positive pressure caused by venous resistance on the blood side of the filter and the negative pressure generated by gravity as determined by the height of the drain bag on the ultrafiltrate side. When the rate of ultrafiltration exceeds the desired rate of fluid removal, replacement fluid is given. A wide range of sophisticated ultrafiltration controls are available for continuous venovenous hemofiltration (CVVH) or CAVH, with new refinements being introduced regularly. For all continuous therapies, toxins are removed by convection in concentrations approximately equal to the unbound blood level, but the serum concentration does not change until replacement solution is given. Continuous therapies are relatively inefficient for solute (and thus toxin) removal. Efficiency can be increased by circulating dialysate on the outside of the dialysis membranes. Because the membrane is permeable enough to allow the passage of larger molecules, including inflammatory mediators, the dialysate solution must be sterile. One of a number of specifically formulated dialysis fluids, including peritoneal dialysate, can be used. Many of the fluids designed for continuous systems use lactate as the base precursor, which needs to be changed to a bicarbonate-containing solution in patients with lactic acidosis. The dialysate flow rate with continuous therapies is usually no more than 4 L/h (more commonly 1 or 2 L/h), rather than the 30 L/h used in hemodialysis.

Continuous methods have several advantages. The larger pore size allows removal of molecules up to 50,000 daltons. These methods are better tolerated in hemodynamically unstable patients. For conditions in which there is endogenous production of a toxic substance, such as lactate, or ongoing absorption from an inadequately decontaminated gastrointestinal tract, continuous therapies provide ongoing removal. Finally, they avoid the problem of rebound toxicity by removing the toxin continuously as it reenters the intravascular space.

Peritoneal Dialysis

Peritoneal dialysis involves instillation of a dialysate of electrolytes, glucose, calcium, and magnesium into the peritoneal space through a percutaneously placed peritoneal catheter. Toxins from the splanchnic circulation diffuse across the abdominal mesentery into the dialysate, which is then drained from the body. The efficiency of dialysis depends largely on dialysate flow rate. When acute dialysis is performed, the fluid is usually changed hourly. Peritoneal dialysis is much less efficient than hemodialysis in the removal of toxins, and it is generally used only when hemodialysis is not available. According to Fine and co-workers, peritoneal dialysis is more efficient in children than in adults because the peritoneal surface area in children is larger than in adults relative to body surface area. The base precursor in most peritoneal dialysis solutions is lactate, which precludes its use in intoxications associated with lactic acidosis. When dialysis is instituted for the treatment of toxin-induced renal failure, rather than for toxin removal, peritoneal dialysis is an acceptable alternative in all but the most catabolic patients.

Plasmapheresis

Plasmapheresis is the removal of plasma in exchange for albumin or fresh frozen plasma. It removes toxins only from the intravascular space. The plasma concentration of toxins is lowered by the plasma volume exchanged. Double-lumen central access is required, as well as a centrifugal separator to remove the plasma. Specifically trained technicians are required for monitoring plasma removal, with appropriate physician-directed replacement. Complications include hypotension, bleeding, hypocalcemia, alkalosis secondary to the citrate preservative in the blood products, and complications of central venous access. Bleeding complications are exacerbated when albumin is used for replacement because the patient's clotting factors are removed along with plasma and the toxin. Plasmapheresis is most useful for removing protein-bound toxins, such as phenytoin, that are not removed by hemodialysis and are inefficiently removed by hemoperfusion (Table 18–6).

Exchange Transfusion

Exchange transfusion is the technique of removing blood from a patient, followed by transfusions of the similar quantity of blood from a donor. The process is usually repeated several times to remove a sufficient quantity of the toxin. This technique is theoretically helpful in situations of hemoglobin toxicity (Table 18–7). This technique is rarely used except in neonates, as described by Osborn and colleagues. The complications are those associated with the risk of transfusions.

Extracorporeal Removal Combined With Chelation Therapy

Occasionally, metals such as iron and aluminum accumulate in the body in quantities sufficient to cause neurologic and hematologic toxicity, severe bone disease, or

Table 18–6. Removal of Toxicants via Plasmapheresis

Enhanced Elimination	Ineffective Elimination
Phenytoin	Vancomycin
Mercury	Organophosphate agents
Paraquat (decreased level by 80%)	Thyroxin
Vanadate	Digoxin
Propranolol	Gentamicin
Maprotyline	Carbamazepine (significant rebound effect)
Tobramycin	Tacrolimus
Amanita phalloides (mortality: 18%)	
Verapamil	
Diltiazem	

Source: Based on work by Nenov VD, Marinov P, Sabeva J, et al: Current applications of plasmapheresis in clinical toxicology. *Nephrol Dial Transplant* 18:V56–V58, 2003 and Mokrzycki MH, Kaplan AA: Therapeutic plasma exchange: Complications and management. *Am J Kidney Dis* 23:817–827, 1994.

liver disease. Patients with renal failure are at particular risk for the accumulation of metals. The neurologic complications of aluminum accumulation include myoclonus, dementia, and coma. Aluminum can also cause amicrocytic anemia and osteomalacia. Iron accumulates in patients receiving frequent blood transfusions. Patients with renal failure who receive frequent transfusions or

Table 18–7. Toxicants for Which Exchange Transfusions May Be Helpful

Parathion
Acetaminophen
Iron (serum levels >1000 μg/dL)
Caffeine
Methyl salicylate
Propafenone
Ganciclovir/acyclovir
Methemoglobin producers[a]
Lead
Phenazopyridine hydrochloride
Pine oil
Theophylline (serum levels >90 mg/L)
E. coli 0157: H7-associated hemolytic–uremic syndrome

[a]Especially patients with G-6-PD– or NADPH-dependent methemoglobin reductase deficiency and/or to methylene blue therapy with methemoglobin levels >70%.

intravenous infusions of iron as part of treatment with erythropoietin are at particular risk for iron accumulation, with its associated liver and heart disease. Removal from the body is achieved only after combination of these metals with chelating agents. Chelation therapy may be effective in patients with normal renal function, but in patients with renal failure chelation of some metals must be combined with hemodialysis to have effective removal. Caution must be taken when one uses chelating agents to avoid precipitating acute toxicity because of an increase in serum levels due to mobilization from tissues. This therapy is also associated with anaphylactic reactions and severe hypotension. Long-term therapy with deferoxamine can predispose to fungal infections.

Liver or Albumin Dialysis

Extracorporeal liver assistance methods utilizing an albumin dialysate (molecular absorbent recycling system [MARS]) has been utilized in Europe to remove protein-bound and water-soluble substances in patients with liver failure and grade III or IV hepatic encephalopathy. Successful results with avoidance of orthotopic hepatic transplantation have been noted with patients exposed to *Amanita phalloides* and paracetamol. It has been safely utilized in children as young as 7 years old. Complications include decreases in platelet counts by 15% and prolongation of activated prothrombin time by 21%. According to Klammt and associates, blood pressure, hemoglobin, white blood cell count, electrolytes, transaminases, and albumin levels do not appear to be significantly affected. There is a recent report of a severe case of phenytoin toxicity associated with acute renal failure, cardiac arrhythmia, hepatotoxicity, and alerted mental status that was successfully treated with the MARS system.

OVERDOSES COMMONLY TREATED WITH EXTRACORPOREAL THERAPY

Because of the characteristics required for effective removal of a drug or toxin by extracorporeal techniques, the number of drugs for which hemodialysis is useful is relatively small. For the drugs that are removed well by both hemoperfusion and hemodialysis, hemodialysis is usually preferred because of the greater experience with its use and because it simultaneously corrects associated electrolyte abnormalities. For drugs and toxins for which hemoperfusion is superior, hemodialysis should be used only hemoperfusion is not available.

Barbiturates

Most patients with barbiturate overdose do well with supportive care. Chronic users of these drugs may tolerate very high levels with minimal symptoms, so that a decision to dialyze a patient with barbiturate overdose should be based on evidence of severe toxicity unresponsive to conservative management, rather than on blood levels. Phenobarbital can be removed by hemoperfusion or hemodialysis because of its low volume of distribution, its adsorbency to activated charcoal, and its slow intrinsic elimination rate. It is the barbiturate most frequently considered for extracorporeal removal. Hemoperfusion (more effective) or hemodialysis should be considered for toxicity associated with hypotension, respiratory depression, or deep and prolonged coma. When extracorporeal removal is instituted for barbiturate overdose, the treatment may precipitate a state of acute withdrawal manifested by seizures or delirium tremens in the chronic user. Porto and associates described the effective removal of phenobarbital with chronic peritoneal dialysis in a 2.5-year-old child. Forty percent to 50% of total doses were removed with this therapy. Constant low-flux hemodialysis successfully removed phenobarbital from a 9-month-old infant according to Soylemezoglu and associates.

Ethylene Glycol

Ethylene glycol is converted by multiple enzymatic reactions to metabolites that cause metabolic acidosis, renal failure, pulmonary edema, and central nervous system damage, including cerebral edema. The treatment for ethylene glycol poisoning consists of inhibiting alcohol dehydrogenase, the initial enzyme in the metabolic pathway, and instituting hemodialysis to remove the parent compound and its metabolites, to treat the metabolic acidosis and to treat the renal failure. The indications for dialysis include an ethylene glycol level of at least 50 mg/dL or evidence of ongoing metabolic acidosis with end-organ failure, such as rising serum creatinine, decreased urine output, pulmonary edema, and cerebral edema, regardless of the serum level. Hemodialysis clearance rates of 156 m^2/min and 210 mL/min have been achieved for ethylene glycol. These clearances are significantly greater than the normal renal clearance rate reported at 27.5 ± 4.1 mL/min. Glycolate, the metabolite responsible for the acidosis, is also cleared by hemodialysis. In 10 patients studied as part of a multicenter, prospective trial by Moreau and colleagues, the hemodialysis clearance of glycolate was 170 ± 23 mL/min (flow rates 250 to 400 mL/min) with an elimination half-time of 155 ± 42 minutes. This compared favorably to a nonhemodialysis elimination rate of 1.08 ± 0.67 mmol/L/h with an elimination half-time of 626 ± 474 minutes. Prior to the use of extracorporeal removal, treatment with fomepizole (4-methylprazole) intravenously should be considered. Successful treatments in children have been documented.

Lithium

Lithium is ideally suited to removal by hemodialysis. With a weight of 74 daltons, it passes readily across virtually all dialysis membranes. It has a volume of distribution of 0.8 L/kg of body weight and is not protein bound. Extraction by dialysis is 90%. In a series of 14 patients, hemodialysis clearances in three patients ranged from 63.2 to 114.4 mL/min. In a study of 14 patients by Hansen and co-workers, the mean renal clearance was 17.2 ± 5.4 mL/min. In patients in whom renal function is preserved, dialysis and renal excretion are additive. Hemodialysis should be instituted regardless of serum levels if moderate to severe central nervous system abnormalities such as confusion, stupor, coma, or seizures are present. The serum lithium level is effectively lowered by hemodialysis. However, a rebound in serum lithium levels that peaks at 6 to 8 hours after a treatment occurs as lithium enters the blood from the interstitial and intracellular spaces. This rebound often necessitates repeated treatments until the serum lithium level remains below 1.0 mEq/L. Lithium is also removed via continuous hemofiltration. In a study of seven patients treated with CAVH or CVVH for 18 to 44 hours by LaBlanc and associates, the mean lithium clearances were 41.4 ± 4.6 m^2/min (CAVH, flow rate 4 L/h) and 48.4 ± 1.4 to 61.9 ± 2.3 mL/min (CVVH, flow rate 1 to 2 L/h). No significant rebound in the serum lithium levels occurred. This technique may also be employed after initial hemodialysis. Meyer and co-workers reported successful treatment of lithium toxicity in two children who presented with lithium levels three times the therapeutic levels. Each child was initiated on hemodialysis and subsequently treated for 34.5 hours (patient 1) and 26 hours (patient 2) with continuous venous hemofiltration with dialysis. Both children had return of normal mental status and suffered no complications of dialysis.

Methanol

Methanol toxicity causes blindness, severe metabolic acidosis, central nervous system toxicity, and death. Formic acid is responsible for the toxic manifestations and acidosis. It is produced when methanol is metabolized to formaldehyde by alcohol dehydrogenase and then to formic acid by aldehyde dehydrogenase. Like ethylene glycol, methanol poisoning is treated by infusion of an alcohol dehydrogenase inhibitor to block metabolism, followed by hemodialysis.

Hemodialysis indications mirror those for ethylene glycol listed earlier, and include a plasma level of 50 mg/dL or greater or evidence of ongoing metabolic acidosis with end-organ failure. Hemodialysis clearance rates of 142 to 286 mL/min have been reported for methanol; formic acid clearances range from 148 to 203 mL/min. However, the hemodialysis elimination half-time of formic acid does not vary appreciably from the nonhemodialysis half-time. In a prospective multicenter trial involving 11 patients poisoned with methanol, 7 of whom underwent hemodialysis, the nonhemodialysis half-time of formic acid was 205 ± 25 minutes, and the hemodialysis half-time was 185.0 ± 62.7 minutes. According to Kerns and associates, overall, the hemodialysis clearance for formic acid was 223.0 ± 24.5 mL/min.

When hemodialysis is used to treat methanol or ethylene glycol intoxication, the dose of fomepizole or ethanol should be increased during dialysis to offset the removal of these alcohol dehydrogenase inhibitors (see Chapter 47).

Salicylates

Salicylates are poorly removed by dialysis at therapeutic levels because protein binding exceeds 90%. However, at toxic levels, protein binding saturates and decreases to 50% to 75%, leaving a large free fraction that can be readily removed. Hemodialysis should be instituted when the serum level is 100 mg/dL or greater or when altered mental status, noncardiogenic pulmonary edema, noncorrectable severe acid–base disturbances, renal failure, or a deteriorating clinical condition occur at lower levels. Hemoperfusion removes salicylates more effectively; however, hemodialysis facilitates correction of the associated acid–base disturbances while also removing the toxin.

Theophylline

Hemoperfusion is the preferred method for removal of theophylline, which is more than 50% protein bound, but hemodialysis is also effective. Theophylline avidly binds to the activated charcoal cartridges. The level at which extracorporeal removal should be instituted depends on whether the poisoning results from acute ingestion or chronic toxicity. With acute ingestion, extracorporeal removal is usually instituted if the serum levels is 90 mg/L or more. According to Garella, in the setting of chronic ingestion, hemoperfusion or hemodialysis is instituted if serum levels are more than 40 mg/L and the patient manifests serious toxicity. Extracorporeal removal should be used in the presence of ventricular dysrhythmias, metabolic acidosis, refractory hypotension, or seizures. See Chapter 38 for a more extensive discussion of the indications for extracorporeal therapy and extracorporeal elimination rates in theophylline toxicity.

COMPLICATIONS OF EXTRACORPOREAL REMOVAL OF TOXINS

Although in the United States only 900 to 1000 poisoned patients are treated with hemodialysis yearly, the total number of hemodialysis treatments performed annually has reached the tens of millions. Extensive experience has made it a relatively safe procedure, particularly when only a few treatments are needed. The use of dialysis in the pediatric population remains static, unlike the expanding adult end-stage renal disease population. Experience with pediatric dialysis remains limited to specialized centers. Pediatric dialysis volumes, blood rates, and permissible dialysis surface area are all factors requiring a pediatric nephrologist or nephrologist with pediatric experience. Although it is rational to use extracorporeal techniques in cases of severe poisoning when these techniques can remove significant amounts of toxin, there are few data that clearly demonstrate decreases in mortality and long-term disability produced by these interventions.

Vascular Access

With the exception of peritoneal dialysis, all the aforementioned therapies require access to the intravascular space with a large-bore catheter. For hemodialysis or CVVH, a large-bore catheter is placed in either the femoral, subclavian, or jugular vein. Rarely, umbilical vessels can be used for infants. For poisoned patients who do not have renal failure, treatment is limited to one or two treatments and the problems of long- or intermediate-term vascular access are usually not of concern. If short-term treatment is anticipated, placement of the catheter in the femoral vein carries the lowest risk of complications. Perforation of an artery or of the opposite side of the vein is a risk associated with placement of a

line in any of these vessels, but control of bleeding is easiest with femoral placement. Placement in the subclavian vein also carries the risk of pneumothorax, hemothorax, hemopericardium, and laceration of the thoracic duct. A later complication of subclavian lines is stenosis of the subclavian vein. CAVH requires the placement of a catheter in a large artery, and the patient must be monitored for signs of arterial occlusion distal to the catheter. As with any intravenous access, catheters placed for hemodialysis or hemoperfusion can introduce infection. This risk increases with the length of time the catheter is in place.

Hypotension

Hypotension, the most common complication of dialysis, is most often precipitated by fluid removal. The extracorporeal circuit itself contains 70 to 175 mL in the dialyzer and 100 to 150 mL in the blood lines for adult patients. Pediatric systems limit this to 100 mL. In an otherwise stable patient, dialysis without the removal of fluid causes hemodynamic demands that are easily met. In the patient with a drug overdose, dialysis may exacerbate hypotension in a patient with hemodynamic instability from the effects of the drug. If the intoxication involves a drug that causes renal failure, the patient may have received large quantities of fluid during an attempt at conservative treatment that must now be removed by dialysis. When hemodynamic instability is a limiting factor, a continuous therapy such as CVVH may be used, although the efficacy of these modalities is unknown. Hypotension may also be caused by sepsis, bleeding, pericardial tamponade or by toxin-induced sympathetic blockade, acidosis, myocardial depression, or dysrhythmia.

Bleeding

The performance of hemodialysis, CAVH, and CVVH are facilitated by the use of heparin or other anticoagulants, although hemodialysis can be performed without anticoagulation. When heparin is not used, there is an increased risk of clotting of the extracorporeal circuit, but the risk of late bleeding is minimal. Hemoperfusion cannot be done without full anticoagulation. The bleeding tendency increases during hemoperfusion because of thrombocytopenia. Bleeding may occur at any site, and severe bleeding into the retroperitoneum may occur without clinical manifestations until hypotension in develops.

Citrate has been used as an anticoagulant in continuous therapies that combine diffusive and convective clearance. It is associated with fewer bleeding complications, but with a higher risk of disturbances of calcium metabolism and metabolic alkalosis.

Accidental disconnection of blood lines in any of these therapies can result in death from exsanguination. Hemodialysis machines are equipped with alarms that will detect a change in pressure associated with disconnection, stop the blood pump, and clamp the blood lines. The most sophisticated machines will not run if the alarms are disarmed. Most pumps for CVVH are similarly equipped with pressure monitors and air detectors. CAVH, which does not employ a blood pump, requires that the connections always be exposed so that accidental disconnection is immediately detected. The use of Luer lock connections minimizes this risk.

Other Complications

The use of intermittent hemodialysis on a widespread basis for acute and chronic renal failure has led to technology that minimizes many of the risks. Several of the most feared complications of dialysis have become uncommon. Virtually all dialysis machines are equipped with air detectors that shut off the blood pump and prevent air emboli. Many machines will not function unless the air detector is armed. On the outflow path of the dialysate, there is a colorimetric blood leak detector that will detect small quantities of blood in the dialysate exiting the dialyzer. If small quantities of blood are detected, the blood pump is shut off, preventing the return of blood contaminated by nonsterile dialysate to the patient. The amount of blood loss with rupture of the membrane in a hollow-fiber kidney is trivial.

There are monitoring systems that detect changes in the osmolality of dialysate and shunt blood away from the dialysate to prevent exposure to very hypotonic or hypertonic solution. A temperature monitor prevents exposure to overheated dialysate that may result in hemolysis.

Some dialyzers, particularly with membranes made of cuprophane, have occasionally been associated with anaphylactic reactions. These membranes have been replaced largely by more biocompatible synthetic membranes, particularly in the hospital setting, which have been associated with a more rapid recovery from acute renal failure.

Removal of Therapeutic Agents

During dialysis it should be remembered that some drugs will be removed and must be supplemented. Categories of drugs removed by extracorporeal therapy are listed in Table 18–4. Not every drug in a category is removed equally well. As new drugs in each category are introduced, the need for replacement during or after extracorporeal therapy should be checked. For some drugs, removal with extracorporeal therapy may be sufficient to interfere with therapeutic levels, but such therapy may not be good enough to reliably treat overdose. When dialysis is used in the absence of renal failure, the loss of some solutes generally present in excess in renal failure may become a problem. These include phosphorus and magnesium.

Chronic Dialysis-Induced Toxicity

Chronic dialysis patients have received significant toxic exposures via contaminated dialysis equipment. The primary vehicle of toxic exposure is contaminated water used in the dialysis process. Elevated water levels of calcium, copper, fluoride, chloramines, hydrogen peroxide, sodium, formaldehyde, sodium azide, sodium hypochlorite, aluminum, and zinc all have been reported to cause toxicity in dialysis patients, Recently, 50 deaths were reported by Jochimsen and co-workers in Brazil when microcystins produced by Cyanobacteria in the public water system caused acute hepatic failure in dialysis patients at one dialysis center.

SUMMARY

Extracorporeal removal of drugs and toxins is an essential although infrequently utilized tool in the management of the poisoned pediatric patient. Specific criteria related to the physical characteristics of the toxin, the efficacy of alternative therapies, and the severity of poisoning guide decisions regarding the utilization of these techniques. These are not last-ditch heroic maneuvers, but essential modalities for toxin removal that have an important role in the treatment of selected poisoned patients.

SUGGESTED READINGS

Alvan G, Bergman U, Gustafsson LL: High unbound fraction of salicylate in plasma during intoxication. *Br J Clin Pharmacol* 11:625–626, 1981.

Aronoff PM, Bland LA, Garcia-Houchins S, et al: An outbreak of fatal fluoride intoxication in a long-term hemodialysis unit. *Ann Intern Med* 121:339, 1994.

Aronoff GR, Bems JS, Brier ME, et al: *Drug Prescribing in Renal Failure*. Philadelphia: American College of Physicians; 1999.

Bellomo R, Kearly Y, Parkin G, et al: Treatment of life-threatening lithium toxicity with continuous arterio-venous hemodiafiltration. *Crit Care Med* 19:836, 1991.

Boyers EW, Mejia M, Woolf A, et al: Severe ethylene glycol ingestion treated without hemodialysis. *Pediatrics* 107:172–173, 2001.

Brent J, McMartin K, Phillips S, et al: Fomepizole treatment of ethylene glycol poisoning. Methylpyrazole for Toxic Alcohols Study Group. *N Engl J Med* 340:832–838, 1999.

Brophy PD, Tenenbein M, Gardner J, et al: Childhood diethylene glycol poisoning treated with alcohol dehydrogenase inhibitor fomepizole and hemodialysis. *Am J Kidney Dis* 35:958–962, 2000.

Burwen DR, Olsen SM, Bland LA, et al: Epidemic aluminum intoxication in hemodialysis patients traced to use of an aluminum pump. *Kidney Int* 48:469, 1995.

Catalilna MV, Nunez O, Ponferrada A, et al: Liver failure due to mushroom poisoning: Clinical course and treatment perspectives. *Gastroenterol Hepatol* 26:417–420, 2003.

Cohen BL, Bovasso GJ Jr: Acquired methemoglobinemia and hemolytic anemia following excessive pyridium (phenazopyridine hydrochloride) ingestion. *Clin Pediatr* 10:537, 1971.

Covic A, Goldsmith DJA, Gusbeth Tatomir P, et al: Successful use of molecular absorbent regenerating system (MARS) dialysis for the treatment of fulminant hepatic failure in children accidentally poisoned by toxic mushroom ingestion. *Liver Int* 23(Suppl 3):21–27, 2003

Cutler RE, Fodand SC, St. John Hammond PG, et al: Extracorporeal removal of drugs and poisons by hemodialysis and hemoperfusion. *Annu Rev Pharmacol Toxicol* 27:169–191, 1987.

Dasgupta A, Cao S, Wells A: Activated charcoal is effective but equilibrium dialysis is ineffective in removing oleander leaf extract and oleandrin from human serum: Monitoring the effect by measuring apparent digoxin concentration. *Ther Drug Monit* 25:323–330, 2003.

De Monchy JGR, Snoek WJ, Sliviter HJ, et al: Treatment of severe parathion intoxication. *Vet Hum Toxicol* 21(suppl 1):115–117, 1979.

Eaton JW, Kolpin CF, Swofford HS, et al: Chlorinated urban water. A cause of dialysis-induced hemolytic anemia. *Science* 181:463, 1973.

Ekins BR, Rollins DE, Duffy DP, et al: Standardized treatment of severe methanol poisoning with ethanol and hemodialysis. *West J Med* 142:337, 1985.

Faybik P, Hetz H, Baker A, et al: Extracorporeal albumin dialysis in patients with *Amanita phalloides* poisoning. *Liver Int* 23(suppl 3):28–33, 2003

Fine RN, Tejani A: Dialysis in infants and children. In: Daugirdas JT, Ing TS, eds: *Handbook of Dialysis*. Boston: Little, Brown; 1994:553–568.

Ford MD, Sivilotti MLA: Alcohols and glycols. In: Irwin RS, Cem RS Cerra FB, et al, eds: *Irwin and Rippe's Intensive Care Medicine*. 4th ed. Philadelphia: Lippincott–Raven; 1999:1478–1493.

Freeman RM, Lawton RL, Chamberlain MA: Hard-water syndrome. *N Engl J Med* 276:1113, 1967.

Garella S: Extracorporeal techniques in the treatment of exogenous intoxications. *Kidney Int* 33:735, 1988.

Garrettson LK, Geller RJ: Acid and alkaline diuresis: When are they of value in the treatment of poisoning. *Drug Safety* 5:220, 1990.

Gentilello LM, Cobean RA, Offner PJ, et al: Continuous arteriovenous rewarming: Rapid reversal of hypothermia in critically ill patients. *J Trauma* 32:316, 1992.

Gordon SM, Bland LA, Alexander SR, et al: Hemolysis associated with hydrogen peroxide at a pediatric dialysis center. *Am J Nephrol* 10:123, 1990.

Gordon SM, Drachman J, Bland LA, et al: Epidemic hypotension in a dialysis center caused by sodium azide. *Kidney Int* 37:110–115, 1990.

Groleau G: Lithium toxicity. *Emerg Med Clin North Am* 12:511–531, 1994.

Gualideri JF, DeBoer L, Harris CR, et al: Repeated ingestion of 2-butoxy-ethanol: Case report and literature review. *J Toxicol Clin Toxicol* 41:57–62, 2003.

Gurland H, Samtleven W, Lysacht MJ, et al: Extracorporeal blood purification techniques: Plasmapheresis and hemoperfusion. In: Jacob C, Kjellstrand CM, Kock KM, et al, eds: *Replacement of Renal Function by Dialysis*. Dordrecht: Kluwer Academic; 1996:2.

Hansen HE, Amdisen A: Lithium intoxication: Report of 23 cases and review of 100 cases from the literature. *Q J Med* 186:123, 1978.

Hoy RH: Accidental systemic exposure to sodium hypochlorite (Chlorox) during hemodialysis. *Am J Hosp Pharm* 38:1512, 1981.

Hughes, RD: Review of methods to remove protein-bound substance liver failure. *Int J Artif Organs* 25:911–917, 2002.

Jacobsen D, Jansen H, Wilk-Larsen E, et al: Studies on methanol poisoning. *Acta Med Scand* 212:5, 1982.

Jacobsen D, McMartin KE: Antidotes for methanol and ethylene glycol poisoning. *J Toxicol Clin Toxicol* 35:127, 1997.

Jacobsen D, Ovrebo S, Sejersted OM: Toxicokinetics of formate during hemodialysis. *Acta Med Scand* 214:409, 1983.

Jacobsen D, Webb R, Collins TD, et al: Methanol and formate kinetics in late diagnosed methanol intoxication. *Mod Toxicol* 3:418, 1988.

Jacobsen D, Wilk-Larsen E, Dahl T, et al: Pharmacokinetic evaluation of haemoperfusion in phenobarbital poisoning. *Eur J Clin Pharm* 26:109, 1984.

Jochimsen EM, Carmichael WW, An JS, et al: Liver failure and death after exposure to microcystins at a hemodialysis center in Brazil. *N Engl J Med* 338:873, 1998.

Johnson LZ, Martinez I, Fernandez MC, et al: Successful treatment of valproic acid overdose with hemodialysis. *Am J Kidney Dis* 33:786, 1999.

Kerns W, Tomaszewski C, McMartin K, et al: Formate kinetics in methanol poisoning [abstract]. *J Toxicol Clin Toxicol* 37:669, 1999.

Klammt, S, Stange, J, Mitzner, SR et al: Extracorporeal liver support by re-circulating albumin dialysis: Analyzing the effect of the first clinically used generation of the MARS system. *Liver* 22(suppl 2):30–34, 2002.

Koivusal AM, Yildrim Y, Vakkuri A, et al: Experience with albumin dialysis in five patients with severe overdoses of Paracetamol. *Acta Anasthesiol Scand* 47:1145–1150, 2003.

Larsen LS, Sterrett JR, Whitehead B, et al: Adjunctive therapy of phenytoin overdose: A case report using plasmapheresis. *J Toxicol Clin Toxicol* 24:37, 1996.

Leblanc M, Raymond M, Bonnardeaux A, et al: Lithium poisoning treated by high-performance continuous arteriovenous and venovenous hemodiafiltration. *Am J Kidney Dis* 27:365, 1996.

Lim PS, Lim JL: Continuous arteriovenous hemoperfusion in acute poisoning. *Ann Emerg Med* 26:725, 1995.

Litovitz TL, Schwartz-Klein W, Rodgers GC, et al: 2001 annual report of the AAPCC Toxic Exposure Surveillance System. *Am J Emerg Med* 20:391–452, 2002.

McDonald LK, Taraglione TA, Mendelman PM, et al: Lack of toxicity in two cases of neonatal acyclovir overdose. *Pediatr Infect Dis J* 8:529–532, 1989.

Malluche HH, Smith AJ, Abreo K, et al: The use of desfero examine in the management of aluminum accumulation M bone in patients with renal failure. *N Engl J Med* 311:140, 1984.

Manns M, Sigler MH, Teehan BP: Continuous renal replacement therapies: An update. *Am J Kidney Dis* 32:185, 1998.

Manzler AD, Schreiner AW: Copper-induced acute hemolytic anemia: A new complication of hemodialysis. *Ann Intern Med* 73:409, 1970.

Mehta RL, Dobos GJ, Ward DM: Anticoagulation in continuous renal replacement therapy. *Semin Dial* 5:61, 1992.

Meyer RJ, Flynn JT, Brophy PD, et al: Hemodialysis followed by continuous hemofiltration for treatment of lithium intoxication in children. *Am J Kidney Dis* 37:1044–1047, 2001.

Mokrzycki, MH, Kaplan, AA: Therapeutic plasma exchange: Complications and management. *Am J Kidney Dis* 23:817–827, 1994

Molina R, Fabian C, Cowley B: Use of charcoal hemoperfusion with sequential hemodialysis to reduce serum methotrexate levels in a patient with acute renal insufficiency. *Am J Med* 82:350, 1987.

Moreau CL, Kerns W, Tomaszewski CA, et al: Glycolate kinetics and hemodialysis clearance in ethylene glycol poisoning. *J Toxicol Clin Toxicol* 36:659, 1998.

Nenov VD, Marinov P, Sabeva J, et al: Current applications of plasmapheresis in clinical toxicology. *Nephrol Dial Transplant* 18:V56–V58, 2003.

Nickey WA, Chinitz VL, Kim DE, et al: Hypernatremia from water softener malfunction during home dialysis. *JAMA* 214:915, 1970.

Orlowski JM, Hou S, Leikin J: Extracorporeal removal of drugs and toxins. In: Ford M, Delaney K, Ling L, et al, eds: Philadelphia: Saunders; 2001:43–50.

Orriger EP, Mattern WD: Formaldehyde-induced hemolysis during chronic hemodialysis. *N Engl J Med* 294:1416, 1976.

Osborn HH, Henry G, Wax P, et al: Theophylline toxicity in a premature neonate—Elimination kinetics of exchange transfusion. *J Toxicol Clin Toxicol* 31:639, 1993.

Perrin C, Debrugne D, La Cotte J, et al: Treatment caffeine intoxication by exchange transfusion in a newborn. *Acta Paediatr Scand* 76:679–681, 1987.

Peterson CD, Collins AJ, Himes JM, et al: Ethylene glycol poisoning: Pharmacokinetics during therapy with ethanol and hemodialysis. *N Engl J Med* 304:21, 1981.

Petrie JJB, Row PG: Dialysis anemia caused by subacute zinc toxicity. *Lancet* 1:1178, 1977.

Pond SM: Extracorporeal techniques in the treatment of poisoned patients. *Med J Aust* 154:617, 1991.

Porto I, John EG, Heilliczer J: Removal of phenobarbital during continuous cycling peritoneal dialysis in a child. *Pharmacotherapy* 17:832–835, 1997.

Roberts M, Daugirdas JT: REDY sorbent hemodialysis. In Daugirdas JT, Ing TS, eds: *Handbook of Dialysis.* Boston: Little, Brown; 1994.

Sabeel AI, Kurkus J, Lindholm T: Intensified dialysis treatment of ethylene glycol intoxication. *Scand J Urol Nephrol* 29:125–129, 1995.

Sancak R, Kucukoduk R, Tagdemir HA, et al: Exchange transfusion treatment in a newborn with phenobarbital intoxication. *Pediatr Emerg Care* 15:268–270, 1999.

Sen S, Ratnaraj N, Davies NA, et al. Treatment of phenytoin toxicity by the molecular absorbents recirculating system (MARS). *Epilepsia* 44:265–267, 2003.

Shannon, M, Wernovsky, G, Morris, C: Exchange transfusion in the treatment of severe theophylline poisoning. *Pediatrics* 89:145–147, 1992.

Shi Y, He J, Chen S, et al: MARS: Optimistic therapy method in fulminant hepatic failure secondary to cytotoxic mushroom poisoning—A case report. *Liver* 22(suppl 2):78–80, 2002.

Soylemezoglu O, Bakkaloglu A, Yigit S, et al: Hemodialysis treatment in phenobarbital intoxication in infancy. *Int Urol Nephrol* 25:111–113, 1993.

Swartz RD, Millman RP, Blli JE, et al: Epidemic methanol poisoning: Clinical and biochemical analysis of a recent episode. *Medicine* 60:373–382, 1981.

Tauscher JW, Polich JJ: Treatment of pine oil poisoning by exchange transfusion. *J Pediatr* 55:571–575, 1959.

U.S. Department of Health and Human Services: *Hemoperfusion in Conjunction with Desferoxmine for the Treatment of Aluminum Toxicity and Iron Overload in Patients with End-Stage Renal Disease.* Rockville, MD: USDHHS; 1986.

Vaziri ND, Upham T, Barton CH: Hemodialysis clearance of arsenic. *J Toxicol Clin Toxicol* 17:451, 1980.

Winchester JF: Use of dialysis and hemoperfusion in treatment of poisoning. In: Daugirdas JT, Ing TS, eds: *Handbook of Dialysis.* Boston: Little, Brown; 1994.

Woo OF, Pond SM, Benowitz NL, et al: Benefit of hemoperfusion in acute theophylline intoxication. *J Toxicol Clin Toxicol* 22:411–424, 1984.

Wright RO, Lewander WJ, Woolf AD: Methemoglobin: Etiology, pharmacology, and clinical management. *Ann Emerg Med* 34:646–656, 1999.

Yip L, Dart RC, Gabow PA: Concepts and controversies in salicylate toxicity. *Emerg Med Clin North Am* 12:351, 1994.

19

Pediatric Toxicology in the Pediatric Intensive Care Unit

William Banner, Jr.
R. Philip Barton

HIGH-YIELD FACTS

- Airway management is critical and is best accomplished when the patient has an empty stomach.
- Ventilator support for critically ill patients is best approached in a systematic, step-wise fashion, and may include high-frequency techniques.
- Continuous replacement therapies may accomplish many of the goals of dialysis in a wider variety of settings.
- Cardiovascular support for poisoned patients should progress from preload to cardiac output and finally to correction of afterload.
- Toxic exposures may cause critical illness that requires extracorporeal membrane oxygenation (ECMO) to provide support for both the pulmonary and cardiac systems.

There have been significant strides in the delivery of intensive care to children over the past decades. There has also been as a great deal of research into the area of management of intoxicated patients, focusing primarily on adults. The interface of intensive care and toxicology for the pediatric patient is largely unexplored. The toxicologist must be familiar with the modalities available to the intensive care practitioner to guide the care of the pediatric patient.

There is no question that initiation of endotracheal (ET) intubation and mechanical ventilation is the single most critical decision in the management of any poi-

soned patient. In that regard, specialists in pediatric critical care have the technical capabilities to improve outcome dramatically. Rapid-sequence induction (RSI) using neuromuscular blockers has now become a standard of care outside the operating room. The traditional modalities of decontamination—especially the instillation of activated charcoal—are sometimes in conflict with the more basic need to provide airway support. The patient whose stomach contains charcoal may be at risk for aspiration pneumonia. Similarly, toxicologic mainstays such as repeated doses of activated charcoal and urinary alkalinization may present difficulties in very young children or in those with multisystem organ failure. Despite the benefits of gastrointestinal decontamination and enhanced elimination, the critical care practitioner may be more comfortable focusing on respiratory and cardiovascular support. Reversal of benzodiazepine intoxication with flumazenil, for example, may be more problematic than providing respiratory support while the patient clears the drug via metabolism. These issues should be relatively simple to resolve if one carefully considers which modalities are most likely to really alter outcome in the face of good supportive care.

CHOICES OF AGENTS FOR RAPID-SEQUENCE INDUCTION

ET intubation is generally most successful under controlled circumstances. Before the procedure is attempted, the individual assigned to manage the airway should ensure that all equipment is available and functioning properly to minimize sequelae. Ideally, the patient should have an empty stomach and be adequately sedated. An intact gag reflex in a partially sedated patient may provoke inopportune vomiting.

In patients with caustic ingestions, emesis of an acid or alkali may also pose a risk to medical personnel; face covering, especially of the eyes, is important. Special considerations in the poisoned patient may include inhibition of drug metabolism and airway damage from the ingested poison.

Succinylcholine has a limited role in neuromuscular blockade in children because of possible adverse events, including increased intragastric pressure, increased intraocular pressure, increased intracranial pressure, hyperkalemia, and bradycardia. Certain toxins may further limit its use. The presence of insecticides or nerve agents that inhibit cholinesterase will prolong its duration. In cases of tricyclic antidepressant poisoning, transient hyperkalemia of succinylcholine depolarization may counter the otherwise protective effect of increased extracellular sodium and worsen dysrhythmias. In theory, muscle fasciculations may exacerbate disorders such as the neuroleptic malignant syndrome with rhabdomyolysis. Pretreatment with defasciculating doses of nondepolarizing agents may mitigate the latter, but given the availability of rapid-onset neuromuscular blockers such as rocuronium, it seems difficult to justify even minor risks associated with succinylcholine. If succinylcholine is administered, pretreatment with atropine minimizes secretions and prevents bradycardia. This would obviously be inappropriate in the setting of anticholinergic toxicity.

Choices of adjunct sedatives in the poisoned patient are relatively straightforward. Even in the presence of an ingested benzodiazepine, the addition of a single dose of midazolam or lorazepam is not likely to alter outcome. Barbiturates or propofol are rarely needed.

Patients with epiglottic or tracheal swelling from caustic burns may lose airway integrity and not respond to bag–mask ventilation. In this setting of upper airway obstruction, the use of neuromuscular blockers is relatively contraindicated. Anesthetic gases may be useful but are not likely to be readily available. An alternative is ketamine, which generally maintains airway integrity during intubation. The issue of pretreatment with atropine should be considered as above.

RESPIRATORY FAILURE

A large number of drugs contribute to respiratory failure, generally through central nervous system depression rather than direct lung injury. In either scenario, resultant aspiration pneumonia may progress to the acute respiratory distress syndrome (ARDS), requiring advanced modes of mechanical ventilation. The intense inflammatory response and decreases in both surfactant production and function associated with hydrocarbon aspiration may resemble classic ARDS and require aggressive intervention. Paraquat is unusual in that it injures type II cells of the lungs to produce ARDS.

Management of respiratory failure should be viewed as a continuum of care that begins with the least invasive support and progresses to more aggressive techniques while minimizing risks such as pneumothorax. The goal of mechanical ventilation may not always be to achieve normal blood gases. Maintaining minimal ventilation to avoid barotrauma and allowing pH to decrease closer to 7.20 with $PaCO_2$ increasing to 50 to 60 mmHg may be safe in most disease states. Poisoned patients, however, may pose additional challenges. Intoxication with weakly acidic compounds such as salicylates may be more complex. Systemic acidemia may allow the pH of cerebrospinal fluid to be higher than that of blood, creating ion trapping in the central nervous system. Given the propensity for central hyperventilation and the potential for sudden pulmonary edema in salicylate poisoning, mechanical ventilation of these patients may present significant challenges.

CONVENTIONAL MODES OF VENTILATION

In general, mechanical ventilation may be initiated using a volume-cycle mode at a rate and tidal volume designed to somewhat mimic natural respiration. End-expiratory pressure may be used to improve functional residual capacity and maintain alveolar distension. Unfortunately, many ventilators use volume-control modes that deliver continuous flow that yields higher peak-inspiratory pressures at a specific tidal volume. The evidence suggests that this causes airway damage; thus, as lung compliance decreases and peak-inspiratory pressures increase, it is desirable to avoid this flow pattern.

Changing to a pressure-control mode allows airflow to be delivered in a decelerating pattern, increasing the mean airway pressure while decreasing the peak-inspiratory pressure, minimizing damage to the airway. As compliance changes, however, the delivered tidal volumes deteriorate, and ventilation is severely compromised. Thus, neither mode is ideal. State-of-the-art ventilators now include modes such as pressure-regulated volume control (PRVC), for which a pressure-controlled breath is delivered in a decelerating flow pattern to guarantee a fixed tidal volume delivery. This mode generally requires that the patient be sedated and not in competition with the ventilator (frequently not an issue for overdose patients). In addition, the latest generation of ventilators allows for synchronous breathing in a so-called PRVC mode, thus an SIMV-PRVC. Even given these modalities, peak airway pressures may rise; as pressures exceed a total of 40 cm H_2O, the risks of lung damage such as pneumothorax begin to increase. Although conventional mechanical ventilation is the mainstay of ventilatory support for patients with diffuse alveolar disease or ARDS, there are potential pitfalls that the clinician must avoid. This process is generally referred to as barotrauma.

Barotrauma is defined as air leaks that usually occur in terminal bronchioles with high peak-inspiratory pressures. Studies have shown that peak-inspiratory pressures >40 cm H_2O increase the risk of barotrauma tremendously in patients with diffuse alveolar disease. *Volutrauma* is defined as air leaks that typically occur in overdistended normal alveoli with excessive tidal volumes. Delivered tidal volumes >15 cc/kg are associated with a high risk of volutrauma in patients with diffuse alveolar disease. High concentrations of inspired oxygen may generate free radicals to damage alveolar endothelium and surfactant production/function in type II cells. Free radical formation is enhanced with inspired oxygen concentrations above 60%. Studies in healthy volunteers have shown that surfactant production and function decrease with exposure to inspired oxygen levels over 60% for as few as 6 to 8 hours. A toxin like paraquat will exaggerate this toxic effect.

HIGH-FREQUENCY MODES OF VENTILATION

There are patients for whom clinically tolerable gas exchange is acceptable only with conventional ventilator settings that promote barotrauma, volutrauma, or oxygen toxicity despite the use of the advanced methods described. It is in these settings that high-frequency forms of mechanical ventilation are indicated.

High-frequency ventilation has been used in two relatively different patient populations: neonatal and pediatric. The goal of high-frequency ventilation is to maximize oxygenation and ventilation while minimizing barotrauma, volutrauma, and oxygen toxicity. The two most widely used modalities are high-frequency oscillatory ventilation (HFOV) and high-frequency jet ventilation (HFJV). HFOV and HFJV are applied with two different strategies.

High-Frequency Jet Ventilation

During the inspiratory phase, HFJV provides a high-pressure gas flow through a small-bore cannula adapter attached to the ET tube. A gas-flow interrupter system regulates the connection between the cannula adapter and a high-pressure gas source. The small diameter of the cannula generates resistance that reduces pressure in the distal pulmonary bed. The regular portion of the ET tube is connected to a conventional ventilator to generate mean airway pressure through the application of positive end-expiratory pressure (PEEP). The typical HFJV tidal volumes generated are 3 to 5 cc/kg, and unlike HFOV, the exhalation phase is a passive process. Compared with conventional mechanical ventilation and HFOV, HFJV usually requires a significantly lower mean airway pressure to achieve similar levels of oxygenation. HFJV alone cannot maintain adequate lung volumes, and therefore requires the concomitant use of a conventional ventilator to generate PEEP and to provide periodic tidal-breath volumes. Thus, baro- or volutrauma may still occur. The benefits may be particularly desired when right ventricular function is poor or right ventricular venous return cannot be tolerated. HFJV also improves access to the airways during diagnostic bronchoscopy.

High-Frequency Oscillatory Ventilation

HFOV devices require a source for gas flow, a diaphragm capable of generating high-frequency oscillations of a gas column and a specialized exhalation port that maintains a preset mean airway pressure. The HFOV circuit and the patient's airways dampen the high peak pressures generated during inspiration in the large airways. As a result, alveoli are exposed to significantly lower pressure. In addition, the continuous flow of gas washes out CO_2.

The back-and-forth movement of the HFOV piston transmitted through the gas column generates a positive inspiratory pressure and a negative or active expiratory pressure. HFOV tidal volume is less than that of HFJV and is usually well below anatomic dead space volume, typically 1 to 3 cc/kg.

Compared to conventional mechanical ventilation and HFJV, HFOV usually requires significantly higher mean airway pressures to achieve similar levels of oxygenation, but at lower peak airway pressures (to limit barotrauma) and lower tidal volumes (to limit volutrauma). With adequate lung expansion, a more favorable pressure–volume relationship occurs, along with improved compliance and improved gas exchange.

Initially reserved for small infants, the latest generation of high-frequency ventilators may be used on adults. Although HFJV has been used to support neonates and adults for several years, information about its pediatric application is scarce. There are far more pediatric data regarding HFOV, as its application in diffuse alveolar disease gains widespread acceptance in this population.

Contraindications

Obstructive airway disease is usually considered a contraindication to most high-frequency devices. All have limited expiratory times and should be avoided in conditions such as emphysema and asthma.

Patients with severe intravascular volume depletion may not be able to maintain an adequate blood flow at high mean airway pressures needed to recruit or reexpand severely diseased lung. Conditions such as severe dehydration or distributive vasodilation as seen in sepsis or tricyclic overdose require adequate preload prior to initiation of high-frequency ventilation. Various agents may induce cardiogenic shock; contractility must also be maximized before high-frequency ventilation.

The most expeditious approach to the use of mechanical ventilation is to have fixed endpoints for moving to more invasive support. When high-frequency ventilation is unable to achieve adequate gas exchange and mean airway pressures reach 40 cm H_2O, or the patient has a combination of cardiogenic shock unresponsive to aggressive inotropic support with diffuse alveolar disease, consideration of extracorporeal support is indicated.

NITRIC OXIDE

Nitric oxide (NO) is a locally active vasodilator that is administered via inhalation for the treatment of pulmonary hypertension. It is a compound that was explored initially in the neonatal intensive care unit. NO is now a readily available modality for the pediatric intensive care unit, but its role in the management of poisonings has not been well established. One possible application would be mitigation of pulmonary hypertension that follows chronic exposure to paraquat.

SURFACTANT

Surface-active agents or *surfactants* that allow easier expansion of the alveolar bubble exist in a variety of forms.

They vary primarily by species derivation and preparation technique. They have been used extensively in premature neonates whose lungs are surfactant deficient. Surfactant use in older children and adults has been less widely studied and accepted. For example, although hydrocarbons induce an inflammatory response that would not be expected to benefit from surfactant use, animal studies have varied in outcome; the therapy has minimal side effects and may allow oxygenation at more acceptable airway pressures. Paraquat is a toxin that damages type II cells to reduce surfactant, and animal studies have shown short-term improvement with replacement therapy. Human use seems rational but is not yet evidence based.

CARDIOVASCULAR FAILURE
Mechanisms

Poisoning may affect the cardiovascular system through a variety of mechanisms. Most commonly, narcotics, benzodiazepines, and barbiturates cause global cardiac depression and may cause progressive changes in preload, cardiac output, and afterload. Even therapeutic doses of narcotics and anesthetic agents produce some venous pooling and a decrease in preload, with a compensatory increase in heart rate. Additional intravascular volume supports the patient in this circumstance. Drugs that produce cardiac arrhythmias may also decrease cardiac output on the basis of these mechanisms. Drugs that directly depress myocardial function, however, are of greater concern. In extreme situations, the arterial system may lose integrity, severely decreasing afterload and blood pressure. In reality, these effects may overlap, and require frequent clinical reassessment.

Assessment

The early assessment of cardiovascular alterations in pediatric patients consists of the usual clinical parameters. Pulse rate, blood pressure, and subjective measures such as peripheral perfusion and capillary refill are useful in the short term, but are no substitute for measurements of central venous pressure. More invasive direct measurements require the placement of a Swan–Ganz catheter.

Choices of Inotropes and Vasopressors

The choices of agents for cardiovascular support are more frequently made on the basis of habit than pharmacology. It is critical to remember that agents such as dobutamine support a patient with low cardiac output, but also produce a decrease in preload and afterload. It would be an extremely unusual poisoning for which this agent would be appropriate. Although dopamine may be useful as a first-line drug, the relative α-adrenergic receptor blockade of drugs like tricyclic antidepressants may respond only to potent α-adrenergic agents such as phenylephrine, norepinephrine, and epinephrine. Although a patient with progressive cooling of the extremities and poor distal pulses may appear to be vasoconstricted, invasive assessment of cardiac output may reveal shunting that diminishes systemic vascular resistance. Aggressive use of vasoconstrictor agents may prove more beneficial in maintaining organ perfusion. Invasive data can guide the safe use of agents such as phenylephrine, epinephrine, and norepinephrine.

Extracorporeal Membrane Oxygenation

The use of extracorporeal membrane oxygenation (ECMO) to support poisoned patients with either respiratory or cardiac failure would appear to be a logical modality. Anecdotal reports of survival following the institution of ECMO in poisoned patients, however, remain the basis for its use. There are two basic modes of ECMO: venovenous (VV) and venoarterial (VA). In VV mode, deoxygenated blood is drained from a large vein, oxygenated, and returned to another large vein so that venous blood entering the right heart has increased oxygen content. Toxins that produce severe respiratory failure without affecting myocardial function are candidates for VV ECMO.

In VA mode, blood is drained from a large vein, oxygenated, and returned under pressure to the aortic arch. VA mode thus generates an arterial blood pressure with oxygenated blood. Patients who ingest overdoses of β-adrenergic antagonists or calcium channel antagonists may have depressed myocardial function or disrupted cardiac conduction, and may require cardiac output support from VA ECMO. It is unlikely that use of these modalities will occur frequently enough to base any decisions on conclusive evidence.

Overall, ECMO appears to reduce mortality effectively in selected situations and thus must be entertained cautiously when other supportive care is failing to sustain life. Case reports of poisoned patients who survived after ECMO treatment are increasingly common. Two caveats concerning this extreme measure should be emphasized. First, long-term survival following ECMO improves dramatically when the decision to initiate care is made early in the course of respiratory failure, in part because sustained high pressures and oxygen concentrations from mechanical ventilation are mitigated; ECMO cannot be viewed as a rescue after a sustained failure of ventilator management. Second, the decision to initiate ECMO must consider reversibility of the toxic effect. One example would be the decision to withhold ECMO from a patient who ingests paraquat and develops potentially irreversible pulmonary disease.

RENAL FAILURE

In the poisoned patient, deteriorating cardiopulmonary function may lead to multisystem organ failure and ultimately renal failure. In this respect, the management of toxin-associated renal failure is no different from that of other causes. In addition, some toxins such as mercury, chromium, and boron may present a direct effect on the kidney. Dialysis may be required to enhance elimination of certain drugs or toxins, particularly if renal failure exists.

Altering Nephrotoxicity

The management of any critical care patient is greatly simplified if anuria is avoided and adequate urine output is maintained. One of the most common approaches is the use of high-dose loop diuretics. In renal failure, these drugs produce an increase in renal blood flow and glomerular filtration that is beneficial in the short term without altering chronic outcome. In a study of animals poisoned with chromium and boron, treatment with *N*-acetylcysteine improved urine output, suggesting a nephroprotective effect.

Renal Replacement Therapy: Intermittent Versus Continuous Techniques

Intermittent and continuous techniques include the following:

- CVVH: Continuous venovenous hemofiltration
- CVVHD: Continuous venovenous hemodiafiltration
- Dialysis: A general term usually reserved for intermittent hemodialysis
- PD: Peritoneal dialysis
- SCUF: Slow continuous ultrafiltration

CVVH involves the passive filtration of blood across a filter that has a molecular weight cut-off around 50,000 daltons. The process removes fluid and replaces it with an electrolyte-containing fluid infused on the inflow side of the filter cartridge. Dilution occurs, allowing greater flux of toxins across the filter. In an animal model, a chelating agent infused with the replacement fluid increased iron removal. CVVHD uses the same technology as CVVH, but additional dialysis fluid is infused around the filter fibers to further increase the removal of toxins.

In general, the clearance of urea nitrogen is the standard for assessing these techniques. Dialysis is the most effective technique for rapid removal of many toxins, although technical capabilities of the hospital and hemodynamic stability of the patient may limit its use. There is also a limit to the amount of fluid that may be removed over a short period of time without replacement. In situations requiring massive blood product replacement, vascular volumes may become excessive as intermittent hemodialysis fails to remove sufficient fluid. The clearance of toxins is second greatest for CVVHD, followed by CVVH, with peritoneal dialysis being the least effective approach.

Slow continuous ultrafiltration (SCUF) is the passive removal of fluid without replacement. It has limited clinical utility for drug removal.

Using a charcoal cartridge in place of a membrane cartridge is a technique called *charcoal hemoperfusion.* In theory it overcomes the limitation of toxin/protein binding in serum to allow greater removal of drug. There are rare situations where drugs with a high degree of protein binding do not also have a large volume of distribution, but for the majority the limiting factor is the net clearance of drug and not removal from the blood compartment. Thus, the initial promise of the charcoal cartridge use has in reality met with limited application. It has been used on dialysis machines and also on continuous machines. The most concerning problem with this approach is the effect of aggregating platelets, requiring monitoring and replacement.

CVVH may be added easily to an ECMO circuit, allowing supportive care while enhancing elimination.

HEPATIC FAILURE

Plasmapheresis Versus Continuous Venovenous Hemofiltration

Drugs such as acetaminophen are metabolized to hepatic toxins that may induce striking changes in liver function. In addition, endogenous toxins such as ammonia may accumulate. Untreated acetaminophen poisoning may evolve rapidly to hepatic failure, requiring consideration of hepatic transplantation. Limited organ availability and the possibility of recovery following acute toxic hepatic failure may lead to greater attempts at supportive care before transplantation. Removal of ammonia becomes a critical form of support; because renal removal is minimal, alternative methods are required. The two principal modalities for long-term support are plasmapheresis and CVVH or CVVHD. All require the placement of large venous catheters capable of relatively high blood-flow rates. The literature generally supports the use of intermittent plasmapheresis to lower ammonia levels, although continuous dialysis techniques have the advantage of milder inflammatory activation. Because many of these children are critically ill and may exhibit the systemic inflammatory response syndrome (SIRS), further activation of this response by plasmapheresis may be counterproductive.

HEMATOLOGIC DISORDERS

Disseminated Intravascular Coagulation

Potassium dichromate is an example of a toxin that may provoke SIRS, leading to disseminated intravascular coagulation (DIC). Traditional management of DIC has consisted primarily of replacement of clotting factors and platelets consumed in the process. Research in the area of DIC associated with septic shock has led to the development of activated recombinant protein C to interrupt the process. Clinical observation in those rare cases of toxin-induced DIC may suggest whether this process can be similarly interrupted.

CONCLUSION

The admission of children to the PICU for management of poisoning offers them the advantage of many advanced modes of life support. The decision to institute airway management and mechanical ventilation is the single most important act that will alter the outcome of these patients. The inflammatory effects of hydrocarbons or gastric acid in the lungs may lead to diffuse alveolar disease that may require the advantages of high-frequency ventilation. Advanced technology like extracorporeal support may be the last resort to support the more critically ill child. As a frequent first-line provider of care, the toxicologist is in a unique position to triage children to settings where they will receive optimal care. Recognition of poisoning that may require advanced critical care is important because of the time factors involved in delivering care and the risks of transporting a child who has already deteriorated. Communication between the poison management and the critical care teams requires some understanding of the modalities available and the relative risks of standard toxicology treatments and critical care treatments.

SUGGESTED READINGS

Auzinger GM, Scheinkestel CD: Successful extracorporeal life support in a case of severe flecainide intoxication. *Crit Care Med* 29:887–890, 2001.

Banner W Jr: Risks of extracorporeal membrane oxygenation: Is there a role for use in the management of the acutely poisoned patient? *J Toxicol Clin Toxicol* 34:365–371, 1996.

Banner W Jr, Timmons OD, Vernon DD: Advances in the critical care of poisoned paediatric patients. *Drug Saf* 10:83–92, 1994.

Banner W Jr, Vernon DD, Ward RM, et al: Continuous arteriovenous hemofiltration in experimental iron intoxication. *Crit Care Med* 17:1187–1190, 1989.

Bysani GK, Rucoba RJ, Noah ZL: Treatment of hydrocarbon pneumonitis. High frequency jet ventilation as an alternative to extracorporeal membrane oxygenation. *Chest* 106:300–303, 1994.

Chyka PA: Benefits of extracorporeal membrane oxygenation for hydrocarbon pneumonitis. *J Toxicol Clin Toxicol* 34:357–363, 1996.

Goodwin DA, Lally KP, Null DM Jr: Extracorporeal membrane oxygenation support for cardiac dysfunction from tricyclic antidepressant overdose. *Crit Care Med* 21:625–627, 1993.

So KL, de Buijzer E, Gommers D, et al: Surfactant therapy restores gas exchange in lung injury due to paraquat intoxication in rats. *Eur Respir J* 12:284–287, 1998.

Tecklenburg FW, Thomas NJ, Webb SA, et al: Pediatric ECMO for severe quinidine cardiotoxicity. *Pediatr Emerg Care* 13:111–113, 1997.

Widner LR, Goodwin SR, Berman LS, et al: Artificial surfactant for therapy in hydrocarbon-induced lung injury in sheep. *Crit Care Med* 24:1524–1529, 1996.

DIAGNOSTIC TESTING AND PHYSICAL ASSESSMENT

20

Laboratory Testing

Robert J. Hoffman

HIGH-YIELD FACTS

- Any patient with altered mental status or the potential to develop hypoglycemia from a poisoning should have a bedside glucose assessment.

- Serum chemistry assessment, calculation of an anion gap, and blood gas assessment can be used in poisonings by agents known to cause elevated anion gap metabolic acidosis.

- Classic toxicologic causes of elevated osmolal gaps include ethylene glycol, ethanol, and isopropanol poisoning.

- For unknown ingestions, a routine quantitative serum acetaminophen level is recommended; this agent is common in over-the-counter preparations and, in overdose, may not exhibit early diagnostic clues.

- A pregnancy test is recommended in female patients of childbearing age who present with overdose.

- Quantitative blood tests are useful only for those drugs for which clinical effects and toxicity correlate with the serum level of drug.

- Toxicology screens have limitations. Most immunoassays are capable of screening for commonly abused drugs such as marijuana, amphetamines, benzodiazepines, and cocaine.

INITIAL EVALUATION AND LABORATORY TESTING

In the poisoned pediatric patient, there is often a role for laboratory testing. An understanding of laboratory assays, their indications, and their limitations is an important aspect of patient management (Table 20–1).

Glucose and Serum Chemistry, Blood Gas, and Osmolality

One of the most commonly ordered test for poisoned patients is a blood glucose concentration. Of the deleterious effects of poisons, hypoglycemia is one the most easily detected and readily treated. Any patient with altered mental status or the potential to develop hypoglycemia from a poisoning should have a bedside blood glucose assessment.

Serum chemistry assessment, calculation of an anion gap, and blood gas assessment can be used in poisonings by unknown agents or agents known to cause elevated anion gap metabolic acidosis. The anion gap is calculated using the equation:

$$(Na) - (Cl + HCO_3)$$

A metabolic acidosis with an increased anion gap results from the presence of organically active acids and is characteristic of several toxins and various other disease states. Although 8 to 12 mEq/L is traditionally accepted as the normal range for an anion gap, the measured and calculated anion gap can vary considerably. When a patient presents with an elevated anion gap, the mnemonic METALACID GAP will assist in identifying most of the

Table 20–1. General Tests for Poisoned Patients

Bedside serum glucose determination[a]
ECG[b]
Pulse oximetry[a]
Serum electrolytes and calculation of anion gap[a]
Serum osmolality and calculation of osmolal gap[c]
Serum acetaminophen level[b]
Hemoglobin co-oximetry[c]
Focused toxicology lab testing[c]

[a]Indicated for all patients
[b]Indicated in certain instances
[c]Only indicated by unique, specific circumstances

common toxic causes. These poisons include salicylates, ethanol, ethylene glycol, methanol, isoniazid, and iron (Table 20–2). A normal anion gap is expected early in the course of poisoning because it takes 6 to 12 hours to metabolize toxins such as ethylene glycol and methanol or to absorb adequate concentrations of salicylate or iron to cause acidosis.

Another valuable clue in establishing the diagnosis is the presence of an elevated osmolal gap. The *osmolal gap* is the difference between measured and calculated serum osmolarity. An elevated osmolal gap indicates that a low-molecular-weight, highly osmotic compound not normally found in the serum, is present in a significant quantity.

$$\text{Calculated Osmolal} = 2(\text{Na}) + \text{Glucose}/18 + \text{BUN}/2.8 + \text{ETOH}/4.6$$
$$\text{Osmolal Gap} = \text{Measured Osmol} - \text{Calculated Osmol (normal} < 10)$$

Table 20–2. Agents Causing an Elevated Anion Gap (Metalacid Gap) (Metal Acid Gaps)

Methanol, Metformin
Ethylene glycol
Toluene
Alcoholic ketoacidosis
Lactic acidosis
Aminoglycosides, other uremic agents
Cyanide, carbon monoxide
Isoniazid, iron
Diabetic ketoacidosis
Generalized seizure-producing toxins
ASA or other salicylates
Paraldehyde, phenformin

Abbreviation: ASA, aspirin.

Classic toxicologic causes of elevated osmolal gaps include ethylene glycol, ethanol, and isopropanol poisoning, all of which are highly osmotically active compounds. The most accurate measurement of serum osmolarity is determined by a freezing point depression method; standard vapor pressure analysis volatilizes alcohols and can lead to erroneous results. An elevated osmolar gap has been rather arbitrarily defined as greater than 10 mosm/kg H_2O. The mnemonic ME DIE includes the major toxins that produce an increased osmolar gap (Table 20–3).

It is important to realize that a normal osmolar gap does not absolutely exclude substances known to be osmotically active. For example, ethylene glycol has such a high molecular weight that even toxic amounts may contribute minimally to a patient's overall osmolality. Furthermore, depending on the time of ingestion, little of the osmotically active parent compound may be present when a patient presents with toxicity. As a result, the range of a normal gap may actually vary from −5 to 15 mOsm, depending on the equation used to determine the gap, and the time the calculation was made post-ingestion. Thus, the sensitivity and specificity the osmolar gap is variable following a toxic ingestion.

As with the above calculation of ETOH/4.6, if quantitative serum levels of the other toxic alcohols are not readily available, these levels can also be estimated by using the following denominators in the above equation: methanol = 3.2; ethylene glycol = 6.2; and isopropanol = 6.0.

Hemoglobin Co-Oximetry

Carboxyhemoglobin or methemoglobin levels should be should be performed in any circumstance in which exposure to these toxins is suspected. These levels are usually measured with a co-oximeter using arterial blood, although studies have demonstrated that venous blood levels following carbon monoxide exposure are comparably accurate.

Dyshemoglobinemia can cause misleading pulse oximetry determinations. Carboxyhemoglobin typically results in a falsely elevated SpO_2, usually at or near 100%. Methemoglobinemia typically causes the pulse oximetry reading to

Table 20–3. Agents Increasing the Osmolar Gap (ME DIE)

Methanol
Ethylene glycol
Diuretics (mannitol)
Isopropyl alcohol
Ethanol

either increase or decrease to a range of 75% to 85% oxygen saturation. Supplemental oxygen to patients with carbon monoxide poisoning or methemoglobinemia characteristically fails to result in concomitant rise in SpO_2.

Co-oximetry, in contrast, is able to make the distinction between these species and quantify the percentage of carboxyhemoglobin or methemoglobin. Although carboxyhemoglobin levels do not always correlate well with clinical signs and symptoms, they may help to guide patient management and disposition.

For any patient having been in a closed-space fire, a serum lactate level should be obtained in cases where there is an elevated carboxyhemoglobin level in patients demonstrating profound metabolic acidosis. Elevated serum lactate levels, particularly levels greater than 10 mmol/L, are suggestive of cyanide poisoning. Rapid assessment and treatment may be necessary to save cyanide-poisoned patients. Because real-time determination of serum cyanide levels is not always possible, serum lactate levels serve as a surrogate marker of cyanide poisoning.

Acetaminophen Levels

For unknown ingestions, a routine quantitative serum acetaminophen level is recommended; this agent is common in over-the-counter preparations and, in overdose, may not exhibit early diagnostic clues. Determination of a serum acetaminophen concentration with subsequent plotting on the Rumack-Matthew nomogram (see Chapter 28) should be a routine step in the assessment of any acute acetaminophen ingestion or polydrug ingestion. Although unintentional childhood ingestions of acetaminophen are unlikely to result in hepatotoxicity, there is no clear evidence demonstrating the safety of managing acetaminophen ingestions without laboratory assessment of serum acetaminophen levels.

Pregnancy Testing of the Poisoned Patient

A pregnancy test is recommended in female patients of childbearing age who present with overdose, because of the possibility that the ingestion may have been prompted by a wish to abort a fetus. Fortunately, the fetus is rarely affected by a one-time toxic exposure in such cases.

Certain exposures do warrant counseling regarding the potential for fetal loss or malformation, including hormones, retinoids, anti-neoplastic agents, anticonvulsants, and coumadin. A positive pregnancy test may also prompt a more aggressive intervention, such as hyperbaric oxygen therapy for carbon monoxide poisoning.

Urine Analysis

Detailed laboratory urine analysis may reveal important diagnostic clues concerning the overdosed patient. For example, calcium oxalate crystals are considered virtually pathognomonic for ethylene glycol poisoning. These crystals are usually discovered late in the clinical course, and may be absent in the urine if testing occurs early after ethylene glycol ingestion. Additionally, some sources suggest using a Wood's lamp to detect urine fluorescence following an ethylene glycol ingestion. However, a more recent pediatric trial refutes the utility of this technique, citing numerous false-positive results. A urinalysis showing occult blood, with no evidence of red blood cells, suggests myoglobinuria or hemolysis. A positive ferric chloride test usually indicates the presence of phenothiazines, salicylates, or ketones.

Urine color may also provide a diagnostic clue. For example, an orange to red-orange hue is seen with phenazopyridine, rifampin, deferoxamine, mercury, or chronic lead poisoning; pink with cephalosporin or ampicillin overdose; brown with chloroquine or carbon tetrachloride; and greenish-blue with copper sulfate or methylene blue.

FOCUSED QUANTITATIVE ASSAYS

Drug and Toxin Levels

Commonly referred to as *levels,* precise quantitative drug assays are used to measure the concentration of a particular drug or toxin. Substances for which assays are used are in Table 20–4.

Quantitative blood tests are useful only for those drugs for which the clinical effects and toxicity correlate with the serum level of drug. Examples of specific management interventions are hemodialysis, hemoperfusion, or chelation therapy based on the presence of a toxic serum concentration of a particular poison.

Assays for Heavy Metals

Lead

Screening for lead exposure is a routine part of pediatric care. Health care institutions as well as state and local health care authorities are equipped to handle lead screening children with blood lead levels above 10 μg/dL. Patients with elevated serum lead levels should have a physical examination to detect clinical signs of lead toxicity as well as repeat laboratory testing to confirm the trend of increasing or decreasing levels. The most common

Table 20–4. Useful Quantitative Drug and Toxin Assays

Acetaminophen
Anticonvulsants (carbamazepine, phenytoin, valproic acid)
Barbiturates
Carbon monoxide (COHb)
Digoxin
Ethanol
Ethylene glycol
Iron
Lead and other heavy metals
Lithium
Methanol
Methemoglobinemia
Salicylate
Theophylline

---

cause for spurious results blood lead screening is failure to adequately scrub lead-containing dirt from the skin before performing blood sampling. Typically, any patient with elevated lead levels should undergo assessment of their erythropoietic status with a complete blood count.

Iron

Typically performed after ingestion of iron tablets or multivitamins containing iron, determination of serum iron level is useful for prognostic value and to guide management. The serum iron level is ideally assessed 4 hours after suspected exposure. After this time, the serum iron level may decrease as a result of redistribution of iron from the vascular space. For this reason, the utility of iron levels decreases and late iron levels in a seemingly nontoxic range should not delay antidotal therapy or medical management of patients with clinical symptoms consistent with iron toxicity. When an iron level is not available, serum glucose level >150 and white blood cell count >15,000 suggest elevated iron levels. However, one cannot rule out iron toxicity if these baseline parameters are normal. Total iron binding capacity, although commonly ordered in the past, has poor clinical correlation and is therefore an unnecessary test in the setting of acute iron poisoning.

Mercury and Other Metals

Circumstances warranting laboratory assay for mercury are rare, but include illness suggestive of or consistent with mercury toxicity, such as peripheral neuropathy and

renal disease following initial gastrointestinal symptoms, or suspected exposure to toxic forms of mercury. In children, this exposure may include inhalation of volatilized elemental mercury, exposure to mercury in chemicals or industrial products, or even confirmed mercury toxicity in a family member without clear exposure risk. Recent concern about potential toxic exposures to mercury from mercury amalgam in dental filling or thiomersal in vaccines has prompted parents and clinicians to seek laboratory mercury assays for children. There is no need or justification for mercury testing in such circumstances. Inappropriate testing regularly yields false-positive results or results that are difficult to interpret because there is considerable overlap among mercury concentrations found in the normal population, asymptomatic exposed individuals, and patients with clinical evidence of poisoning. There is no definitive correlation between blood or urine mercury levels and mercury toxicity. The most rapid and sensitive method of mercury detection, cold atomic absorption spectrometry, cannot distinguish between organic and inorganic mercury; this differentiation must be analyzed by thin-layer or gas chromatography.

With expansion of alternative medicine, there has been an increase in patients interested in their exposure to metals, including aluminum, arsenic, cadmium, chromium, manganese, mercury, selenium, and thallium, and others. Parents with children with disorders such as autism, attention deficit hyperactivity disorder, or mental retardation are most likely to seek testing in attempt to diagnose heavy metal toxicity.

Toxicologists are regularly consulted in cases of elevated heavy metal levels only to discover fundamental flaws in testing procedure. Common spurious causes of toxic heavy metal levels include urine collected in a container with a metal lid, patients failing to maintain a seafood-free diet for a week prior to testing, and laboratories assessing nontoxic species of heavy metals or with inappropriate reference ranges for normal values. Because of these and other issues, laboratory testing for heavy metals should be performed under the guidance of a toxicologist or other specialist with training and experience in conducting and interpreting these assays.

TOXICOLOGY SCREENING OF THE ACUTELY POISONED PATIENT

There is no standard definition of what constitutes toxicology screening. Generally speaking, a *tox screen* usually comprises qualitative detection of specific drugs in the urine or blood. The majority of toxicologic diagnoses and therapeutic decisions are made on a clinical or historical basis, even though technology has provided the ability to measure many toxins. The applications of these laboratory measurements are limited by practical considerations. Analytic turnaround time is often longer than the critical time course of an overdose, and laboratories cannot support the cost of maintaining the procedures, instruments, training, and specialized labor that would be needed to analyze every toxin.

Toxicology screens have limitations. Most immunoassays are capable of screening for commonly abused drugs such as marijuana, amphetamines, benzodiazepines, and cocaine. However, many dangerous drugs and poisons, such as isoniazid, digitalis glycosides, calcium antagonists, β-blockers, heavy metals, and pesticides are not detected by routine screening. On the other hand, some drugs with legitimate therapeutic use, such as opioids and benzodiazepines, may be detected by the screen even though they are causing no contributing clinical symptoms. Some laboratories can perform highly specific assays for hundreds of drugs on urine and blood specimens. It is important for the health care provider to understand the specific testing available at their facility.

Drug of Abuse Screening

Testing for illicit drugs is a two-step process. The first step is a screening enzyme immunoassay method. The enzyme-multiplied immunoassay technique is a relatively fast and cost-effective screening tool used by many testing hospitals and laboratories. In some hospital laboratories, positive samples are sent for a second analytical procedure or *confirmation test*. In the emergency setting, most hospitals only run the initial screening immunoassay method.

The toxicology screen may have little clinical correlation if specimens are collected too early or late for detection. In general, urine specimens are more useful than blood, because drug metabolites in the urine can be detected as many as 2 to 3 days after exposure, compared with 6 to 12 hours in the blood. The disadvantages to urinary screening include lack of correlation of test results with impairment or time of drug use. Also, metabolites rather than parent drugs are usually measured.

A comprehensive urine toxicology screen is labor intensive, and intended to detect as many drugs as possible. Usually detected are the alcohols, sedative-hypnotics, barbiturates, benzodiazepines, anticonvulsants, antihistamines, antidepressants, antipsychotics, stimulants, opioids, cardiovascular drugs, oral hypoglycemics, and methylxanthines. Unexpected findings on urine drug screening that lead to changes in management are uncommon.

Routine comprehensive toxicology screening adds significantly to the cost of care. Focused toxicology screening based on historical and clinical suspicion of exposure to a particular drug that can be quantitatively assayed is more useful. Substances for which such assays are used are in Table 20–5.

Table 20–5. Toxic or Action Levels for Common Poisons

	Normal or Therapeutic Level		Toxic or Action Level	
	Conventional Units	**SI Units**	**Conventional Units**	**SI Units**
Acetaminophen	10–33 μg/mL	66–199 μmol/L	150 μg/mL (4 h)	993 μmol/L (4 h)
Caffeine	1–10 μg/mL	5.2–51 μmol/L	25 μg/mL	129 μmol/L
Carbamazepine	4–12 mg/L	17–51 μmol/L	12 mg/L	51 μmol/L
Carboxyhemoglobin	1–2%		10%	
Digoxin	0.8–2.0 ng/mL	1.1–2.6 nmol/L	2.0 ng/mL	2.6 nmol/L
Ethylene glycol	0 mg/dL	0 mmol/L	25 mg/dL	4 mmol/L
Iron	80–180 μg/dL	14–32 μmol/L	500 μg/dL	90 μmol/L
Lead	<10 μg/dL	<0.48 μmol/L	10–45 μg/dL	0.48–2.16 μmol/L
Lidocaine	1.5–5.0 μg/mL	6.4–21.4 μmol/L	5 μg/mL	21.4 μmol/L
Lithium	0.6–1.2 mEq/L	0.6–1.2 mmol/L	2.0 mEq/L	2 mmol/L
Methanol	0 mg/dL	0 mmol/L	25 mg/dL	7.8 mmol/L
Methemoglobin	<1%		>15%	
Phenobarbitol	15–40 mg/L	65–172 μmol/L	40 mg/L	172 μmol/L
Phenytoin	10–20 mg/L	40–79 μmol/L	20 mg/L	79 μmol/L
Salicylates	15–30 mg/dL	1.1–2.2 mmol/L	100 mg/dL	7.2 mmol/L
Theophylline	5–15 mg/mL	27.8–83 μmol/L	20 mg/mL	111 μmol/L
Valproic acid	50–120 mg/L	347–833 μmol/L	120 mg/L	833 μmol/L

There is a tremendous appeal to the idea that toxicology screening can allow clinicians to make toxicologic diagnoses. This idea, however, is in part the basis for the widespread misunderstanding of toxicology screening.

False-Negative Results

Negative toxicology screening tends to be unhelpful clinically because of the limited ability of screens to detect some drugs, and the limited window of time after which exposure to a drug will be detectable. Many assays do not detect all drugs in their specific class. For example, benzodiazepine screening typically detects oxazepam, which is a common metabolite of most benzodiazepines. Because lorazepam (Ativan) and alprazolam (Xanax) are not metabolized to oxazepam, exposure to these benzodiazepines will not be detected by most benzodiazepine screening. Amphetamine screening tests may not detect commonly abused amphetamines such as methamphetamine or methylenedioxymethamphetamine (MDMA, ecstasy) and opioid screening may not detect synthetic opioids such as methadone or fentanyl. Furthermore, many drugs of abuse, such as γ–hydroxybutyrate (GHB), ketamine, flunitrazepam (Rohypnol), D-lysergic acid diethylamide (LSD), are not assayed for by routine drug of abuse screening tests. (Table 20–6)

Toxicology screening assays only reflect the presence or absence of drugs or metabolites at or above a threshold concentration at the time of the assay. It does not exclude the presence of drug or metabolite, but only concludes that the substance assayed was not present in a minimum threshold quantity. Savvy drug users know to abstain from using drugs for a period of time before submitting a sample. A negative toxicology screening may be misinterpreted as meaning that the patient has not used the drugs. A negative result only means that the drug in question has not been used recently enough to cause a positive result.

False-Positive Results

In some situations toxicology screening can yield false-positive results. Many substances can interfere and cross-react with various drug of abuse screening assays. Over-the-counter cough and cold preparations cause positive tests for amphetamines and phencyclidine (PCP), and poppy seeds may result in a positive screening test for opioids (Table 20–7).

Also, screening tests are not intended to determine if there is a clinically significant quantity of drug in exposed patients. Government and industry have established the

Table 20–6. Commonly Abused Drugs Not Detected by Most Drugs of Abuse Screening Assays

Benzodiazepine analogs
Dextromethorphan
Herbal and plant products:
    Ayahauasca
    Ephedra
    Ibogaine
    Jimsonweed
    Kava-kava
    Khat
    Morning Glory seeds
    Nutmeg
    Psylocibin mushrooms
    Salvia divinorum
GHB
Ketamine
LSD, Mescaline
MDMA (ecstasy) and similar amphetamines
Methaqualone
Nitrous oxide, amyl nitrite (poppers), isobutyl nitrite and analogs
PCP analogs
Synthetic opioids and opioid analogs
Volatile hydrocarbons

Abbreviations: GHB, γ-hydroxybutyrate; LSD, D-lysergic acid diethylamide; MDMA, methylenedioxymethamphetamine; PCP, phencyclidine.

standards of toxicology screening assays for a variety of drugs of abuse to detect casual drug use in employees. Routinely assayed drugs of abuse, including amphetamines, benzodiazepines, cocaine, opioids, and PCP, are typically detectable for several days after exposure. Barbiturates, methadone, and marijuana may be detected for much longer periods. Trace amounts of drug will not cause clinically significant symptoms. Qualitative detection without quantitative data may be both unhelpful and misleading when such results are applied clinically.

The most concerning pitfall of toxicology screening is the misinterpretation of a positive assay. Altered mental status is often the impetus for clinicians to perform toxicology screening. A positive toxicology screening assay cannot be used solely to explain altered mental status for several reasons. A positive screening cannot rule out the existence of other treatable causes of altered mental status such as intracranial hemorrhage, cerebrovascular accident, meningitis, encephalitis, or a metabolic disturbance. Thus, it is important to consider all possible eti-

Table 20–7. Drug of Abuse Screening Assay Characteristics

Drug/Group	What Is Detected	False Positive	Comments
Amphetamine	Amphetamine	Many cough/cold preparations containing ephedrine, pseudoephedrine, phenylpropanolamine, and other similar drugs.	Typically may not detect methamphetamine, or MDMA (ecstasy), which are more commonly abused than amphetamine.
Barbiturates	Barbiturate	Some NSAIDs.	Barbiturates are relatively infrequently abused by pediatric patients.
Benzodiazepines	Oxazepam, a benzodiazepine metabolite	Some NSAIDs.	Many do not detect alprazolam (Xanax), flunitrazepam (Rohypnol), lorazepam (Ativan), midazolam (Versed), triazolam (Halcyon).
Cocaine	Benzoylecgonine, a cocaine metabolite	Consumption of tea made from coca leaves.	Very sensitive and specific test.
Marijuana	Tetrahydrocannabinol, an active ingredient in marijuana	NSAIDs in the past.	Secondhand smoke may cause positive result.
Opioids	Morphine, a metabolite of heroin and many opioids	Poppy seeds, rifampin.	Does not detect synthetic opioids fentanyl (Sublimaze), meperidine (Demerol), methadone, propoxyphene (Darvon), or tramadol (Ultram).
PCP	PCP	Dextromethorphan, diphenhydramine, doxylamine, ketamine.	Dozens of analogs of PCP exist; these are not reliably detected by PCP assay.

Abbreviations: MDMA, methylenedioxymethamphetamine; NSAIDs, nonsteroidal anti-inflammatory drugs; PCP, phencyclidine.

ologies of a clinical presentation and to evaluate for those conditions that may require specific interventions, using toxicology screening only as an adjunctive diagnostic to help confirm a diagnosis.

Assent and Consent for Drug of Abuse Screening

Acknowledgment of the rights of minor patients has ramifications for drug of abuse screening. The American Academy of Pediatrics has a specific practice guidelines, which state that a patient suspected of voluntarily using substances of abuse has a right to be informed of a clinician's desire to perform drug of abuse screening, and

should be informed that they have the right to refuse such testing without penalty. Screening for drugs of abuse should only proceed if the patient understands and grants consent. The exception to this would be children or adolescents with altered mental status impairing their judgment or competency.

In the common circumstance of parents seeking drug of abuse testing in a child they suspect of abusing drugs, testing should only occur if there is a clear medical need. In the preponderance of cases, such a need rarely exists. Unfortunately, it may be very difficult for parents to understand this concept.

In the extremely rare circumstances in which provision of urgent or emergent medical care is predicated upon the results of drug of abuse screening, a patient's refusal to submit to such testing may be overridden, but should be thoroughly documented. The American Academy of Pediatrics' policy statement clearly states that only in exceptional cases should patients be tested unknowingly or against their will.

Forensic Testing

An important exception to the preceding discussion relates to suspected child abuse or neglect. For patients incapable of intentionally using drugs of abuse volitionally and in cases of malicious poisoning, laboratory assays might be helpful in confirming the presence of illicit substances, providing valuable forensic evidence. A chain of custody should be maintained for such samples.

Date-Rape Drug Screening

In recent decades, use of drugs to incapacitate for the purpose of sexual assault has paralleled the rise of contemporary drugs of abuse. When suspicion of drug-facilitated sexual assault exists, screening for date-rape drugs may be employed. Many commercial laboratories have a screening panel for date-rape drugs, but before ordering them, clinicians should be aware of what specific testing is available. Agents commonly used in sexual assault that can be detected include GHB, benzodiazepines (including flunitrazepam [Rohypnol], Zolpidem [Ambien]), and zalepon [Sonata]). Barbiturates, chloral hydrate, dextromethorphan, ketamine, PCP, and opioids are also detectable.

There are several difficulties with date-rape drug screening. First and foremost, drugs used to facilitate sexual assault are most frequently used knowingly by individuals recreationally. The use of these drugs to facilitate date-rape accounts for only a small fraction of their use. Laboratory testing for date-rape drugs can only confirm the presence of such drugs; it does not confirm that the patient was slipped the drug unknowingly or took it unwillingly. In addition, screening may detect drugs such as cocaine, marijuana, or amphetamines that are not considered date-rape drugs. Detection of drugs other than date-rape drugs may prejudice a jury against a rape victim in the event it is used as evidence.

Negative date-rape drug screening may mislead law enforcement officials or a jury as well. GHB, probably the most widely recognized date-rape drug, has a half-life so brief that it is reliably present in urine in detectable quantities only within several hours of ingestion. Therefore, even in cases where the patient relates a very convincing history of GHB poisoning, the substance might not be detected by laboratory screening. Additionally, laboratory screening for date-rape drugs can never be broad enough to include all incapacitating agents. Esoteric medicines, such as eye drops containing bromonidine, clonidine, or scolpolamine may be used as incapacitating agents that would only be discovered if the laboratory specifically knew to assay for them. The risk of date-rape drug screening is that a negative result may be misinterpreted as indicating that no such agent was used.

A formulated plan should be in place to determine in what circumstances date-rape drug screening should be utilized. Adherence to a previously determined plan avoids the need for a hurried or improvised plan of action when a victim of sexual assault arrives.

Hair Sampling

Hair sampling for toxicology screening is an excellent tool because as a hair grows, traces of drugs present in the body at a given time are incorporated into it. Hair is essentially a diary of drug exposure, providing a chronological reference correlated with the areas of the hair strand that contain drug. This analysis can differentiate between one-time exposure and repeated drug use. Short-term abstinence from drug use just to pass a urine or blood drug test is not an issue when hair is sampled. Hair testing is not relevant to the emergent management of poisoning, but can be used to confirm drug exposures for forensic purposes. Examples include assessing neonates for prenatal exposure to drugs of abuse, detecting repeated malicious drug exposure, or determining the extent and duration of drug abuse. In neonates, use of meconium may also be an excellent sampling method to detect exposure to illicit drugs in utero.

Special Considerations in the Neonate

Neonates have important differences in the normal range for certain toxicology laboratory measurements that may falsely indicate poisoning has occurred. This may cause significant difficulties when attempting to identify specific toxins. Carboxyhemoglobin levels in neonates typically range from 2% to 5%, because carbon monoxide is a byproduct of protoporphyrin metabolism. In the absence of exposure to exogenous toxins, neonates may develop severe methemoglobinemia and metabolic acidosis from gastroenteritis. Neonates also have a lower baseline cholinesterase activity that may interfere with the interpretation of plasma pseudocholinesterase and red blood cell cholinesterase levels. Finally, the abnormal metabolic products present in the disease methylmalonic acidemia may be mistaken for ethylene glycol. Those investigating poisoning in the neonate must be aware of these important age-related differences in laboratory measurements.

SUMMARY

No laboratory assays should be routinely ordered in every poisoned patient, but rather tests should be performed based on the type of poisoning and clinical status of the patient. Routine toxicology screening, particularly for drugs of abuse, has repeatedly been demonstrated not to be helpful in the management of poisoned patients. Focused, quantitative assessment of specific poisons such as salicylates, acetaminophen, and anticonvulsants, for which quantitative serum levels assist in management, is the most helpful type of toxicology lab testing. A lack of understanding of the capabilities, limitations, and indications for laboratory testing frequently results in the ordering of unnecessary and unhelpful laboratory tests. Understanding available laboratory assays and how these tests can and cannot assist in diagnosis and management should allow the clinician to rationally use toxicology tests.

SUGGESTED READINGS

Avner JR, Henretig FM, McAneney CM: Acquired methemoglobinemia: The relationship of cause to course of illness. *Am J Dis Child* 144:1229–1230, 1990.

Belson MG, Simon HK: Utility of comprehensive toxicologic screens in children. *Am J Emerg Med* 17:221–224, 1999.

Brett AS: Implications of discordance between clinical impression and toxicology analysis in drug overdose. *Arch Intern Med* 148:437, 1988.

Cassavant MJ, Shah MN, Battles R: Does fluorescent urine indicate antifreeze ingestion by children? *Pediatrics* 107:113–114, 2001.

Erickson T, Aks S, Gussow L, et al: Toxicology diagnosis and management: A rational approach to the poisoned patient. Emergency Medicine Practice 8:1–25, 2001.

Fabbri A, Marchesini G, Morselli-Labate AM, et al: Comprehensive drug screening in decision making of patients attending the emergency department for suspected drug overdose. *Emerg Med J* 20:25–28, 2003.

Glaser DS: Utility of serum osmol gap in the diagnosis of methanol or ethylene glycol ingestion. *Ann Emerg Med* 27:343–346, 1996.

Karlsen RL, Sterri S, Lyngaas S, et al: Reference values for erythrocyte acetylcholinesterase and plasma activities in children: implications for organophosphate intoxications. *Scand J Clin Lab Invest* 4:301–302, 1981.

Kellerman AL, Fihn SD, Logerfo JP, et al: Utilization and yield of drug screens in the emergency department. *Am J Emerg Med* 6:14, 1988.

Osterloh JD: Utility and reliability of emergency toxicologic testing. *Emerg Med Clin North Am* 8:693–723, 1990.

Osterloh JD: Laboratory testing in emergency toxicology. In: Ford M, Delaney K, Ling L, et al, eds: *Clinical Toxicology.* Philadelphia: Saunders; 2001:51–60.

Perrone J, De Roos F, Jayaraman S, et al: Drug screening versus history in detection of substance use in ED psychiatric patients. *Am J Emerg Med* 19:49–51, 2001.

Perrone J, Hoffamn RS: Toxic ingestions in pregnancy: Abortifacient use in a case series of pregnant overdose patients. *Acad Emerg Med* 4:206–209, 1997.

Roberts WL, Paulson WD: Method-specific reference intervals. *Lab Med* 29:261–262, 1998.

Shoemaker JD, Lynch RE, Hoffman JW, et al: Misidentification of proprionic acid as ethylene glycol in a patient with methylmalonic acidemia. *J Pediatr* 120:417–421, 1992.

Steinhart B: Severe ethylene glycol intoxication with normal osmolal gap "a chilling thought." *Emerg Med* 8:583, 1990.

Trummel J, Ford M, Austin P: Ingestion of an unknown alcohol. *Ann Emerg Med* 27:368–374, 1996.

Winter ML, Ellis MD, Snodgrass WR: Urine fluorescence using a Wood's lamp to detect the antifreeze additive sodium fluorescein: A qualitative adjunctive test in suspected ethylene glycol ingestions. *Ann Emerg Med* 19:663–667, 1990.

Wright GR, Shephard RJ: Physiological effects of carbon monoxide. *Int Rev Physiol* 20:311–368, 1979.

21

Fluids, Electrolytes, and Acid–Base Management

Susan A. Kecskes

HIGH-YIELD FACTS

- Fluid resuscitation may be necessary in pediatric poisoning due to hypovolemia or relative hypovolemia related to vasodilation.
- Fluid requirements are divided into three parts:
  - Maintenance fluids
  - Deficit replacement
  - Replacement of ongoing losses
- Correction of circulatory failure with isotonic crystalloid or appropriate colloid is the first step in fluid management.
- Elevated anion gap acidosis is associated with ingestion of the alcohols, salicylate, and poisonings resulting in lactic acidosis.
- Correction of metabolic acidosis includes restoration of oxygen delivery, sodium bicarbonate, and dialysis.
- The osmolar gap is a useful tool in estimating alcohol toxicity.
- Hypernatremia should be corrected gradually to avoid the complications of cerebral edema.
- Therapy for hyperkalemia is aimed at halting intake, stabilizing cellular membranes, intracellular translocation, and enhancing elimination.
- Alkaline diuresis may enhance elimination of toxins that are renally excreted, poorly protein bound, and have a pK between 3.0 and 7.2.

There are many fluid and electrolyte abnormalities associated with poisoning in the pediatric patient. Some are directly or indirectly related to the toxin and others are related to the treatments employed to combat the toxin. Awareness of these issues and the appropriate interventions reduce morbidity and mortality in these patients.

FLUIDS

Many patients with poisoning experience hypotension as part of their toxic state. Nausea, vomiting, and diarrhea associated with the toxin itself or efforts to eliminate the toxin may lead to hypovolemia. Some toxins, such as iron, may cause acute third-space volume losses through the gastrointestinal system. Other patients may experience relative hypovolemia owing to vasodilatation from toxins such as opioids. Appropriate response to hypotension requires an understanding of the fluid compartments of the body and of movement of fluid within those compartments.

Fluid Compartments

Total body water (TBW) is divided into the intracellular and extracellular compartments, with the extracellular compartment subdivided into intravascular and extravascular compartments. By the time the child is 1 year of age, TBW comprises approximately 60% of body weight and is approaching the adult distribution of one third in the extracellular and two thirds in the intracellular compartments. The intravascular compartment is primarily responsible for perfusion.

Movement of Fluid

Cellular membranes form the barrier between the extracellular and intracellular spaces. They are freely permeable to water, but impermeable to electrolytes and proteins except by active transport. Although the specific osmoles differ in the two compartments, the osmolality is equal. Water distributes across this barrier by osmotic pressure. A rise in extracellular osmolality, as occurs with a sodium load, results in movement of water from the intracellular space to the extracellular space. Conversely, water intoxication leads to a movement of water from the extracellular space to the intracellular space.

The vascular endothelium forms the barrier between the intravascular and interstitial spaces. It is permeable to water and electrolytes, but not to protein. Two forces regulate fluid movement. *Hydrostatic pressure* created by the propulsion of blood through vessels favors movement of fluid from the intravascular space to the interstitial space. This pressure falls as blood travels from the arterioles through the capillary bed to the lower pressure veins. *Oncotic pressure,* exerted primarily by albumin found in the vascular space, favors water movement from the interstitium into the vascular space. Under normal conditions, there is a balance in the movement of water and electrolytes from the vascular space to the endothelium at the arteriolar side and in the reverse direction at the venous side.

These factors guide the selection of fluid to be administered to a patient. Free water added to the vascular space distributes proportionally to all three compartments. Isotonic crystalloid distributes throughout the extracellular space. Isoncotic fluid remains in the vascular space with the exception of a small distribution to the interstitial space because of the increase in hydrostatic pressure.

Fluid Requirements

Fluid requirements can be divided into three categories. First, there are maintenance fluids, which replace routine daily fluid losses. Some patients may also require replacement of a fluid deficit or ongoing excessive losses.

Maintenance fluids include insensible losses and routine outputs of urine and stool. These are proportional to the body surface area. Because infants and children have a higher body surface area per kilogram, they also have proportionally higher fluid requirements. There are four common methods to calculate maintenance fluids (Table 20–1). Common maintenance fluids are D_5 0.2 NaCl with 20 mEq/L of KCl in infants and young children and D_5 0.45 NaCl with 20 mEq/L of KCl in older children

Table 20–1. Four Methods for Maintenance Fluid Calculations

Body Surface Area Method	
1500 mL/BSA (m^2)/day	

100/50/20 Method	
Weight	**Fluid**
0–10	100 mL/kg/d
11–20	1000 mL + 50 mL/kg/d for every kg >10 kg
>20	1500 mL + 20 mL/kg/d for every kg >20 kg

4/2/1 Method	
Weight	**Fluid**
0–10	4 mL/kg/h
11–20	40 mL + 2 ml/kg/h for every kg >10 kg
>20	60 mL + 1 mL/kg/h for every kg >20 kg

Insensible + Measured Losses Method
400–600 mL/BSA (m^2)/d + Urine Output (mL/mL) + Other measured losses (mL/mL)

Source: As modified from Kecskes SA: Fluids and Electrolytes, in Strange GR, Ahrens WR Lelyveld S, et al. (eds.): *Pediatric Emergency Medicine: A Comprehensive Study Guide,* 2nd ed. New York, McGraw-Hill, 2002, p 400, with permission.

and adults. Patients in renal failure should have maintenance fluids calculated as insensible loss plus urine replacement.

Many victims of poisoning have fluid deficits that require replacement. Toxins can cause nausea and vomiting directly. Treatment with emetics and cathartics to hasten elimination of the toxin also contributes to the fluid deficit. Some toxins, such as iron, may cause massive third-space losses creating intravascular volume deficit. The first priority in patients with fluid deficits is to restore circulation. To begin, the adequacy of the patient's perfusion is determined (Table 20–2). Mental status, urine output, skin character, capillary refill, and vital signs are assessed. Serum electrolytes, blood urea nitrogen, creatinine, acid–base status, urinalysis, and urine sodium concentration may be useful. If the patient's perfusion is inadequate, fluid resuscitation should be initiated. An initial bolus of 20 mL/kg of isotonic crystalloid

Table 20–2. Signs and Symptoms of Dehydration

	Mild (5% TB Wt)	Moderate (10% TB Wt)	Severe (15% TB Wt)
Mental status	Alert	Irritable; drowsy	Lethargic
Skin turgor	Brisk retraction	Mild delay	Prolonged retraction
Anterior fontanel	Normal	Minimally sunken	Sunken
Eyes	Moist; + tears	Dry; −tears	Sunken; −tears
Mucous membranes	Moist	Dry	Very Dry
Pulses	Normal	Rapid; weak peripherally	Rapid; Weak centrally
Capillary refill	<2 sec	2–5 sec	>5 sec
Respiration	Normal	Rapid	Deep and rapid
Urine output	>1 mL/kg/h	<1 mL/kg/h	Minimal or absent
Blood pressure	Normal	Low normal	Hypotension

Source: As modified from Kecskes SA: Fluids and Electrolytes, in Strange GR, Ahrens WR Lelyveld S, et al. (eds.): *Pediatric Emergency Medicine: A Comprehensive Study Guide,* 2nd ed. New York, McGraw-Hill, 2002, p 400, with permission.

[0.9% NaCl or lactated Ringer's (LR) solution] is given intravenously over <20 minutes. The patient is reassessed and further boluses are given until perfusion is adequate. Pediatric patients commonly require >60 mL/kg of resuscitation fluid to restore perfusion. If required, blood products may be substituted for some of the bolus fluid. Central venous pressure (CVP) may be used to guide fluid therapy if there is concern regarding fluid overload. It is generally safe to continue fluid resuscitation until the CVP exceeds 10 cm H_2O. Additional therapy, such as inotropes or pressors, may be added if the circulatory failure is not solely related to fluid deficit. This may be the case with toxins such as opioids that cause vasodilation.

Once circulation has been stabilized, the remaining deficit needs to be replaced. The magnitude of dehydration is divided into mild (water loss <5% TBW), moderate (water loss 5% to 10% TBW), and severe (water loss >10% TBW). Resuscitation fluids may be subtracted from the calculated deficit and the remainder replaced over 24 hours if the patient is in a normal osmotic state. Typically, the remaining deficit is replaced with a hypotonic fluid such as D_5 0.45% NaCl with 20 mEq/L of KCl. Replacement solutions should be adjusted to the electrolyte status of the individual patient.

Some patients may require replacement of ongoing fluid losses not included in normal maintenance requirements (Table 20–3). Continuing emesis and diarrheal

Table 20–3. Adjustments to Maintenance Fluids

Fever	Increase maintenance fluids by 10% for each degree >37.8°C.
Tachypnea (nonhumidified environment)	Increase maintenance fluids by 5–10%.
Vomiting/gastric loss	Replace with 0.45% NaCl with 10 mEq/L KCl.
Stool loss	Replace with LR with 15 mEq/L KCl or 0.45%NaCl with 20 mEq/L KCl and 20 mEq/L $NaHCO_3$.
Blood	<25% *TBV*: Replace with LR or 0.9% NaCl; assess hematocrit and physiologic status for administration of blood.
	>25% *TBV*: Replace ½ to ⅔ of loss as whole blood and reassess. Alternatively, use three-for-one rule and replace 3× the blood loss with LR or 0.9% NaCl.
Third-space losses	Estimate based on patient's physiologic status. Replace with LR or 0.9% NaCl.

Abbreviations: TBV, total blood volume; RL, Ringer's lactate.
Source: As modified from Kecskes SA: Fluids and Electrolytes, in Strange GR, Ahrens WR Lelyveld S, et al. (eds.): *Pediatric Emergency Medicine: A Comprehensive Study Guide,* 2nd ed. New York, McGraw-Hill, 2002, p 401, with permission.

losses require replacement along with losses through external drains such as nasogastric (NG) tubes. Fever increases the water requirement by 10% for each degree elevation over 37.8°C. Ongoing third-space loss should be estimated and replaced. The type of fluid should be tailored to the content of the fluid lost. A standard solution with a composition close to the fluid being replaced is usually adequate to maintain homeostasis in patients with intact renal function. If more precision is required, the electrolyte content of the fluid being lost may be measured and replaced.

ACID–BASE ABNORMALITIES

Many patients with poisoning have acid–base abnormalities as a direct effect of the toxin, as is the case with methanol or ethylene glycol. Others may be indirectly related, such as lactic acidosis associated with shock or respiratory acidosis associated with hypoventilation.

The body generally tries to maintain a neutral pH of 7.35 to 7.45. Buffering systems in the intracellular and extracellular fluid (ECF) compartments are the first line of defense in maintaining acid–base homeostasis. This is followed by an effort by the kidneys and lungs to compensate for the imbalance. The carbonic acid–bicarbonate system links carbon dioxide regulated by the lung to bicarbonate regulated by the kidney:

$$H_2O + CO_2 \leftrightarrow H_2CO_3 \leftrightarrow H^+ + HCO_3^-$$

If metabolic acidosis is present, the lungs try to excrete more carbon dioxide (CO_2), driving the equation to the left. If respiratory acidosis is present, the kidneys try to eliminate bicarbonate (HCO_3^-), driving the equation to the right. Factors that impair the ability of the compensatory organ to function impede homeostasis.

Metabolic Acidosis

Metabolic acidosis results from an increase in hydrogen (H^+) or a decrease in HCO_3^-. Initially, the body buffers the resulting excess H^+ in the ECF and intracellular fluid (ICF). The respiratory system increases excretion of CO_2, creating a compensatory respiratory alkalosis. The kidney responds more slowly by increasing excretion of H^+ and resorption of HCO_3^-. When compensatory mechanisms are exceeded, the pH falls.

Many toxins cause a direct metabolic acidosis. The acid metabolites of methanol, ethylene glycol, and toluene, or the mixed organic acids associated with iron and salicylate intoxication are representative of this state.

Others, such as cyanide or carbon monoxide, may cause tissue hypoxia or ischemia resulting in lactic acidosis. A useful tool for detecting these problems is calculation of the anion gap:

$$\text{Anion Gap} = Na^+ - (Cl^- + HCO_3^-)$$

The normal anion gap is 8 to 12 mEq/L. Normal anion gap acidosis results from the loss of HCO_3^- or from the addition of chloride (Cl^-). Elevated anion gap metabolic acidosis occurs with increases of organic acids including lactic acid. A lactate level may be helpful to identify the origin of the elevated anion gap. Low anion gaps can occur with an increase in unmeasured cations or a decrease in unmeasured anions. Lithium, iodine, and bromide intoxications may have this finding.

Appropriate clinical response to the metabolic acidosis depends on the origin. If the cause is lactic acidosis as a result of anaerobic metabolism, efforts should be directed to optimize oxygen delivery and utilization. Circulation should be restored with volume, inotropes, and pressors. Fluid is the mainstay of therapy. The patient should be provided with oxygen and ventilation as necessary. Circulating hemoglobin should be normalized. If there is a problem at the oxygen dissociation or utilization points as occur with carbon monoxide or cyanide toxicity, hyperbaric oxygen therapy may be considered. Exogenous administration of sodium bicarbonate is usually reserved for those with organ system failure related to the acidosis (i.e., myocardial failure) or those requiring alkalinization to promote excretion of the toxin. Sodium bicarbonate may be administered in an initial dose of 1mEq/kg over 10 to 30 minutes (not to exceed 10 mEq/min) intravenously (IV). Subsequent dosing is 0.5 mEq/kg IV over 10 to 30 minutes. A continuous infusion may be given at a rate not exceeding 1 mEq/kg/h. Repeated measurements are necessary as the patient's ongoing production of acid and their buffering capabilities change over time. For lactic acidosis unresponsive to these measures or patients developing hypernatremia from sodium bicarbonate administration, hemodialysis may be considered. Hemodialysis is also useful to eliminate other acids contributing to elevated anion gap acidosis. Toxins amenable to this therapy include methanol, ethylene glycol, isopropanol, and salicylates.

Respiratory Alkalosis

Respiratory alkalosis results from a decrease in CO_2 to less than 30 mmHg by elimination from the lungs. The kidney compensates by increased elimination of HCO_3^-

and retention of H^+. When the compensatory mechanisms are exceeded, pH rises. Tachypnea and hyperpnea are the clinical hallmarks of respiratory alkalosis. In some patients, the respiratory alkalosis is primary, as in salicylate toxicity. In others, it is compensatory for a primary metabolic acidosis. Correction requires treatment of the underlying toxicity.

Respiratory Acidosis

Respiratory acidosis results from inadequate elimination of CO_2 by the respiratory system. When ventilation is inadequate, P_{CO_2} exceeds the normal range of 35 to 45 mmHg. Acutely, pH falls. Over the next 24 hours, the kidney begins to compensate by increasing elimination of H^+. The pH may rise as high as the normal range with effective compensation. Toxins that depress respiration are classically associated with respiratory acidosis. These include opioids, benzodiazepines, barbiturates, and alcohols. If the toxicity cannot be immediately reversed, mechanical ventilation should be instituted.

ELECTROLYTE DISTURBANCES

Alterations in electrolyte homeostasis are common in pediatric poisoning. Common patterns suggest specific toxins. Treatment is targeted at both the underlying poisoning and at the specific electrolyte disturbance.

Osmolar Gap

The osmolar gap is a useful tool to diagnose alcohol ingestions. The osmolar gap is defined as the difference between calculated and measured osmolality:

Calculated osmolality =
$$(2 \times Na^+) + BUN/2.8 + Glucose/18$$

Osmolar Gap =
$$\text{Measured Osmolality} - \text{Calculated Osmolality}$$

where BUN = blood urea nitrogen. A normal osmolar gap is less than 10. The measured osmolality must be done by freezing point depression technique rather than vapor pressure method to avoid loss of alcohol by boiling off. An elevated osmolar gap may indicate poisoning with methanol, ethanol, isopropyl alcohol, ethylene glycol, or acetone. It may also be seen with use of mannitol or glycerol. The osmolar gap can be used to estimate the alcohol level by a conversion factor specific to each alcohol (Table 20–4). For ethanol, each 1 mOsm increase in

Table 20–4. Estimation of Alcohol Level by Osmolar Gap

Alcohol	Conversion Factor
Ethanol	4.6
Methanol	3.2
Ethylene glycol	6.2
Isopropyl alcohol	6.0

Estimated blood alcohol level (mg/dL) = Conversion Factor $\times$ Osmolar Gap (mOsm/kg).

the osmolar gap corresponds to a blood ethanol increase of 4.6 mg/dL. This is primarily useful in the early phase after ingestion, as most of the metabolites of the alcohols do not contribute to the osmolar gap.

Sodium

The concentration of sodium reflects the total body store of sodium and its relation to TBW. In both hyponatremia and hypernatremia, the total body store of sodium may be high, low, or normal. It is the amount of TBW relative to total body sodium that determines sodium concentration. Sodium is found in highest concentration in the ECF and is normally maintained between 135 and 145 mEq/L.

Hypernatremia is defined as serum sodium greater than 150 mEq/L. It can result from intake of sodium in excess of water or from loss of water in excess of sodium. In pediatric poisoning, sodium excess may be associated with administration of sodium bicarbonate to treat acidosis or alkalinize urine to enhance elimination of the toxin. Salicylate intoxication is an example of a toxic ingestion that may manifest hypovolemic hypernatremia, in which water loss exceeds sodium loss. Patients have increased insensible water loss from fever, perspiration, and hyperventilation. They have decreased water input related to nausea and vomiting. They may have inappropriately high urine output relative to sodium owing to an enhanced renal solute load. The result is hypernatremic dehydration.

As the serum sodium rises, ECF becomes relatively hyperosmolal compared to ICF. Water moves from the intracellular space to the extracellular space to equilibrate the osmolality. Assessment of decreased intravascular volume status is associated with a greater TBW deficit in hypernatremia than in isotonic or hypotonic states. The brain attempts to conserve water by an increase in glucose, electrolytes, and idiogenic osmoles. This process occurs over approximately 48 hours. Thus, although the intracellular space is relatively volume depleted in hypernatremia, the brain preserves its volume status.

Initial therapy of hypovolemic hypernatremia is focused on correction of circulatory failure, if present. Subsequent restoration of TBW should be gradual, over 48 hours or longer. Fatal cases of cerebral edema have occurred with correction over 24 hours, as fluid enters the already volume-replete brain. A gradual correction allows the brain to reduce the idiogenic osmoles and equilibrate with the ECF. The goal is to reduce the serum sodium at a rate of 0.5 to 1.0 mEq/L/h. The higher the serum sodium, the slower the rate of correction should be. Typically, the correction is started with isotonic crystalloid for stabilization of the circulatory system and completed with hypotonic crystalloid such as $D_5 0.45\%$ NaCl. Maintenance fluids and replacement of ongoing losses must be provided in addition to the deficit correction. Plasma electrolytes and osmolality should be monitored frequently.

Primary sodium excess is treated by removal of excess sodium. First, sodium intake is curtailed. Diuretics, in combination with hypotonic fluid administration, diminish sodium concentration in patients with intact renal function. Patients with renal failure or who are inadequately responsive to the above measures require dialysis.

Hyponatremia is defined as a serum sodium concentration <130 mEq/L and reflects excess body water relative to body sodium. Depending on etiology, total body sodium may be decreased, increased, or normal. Hyponatremia with decreased total body sodium occurs when sodium loss exceeds water loss. These losses may be extrarenal or renal. The most common extrarenal losses in poisoned children are vomiting and diarrhea. Extrarenal etiologies are associated with renal sodium conservation (urine Na^+ <20 mEq/L). Renal losses are associated with diuretic ingestions, osmotic diuresis (mannitol), and glucosuria.

The clinical manifestations of hyponatremia depend on the volume status of the patient, the rapidity of development, and degree of hypoosmolality. In hypovolemic hyponatremia, symptoms of dehydration and acute circulatory failure prevail. Hyponatremia produces a decrease in the osmolality of the ECF. Water flows into the ICF to maintain homeostasis. Rapid changes result in brain edema and central nervous system pathology. Symptoms range from lethargy to coma. Brain herniation may occur in the most severe cases.

Treatment of hyponatremia begins with an assessment of the patient's volume status and correction of hypovolemic shock, if present. Correction of hyponatremia requires a loss of water in excess of sodium. This must be undertaken with care, because aggressive correction can lead to osmotic demyelination syndrome. Just as the brain can generate idiogenic osmoles to maintain cellular volume in hyperosmolal states, it can rid itself of osmoles in hypoosmolal states to prevent brain edema. Once rid of these osmoles, too rapid a correction of sodium can result in cell desiccation and myelinolysis. Gradual correction allows the brain time to equilibrate with a reduction in neurologic sequelae. In hyponatremia of acute onset (<48 hours), it appears safe to correct the sodium over 24 hours. In hyponatremia of more gradual onset, sodium correction should not exceed a rate of 0.5 mEq/L/h. Therapy can be initiated with isotonic crystalloid at rates determined by the volume status of the patient. In euvolemic or hypervolemic patients, this may be at maintenance or fluid-restricted rates. In hypovolemic patients, the deficit needs to be assessed and the correction timed to the desired rise in sodium concentration (approximately 10 mEq/L/24 h). Although most patients will correct gradually with isotonic crystalloid, more aggressive partial correction may be desired in patients with severe neurologic symptoms such as seizures. A rise in serum sodium of 5 mEq/L can be produced by IV infusion of 6 mL/kg of 3% sodium chloride over 20 to 60 minutes. A single bolus is usually sufficient to reduce acute symptoms and the remainder of the correction can be undertaken more gradually. Loop diuretics, such as furosemide, have been used as an adjunct to therapy to increase free water clearance.

Potassium

Although only 2% of total body potassium is in the ECF, potassium is the main cation in ICF. Normal potassium concentration in the ECF is 3.5 to 5.5 mEq/L compared to approximately 150 mEq/L in the ICF. The sodium–potassium ATPase pump in the cell membrane maintains this large concentration gradient.

Potassium homeostasis is managed by both excretion and translocation. The majority of potassium excretion occurs in the kidney. The kidney can adjust urinary potassium excretion from less than 5 mEq to more than 1000 mEq/24 h. Approximately 10% of daily potassium intake is lost through the gastrointestinal tract in stool. Because only 50% of a potassium load is excreted in the first 4 to 6 hours, translocation allows the body to maintain stable ECF potassium. In the first hours after ingestion, potassium is translocated into cells, primarily in the liver and muscle. Acid–base changes also result in potassium shifts. Acidemia promotes movement of potassium to the ECF, and alkalosis favors movement of potassium to the ICF.

Hyperkalemia

Hyperkalemia is defined as serum potassium >5.5 mEq/L and can result from increased potassium intake, decreased potassium loss, or from redistribution from the ICF. In pediatric poisoning, potassium is shifted to the ECF from the ICF as part of the body's buffering response to metabolic acidosis. Other mechanisms include the release of intracellular potassium associated with rhabdomyolysis and decreased excretion with acute renal failure. Ingestion of digitalis, a potassium supplement, or a potassium-sparing diuretic may also be responsible.

Most patients with hyperkalemia are asymptomatic. Neuromuscular symptoms begin with paresthesias and progress to muscle weakness and, ultimately, flaccid paralysis. Cardiac abnormalities are much more likely to produce life-threatening situations. Characteristic changes in the electrocardiogram (ECG) include peaked T waves, prolongation of the PR interval, and progressive widening of the QRS complex. As potassium continues to rise (typically >8 mEq/L), the classic sine wave of hyperkalemia appears. This may rapidly degenerate to asystole or ventricular fibrillation.

An ECG should always be obtained when hyperkalemia is suspected. Serum electrolytes, renal indices (BUN, creatinine, and urinalysis), a complete blood count (CBC), and acid–base status should be obtained. All patients with serum potassium levels >6.5 mEq/L should have continuous ECG monitoring and frequent laboratory follow up.

Treatment of hyperkalemia depends on the level of serum potassium, along with the clinical symptoms and renal status of the patient. In all cases, intake of potassium and potassium-sparing medication should be halted. In asymptomatic patients with intact renal function and modest (<7 mEq/L) levels of serum potassium, halting intake and follow up of serum potassium levels may be all that is required (Table 20–5). In patients with renal dysfunction, the addition of the potassium-binding agent, sodium polystyrene sulfonate (Kayexalate, 1 to 2 g/kg PO, NG, or PR), or dialysis should be considered to enhance elimination.

Those patients with serum potassium levels >7 mEq/L or who are symptomatic require aggressive intervention to stabilize the cellular membrane, shift potassium intracellularly, and increase potassium elimination. Membrane stabilization is effected by IV administration of calcium. Calcium gluconate, 10%, in a dose of 60 to 100 mg/kg (maximum 3 g/dose) or calcium chloride, 10%, in a dose of 20 mg/kg, may be administered over 5 to 10 minutes with continuous ECG monitoring. Onset of

Table 20–5. Treatment of Hyperkalemia

Halt potassium intake

- Eliminate high potassium food/drink.
- Discontinue intravenous potassium-containing solutions.
- Discontinue medications high in potassium or cause increased potassium.

Stabilize cell membranes

- Calcium chloride, 10%, 20 mg/kg, IV, over 5–10 min *or* calcium gluconate, 10%, 60–100 mg/kg (maximum 3 g/dose), IV, over 5–10 min (*Note:* Avoid with acute digitalis toxicity)

Translocate potassium intracellularly

- Sodium bicarbonate, 1–2 mEq/kg IV over 5–10 min
- Regular insulin, 0.25 U/kg, with Dextrose, 1g/kg, administered as a continuous infusion over 2 hours
- Albuterol, 2.5 mg for patients <25 kg and 5.0 mg for patients >25 kg, nebulized with 2.5 mL 0.9% NaCl

Eliminate potassium

- Sodium polystyrene sulfonate, 1–2 g/kg, PO, NG, or PR
- Diuretics
- Furosemide, 1–2 mg/kg, IV or PO
- Hydrochlorothiazide, 1 mg/kg (maximum 200 mg), PO
- Dialysis

Source: As modified from Kecskes SA: Fluids and Electrolytes, in Strange GR, Ahrens WR Lelyveld S, et al. (eds.): *Pediatric Emergency Medicine: A Comprehensive Study Guide,* 2nd ed. New York, McGraw-Hill, 2002, p 406, with permission.

action is immediate and the stabilizing effects last 30 to 60 minutes. Potassium may be shifted intracellularly to temporarily reduce serum potassium levels. Administration of calcium is contraindicated in cases of hyperkalemia induced by acute digoxin or digitalis poisoning. In this setting, hyperkalemia is optimally treated with digibind FAB fragments (see Chapter 37).

Administration of sodium bicarbonate (1 to 2 mEq/kg IV over 5 to 10 minutes) has an immediate onset of action and duration of up to 1 hour. The dose may be repeated if necessary. Insulin administered in conjunction with glucose effectively shifts potassium to the ICF as well. Dextrose (1 g/kg) may be combined with insulin

(0.25 U/kg) and infused over 2 hours. Inhalation of β-2 agonists is an attractive alternative for patients with delayed IV access. Nebulized albuterol, in a dose of 2.5 mg for patients <25 kg and 5 mg for patients >25 kg, has been reported to reduce potassium in adult patients with chronic renal failure and is likely to have a similar effect in pediatric patients. It should not be a substitute for appropriate IV therapy, but may be used while access is obtained.

None of these methods alter total body potassium, so the time they buy should be utilized to enhance elimination of potassium from the body. In the absence of renal failure, loop diuretics and/or thiazides enhance renal elimination of potassium. Sodium polystyrene sulfonate is a resin that exchanges sodium for potassium at a 1:1 ratio. It is administered through the gastrointestinal tract and may be used in patients with and without renal failure. In patients with renal failure or severely symptomatic cases, dialysis is the definitive therapy.

Hypokalemia

Hypokalemia is defined by a serum potassium level <3.5 mEq/L and can result from decreased intake, increased renal excretion, increased extrarenal losses, or a shift of potassium from the ECF to the ICF. In pediatric poisoning, increased renal excretion may result from ingestion of diuretics or diuresis used to enhance elimination. Extrarenal losses occur primarily through the gastrointestinal system. Diarrhea, in particular, is associated with large potassium losses. Movement of potassium into the cells from the ECF can occur with correction of acidosis with sodium bicarbonate, alkalinization of the urine to enhance toxin elimination, or respiratory alkalosis (i.e., salicylate intoxication).

Clinical manifestations of hypokalemia are related to its rapidity of onset and degree of severity. Muscle contraction is dependent on membrane polarization and requires a rapid influx of sodium into cells and a comparable efflux of potassium. Hypokalemia impairs this process. The result is alteration of nerve conduction and muscle contraction. Clinical symptoms include muscle weakness, ileus, areflexia, and autonomic instability, often manifested as orthostatic hypotension. Respiratory arrest and rhabdomyolysis can occur. The ECG can show flattening of the T wave, ST-segment depression, U waves, premature atrial and ventricular contractions, and dysrhythmias. Hypokalemia can also be associated with chronic digoxin therapy, particularly if the patient is concomitantly on a potassium-wasting diuretic agent. The kidney has a re-

duced ability to concentrate urine in hypokalemia, resulting in polyuria.

Laboratory data should include serum electrolytes including magnesium, serum pH, and urine K^+. Urine K^+ concentration of <15 mEq/L indicates renal conservation and suggests extrarenal loss. An ECG should be performed, looking for the alterations noted above.

In patients without life-threatening complications, hypokalemia should be corrected gradually with oral supplementation or, in patients with a contraindication to oral intake, an increase in the maintenance potassium concentration in the IV fluids. Underlying conditions that accompany the hypokalemia, such as alkalosis or hypomagnesemia, should be corrected. Sources of ongoing potassium loss are identified. The loss is measured and replaced. If life-threatening complications occur from hypokalemia, such as cardiac dysrhythmias, rhabdomyolysis, extreme muscle weakness, or respiratory arrest, IV therapy is required. Extreme care should be exercised in the ordering, preparation, and administration of IV potassium. Recommendations for dosage in pediatric patients range from 0.5 to 1 mEq/kg/dose (maximum dose: 30 mEq) to infuse at 0.3 to 0.5 mEq/kg/h (maximum rate: 1 mEq/kg/h). Potassium must be diluted prior to IV administration. In peripheral lines, the maximum concentration is 80 mEq/L. The maximum recommended central line concentration is 200 mEq/L. Continuous ECG monitoring, along with frequent assessment of serum potassium levels, is essential during IV correction of hypokalemia.

Calcium

Calcium is one of the most abundant and important minerals in the body, with 99% of body calcium stored in bone. Of the 1% present in the circulation, 40% is bound to proteins such as albumin, 15% is complexed with anions such as phosphate and citrate, and 45% is physiologically free and ionized. Calcium is responsible for cellular depolarization, muscle excitation/contraction, neurotransmitter release, hormonal secretion, and the function of both leukocytes and platelets.

A serum calcium level measures both ionized and protein-bound calcium. Because approximately half of serum calcium is bound to albumin, the serum calcium level may need to be adjusted for alterations in the albumin level. For every 1 g/dL decrease in serum albumin, true serum calcium may be estimated by adding 0.8 mg/dL. Alternatively, ionized calcium levels are widely available.

Hypocalcemia is defined as serum calcium <9 mg/dL. Hypocalcemia is a characteristic finding in ethylene glycol toxicity. The oxalic acid metabolite of ethylene glycol precipitates as calcium oxalate crystals in various tissues of the body, which are excreted in the urine. Other etiologies of hypocalcemia in pediatric poisoning patients is toxicity related to phosphate enema use and hydrofluoric acid toxicity.

Nonspecific symptoms, including nausea, weakness, paresthesias, and irritability, are typical. Classic physical findings of neuromuscular irritability are Chvostek and Trousseau's signs. In more severe cases, tetany, seizures, laryngospasm, and psychiatric manifestations may be seen. The ECG may show prolongation of the QT interval, bradycardia, and dysrhythmias. Laboratory tests should include ionized and total calcium, magnesium, phosphorus, albumin and total protein, BUN, creatinine, and alkaline phosphatase.

For significant or symptomatic hypocalcemia, IV calcium may be administered cautiously with continuous ECG monitoring. Calcium gluconate, 10%, (60 to 100 mg/kg/dose) or calcium chloride, 10% (10 to 20 mg/kg/dose) may be administered at a maximum rate of 50 to 100 mg/min. IV calcium is very irritating to tissues and veins, and should be diluted prior to administration. The maximum concentration of calcium gluconate should be 50 mg/mL and calcium chloride, 20 mg/mL. It is preferably given through a central line or very secure peripheral venous access. It should never be given intramuscularly, subcutaneously, or via an endotracheal route, as tissue necrosis and sloughing will occur. IV calcium predisposes to digoxin toxicity and precipitates when mixed with bicarbonate. Hyperphosphatemic patients are at risk of metastatic calcium deposition with calcium administration and require treatment aimed at lowering phosphorus levels. When hypomagnesemia is also present, oral or IV correction should be undertaken. Magnesium sulfate may be administered IV at a dose of 25 to 50 mg/kg, diluted to a maximum concentration of 200 mg/mL, over 2 to 4 hours.

GLUCOSE

Glucose is an essential source of fuel for the body. It is an immediate source of energy providing 38 mol of adenosine triphosphate (ATP) for every 1 mmol of glucose metabolized. The brain is particularly dependent on glucose in the blood as a source of energy. To maintain the adequate blood glucose levels for cerebral energy requirements, the body employs a complex regulatory system. The autonomic nervous system and hormones such as insulin, glucagon, growth hormone, and cortisol regu-

late glycogenolysis and gluconeogenesis. This allows the body to store fuel and utilize it for glucose production when glucose intake is low.

Hypoglycemia is defined as blood glucose <40 mg/dL. It is characteristic of ethanol and isopropanol toxicity. The liver metabolizes alcohol as a preferred fuel. This metabolism alters the NADH/NAD ratio essential for gluconeogenesis. In a child with limited glycogen stores who may not have fed recently, hypoglycemia is precipitated. Other causes of hypoglycemia in pediatric poisoning include ingestion of oral hyperglycemic agents and salicylates. Patients with salicylate ingestion may develop hypoglycemia in later phases owing to increased insulin production and impaired gluconeogenesis. Hypoglycemia is commonly seen in young children with shock and liver failure. Decreased intake owing to nausea and vomiting may exacerbate hypoglycemia in a young infants and toddlers. Symptoms include anxiety, diaphoresis, headache, lethargy, seizures, and coma. Treatment is the administration of dextrose. A bolus of 0.5 to 1.0 g/kg/dose of 25% dextrose (2 to 4 mL/kg/dose) may be given IV over a minimum of 5 minutes. Blood glucose should be closely followed.

Hyperglycemia is a less common finding in pediatric poisoning victims. It may be seen early in the course of salicylate and iron toxicity. Salicylate causes increased absorption of glucose from the intestinal tract and the uncoupling of oxidative phosphorylation leads to ineffective utilization of glucose by the cells. Generally, no treatment is necessary for hyperglycemia other than limiting intake of carbohydrates until the blood glucose normalizes. In critically ill patients, it may be desirable to control the blood glucose to below 110 to 130 mg/dL with insulin therapy. Frequent blood glucose monitoring and adjustments are required to avoid hypoglycemia.

FLUID AND ELECTROLYTE ISSUES ASSOCIATED WITH TREATMENT

The mainstays of treatment in the poisoned patient are decontamination, hastening elimination, and antidote administration. Several of these may be complicated by fluid and electrolyte issues.

Decontamination

Activated charcoal and gastric lavage are among the earliest modalities used to treat the poisoned patient. Ipecac-induced emesis can cause dehydration and hypokalemia when used chronically or in vulnerable patients. Gastric lavage may be indicated following recent life-threatening poisonings. There is a risk of absorption of large amounts of free water in the course of lavage, particularly in younger patients. Clinically significant hyponatremia may result. This complication may be avoided by using 0.45% or 0.9% saline instead of water as the lavage fluid. Electrolytes should be closely monitored in young children undergoing gastric lavage.

Cathartics are administered to patients with toxic ingestions to reduce drug absorption by shortening intestinal transit time, but have never been well studied as a sole agent of gastrointestinal decontamination. Sorbitol, magnesium citrate, and magnesium sulfate are the most commonly used cathartics in the treatment of the poisoned patient. Although generally safe if used within the recommended dosing guidelines, fluid and electrolyte complications can occur. Sorbitol has been reported to induce severe intravascular volume depletion, metabolic acidosis, and hypernatremia in young infants and is not recommended for those under 1 year of age. Hypermagnesemia does not usually occur after single doses in patients with normal renal function, but may occur with multiple doses. Magnesium citrate and magnesium sulfate should be avoided in patients with renal failure. Hyperphosphatemia, hypocalcemia, and hypernatremia may occur after use of hypertonic phosphate enemas.

When toxins are not well absorbed by activated charcoal, whole-bowel irrigation may be used to decrease time for drug absorption in the intestine. Isotonic polyethylene glycol electrolyte solutions (e.g., Golytely) are administered to flush out the intestinal tract. Although generally safe, electrolytes should be closely monitored, particularly in younger children.

Hastening Elimination of Poisons

Techniques to hasten elimination of poisons are commonly undertaken after decontamination and appropriate supportive care have been provided. These techniques include diuresis with and without alteration of urinary pH, gastrointestinal diuresis with activated charcoal, dialysis, hemoperfusion, and plasmapheresis. All of these techniques have associated fluid and electrolyte issues.

Many drugs and toxins are eliminated from the body by the kidney. Drugs that are not protein bound are filtered by the glomerulus. There is active transport of some drugs into the proximal convoluted tubules. Lipid-soluble, unionized drugs undergo passive bidirectional diffusion along a concentration gradient along the length of the nephron. As H_2O and Na^+ are resorbed, the concentration of intraluminal drug increases. The gradient

favors resorption, not elimination. However, by promoting urine flow of 2 to 5 mL/kg/h, the concentration of the drug in the distal segment is decreased, resorption is decreased, and elimination is enhanced. This may be combined with techniques to alter the pH of urine and trap the drug intraluminally. Efficient reabsorption of drugs across the renal tubule only occurs when the drug is unionized and lipid soluble. The proportion of the drug in the unionized form depends on the pK of the drug and the pH of the solution. By altering the pH of the urine, the proportion of the ionized drug is enhanced, trapping the poorly reabsorbed compound in the tubular lumen.

This technique is most applicable to drugs predominantly eliminated by the kidney. The drug must be poorly protein bound to allow for glomerular filtration. The pK_a of the drug should be such that altering urinary pH will allow ionization and produce trapping. Alkalinization of the urine is effective for drugs with a pK_a of 3.0 to 7.2 (isoniazid, salicylate, phenobarbital). Acidification is potentially effective for drugs with a pK_a of 7.2 to 9.5 (quinidine, phencyclidine, amphetamine), although the risks of acidification almost always outweigh the benefits.

Diuresis is initiated with IV fluids at one to three times maintenance to achieve a urine output of 2 to 5 mL/kg/h. Preexisting fluid deficits must be restored and ongoing losses must be replaced. Blood glucose should be monitored and the dextrose content of the fluid adjusted to achieve normalization. Bladder catheterization allows assessment of urine output, as well as pH. Diuretics such as mannitol and furosemide may be added to enhance diuresis. Complications of enhanced diuresis include fluid overload, pulmonary edema, cerebral edema, hypokalemia, and hyponatremia. Careful monitoring of the patient and their acid–base and electrolyte status are required when employing these techniques.

Sodium bicarbonate is administered to produce urine alkalinization to a target pH of 7 to 8. It may be given in the IV fluid by adding 50 to 75 mEq/L $NaHCO_3$ to a D_5W or 0.45% saline solution. Hypernatremia, alkalosis, and hypokalemia should be anticipated. Hypokalemia may cause resistance to alkalinization. Careful supplementation of potassium may alleviate the situation.

Gastrointestinal diuresis with activated charcoal is used to create a diffusion gradient from the systemic circulation to the gut and hasten gastrointestinal elimination of the drug. The activated charcoal dose is 1 g/kg (maximum 50 g) administered orally or by nasogastric tube every 2 to 4 hours. It is generally safe if airway protection is ensured. Care should be taken to avoid activated charcoal in sorbitol in children younger than 1 because of the risk of hypernatremic dehydration and shock.

Dialysis, charcoal hemoperfusion, and plasmapheresis techniques may be employed to hasten elimination of toxins in high-risk patients (see Chapter 18). These techniques require special equipment and expertise. Fluid and electrolyte shifts are common with these techniques and are anticipated in the execution of the procedures.

SUGGESTED READINGS

Adelman RD, Solhaug MJ: Pathophysiology of body fluids and fluid therapy. In: Behrman RE, Kliegman RM, Jenson HB, eds: *Nelson Textbook of Pediatrics.* 16th ed. Philadelphia: Saunders; 2000:197.

Adrogue HJ, Madias NE: Hyponatremia. *N Engl J Med* 342: 1581, 2000.

Allon M, Dunlay R, Copkney C: Nebulized albuterol for acute hyperkalemia in patients on hemodialysis. *Ann Intern Med* 110:426, 1989.

Davis RF, Eichner JM, Bleyer WA: Hypocalcemia, hyperphosphatemia, and dehydration following a single hypertonic phosphate enema. *J Pediatr* 90:484, 1977.

Farley TA: Severe hypernatremic dehydration after use of an activated charcoal-sorbitol suspension. *J Pediatr* 109:719, 1986.

Finberg L: Hypernatremia (hypertonic) dehydration in infants. *N Engl J Med* 289:196, 1973.

Kecskes SA: Fluids and electrolytes. In: Strange GR, Ahrens WR, Lelyveld S, et al, eds: *Pediatric Emergency Medicine: A Comprehensive Study Guide.* 2nd ed. New York: McGraw-Hill; 2002:398.

Kelleher SP, Raciti A, Arbeit LA: Reduced or absent serum anion gap as a marker of severe lithium carbonate intoxication. *Arch Intern Med* 146:1839, 1986.

Lee JH, Arcinue E, Ross BD: Brief report: Organic osmolytes in the brain of an infant with hypernatremia. *N Engl J Med* 331:439, 1994.

Lynch RE: Ionized calcium: Pediatric perspective. *Pediatr Clin North Am* 37:373, 1990.

McGuigan MA: Two-year review of salicylate deaths in Ontario. *Arch Intern Med* 147:510, 1987.

Rosansky SJ: Isopropyl alcohol poisoning treated with hemodialysis: Kinetics of isopropyl alcohol and acetone removal. *J Toxicol Clin Toxicol* 19:265, 1982.

Rothenberg DM, Berns AS, Barkin K, et al: Bromide intoxication secondary to pyridostigmine bromide therapy. *JAMA* 263:1121, 1990.

Sterns RH, Riggs JE, Schochet Jr SS: Osmotic demyelination syndrome following correction of hyponatremia. *N Engl J Med* 314:1535, 1986.

Taketomo CK, Hodding JH, Kraus DM: *Pediatric Dosage Handbook.* 10th ed. Hudson, OH: Lexi-Comp; 2003.

Van den Berghe G, Waters P, Weekers F, et al: Intensive insulin therapy in the critically ill patients. *N Engl J Med* 345:1359, 2001.

Woolf AD, Berkowitz ID, Liebelt E, et al: Poisoning and the critically ill child. In: Rogers MC, ed: *Textbook of Pediatric Intensive Care.* 3rd ed. Baltimore: Williams & Wilkins; 1996:1339.

Younossi-Hartenstein A, Roth B, Iffland R, et al: Short term hemodialysis for ethylene glycol poisoning. *J Pediatr* 109:731, 1986.

22

Thermoregulation

Erica L. Liebelt
Michele K. Nichols

A variety of drugs, chemicals, and toxins may disrupt thermoregulation in children. Unique aspects of their physiology and environment render children more susceptible than some adults to the adverse effects of these substances. Vital signs often provide clinical clues to poisonings, and temperature measurement is a critical part of the overall assessment. Elevation or depression of normal core body temperature can occur when drugs or chemicals interfere with normal thermoregulatory mechanisms that lead to inadequate heat production (*hypothermia*) or heat dissipation (*hyperthermia*).

Thermoregulation is the complex physiologic process that serves to maintain hypothalamic temperature within a narrow range of $37.0 \pm 0.4°C$ ($98.6 \pm 0.8°F$), which is known as the *set point*. The primary thermoregulatory center resides in the preoptic area of the hypothalamus, and controls the balance between heat gain and heat loss. Additional thermosensitive neurons are present in the skin, spinal cord, abdominal viscera, and large veins; all are capable of sending signals to the hypothalamic center. Responding to cold and heat, the hypothalamic neurons send signals to the autonomic nervous system that cause many outwardly visible physiologic manifestations, such as sweating, shivering, and peripheral vasoconstriction/vasodilation.

Many neurotransmitters are involved in thermoregulation, including serotonin, norepinephrine, acetylcholine, dopamine, prostaglandins, and β-endorphins. Hypothalamic peptides include arginine vasopressin, adrenocorticotrophic hormone, and thyrotropin releasing hormone. Although the effects of individual neurotransmitters on thermoregulation are not entirely clear, classes of drugs that affect certain neurotransmitters have demonstrated patterns of thermoregulatory disruption. Specifically, drugs that affect acetylcholine, dopamine, norepinephrine, and serotonin are associated with various hyperthermic syndromes. Both a lack of central dopaminergic activity and serotonergic hyperstimulation have been associated with altered hypothalamic thermoregulatory control. In addition, abnormal central sympathetic and motor activity may influence peripheral body heat production and dissipation.

DEVELOPMENTAL CONSIDERATIONS

Because of differences in heat production and heat loss, infants and children are less tolerant than adults to extremes of temperature. Neonates, infants, and children younger than 2 have underdeveloped thermoregulatory controls. Children, especially infants and toddlers, have higher surface area to body mass ratios than adults, allowing more efficient transfer of heat between the environment and their bodies. In addition, children produce more endogenous heat per kilogram of body weight than adults, especially during physical activity. Compared to adults, children are less efficient at evaporative heat loss, because their capacity to sweat is lower and the temperature at which they begin to sweat is higher. Finally, obese children are less tolerant of heat than children of normal body weight.

There are other physiologic factors that may predispose children to thermoregulatory dysfunction when exposed to drugs and other substances. Febrile illnesses, common among children, increase the metabolic rate and endogenous heat production, and can increase the risk of drug-related hyperthermic syndromes. Illnesses that cause dehydration are relatively common in children; dehydration itself leads to an increase in core body temperature, an effect that is more pronounced in children than adults. In addition, children are vulnerable to dehydration because they or their caregivers may not recognize the need to increase water consumption during diarrheal illnesses.

Drugs and other substances that alter thermoregulation can disproportionately affect children and adolescents with certain chronic diseases. Children with spina bifida, sweating insufficiency syndrome, quadriplegia, and severe eczema have decreased sweat production, which limits evaporative heat loss. Children with cystic fibrosis can have excessive sweating that increases fluid loss and/or diminishes thirst, which in turn increases the likelihood of dehydration. Young children or children with mental retardation can have inadequate fluid intake. Anorexia nervosa and malnutrition cause abnormal hypothalamic thermoregulatory function that can predispose to hypo- or hyperthermic syndromes.

DRUG, CHEMICAL, AND TOXIN EFFECTS

Numerous drugs, chemicals, and toxins have pharmacologic effects that interfere with normal thermoregulatory responses. α-Adrenergic–mediated vasoconstriction that can occur with the use of cocaine, ephedrine, and amphetamines, and sweat gland dysfunction that can occur with anticholinergic agents, can impair cutaneous heat loss. Temperature can be affected by drugs that cause myocardial depression and reduce circulating blood volume, as well as agents such as antipsychotics that cause hypothalamic depression. An impaired behavioral response to temperature stress can occur in drugs that impair judgment, such as phencyclidine and cocaine. Hyperthermia can occur from uncoupling of oxidative phosphorylation, as is seen in toxicity from salicylates and dinitrophenol. Drugs that cause agitation or an increase in muscle activity can result in hyperthermia; these include sympathomimetic agents, phencyclidine, caffeine, and lithium. Severe withdrawal from dopamine agonists, ethanol, or other sedative-hypnotics can also increase body temperature (Table 22–1).

Mechanisms that predispose to hypothermia include impaired nonshivering thermogenesis, which can occur with β-adrenergic antagonists, cholinergic agents, and hypoglycemic agents. Impaired perception of cold can result from exposure to ethanol, hypoglycemic agents, and opioids. Shivering can be impaired by hypothalamic depression that can occur with opioids, phenothiazines, and ethanol, and impaired vasoconstriction can result from α-adrenergic antagonists, ethanol, and phenothiazines (Table 22–2).

SPECIFIC HYPERTHERMIC SYNDROMES

Numerous drugs or drug classes may give rise to several specific hyperthermic syndromes. Significant clinical

Table 22–1. Common Drug Causes of Hyperthermia

α-Adrenergic agonists
Amphetamines
Antihistamines
Belladonna alkaloids (atropine, scopolamine)
Butyrophenones (haloperidol, droperidol)
Caffeine
Cocaine
Cyclic antidepressants
Dinitrophenol
Diuretics
Ephedrine/pseudoephedrine
Isoniazid
Lithium
Methamphetamines/Ecstasy
MAOIs
Pentachlorophenol
Phenothiazines
Salicylates
Sympathomimetic agents
Strychnine
Withdrawal of ethanol, dopamine agonists, sedative-hypnotics

Abbreviation: MAOIs, monoamine oxidase inhibitors.

manifestations of hyperthermia include central nervous system dysfunction, which can be severe, rhabdomyolysis, disseminated intravascular coagulation, acute tubular necrosis with associated hyperkalemia, cardiac dysfunction, and dysrhythmias. In theory, these represent unique syndromes, although there may be many overlapping symptoms and signs.

Table 22–2. Common Drug Causes of Hypothermia

α-Adrenergic antagonists
β-Adrenergic antagonists
Calcium channel antagonists
Cholinergic agents
Clonidine
Ethanol
Hypoglycemic agents
Lithium
Opioids
Phenothiazines
Sedative-hypnotics

Serotonin Syndrome

Central serotonin syndrome (CSS) is an iatrogenic complication of the use of drugs and dietary supplements that have central nervous system serotonin (5-HT) activity. The *serotonin receptor neurotransmitter hypothesis* describes a cascade of events leading to increased synaptic and postsynaptic 5-HT. CSS most commonly results when a monoamine oxidase inhibitor (MAOI) is combined with a tricyclic antidepressant, a selective serotonin reuptake inhibitor (SSRI), meperidine, dextromethorphan, or L-tryptophan. Methylenedioxymethamphetamine (Ecstasy) may also cause CSS, because this drug is often consumed with amino-acid drinks while in a hot environment such as a dance club. CSS is a toxidrome of symptoms and signs that is similar to the anticholinergic, sympathomimetic, and salicylate toxidromes, as well as the neuroleptic malignant syndrome (NMS). The triad of cognitive/behavioral, autonomic, and neuromuscular abnormalities characterizes CSS. At least 3 of the 11 clinical features listed in Table 22–3 must be present after the addition or increase of a known serotonergic agent. In one review of 127 patients, 46% of patients developed hyperthermia. Onset of symptoms usually occurs minutes to hours after the drug change.

Neuroleptic Malignant Syndrome

NMS is an idiosyncratic reaction to certain medications. The most common causative agents are the neuroleptics; the most common offenders reported are haloperidol and fluphenazine. An acute alteration and reduction of central dopaminergic activity in the basal ganglia and the hypothalamus is generally regarded as the cause of NMS.

The reported incidence of NMS has varied from 0.02% to 3.32% in patients taking neuroleptic medication.

Table 22–3. Clinical Criteria for Diagnosis of CSS

Mental status changes
Agitation
Myoclonus
Muscle rigidity
Hyperreflexia
Diaphoresis
Shivering
Tremor
Diarrhea
Incoordination
Fever

Abbreviation: CSS, central serotonin syndrome.

Characteristics of NMS include hyperthermia, muscle rigidity, autonomic instability, and altered mental status. Increased muscle activity is presumed to be the cause of hyperthermia, although severe NMS may present without muscular rigidity or hyperthermia. Initial symptoms usually occur within the first 3 to 9 days of therapy, but may occur years after its initiation. Resolution of symptoms require up to 10 days. Although the mortality rate is approximately 10%, early recognition of NMS has contributed to a declining incidence.

Distinguishing NMS from CSS is often difficult. NMS presents with hyperthermia, altered mental status, autonomic changes, and lead pipe muscle rigidity in more than 90% of cases, whereas CSS presents with these symptoms in about 50%. One distinguishing symptom that helps to differentiate the two syndromes is myoclonus, which is rare in NMS, but common in CSS (60%).

Malignant Hyperthermia

Malignant hyperthermia (MH) is a rare idiosyncratic clinical syndrome often seen in genetically susceptible individuals undergoing general anesthesia. Inhaled volatile anesthetics and depolarizing muscle paralytics are the chief triggers. Patients with certain muscular disorders, such as muscular dystrophies, are at an increased risk of MH. The classic clinical triad includes hyperthermia, muscle rigidity, and metabolic acidosis. Other symptoms include jaw and chest pain, tachycardia, arrhythmias, hypotension, fatigue, and weakness. Hyperthermia in this setting is often delayed and may not occur in all cases. Increased sympathetic tone and skeletal muscle hyperactivity have been implicated in the etiology of MH. Severe cases that produced body temperature elevations of 1°C every 5 minutes and temperatures as high as 46°C have been reported in children. Early recognition and appropriate treatment have contributed to a decline in mortality rate over the years.

Anticholinergic Poisoning Syndrome

Blockade of muscarinic acetylcholine receptors gives rise to the anticholinergic poisoning syndrome. Agitation and seizures create muscular hyperactivity, and peripheral muscarinic blockade impairs sweating that might otherwise mitigate hyperthermia. Hyperthermia can persist for several days until normal thermoregulation resumes. The presence of dry axillae often assists in differentiating anticholinergic toxicity from sympathomimetic poisoning, which is associated with diaphoretic skin (Table 22–4). Body temperatures in excess of 43°C have been reported in

Table 22–4. Clinical Clues in Hyperthermia and Poisonings

Hypertension
    Amphetamines
    Cocaine
    Tricyclic antidepressants
Mydriasis
    Anticholinergics
    Hallucinogenics
Miosis (children only)
    PCP
Diaphoresis
    Sympathomimetics
    Amphetamines
Dry skin
    Anticholinergics
Flushing
    Anticholinergics
Delirium
    Anticholinergics
    PCP
    Cocaine
    Amphetamines
Seizures
    Anticholinergics
    Cocaine
    Amphetamines
    Atropine
    PCP
    Salicylates
    Cyclic antidepressants
Rigidity
    Malignant hyperthermia
    Neuroleptic malignant syndrome
    PCP
Dyskinesias
    Cocaine
    PCP
    Anticholinergics
Dystonic reactions
    Phenothiazines
Coma
    Anticholinergics
Hallucinations
    Hallucinogenics
Metabolic acidosis
    Salicylates

Abbreviation: PCP, phencyclidine.

severe poisonings. Children are prone to hyperthermia from anticholinergic medications, even when administered in therapeutic doses.

Sympathomimetic Poisoning Syndrome

Although mild to moderate hyperthermia can occur with recreational or pharmaceutical sympathomimetic use, life-threatening hyperthermia can also occur. Effects of sympathomimetics that predispose to hyperthermia include peripheral vasoconstriction and impaired cutaneous heat loss, agitation, seizures, increased muscle activity, and impaired behavioral responses. Sympathomimetics raise synaptic concentrations of norepinephrine, dopamine, and serotonin to produce their effects. Central thermoregulatory dysfunction can arise from complex interactions between dopamine and serotonin in the brain stem and hypothalamus. Use of adulterants such as diphenhydramine in the manufacture of sympathomimetic drugs can further exacerbate the hyperthermia.

In cocaine intoxication, agitation and α-adrenergic stimulation are responsible, in part, for hyperthermia. Cocaine overdose often resembles NMS, with hyperthermia, altered mental status, tachycardia, muscle rigidity, coagulopathy, and renal and hepatic dysfunction characterizing the clinical presentation. Amphetamine and methamphetamine increase the release of the neurotransmitters from the presynaptic nerve terminals and inhibit their uptake from the synapse. Hyperthermia alone can be responsible for many of the clinical findings seen with amphetamine or cocaine toxicity, such as coma or seizures. Exertional hyperthermia in the setting of sympathomimetic ingestions may produce rhabdomyolysis, coagulopathy, hyperkalemia, myocardial dysfunction, and cardiovascular collapse.

OTHERS

Salicylates

Clinical features of salicylate toxicity occur as a result of uncoupled oxidative phosphorylation and disruption of the Krebs cycle. Hyperthermia is seen in 20% of patients with severe salicylate toxicity; neurologic abnormalities are seen in 61%, metabolic acidosis in 50%, pulmonary complications in 43%, and circulatory effects in 14%.

Dissociative Drugs

Dissociative drugs such as ketamine and PCP act on all neurotransmitter systems and present with a sympatho-

mimetic picture. Dopamine and norepinephrine are released and produce muscle rigidity, agitation, fever, and
central nervous system stimulation.

HYPOTHERMIC SYNDROME

Toxin-induced hypothermia is usually mild unless an environmental exposure has occurred as well. Extreme exposures may produce profound hypothermia in healthy
persons, but mortality is related in part to the cardiac
rhythm at rescue and whether the patient had asphyxia
prior to the onset of hypothermia. Examination of the hypothermic patient should focus on mental status and vital
signs. Because neurologic depression is a direct function
of brain temperature, significant mental status depression
in patients with temperatures above 31.7°C (89°F)
should suggest a complicating condition such as a toxic
exposure. Vital signs may provide a clue to poisonings.
Heart rate normally increases as the body temperature
declines until the temperature falls below 29°C (84.2°F).
If the heart rate or blood pressure is altered disproportionately to the temperature depression, a drug, chemical,
or toxin may account for the vital signs. For instance, a
β-adrenergic blocker or calcium-channel blocker can
cause bradycardia and hypotension that hypothermia
alone cannot explain.

Several toxins, including ethanol, sedative-hypnotics,
barbiturates, opioids, and carbon monoxide, can cause
both hypothermia and coma. Overdoses of phenothiazines, organophosphates, β-adrenergic receptor antagonists, or centrally acting α-adrenergic agonists such as
clonidine depress hypothalamic function and impair central thermoregulation. β-Adrenergic antagonists may interfere with mobilization of substrates required for thermogenesis and thus disrupt mechanisms to maintain
normothermia. Some drugs, such as ethanol and hydra-
lazine, prevent vasoconstriction, whereas others, such as
chlorpromazine, have α-adrenergic receptor blocking effects. Hypoglycemic agents may also lead to hypothermia (see Table 22–2).

MANAGEMENT

Initial management of hyperthermia and hypothermia
relies on the basic principles of pediatric advanced life
support, with specific interventions depending on the etiology. All patients require measurement of rectal temperature. Severe hyperthermia and hypothermia require
continuous temperature monitoring.

Hyperthermia must be treated aggressively to avoid
serious complications. Excessive heat production related
to agitation or increased muscle rigidity can be controlled with benzodiazepines and dantrolene (Figure
22–1). Seizure activity is treated with benzodiazepines or
barbiturates. For patients with refractory status epilepticus, paralysis and mechanical ventilation is an option.
External cooling can be accomplished with strategic ice
pack application to the groin, axillae, and neck; cooling
blankets; and ice water gastric lavage. The most efficient
method of external cooling combines a water spray or
water-soaked sheets to wet the skin with fans used to
cool the patient via evaporative heat loss. Once core
body temperature has decreased to 38°C to 39°C, cooling measures should cease, to prevent iatrogenic hypothermia. Throughout cooling therapy, continuous
monitoring of core temperature is mandatory. Antipyretic medications are not indicated in drug-induced
hyperthermia. Some drugs, such as salicylates, may
worsen hyperthermia. General and specific interventions
are presented in Table 22–5.

For significant hypothermia, basic pediatric advanced
life support principles of airway, breathing, and circulation must be followed very cautiously. Every effort

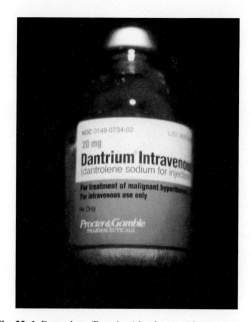

Fig. 22–1. Dantrolene (Dantrium) has been used to treat muscle rigidity associated with malignant hyperthermia and neuroleptic malignant syndrome.

Table 22–5. Treatment of Drug-Induced Hyperthermic Syndromes

General management
   Airway and breathing
   IV fluids
   Benzodiazepines
   Barbiturates
   Paralysis with nondepolarizing neuromuscular
      blocking agent and mechanical ventilation
   External cooling measures
   Internal cooling measures
Malignant Hyperthermia
   Immediate cessation of operative procedures and
      triggering agent
   Dantrolene, 1–2 mg/kg IV every 6–8 h (may be
      increased up to 10 mg/kg)
Neuroleptic malignant syndrome
   Bromocriptine, 2.5 mg up to 10–20 mg PO TID
   Dantrolene (see above dosing)
Severe anticholinergic poisoning syndrome
   Physostigmine, 0.02 mg/kg up to 0.5 mg q5min PRN
      to maximum 2.0 mg

Abbreviations: IV, intravenous; PO, orally; PRN, as needed; TID, three times a day.

should be made to limit patient activity and stimulation during the acute rewarming period, because activity may increase the risk of iatrogenic ventricular fibrillation (VF). There are case reports, for example, of VF occurring during endotracheal intubation performed for airway protection. If VF occurs, cardiopulmonary resuscitation should be initiated despite the possibility that standard therapy for defibrillation may not be effective until rewarming is achieved.

There are several rewarming modalities used in the management of hypothermia. Passive external rewarming is done with blankets; active external rewarming involves the application of heat. Techniques for active internal rewarming include using heated, humidified oxygen, gastric lavage with warmed fluids, peritoneal lavage with warmed dialysate, and extracorporeal warming via cardiopulmonary or femoral–femoral bypass.

Passive or active external warming will reverse most drug- or chemical-induced hypothermia.

SUGGESTED READINGS

Arnold DH: The central serotonin syndrome: Paradigm for psychotherapeutic misadventure. *Pediatr Rev* 23:427–432, 2002.
Baumgartner JF, Janusz MT, Jamieson WR, et al: Cardiopulmonary bypass for resuscitation of patients with accidental hypothermia and cardiac arrest. *Can J Surg* 35:184–187, 1992.
Carone JR: Psychiatric emergencies: The neuroleptic malignant serotonin syndromes. *Emerg Clin North Am* 18:317–325, 2000.
Chan TC, Evans SD, Clark RF: Medical toxicology: Drug-induced hyperthermia. *Crit Care Clin* 13:785–808, 1997.
Clark WG, Lipton JM: Brain and pituitary peptides in thermoregulation. *Pharmacol Ther* 22:249–297, 1983.
Committee on Sports Medicine, American Academy of Pediatrics: Climatic heat stress and the exercising child. *Pediatrics* 106:158–159, 2000.
Dubrow JT, Wackym PA, Abus-Rasool IH, et al: Malignant hyperthermia: Experience in the management of eight children. *J Pediatr Surg* 24:163–166, 1989.
Erickson T, Prendergast H: Procedures pertaining to hypothermia and hyperthermia. In: Robert J, Hedges J, eds: *Clinical Procedures in Emergency Medicine.* 4th ed. Philadelphia: Saunders; 2003:1343–1370.
Hoffman JL: Heat-related illness in children. *Clin Pediatr Emerg Med* 2:203–210, 2001.
Mokhlesi B, Leikin JB, Murray P, et al: Critical care review: Adult toxicology in critical care: Part II: Specific poisonings. *Chest* 123:897–922, 2003.
Schwartz PG, Wehr TA, Rosenthal NE, et al: Serotonin and thermoregulation: Physiologic and pharmacologic aspects of control revealed by intravenous M-CPP in normal human subjects. *Neuropsychopharmacology* 13:105–115, 1995.
Stewart C: The spectrum of heat illness in children. *Pediatr Emerg Med Rep* 4:41–52, 1999.
Torline RL: Extreme hyperthermia associated with anticholinergic syndrome. *Anesthesiology* 76:470, 1992.
Vassallo SU, Delaney KA: Thermoregulatory principles. In: Goldfrank L, Flomenbaum N, Lewin N, et al, eds: *Goldfrank's Toxicologic Emergencies.* 7th ed. New York: McGraw-Hill; 2002.
Yamawaki S, Lai H, Horita A: Dopaminergic and serotonergic mechanisms of thermoregulation: Mediation of thermal effects of apomorphine and dopamine. *J Pharmacol Exp Ther* 227:383–388, 1983.

23

Organ System Toxicity

Sean M. Bryant

It is useful to consider toxicology in light of a drug's effect on individual organ systems, because these may provide important information regarding diagnosis and prognosis. A prototypical example is iron poisoning. Iron is a cellular toxin that affects multiple organ systems; however, without gastrointestinal (GI) manifestation of poisoning, one can predict a healthy prognosis for the pediatric patient.

Although many poisons target a specific organ system, others may disrupt homeostasis in multiple ways. Carbamazepine, for example, is a frequently prescribed medication for seizures, migraine headache prophylaxis, and bipolar disorder. In overdose, patients can present with neurologic depression or excitation in the form of seizures, choreoathetosis, or dystonic reactions. The cardiovascular system is prone to tachycardia, hypotension, and QRS widening that can predispose to ventricular dysrhythmias. In addition, idiosyncratic reactions can result in a drug-induced systemic lupus erythematosus syndrome, hepatitis, rash, and fatal aplastic anemia. The objective of this chapter is to provide the clinician with a brief synopsis of pediatric organ system toxicity, and a list of those poisons that affect corresponding physiology.

NEUROLOGIC

There are a myriad of neurologic manifestations of poisoning. Altered mental status may be the first diagnostic clue to poisoning in a young child. Other neurologic abnormalities include seizures and movement disorders such as tremors, choreiform movements (excessive, random movements), dystonias (sustained muscle spasms), dyskinesia (stereotypical movements), and akasthisia (motor restlessness). Antipsychotic agents are well known for inducing many of these movement disorders. Central nerv-

ous system (CNS) stimulation can manifest secondary to stimulants such as cocaine, ephedra, caffeine, antihistamines, and amphetamines. CNS depression follows ingestion of sedatives like benzodiazepines and barbiturates, ethanol, γ-hydroxybutyurate (GHB), and opioids. Seizures can result from a large number of toxins such as isoniazid (INH), theophylline, and salicylates. Tables 23–1 and 23–2 list selected toxins affecting the nervous system.

Table 23–1. Toxin-Induced Seizures

Antihistamines	Lead
Caffeine	Boric acid
Salicylates	Camphor
Carbamazepine	Fluoride
Digoxin	Organophosphates
Isoniazid/*Gyromitra* mushrooms	Pyrethrins
Lidocaine	Rodenticides
Phenytoin	Carbon monoxide
Quinine	Chlorphenoxy herbicides
Theophylline	Hydrocarbons
Oral hypoglycemics (sulfonylureas)	Inhalants (asphyxiation)
Antipsychotics	Elapid snake envenomation
Tricyclic antidepressants	Scorpion envenomation
Lithium	Amphetamines (MDMA)
Methylphenidate	Cocaine
Opioids (propoxyphene, meperidine)	Phencyclidine
Ethanol withdrawal	Nicotine
Sedative-hypnotic withdrawal	Water Hemlock
	Heavy metals
	GHB

Table 23–2. Toxin-Induced Movement Disorders

Tremor	Chorea	Dystonia	Dyskinesia	Akathisia
Carbon monoxide, cyanide	Anticholinergics	Antipsychotics	Antipsychotics	Antidepressants
Lithium	Anticonvulsants	Antiemetics	Metoclopramide	Antiemetics
Caffeine, theophylline, amphetamines	Antipsychotics	Anticonvulsants	Antipsychotics	
Manganese, mercury, lead	Carbon monoxide			
Metoclopramide	Lithium			
Phenytoin, valproic acid, carbamazepine	Corticosteroids			
Ethanol withdrawal, chloral hydrate	Manganese			
Cocaine, phencyclidine	Toluene			

OPHTHALMIC

Physically examining the eyes is essential in all poisoned patients. However, a detailed ocular exam can be difficult in a frightened, uncooperative child. Many toxins target the ophthalmic system. Eye findings such as pupillary size, ocular movement abnormalities, corneal appearance, and fundoscopic details provide vital clues to diagnosis. Classic agents causing papillary constriction (miosis) include opioids and organophosphates. Mydriatic (dilating) agents include anticholinergics such as antihistamines, sympathomimetics like ephedra-containing products, cocaine, and amphetamines. Movement disorders, such as nystagmus, are common after poisoning. Phencyclidine characteristically can induce vertical or rotary nystagmus.

Corneal disruption is frequent after direct caustic injury to the eye from acid or alkali products. Both are considered ophthalmic emergencies. Acids result in superficial coagulation necrosis and alkalis produce a more severe liquefaction necrosis. Prompt irrigation is pursued to prevent subsequent corneal ulceration and ocular per-

foration. Hydrofluoric acid is of particular concern in light of its ability to penetrate deeply and cause extensive damage. Additional ocular manifestations may result from systemic ingestion of poisons. Optic nerve pathology follows methanol's metabolism to formate resulting in hyperemia of the optic disc. Quinine toxicity can also potentially result in permanent blindness, a syndrome known as *cinchonism*. Toxins affecting the visual system are listed in Table 23–3.

OTOLARYNGOLOGIC

Poisons can exhibit characteristic odors, which clinically may provide helpful hints in diagnosis. The bitter almond odor of cyanide, detectable by 60% of the population, and the smell of wintergreen from methyl salicylate are prime examples (Table 23–4). Tinnitus, or ringing in the ears, is a sensation of sound not produced by external stimuli. Salicylate toxicity is a classic example manifesting as levels reach the toxic range (Table 23–5).

Table 23–3. Ocular Toxicity

Miosis	Mydriasis	Nystagmus	Dysconjugate Gaze
Cholinesterase inhibitors (nerve agents, carbamates, organophosphates)	Antihistamines	Phencyclidine	Botulism
	Tricyclic antidepressants	Carbamazepine	Paralytic shellfish poisoning
	Amphetamines	Phenytoin	Tetrodotoxin
Nicotine	Cocaine	Ethanol	Elapid envenomation
Clonidine	Sympathomimetics	Monoamine oxidase inhibitors (MAOIs)	Scorpion stings
Opioids	Withdrawal (ethanol, benzodiazepine, barbiturate)		
Benzodiazepines			
Barbiturates	Jimson weed, atropine		
Ethanol			

Table 23–4. Toxin-Associated Odors

Odor	Toxin
Acetone	Ethanol, isopropanol, chloral hydrate, lacquer
Bitter almond	Cyanide
Rotten eggs	Hydrogen sulfide, disulfiram
Fish	Phosphides (aluminum, zinc)
Garlic	Organophosphates, selenium, phosphorus, arsenic
Freshly mown hay	Phosgene
Mothballs	Camphor, naphthalene
Burnt rope	Marijuana
Tobacco	Nicotine
Violets	Turpentine
Wintergreen	Methyl salicylate

RESPIRATORY

In a poisoned child, changes in the respiratory rate may be the key to diagnosing the causal agent. With intoxicated children, attention to the respiratory drive and airway are paramount. Hypoxia results in more pediatric poisoning deaths than primary cardiac dysrhythmias compared to adults. Toxins like salicylates can affect respiratory drive by stimulation via direct action on the respiratory center in the brain and by induction of metabolic acidosis. The net result is hyperventilation in the form of tachypnea and/or hyperpnea, with concomitant respiratory alkalosis.

Table 23–5. Toxin-Induced Tinnitus

Carbamazepine
Lithium
Antihistamines
Antibiotics (aminoglycosides, vancomycin, tetracycline, doxycycline, metronidazole, clindamycin)
Haloperidol
Quinine
Salicylates
Nonsteroidal anti-inflammatory agents
Local anesthetics (bupivacaine, lidocaine, mepivacaine)
Oral contraceptives
Caffeine
Theophylline
Albuterol
Methylphenidate
Codeine, oxycodone

Table 23–6. Toxins Affecting Respiratory Drive

Hyperventilation	Hypoventilation
Salicylates	Opioids
Amphetamines	Nicotine
Antihistamines	Sedatives (barbiturates, benzodiazepines)
Caffeine	Botulinum toxin
Camphor	Baclofen
Cocaine	GHB
Iron	Ethanol
Theophylline	Toxic alcohols
Toxic alcohols (secondary to acidosis)	Tetrodotoxin, paralytic shellfish poisoning

Abbreviation: GHB, γ-hydroxybutyrate.

Other poisons act to suppress the respiratory center. Opioids do this by direct suppression of the respiratory center in addition to decreasing chemoreceptor responsiveness to carbon dioxide. Respiratory depression is evident in patients with decreased respiratory rates (bradypnea) and/or hypopnea with decreased tidal volumes (Table 23–6). Other effects of poisons on the lungs include the displacement of oxygen by asphyxiant gases like nitrogen, irritation from chemicals such as ammonia, and direct injury at the alveolar-capillary interface resulting in pulmonary edema (Table 23–7). Noncardiogenic pulmonary edema, or acute lung injury, is classically associated with salicylates and opioids, whereas cardiogenic causes follow overdoses with negative inotropic agents like β-blockers and calcium channel β-blockers (Table 23–7).

Table 23–7. Pulmonary Toxicity

Asphyxiants	Irritants	Toxin-Induced Lung Injury
Nitrogen	Ammonia	Opioids
Carbon dioxide	Chlorine	Salicylates
Ethane	Chloramine	Lidocaine
Methane	Hydrogen chloride	Cocaine
Helium	Nitrogen dioxide	Irritant gases
Hydrogen	Sulfur dioxide	Amphetamines
Propane	Isocyanates	Amiodarone
	Phosphine	Carbon monoxide
	Phosgene	Bleomycin
		Paraquat

CARDIOVASCULAR

It is imperative that the clinician be familiar with the normal range of vital signs in children. Blood pressure and pulse readings that are considered hypotensive or tachycardic in adults may be within the acceptable range for a young pediatric patient. Misinterpretation of pediatric vital signs often results in overly aggressive management by clinicians more familiar with adult parameters. In many mixed adult–pediatric emergency department settings, the most commonly neglected pediatric vital sign parameter is an accurate blood pressure measurement, because an improper cuff size is used, or no blood pressure monitoring is instituted.

Toxins can inflict injury in the cardiovascular system by raising or lowering blood pressure, triggering pump failure, and inducing conduction disturbances and dysrhythmias. These effects are secondary to alterations occurring in arteriolar smooth muscle tone or from direct action on the myocardium and conduction system of the

Table 23–8. Toxin-Induced Blood Pressure Changes

Hypertension	Hypotension
Epinephrine	β-Adrenergic antagonists
Norepinephrine	Calcium channel antagonists
Dopamine	Cardiac glycosides (digoxin)
Ephedra	Ethanol
Immidazolines (oxymetazoline, tetrahydrozoline, naphazoline)	Agents causing volume depletion (methylxanthines, diuretics, salicylates, carbamates and organophosphates, castor beans, mushrooms, iron, arsenic)
Pseudophedrine	Central α₂-adrenergic agonists (clonidine, imidazolines, methyldopa)
Amphetamines	Peripheral α₁-adrenergic antagonists (prazosin)
Cocaine	Cyanide
Phencyclidine	Nitrates/nitrites
Nicotine	Theophylline
Corticosteroids	Cyclic antidepressants, sedative-hypnotics
Yohimbine	
Thyroid supplements	
Ergotamines	
MAOIs	

Abbreviation: MAOIs, monoamine oxidase inhibitors.

Table 23–9. Toxin-Related Changes in Heart Rate

Bradycardia	Tachycardia
α_1-Agonists (reflex)	α_1-Antagonists (reflex)
Central α_2-agonists (clonidine, methyldopa)	Sympathomimetics (cocaine, ephedra, amphetamines)
Antidysrhythmics	Methylxanthines
β-Antagonists	Salicylates
Calcium channel antagonists	Dihydropyridine class of calcium channel antagonists (nifedipine, amlodipine) (reflex)
Cholinergic agents (carbamates, organophosphates)	Carbon monoxide
Opioids	Iron
Baclofen	Phencyclidine
Ciguatera toxin	Theophylline
Digitalis, digoxin	Thyroxin
	Antihistamines
	Anticholinergics
	β-agonists (e.g., albuterol)

heart. Cocaine is an example of a poison causing multiple effects on the cardiovascular system. Cocaine induces cardiotoxicity by blocking fast sodium channels, much like tricyclic antidepressants, with resulting QRS widening predisposing the heart to dysrhythmias. In addition, cocaine directly causes vasoconstriction and initiates catecholamine reuptake inhibition resulting in hypertension and tachycardia. When toddlers inadvertently ingest calcium channel blockers or β-blockers, life-threatening bradycardia and hypotension can follow. In addition, exposure to sustained-release antihypertensives may not manifest signs or symptoms of toxicity until several hours after ingestion which necessitates extended observation and cardiac monitoring. Tables 23–8, 23–9, and 23–10 list agents with potential toxicity to various components of the cardiovascular system.

HEMATOLOGIC

Toxicogenetics play a large role in toxin-induced hematologic disorders. Poisons can lead to decreased formation or increased destruction of cells, and impaired coag-

Table 23–10. Cardiac Conduction Disturbances

Conduction Abnormalities	Cardiac Dysrhythmias
α₁-Antagonists	Carbamazepine
Antidysrhythmics	Chloral hydrate
β-Antagonists	Ciguatera toxin
Bupivacaine	Cocaine
Calcium channel antagonists	Ethanol
Carbamazepine	Heavy metals
Digoxin (cardiac glycosides)	Phenothiazines
Cyclobenzaprine	Halogenated hydrocarbons (inhalants/volatiles)
Tricyclic antidepressants	Propoxyphene
Phenothiazines	Tricyclic antidepressants
Propoxyphene	Methylxanthines
Arsenic	Antidysrhythmics (types IA, IC, III)
	Agents that increase QTc interval
	Scorpion venom

ulation or hemoglobin function. Lead is a classic cause of hematologic disruption that can occur in the pediatric patient. As a result of decreased hemoglobin synthesis and decreased erythrocyte longevity, lead poisoning results in anemia. The anticoagulant rodenticides (brodifacoum) can eventually result in a coagulopathy after a significant ingestion. Table 23–11 lists toxic agents affecting the hematologic system.

IMMUNOLOGIC

Toxins can cause immunologic injury by inducing immunosuppression, autoimmunity, immune-mediated hemolytic anemia, as well as hypersensitivity reactions. A common example of immunosuppression is that caused by carbamazepine. Initially, it produces hypogammaglobulinemia, which is followed by agranulocytosis (Tables 23–12, 23–13, and 23–14).

GASTROINTESTINAL

In addition to the GI tract, this section includes agents that can result in pancreatic toxicity. Emesis, the most

Table 23–11. Toxin-Associated Hematologic Poisoning

Agranulocytosis	Aplastic Anemia	Cellular Impairment	Immunosuppression
Antimicrobials (penicillins, cephalosporins, vancomycin, trimethoprim)	Antineoplastics	DDT	Carbamazepine
Phenothiazines	Arsenic, mercury, copper, cadmium	Chlordane	Corticosteroids
Antithyroid agents	Benzene	Lindane	Phenytoin
Analgesics (acetaminophen, ibuprofen)	Carbamazepine	Phencyclidine	Solvents
Carbamazepine	Phenytoin		
Chlorpropamide	Mercury		
Antipsychotics (e.g., clozapine)	Sulfonamides		
Tricyclic antidepressants	Phenylbutazone		
Sedative-hypnotics	Colchicine		
	Pesticides		
	Cimetidine		
	Penicillin		
	Acetaminophen, ibuprofen		
	Phenothiazines		

Table 23–12. Toxin-Induced Hemolysis

Immune Mediated	Nonimmune Mediated
Cephalosporins	Arsine gas (stibine)
Chlorpromazine	Copper
Insulin	Dapsone
Isoniazid	Lead
Penicillin	Venom (snake, spider)
Rifampin	Methylene blue
Sulfonylureas	Dimercaprol

Table 23–13. Toxin-Induced Thrombocytopenia

Decreased Production	Destruction/Consumption
Ethanol	Amrinone
Alkylating agents	Benzene
Antimetabolite agents	Carbamazepine
Thiazides	Cimetidine
Ionizing radiation	Colchicine
Vinblastine	Crotalid venom
	Glyburide
	Furosemide
	Penicillin
	Sulfonamides

basic form of GI toxicity, and often an excellent marker of toxicity, occurs after ingesting significant amounts of iron, mushrooms, and countless other poisons. In the pediatric patient, fluid losses from vomiting and diarrhea are more profound in relation to body weight when compared to adult patients, resulting in rapid dehydration.

Direct injury in the form of ulcers, strictures, and perforation occur after caustic ingestion (e.g., drain or toilet bowl cleaners). Alkali products produce liquefactive destruction to the esophagus, whereas strong acids induce coagulation necrosis in the stomach and duodenum. A notable exception to typical acid injuries is when hydrofluoric acid is consumed. It similarly affects the stomach; however, it is readily absorbed and often initiates significant systemic toxicity and death. See Tables 23–15, 23–16, and 23–17 for lists of poisons that injure the GI tract.

HEPATIC

Hepatic dysfunction is a common manifestation following a toxic exposure. Functionally, the liver's architecture is designed in such a way that geographic predisposition exists to particular patterns of injury depending on the poison. The acinus consists of the area structured concentrically around the portal triad (hepatic arteriole, portal venule, bile ductile). From here, blood flows through sinusoidal conduits progressively through zones 1 through 3 on its way to the terminal hepatic vein, or center of the liver lobule (Figure 23–1). Each anatomic zone is differentiated metabolically. Zone 1 cells receive blood with high oxygen concentration in addition to a considerable magnitude of poison. In light of this, an excess of oxygen free radicals produce injury such as occurs with iron poisoning. Zone 2 represents a transitional region. Zone 3 is a more hypoxic region that exhibits greater cytochrome P-450 activity. Acetaminophen is a classic example of a poison that causes injury in zone 3, better known as *centrilobular necrosis*. It has been documented that children suffer less acetaminophen-induced hepatotoxicity than adults. This may be due to smaller acute ingestions, less chronic toxicity, and the fact pediatric patients have a larger percentage of hepatic sulfonation, one of the pathways responsible for metabolizing acetaminophen in the liver. This results in less accumulation of the toxic metabolites responsible for hepatic failure in adults via the glucouronidation pathway. Other potential mechanisms of liver injury include steatosis, autoimmune, idiosyncratic, cholestatic, and venoocclusive (Table 23–18).

Table 23–14. Toxin-Induced Autoimmunity

SLE	Scleroderma	Thyroid Disease	Glomerulonephritis
Hydralazine	Anilines	Biphenyls (polychlorinated, polybrominated)	Mercury
Procainamide	Silica	Lithium	Cadmium
Phenytoin	Vinyl chloride	Amiodarone	Gold
Hydrazine		Radiation exposure	

Table 23–15. Oroespohageal Toxicity

Pain	Inflammation	Edema	Drooling	Dry	Dysphagia/ Odynophagia
Caustics	Caustics	Penicillin	Organophosphates	Botulism	Caustics
Paraquat	Metals	ACE inhibitors	Carbamates	Anticholinergics	Botulism
Ciguatera	Phenol	Caustics	Nicotine	Salicylates	Strychnine
Foreign bodies	Phenytoin	Oxalate-containing	Phencyclidine	Lithium	Tetrodotoxin
	Phosphorous	plants (*Diffenbachia*)	Ketamine	Colchicine	Paralytic shellfish
			Drug packets	Antipsychotics	poisoning
			Foreign bodies	Antidepressants	Foreign bodies
			Caustics		Concretions
					Mercuric salts
					Paraquat
					Diquat

Abbreviation: ACE, angiotensin-converting enzyme.

Table 23–16. Gastrointestinal Toxicity

Pain	Emesis	Hematemesis	Diarrhea	Constipation
Caustics	Caustics	Caustics	Caustics	Anticholinergic
Alcohols	Colchicine	Alcohols	Metals	(antihistamines)
Arsenic	Metals	(isopropanol)	Colchicine	Botulism
Iron	Mushrooms	Metals	Mushrooms	Opioids
Salicylates	Iron	Salicylates	Podophyllin	
NSAIDs	Salicylates	NSAIDs	Nicotine	
Colchicine	Nicotine	Anticoagulants	Theophylline	
Metallic salts	Solvents	Iron	Cholinergics	
Mushrooms	Opioids		Organophosphate	
Foreign body/	Methylxanthines		Arsenic	
drug packets	Acetaminophen		Laxatives	
	Syrup of ipecac			
	Cocaine			
	Amphetamines			
	Vitamin A			
	Theophylline			
	Thallium, arsenic			

Abbreviation: NSAIDs, nonsteroidal anti-inflammatory drugs.

Table 23–17. Toxin-Induced Pancreatitis

Alcohols
Acetaminophen
Opioids
Valproic acid
Diuretics
Corticosteroids
Estrogens
Organophosphates
Rifampin
Sulfonamides
Tetracycline
Methanol
Scorpion stings

RENAL

Because the kidneys receive up to 25% of cardiac output, they are particularly vulnerable to toxin-induced injury. An active role in filtering toxic substances and possession of their own intrinsic metabolic activity predispose these organs to dysfunction as a result of poison expo-sure. The majority of toxic renal injury can be classified as acute or chronic renal failure, or nephrotic syndrome. Nonsteroidal anti-inflammatory drugs are classic nephro-toxic agents that may cause prerenal injury, hypersensi-tivity vasculitis, acute interstitial nephritis, or nephrotic syndrome. Heavy metals like lead and arsenic are also capable of inducing several types of renal pathology (Table 23–19). Many toxins are capable of producing characteristic color changes to the urine (Table 23–20).

ENDOCRINE

Many agents affecting the endocrine system act to cause hypoglycemia (Table 23–21). Children have immature hepatic glycogen stores when compared to adult patients. As a result, children are more prone to hypoglycemia fol-lowing a toxic ingestion. Pediatric hypoglycemia is most common after ethanol exposure. Delayed hypoglycemia has occurred after the ingestion of sulfonylureas. Some pediatric patients suffer adverse effects from chronically ingesting glucocorticoids such as obesity, acne, alopecia, hypercholesterolemia, coronary artery disease, decreased height, and psychosis.

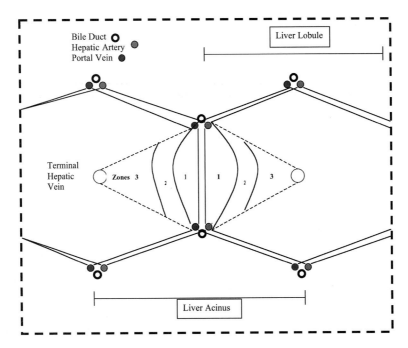

Fig. 23–1. Hepatic architecture. The hepatic lobule is organized around the terminal hepatic vein. Direction of blood flow origi-nates at the base of the acinus and is directed toward the terminal hepatic vein. As blood passes through hepatic sinusoids, it trav-erses across zones 1, 2, and finally 3, which corresponds to the centrilobular region.

Table 23–18. Toxin-Induced Liver Injury

Necrosis	Cholestasis	Steatosis	Tumors	Mitochondrial
Acetaminophen	Rifampin	Ethanol	Estrogens	Valproic acid
Carbon tetrachloride	Nitrofurantoin	Valproic acid	Anabolic steroids	Aflatoxin
Iron	Chlorpromazine	Tetracycline	Vinyl chloride	Hypoglycin
Isoniazid	Chlorpropamide	Corticosteroids	Arsenic	Tetracycline
Arsenic	Erythromycin	Amiodarone		
Phenytoin	Ampicillin	Salicylates		
Tetracycline	Barbiturates			
Cyclopeptide-containing	Naproxen			
mushrooms	Sulfonamides			
Ethanol				

Table 23–19. Toxin-Induced Renal Injury

Prerenal	Vasculitis	IN	NS	ATN	Obstruction
NSAIDs	Amphetamines	Penicillin	Metals (Au, Hg)	Metals (As, Cr, Hg)	Anticholinergics
Iron	Penicillins	Rifampin	NSAIDs	Aminoglycosides	Fluoroquinolones
Cathartics	Sulfonamides	Vancomycin	Heroin	Antineoplastics	Sulfonamides
Antihypertensives	NSAIDs	Sulfonamides	Cocaine	Glycols	Acyclovir
		NSAIDs	Captopril	Hydrocarbons	Ethylene glycol
		Metals (Pb, Cd, Be, Li)		Mushrooms	Chinese herbs

Abbreviation: ATN, acute tubular necrosis; IN, interstitial nephritis; NS, nephrotic syndrome; NSAIDs, nonsteroidal anti-inflammatory drugs.

Table 23–20. Toxin-Induced Urinary Color Change

Red	Yellow	Brown	Black	Blue-Green	Orange
Ibuprofen	Aloe	Iron	Melanin	Amitryptiline	Rifampin
Phenothiazines	Fava beans	Senna	Alcaptonuria	Chlorophyll	Phenazopyridine
Lead	Nitrofurantion	Methyldopa	Homogentisic acid	(breath mints)	Rhabdomyolysis
Phenytoin	Primaquine	Cascara		Indigo blue	Deferoxamine
Doxorubicin	Rhubarb	Phenylhydrazine		Methylene blue	
Beets	Sulfamethoxazole	Chloroquine		Magnesium salicylate	
Blackberries		Carbon tetrachloride		Copper sulfate	
Rhubarb					

Table 23–21. Toxin-Induced Hypoglycemia

Hypoglycin (unripe Ackee fruit)
β-Adrenergic antagonists
Cocaine
Ethanol
Hypoglycemic agents
Opioids
Salicylates
Sulfonamides
Valproic acid
Insulin

DERMATOLOGIC

Various cutaneous reaction patterns arise secondary to a number of agents (Table 23–22). These manifestations can aid the clinician in making diagnostic decisions or commonly can be anticipated after certain exposures. One example is the lobster-red discoloration of the skin after boric acid ingestion in children. Blanching of the finger pads may indicate hydrofluoric acid exposure if there is corresponding history of rust removal or brick cleaning.

CONCLUSION

Many agents induce toxicity in one or more organ systems. Discovering disease patterns in patients may lead the clinician to consider a toxicologic cause for the patient's dysfunction. Although this chapter is by no means comprehensive, its aim is to provide the clinician a framework and to organize the approach to the pediatric patient with organ system toxicity.

Table 23–22. Toxin-Induced Dermatotoxicity

Alopecia	EM	TEN	Photosensitivity	Vasculitis	Other
Thallium	Antibiotics	Bactrim	Ciprofloxacin	Cimetidine	Lobster skin: Boric acid
Anticoagulants	Barbiturates	Nitrofurantoin	Levofloxacin	NSAIDs	Cyanosis: Methemoglobinemia
Chemotherapeutic agents	Carbamazepine	NSAIDs	Naproxen	Penicillin	Slate-discoloration: silver, colloidal silver
Phenytoin	Cimetidine	Penicillin	Furosemide	Phenytoin	Necrotic ulcer: brown recluse envenomation
NSAIDs	Codeine	Phenytoin	Tetracyclines	Quinidine	Bullous lesions: Pit viper envenomation, phenobarbital
Retinoids	Furosemide	Sulfonamides			
Arsenic	NSAIDs				
Radiation	Phenothiazines				
Colchicine	Phenytoin				
	Sulfonamides				

Abbreviations: EM, erythema multiforme; NSAIDs, nonsteroidal anti-inflammatory drugs; TEN, toxic epidermal necrolysis.

SUGGESTED READINGS

Benowitz NL, Rosenberg J, Becker CE: Cardiopulmonary catastrophes in drug-overdosed patients. *Med Clin North Am* 63:127–140, 1979.

Bastuji-Garin S, Rzany B, Stern RS, et al: Clinical classification of cases of toxic epidermal necrolysis, Stevens-Johnson syndrome, and erythema multiforme. *Arch Dermatol* 129:92–96, 1993.

Burns FR, Paterson CA: Prompt irrigation of chemical eye injuries may avert severe damage. *Occup Health Saf* 58:33–36, 1989.

Clive DM, Stoff J: Renal syndromes associated with nonsteroidal anti-inflammatory drugs. *N Engl J Med* 310:563–572, 1984.

Cummins LH: Hypoglycemia and convulsions in children following alcohol ingestion. *J Pediatr* 58:23–26, 1961.

Evans P, Halliwel B: Free radicals and hearing. Cause, consequence, and criteria. *Ann NY Acad Sci* 884:19–40, 1999.

Glassroth J, Adams GD, Schnoll S: The impact of substance abuse on the respiratory system. *Chest* 91:596–602, 1987.

Goldfrank LR, Flomenbaum NE, Lewin NA, et al: *Goldfrank's Toxicologic Emergencies.* 7th ed. New York: McGraw-Hill; 2002.

Gorman RL, Khin-Maung-Gyi MT, Klein-Schwartz W, et al: Initial symptoms as predictors of esophageal injury in alkaline corrosive ingestions. *Am J Emerg Med* 10:189–194, 1992.

Haller JA, Andrews HG, White JJ, et al: Pathophysiology and management of acute corrosive burns of the esophagus: Results of treatment in 285 children. *J Pediatr Surg* 6:578–584, 1971.

Jimenzez-Jimenzez FJ, Garcia-Ruis PJ, Molina JA: Drug-induced movement disorders. *Drug Safety* 16:180–204, 1997.

Karpatkin S: Drug-induced thrombocytopenia. *Am J Med Sci* 262:68–78, 1971.

Kaufman DW, Kelly JP, Jurgelon JM, et al: Drugs in the aetiology of agranulocytosis and aplastic anemia. *Eur J Haematol Suppl* 60:23–30, 1996.

Koren G: The nephrotoxic potential of drugs and chemicals: pharmacologic basis and clinical relevance. *Med Toxicol* 4:59–72, 1989.

Lewis JH: Drug-induced liver disease. *Med Clin North Am* 84:1275–1311, 2000.

Riordan SM, Williams R: Fulminant hepatic failure. *Clin Liver Dis* 4:25–45, 2000.

24

Radiologic Findings

Steven E. Aks
Vivian Harris

The general management of the poisoned child relies primarily on the clinical manifestations and the known pharmacodynamic properties of the toxin ingested. There are, however, some situations where radiologic imaging can be of value in handling these cases. This chapter reviews the situations where one should consider imaging the poisoned child.

ABDOMINAL RADIOGRAPH

The plain abdominal radiograph is one of the most commonly ordered imaging studies in poisoned children. In reality, it is only clinically useful in a small proportion of ingestions. A frequently cited mnemonic for situations where an abdominal radiograph may be of value is CHIPES. This stands for:

- **C**hloral hydrate (and other halogenated hydrocarbons), **C**alcium
- **H**eavy metals
- **I**ron
- **P**henothiazines, **P**ackets (illicit drugs)
- **E**nteric-coated preparations
- **S**ustained-release preparations

Chloral hydrate is a radiopaque liquid; other highly halogenated hydrocarbons can also be seen on abdominal radiographs. Heavy metals such as lead can be seen after a child has ingested paint chips or other lead-containing foreign bodies (Figure 24–1). Lead glaze from ceramics is radiopaque. Lithium is an alkali metal that can also be radiopaque, particularly when ingested in the delayed-release formulation. Other heavy metals that may be seen on an abdominal radiograph include arsenic, bismuth, copper, mercury, and thallium. Bismuth in the form of bismuth subsalicylate can be seen on x-ray.

Iron tablets in prenatal concentrations can be detected on the abdominal radiograph (Figure 24–2). In iron poisoning, this finding can help to guide management with gastrointestinal (GI) decontamination using whole bowel irrigation (see Chapter 68). It is important to note that many pediatric vitamin supplements containing low doses

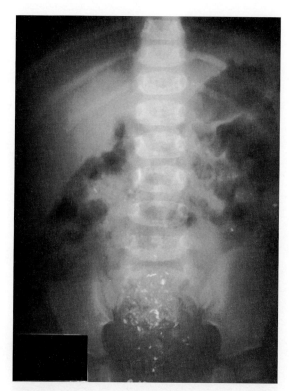

Fig. 24–1. Abdominal radiograph of a child with lead-containing paint chips visible throughout the intestinal tract.

of iron are not as strongly radiopaque as adult iron preparations. Figure 24–3 is an abdominal radiograph in a child who ate a broken thermometer. The elemental mercury from the thermometer is readily visualized throughout the GI tract, whereas the ingested glass is not.

Phenothiazines, although part of the CHIPES mnemonic, are not always visualized, and finding these tablets will generally not change management. Although both enteric-coated and sustained-release preparations have been stated to be radiopaque, this is an unusual finding, and obtaining radiographs for these preparations is generally not useful.

There are other notable findings on abdominal radiographs. Cocaine body packers may have demonstrable packets up to 80% of the time according the literature. A representative example of a body packer is seen in Figure 24–4. In contrast, cocaine body stuffers almost always have a negative abdominal radiographs. In one series by June and colleagues, no abdominal studies were positive. Figure 24–5 shows cecal infarction in a 16-year-old who

ingested cocaine orally. There is an obvious deformity of the cecum in this lower GI study.

Button batteries and cylindrical batteries are easily visualized on plain abdominal studies. Figure 24–6 shows the course of ingested cylindrical (AA) batteries transiting through the GI tract over 48 hours. See Chapter 67 for further discussion on the management of button battery ingestions.

Although not toxic, Figure 24-7 includes images of a large trichobezoar (hair mass) in an adolescent. The plain abdominal radiograph shows a mass in the area of the stomach. The upper GI with contrast shows a filling defect in the same area in the stomach, representing the large trichobezoar.

CHEST RADIOGRAPH

An important chest radiographic finding in pediatric toxicology is pneumonia after hydrocarbon aspiration.

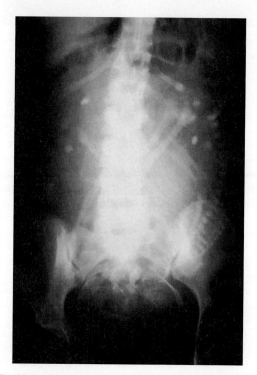

Fig. 24–2. Abdominal radiograph taken in a pregnant patient with iron poisoning.

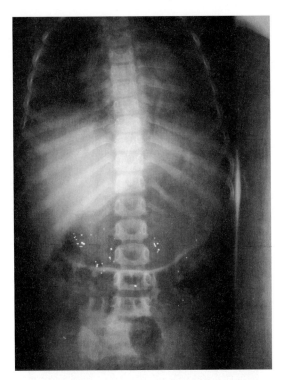

Fig. 24–3. Elemental mercury on abdominal radiograph after thermometer ingestion.

When low-viscosity, high-volatility hydrocarbons are ingested by children, there is a high risk for aspiration pneumonia. Initial findings can include a simple infiltrate, but can progress to large infiltrates, effusions, pneumatocoeles, and pulmonary collapse. The child pictured in Figure 24–8 ingested a hydrocarbon-containing furniture polish. The early chest radiograph shows bilateral lower lobe infiltrates with the right being more severe than the left. This child's condition worsened, and the child eventually died from pulmonary complications.

Several agents can lead to noncardiogenic pulmonary edema (NCPE) or acute lung injury. This will generally appear as diffuse vascular congestion in the absence of cardiomegaly. NCPE may be seen with salicylate toxicity, opioid toxicity, sedative-hypnotic, tricyclic antidepressant, and calcium channel blocker toxicity.

Smoking crack, marijuana, or other inhaled drugs of abuse can lead to pneumomediastinum and pneumothorax. Vigorous inhalation followed by a Valsalva-type maneuver can lead to pneumomediastinum. Figure 24–9 is an excellent example of pneumomediastinum in an 18-year-old after smoking crack. This patient complained of sharp chest and neck pain shortly after smoking.

EXTREMITY RADIOGRAPHS

Lead lines are among the most well-appreciated radiographic manifestations of toxicity. These lines appear in children at the growth plates, and are seen after lead poisoning. It is usually seen after chronic lead toxicity. The lines are due to arrest of the growth plate, and not to heavy metal deposition. Figure 24–9 clearly demonstrates lead lines in two different 3-year-old children. Another important finding on an extremity radiograph is retained bullets in joints or in areas of rapid bone growth. These sites are most highly associated with systemic absorption and the development of lead toxicity.

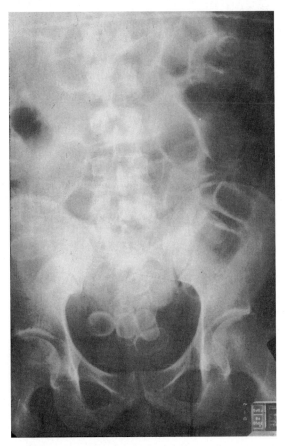

Fig. 24–4. Heroin body packer: note multiple radiopaque foreign bodies throughout the GI tract.

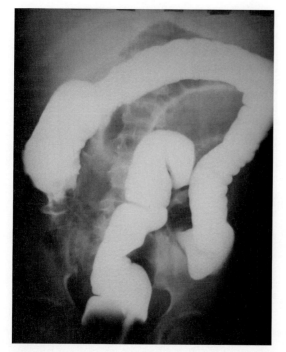

Fig. 24–5. Cecal infarction after cocaine ingestion in a 16-year-old.

Another relevant toxic finding on an extremity radiograph includes subcutaneous hydrocarbon injections. This can be seen after an attempt for abuse, or as a malicious administration. Heavy metals such as mercury have been injected in the subcutaneous tissues and intravenously. These can also appear radiopaque on extremity radiographs.

An unusual skeletal finding is seen with fetal alcohol syndrome. In addition to craniofacial abnormalities there can also be disturbances in bone growth as depicted in Figure 24–10. This radiograph demonstrates hypoplastic phalanges, which are also associated with fetal alcohol syndrome. Hypoplastic nails of the fingers or toes have also been described.

COMPUTED TOMOGRAPHY

Computed tomography (CT) of the head can be of value after various poisonings. After cocaine, amphetamine, or other sympathomimetics of abuse one can observe subarachnoid hemorrhage and ischemic and hemorrhagic strokes. Other poisonings such as carbon monoxide and cyanide can lead to CT findings of globus pallidus and basal ganglia lesions. Cyanide can cause similar findings. Late stages of chronic solvent abuse can lead to

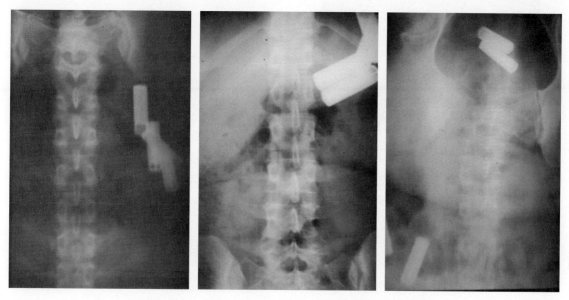

Fig. 24–6. Cylindrical (AA) batteries coursing through the GI tract.

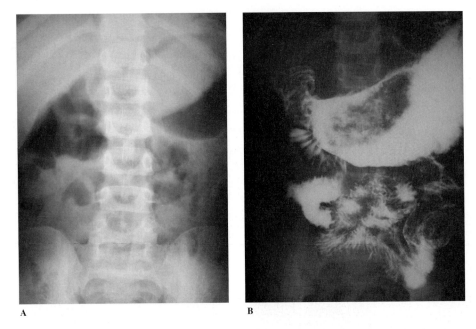

Fig. 24–7. Trichobezoar. **A.** Radiopacity in the stomach. **B.** In the contrast study, a filling defect is seen.

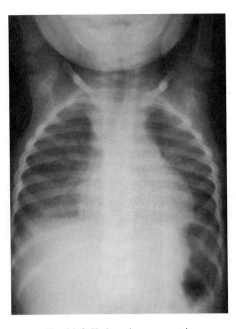

Fig. 24–8. Hydrocarbon pneumonia.

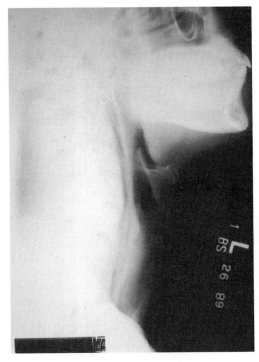

Fig. 24–9. Pneumomediastinum.

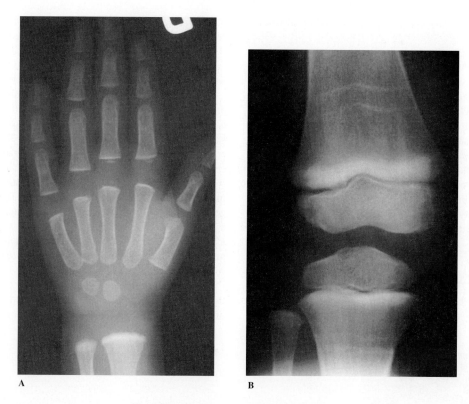

A   B

Fig. 24–10. Lead lines in two 3-year-old children.

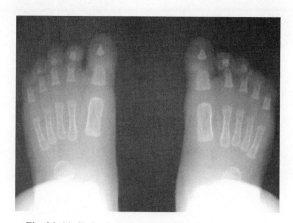

Fig. 24–11. Skeletal changes from fetal alcohol syndrome.

diffuse white matter hypodensity, a finding also seen with MRI.

CT imaging for body packers and stuffers can be a useful technique in a patient without a reliable history. For body packers with radiopaque packets on an abdominal radiograph, they can be followed with serial examinations. If the packets are not visualized, CT may be required. Most cases of body stuffers can be managed without radiographs. However, if the patient is unreliable, symptomatic, has signs of obstruction, or the number of packets ingested needs to be confirmed, then a CT of the abdomen and pelvis is indicated. There has been a false-negative result after CT without oral contrast administration reported. Therefore, using oral contrast with these studies is recommended.

MISCELLANEOUS TECHNIQUES

Ingested foreign bodies are beyond the scope of this chapter, but plain chest radiographs will pick up many of these items (coins, etc.). Occasionally, a contrast study is required to find such a foreign body.

Barium swallow studies are also useful after caustic ingestion to determine the extent of stricture formation, and to assess the viability of esophageal function. Figure 24–12A shows esophageal stricture formation in a 26-month-old after lye ingestion. These strictures can lead to delayed complications, which are demonstrated in Figures 24–12B and 12C. At age 3½, the child ingested a coin that became stuck in the esophagus. At age 10 the child ate meat that also became lodged in the esophagus. Figure 24–12C is a contrast study outlining the meat bolus. Perforation is a disastrous complication of caustic ingestion. Figure 24–13 is a lateral decubitus radiograph of a different child, who developed perforation and free air after an alkaline corrosive ingestion. See Chapter 48 for a detailed discussion of caustic ingestions and esophageal strictures.

Ultrasound has some limited role in the evaluation of the poisoned patient. Figure 24–14 demonstrates cerebral infarction in a neonate whose mother used cocaine

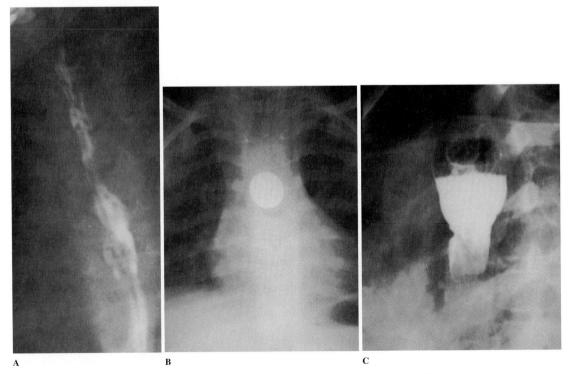

A **B** **C**

Fig. 24–12. A. Barium swallow demonstrating stricture formation in the esophagus of a 26 month-old. **B.** A coin lodged in the esophagus of the same patient, age 3½. **C.** A contrast study with an impacted meat bolus in the same patient aged 10 years.

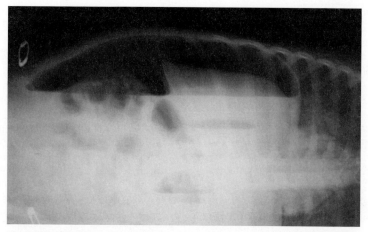

Fig. 24–13. Left lateral decubitus film demonstrating perforation (prominent free air) in a child who ingested a caustic agent.

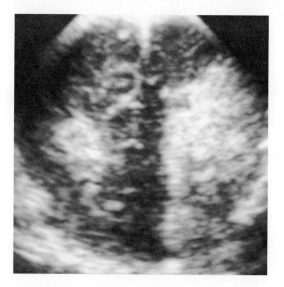

Fig. 24–14. Neonatal ultrasound demonstrating cerebral infarction after maternal cocaine use.

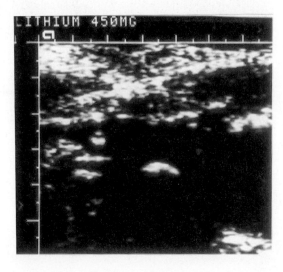

Fig. 24–15. Identification of one lithium tablet in a volunteer (T.B.E.) by ultrasound.

prior to delivery. Ultrasound is also a technique that is emerging in use at the bedside by emergency physicians. Ultrasound has been studies for body packers, and has not been found to be a reliable technique to identify body packets, except when they reside in the stomach. Its utility in the overdose patient has yet to be determined (Figure 24–15).

SUGGESTED READINGS

Amitai Y, Silver B, Leikin JB, et al: Visualization of ingested medications in the stomach by ultrasound. *Am J Emerg Med* 10:18–23, 1992.

Autti-Ramo I, Gaily E, Granstrom M-L: Dysmorphic features in offspring of alcoholic mothers. *Arch Dis Child* 67:712–716, 1992.

Eade NR, Taussig LM, Marks MI: Hydrocarbon pneumonitits. *Pediatr* 54:351–357, 1974.

Eng JG, Aks SE, Waldron R, et al: False-negative abdominal CT scan in a cocaine body stuffer. *Am J Emerg Med* 17:702–704, 1999.

June R, Aks, SE, Keys N, et al: Medical outcome of cocaine bodystuffers. *J Emerg Med* 18:221–224, 2000

Gordon RA, Roberts G, Amin Z, et al: Aggressive approach in the treatment of acute lead encephalopathy with an extraordinarily high concentration of lead. *Arch Pediatr Adolesc Med* 152:1100–1104, 1999.

Kaczorowski JM, Wax PM: Five days of whole-bowel irrigation in a case of pediatric iron ingestion. *Ann Emerg Med* 27:258–263, 1996.

Lang CJ: The use of neuroimaging techniques for clinical detection of neurotoxicity: A review. *Neurotoxicology* 5:847–855, 2000.

Maeder M, Ullmer E: Pneumomediastinum and bilateral pneumothorax as a complication of cocaine smoking. *Respiration* 70:407, 2003.

Marc B, Baud FJ, Aelion MJ, et al: The cocaine body-packer syndrome: Evaluation of a method of contrast study of the bowel. *J Forensic Sci* 35:345–355, 1990.

McCarron M, Wood JD: The cocaine "body packer" syndrome: Diagnosis and treatment. *JAMA* 250:1417–20, 1983.

Miura T, Mitomo M, Kawai R, et al: CT of the brain acute carbon monoxide intoxication: Characteristic features and prognosis. *AJNR* 6:739–742, 1985.

Reed CR, Glauser FL: Drug-induced noncardiogenic pulmonary edema. *Chest* 100:1120–1124, 1991.

Roberge RJ, Martin TG: Whole bowel irrigation in an acute oral lead intoxication. *Am J Emerg Med* 10:577–583, 1992.

Savitt DL, Hawkins HH, Roberts JR: The radiopacity of ingested medications. *Ann Emerg Med* 16:331–339, 1987.

Soo YO, Wong CH, Griffith JF, et al: Subcutaneous injection of metallic mercury. *Hum Exp Toxicol* 6:345–348, 2003.

Tillman DJ, Ruggles DL, Leikin JB: Radiopacity study of extended-release formulations using digitalized radiography. *Am J Emerg Med* 12:310–314, 1994.

25

Lethal Toxins in Small Doses

Leon Gussow

CASE PRESENTATION

A 2-year-old 10-kg boy was brought to the emergency department after becoming lethargic at home. Two hours before, he had developed ataxia. On arrival the child was afebrile, with pulse 136/min. On examination, he was lethargic and sweating. Also noted were increased salivation with drooling, muscle rigidity, torticollis, and nystagmus. The parents mentioned that 1 hour before symptom onset the child was seen playing with an open bottle of clozapine, and that one 100-mg tablet was not accounted for.

INTRODUCTION

Fortunately, the overwhelming majority of toxic exposures in young children are not life threatening. For example, using data from 2002, the Toxic Exposure Surveillance System of the American Association of Poison Control Centers reported nearly 540,000 exposures in children less than 2 years of age, but only 11 fatalities. In addition, most medications that cause serious consequences in toddlers do so only after ingestion of clearly excessive amounts. Because so many accidental pediatric toxic exposures turn out to be innocuous, it is easy for the healthcare provider to become complacent about these cases, especially if by history the child ingested only 1 unit dose of a medication. However, there are a number of prescription and over-the-counter preparations that can cause extreme toxicity, even fatality, in a toddler after ingestion of a single dose. Familiarity with these agents is essential for the practitioner.

This chapter reviews these highly toxic medications. It will not discuss nonmedicinal agents such as hydrocarbons, acetonitrile, caustics, methanol, selenious acid, or environmental toxins that can also be extremely toxic in small amounts. Additionally, this is not an exhaustive discussion of all agents. For example some drugs, such as β-blockers, calcium channel blockers, phenothiazines, and theophylline, are not discussed, but the reader should include these agents in the same lethal category.

For purposes of definition, a *toddler* is a 10-kg child around 2 years of age. At this age, children have developed the motor skills, curiosity, and exploratory behavior that can lead them to sample and taste anything within reach. A *single dose* is considered one tablet, capsule, or swallow of the most potent formulation available as listed in the 2002 *Physicians' Desk Reference*. The average volume of a swallow in children between 2 and 4 years old is 4.5 cc of liquid (0.2 mL/kg) or approximately 1 teaspoon.

BENZOCAINE AND OTHER LOCAL ANESTHETICS

Benzocaine is found in many local anesthetic preparations, including first aid ointments and infant teething formulas. Baby Oragel and Anbesol baby teething gel each contain 7.5% benzocaine, Baby Oragel Nighttime Formula 10%, and Americaine Hemorrhoidal Ointment 20%. Exposure can result from ingestion or dermal absorption. Benzocaine is metabolized to aniline and nitrosobenzene, both of which can cause methemoglobinemia. Infants younger than 4 months are at increased risk because they are deficient in methemoglobin reductase. Methemoglobinemia has occurred in an infant after ingestion of 100 mg of benzocaine, the amount in one-quarter teaspoon of Baby Oragel. Infants have also developed methemoglobinemia from EMLA cream (lidocaine/prilocaine) used topically for analgesia during circumcision.

Onset of toxicity occurs 30 minutes to 6 hours after ingestion, with tachycardia, tachypnea, and a characteristic cyanosis that does not respond to oxygen. In more severe exposures, agitation, hypoxia, metabolic acidosis, lethargy, stupor, and coma may supervene. Seizures can occur.

Because many local anesthetics act by blocking sodium channels in conductive tissue, they can also cause life-threatening cardiac toxicity. Effects on conduction include decreased velocity and slowed ventricular depolarization, leading to ventricular dysrhythmias. Hypotension may result from vasodilatation, myocardial

depression, or dysrhythmias. Dayan and colleagues described three deaths in toddlers who ingested dibucaine ointment or cream. In all three cases, cardiovascular collapse was preceded by seizure activity.

Treatment of toxicity consists of gastric emptying, general support, and administration of antidote if indicated. Induced emesis is contraindicated. The effect of gastric aspiration or lavage on clinical outcome is unknown. Administering a single dose of activated charcoal can be considered. Seizures can be treated with benzodiazepines and phenobarbital.

The antidote for patients with methemoglobinemia is methylene blue. Indications for use include symptoms of respiratory distress or altered mental status, or methemoglobin levels >30%. The methylene dose is 1 to 2 mg/kg IV over 5 minutes. Isolated cyanosis is not an indication for methylene blue, because it often occurs at low methemoglobin levels, is usually well tolerated, and resolves spontaneously. Further discussion of methylene blue therapy is presented in Chapter 74.

CAMPHOR

Camphor can be found in many over-the-counter liniments and cold preparations. Since 1983, the Food and Drug Administration has required that medical products sold in the United States contain less than 11% camphor. Campho-Phenique is 10.8% camphor, Ben-Gay Children's Rub 5%, and Vicks Vaporub 4.18%. A common source of severe toxicity in the past had been camphorated oil, a 20% preparation that was sometimes mistaken for castor oil and administered to children in high doses. Fortunately, this product is no longer available (Figure 25–1).

Camphor is an aromatic cyclic terpene with a ketone group. It has a strong, distinctive odor and a pungent taste that some find appealing. It is highly lipophilic and is a rapidly acting neurotoxin, producing both neurologic excitation and depression. As little as 1 g has been reported to cause death in an 18-month-old child. Major toxicity has not been reported for ingestions <30 mg/kg and is rare in ingestions <50 mg/kg.

Initial clinical symptoms, beginning 5 to 120 minutes after ingestion, include gastrointestinal (GI) discomfort and agitation. Generalized seizure activity may be preceded by muscle twitching and fasciculation, or may occur suddenly without warning signs. The epileptogenic potential of camphor was demonstrated in 1919 by a researcher who administered camphorated oil at a dose of 3.0 to 4.5 g to 20 children between 1 and 4 years of age. All the children developed symptoms and most developed seizures.

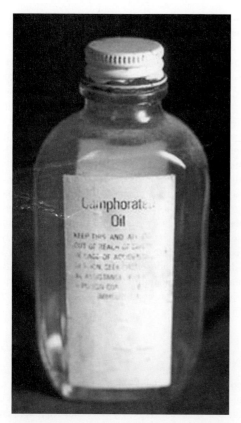

Fig. 25–1. A common source of severe toxicity in the past had been camphorated oil, a 20% preparation that was sometimes mistaken for castor oil and administered to children in high doses. Fortunately, this product is no longer available.

The key to managing serious camphor ingestion is good supportive care. The use of gastric lavage or aspiration in this setting has not been studied, but because camphor is rapidly absorbed it is not likely to be beneficial. Activated charcoal generally does not adsorb hydrocarbons well. Ipecac is never indicated. Seizures not responsive to benzodiazepines can be treated with phenobarbital. Asymptomatic patients should be observed for 6 hours after ingestion prior to discharge from the emergency department.

CHLOROQUINE

Chloroquine has been used since the 1940s for the treatment and prevention of malaria. Additional uses cur-

rently include the treatment of extraintestinal amebiasis and some connective tissue autoimmune diseases. Recently chloroquine has been mentioned in books describing suicide methods. The drug is available in tablets containing 300 mg of chloroquine base. It is a powerful rapidly acting cardiotoxin capable of causing sudden cardiorespiratory collapse. The interval between ingestion and cardiac arrest is often less than 2 hours. Even a small amount can be life threatening in a toddler; Kelly and associates reported the death of an 8-kg girl after ingestion of a single 300-mg chloroquine tablet.

Chloroquine causes myocardial depression and vasodilatation, producing sudden profound hypotension. Automaticity and conductivity of heart muscle is also decreased, resulting in bardycardia and ventricular escape rhythms. The electrocardiogram can show sinus bradycardia, widened QRS complexes, T-wave changes, ST depression, prolonged QT intervals, complete heart block, ventricular tachycardia, or ventricular fibrillation. Neurotoxicity induced by chloroquine often presents as drowsiness and lethargy, followed by excitability. Dysphagia, tremor, hyporeflexia, seizures, and coma can occur.

The physician treating chloroquine toxicity should be prepared to manage sudden cardiac or respiratory arrest. Intubation, ventilation, defibrillation, and cardiac pacing may be required. Blood pressure is maintained with intravenous fluids and pressors. Class IA antiarrhythmics (quinidine, procainamide, disopyramide) are contraindicated. Gastric lavage can be considered if the patient presents within 1 hour of ingestion and the airway is not compromised. Activated charcoal (1 g/kg) can be given by mouth or via orogastric tube. As with theophylline toxicity, hypokalemia can occur because of ion transport into cells. Aggressive repletion of potassium in this setting has in some cases led to severe hyperkalemia. Recent evidence suggests that early mechanical ventilation with high-dose diazepam and epinephrine may be life-saving in severe cases of chloroquine toxicity in adults. However, this therapy has not been well described in the pediatric population.

CLOZAPINE

Clozapine (Clozaril) is an atypical antipsychotic agent used in the management of severe schizophrenia unresponsive to standard therapy. It is considered atypical because it has only weak antidopamine activity, minimizing the risk for dystonic side effects. Additional pharmacologic actions of clozapine include catecholamine blockade and prominent anticholinergic effects. Indications for clozapine use are restricted because with chronic therapy it has a significant risk of causing agranulocytosis. Clozapine should not be confused with the similarly named drug clonazepam (Klonopin), a benzodiazepine anxiolytic, or the antihypertensive medication clonidine.

Signs and symptoms of clozapine overdose seen in reported adult cases include hyperthermia, tachycardia, sedation, seizures, and death. Although experience with unintentional pediatric clozapine overdose is limited, Mady and colleagues described three pediatric clozapine ingestions. The oldest child was a 4-year-old 21-kg girl who ingested a single 100-mg tablet. These children presented variously with lethargy, mydriasis, truncal ataxia, confusion, tachycardia, and unresponsiveness. Motor effects were variable, including both hypotonia and muscular rigidity. Although clozapine has a strong anticholinergic effect, two of the three children in this case series displayed markedly increased salivation with drooling. All three patients recovered normal neurologic status within 24 to 48 hours.

There have been no studies specifically addressing the treatment of clozapine overdose in either adults or children. In addition to aggressive symptomatic and supportive care, Mady and co-workers recommend administering multiple doses of activated charcoal, without citing evidence that it improves clinical outcome or enhances clearance of the drug. In one of the children they describe, treatment with diphenhydramine partially resolved muscular rigidity. However, because clozapine itself has anticholinergic activity, they recommend that this antidote be used judiciously. Clozapine is rapidly absorbed after oral administration. Asymptomatic children who may have ingested clozapine should be observed for 6 hours.

IMIDAZOLINE DECONGESTANTS

Imidazoline decongestants are found in a wide variety of over-the-counter nasal sprays and eye drops. Examples include tetrahydrozoline (Visine), naphazoline (Naphcon), and oxymetazoline (Afrin). Significant toxicity with hypotension, lethargy, and respiratory depression requiring intubation has been reported in a toddler after ingestion of half a teaspoon of Visine eye drops.

Imidazolines are α-2 adrenergic agonists. When applied topically to the nasal mucosa or into the eye, their peripheral α-2 activity produces vasoconstriction. However, after ingestion, these liphophilic agents rapidly enter the central nervous system (CNS) and reduce sympathetic outflow from the vasomotor center, causing hypo-

tension, bradycardia, miosis, CNS depression, and respiratory depression. These opioid-like effects are similar to those caused by the antihypertensive drug clonidine, also an α-2 agonist. Because of the interplay between the central and peripheral actions of the imidazolines, overdose can present with a changing clinical picture. Bradycardia can alternate with tachycardia, hypotension with hypertension, and lethargy with agitation. Hypoglycemia and hypothermia have been reported.

Onset of symptoms is generally within 4 hours of ingestion, with resolution by 24 to 48 hours. Because these products are rapidly absorbed from the GI tract, it is unlikely that aspiration of stomach contents through a nasogastric tube would improve clinical outcome. Inducing emesis with syrup of ipecac is contraindicated. A single dose of activated charcoal can be given but is unlikely to be beneficial. As with clonidine toxicity (see Chapter 35), imidazoline-induced CNS depression may be responsive to naloxone administration. Clinically significant bradycardia can be treated with atropine. Asymptomatic children should be observed for 6 hours.

LINDANE

Lindane is an organochloride insecticide, available as a 1% solution or shampoo for the treatment of scabies and pediculosis. Pediatric toxicity can occur from accidental ingestion or because the child's caregiver does not understand that the medication is for topical use only. Ingestion of lindane causes nausea and vomiting, and either CNS depression or CNS excitation with seizure activity. The key to treating these exposures involves good decontamination and supportive care. Decontamination of the skin, if needed, can be accomplished by irrigating with copious amounts of water. The role of GI decontamination with either aspiration of stomach contents or administration of activated charcoal has not been studied, but there is no reason to think that either of these interventions would improve clinical outcome. Seizures can be treated with benzodiazepines and, if needed, phenobarbital. Phenytoin should be avoided, because in an animal model it increased seizure activity.

LOMOTIL

Lomotil is an antidiarrheal preparation that combines an opioid (diphenoxylate) with an anticholinergic (atropine). Several unique properties make Lomotil poisoning extremely dangerous in the pediatric population. Respiratory depression can occur as late as 24 hours after ingestion, and there appears to be no correlation between the dose ingested and clinical severity. Therefore, any child with known or suspected ingestion of any amount of Lomotil should be admitted and monitored for at least 24 hours, regardless of the initial clinical condition.

Each tablet or 5 mL of liquid Lomotil contains 2.5 mg diphenoxylate hydrochloride and 0.025 mg atropine sulfate. Difenoxine is the major metabolite of diphenoxylate and is both more active and longer acting (half-life, 12 to 24 hours) than its parent drug. This metabolite is probably responsible for the delayed or recurrent respiratory depression often seen in these overdoses.

Ingestions of ½ to 2 tablets have been reported to cause toxic signs and symptoms. Both atropine and diphenoxylate may be rapidly absorbed from the GI tract, but because both drugs delay gastric emptying intact tablets have been recovered from the stomach as long as 27 hours after ingestion.

Although patients often present with a confusing mix of opioid and anticholinergic signs and symptoms, opioid effects are usually seen in overdose and often predominate. Anticholinergic manifestations can occur with varying consistency. Initial presentation of Lomotil overdose in children can include drowsiness or agitation, dyspnea, irritability, miosis, hypotonia or rigidity, and urinary retention. In severe cases the patient may present with coma, respiratory depression, hypoxia, or seizures. Symptoms may not be related to the dose ingested, and can occur as late as 24 hours after ingestion. Death is often accompanied by cerebral edema.

Treatment of Lomotil poisoning includes admission of all patients and careful monitoring for a minimum of 24 hours, with naloxone present at the beside. Syrup of ipecac is contraindicated. In patients with CNS or respiratory depression and a secure airway, gastric lavage may remove some of the medication, even if hours have passed since ingestion. However, there is no literature demonstrating that lavage improves clinical outcome, or that it adds benefit to the administration of activated charcoal alone. If there are bowel sounds, multiple-dose activated charcoal is recommended, because difenoxine undergoes enterohepatic recycling. A cathartic may be given with the first dose of activated charcoal, but is not repeated with subsequent doses. A Foley catheter may be needed to relieve urinary retention. Excessive hydration should be avoided to minimize the risk of cerebral edema. Respiratory depression is treated with intravenous naloxone (0.1 mg/kg), which may have to be repeated frequently. A maintenance dose of naloxone can be given, starting with two-thirds of the bolus dose that initially produced the desired response. This maintenance dose is infused each hour and titrated to clinical condition. When naloxone is given, anticholinergic symptoms may emerge.

METHYL SALICYLATE

Methyl salicylate is a concentrated liquid that is absorbed quickly and can produce early-onset severe salicylate toxicity. It is found in many topical liniments (Ben Gay, Icy Hot Balm). Oil of wintergreen contains 98% methyl salicylate. One teaspoon of oil of wintergreen contains 7 g of salicylate (equivalent to twenty-one 325-mg aspirin tablets). Because ingestion of <1 teaspoon has killed a child, any ingestion of these preparations is potentially serious. Clinical presentation and treatment of this overdose is similar to that of other types of salicylate poisoning (see Chapter 30).

QUININE

Quinine is an alkaloid isolated from the bark of the cinchona tree, which grows in the Amazon rain forest. It has been used to treat malaria since the 1600s. Other therapeutic indications include treatment of nocturnal recumbency leg cramps and babesiosis. It is also used illegally as an abortifacient and as a narcotic adulterant. Quinine is an optical isomer of the Class IA anti-arrhythmic drug quinidine, and shares many of its cardiovascular effects.

Although the medical literature is nearly devoid of descriptions of pediatric quinine overdose, there apparently exists a report of the death of a child after ingestion of 1 g. Quinine is available in a maximum unit dose of 325-mg capsule. The minimal potential fatal dose noted by Koren is 80 mg/kg, but the basis for this figure is not well referenced.

In adults, symptoms of toxicity begin within 3 to 4 hours after ingestion. These initial symptoms are grouped under the toxidrome *cinchonism*, and include nausea, vomiting, diarrhea, tinnitus, hearing loss, dermal flushing, sweating, and headache. In severe ingestions, toxic effects on the heart, CNS, and eye occur. Manifestations of cardiotoxicity include myocardial depression and conduction delays. The ECG can show increased PR, QT, and QRS intervals, as well as ST- and T-wave changes. Ventricular dysrhythmias may occur and result in cardiac arrest. Quinine, like quinidine, is an α-adrenergic blocker and can cause vasodilatation and hypotension. Other possible causes of hypotension in quinine overdose include fluid depletion from vomiting and diarrhea, myocardial depression, and dysrhythmias. In most cases, cardiac toxicity becomes apparent in the first 8 hours after ingestion.

CNS toxicity from quinine includes ataxia, vertigo, syncope, and mental status changes. Coma and seizures occur rarely. The most unusual and dramatic manifestation of quinine toxicity involves the drug's effect on the retina. Along with methanol, it should be considered in the differential diagnosis of bilateral blindness possibly related to a toxin. In adults, visual manifestations start with blurred vision and progress to color changes, visual field defects, and blindness. The onset of these changes is typically delayed up to 6 hours after the initial signs and symptoms of cinchonism. Characteristically the pupils are fixed and dilated, which may be a diagnostic clue in the preverbal child. The retinal exam will be normal when visual changes begin; within the subsequent days, arteriolar narrowing, macular edema, and optic nerve atrophy can be seen. Although it had once been postulated that these retinal effects might be caused by arterial constriction and retinal ischemia, it is now thought that they result from a direct toxic effect of the drug on the retina.

Effective management of quinine toxicity requires careful cardiac monitoring and supportive care. Hypoxia, acidosis, and electrolyte abnormalities should be corrected to minimize occurrence of cardiac dysrhythmias. Repeated doses of activated charcoal, if tolerated, may decrease the half-life of quinine. Other methods of GI decontamination are generally not indicated, because quinine is rapidly absorbed and significant toxicity usually causes profuse vomiting. Hypotension can be treated with fluids, boluses of sodium bicarbonate, and pressors. Slowed ventricular conduction, as manifested by a prolonged QRS interval on the electrocardiogram, is an indication for serum alkalinization with sodium bicarbonate. Although these is no proven treatment for quinine-induced ocular toxicity, in most cases the visual deficits reverse at least partially over time.

TRICYCLIC ANTIDEPRESSANTS

Tricyclic antidepressants, although less used now than in the past, are still prescribed and still cause severe toxicity. The toxic dose is 10 to 20 mg/kg. Because both amitriptyline and desipramine are available in a maximum unit dose of 150 mg, even a single pill can be toxic to a 10-kg toddler. The presentation and treatment of tricyclic antidepressant toxicity are discussed in Chapter 43.

CASE OUTCOME

The child was given 10 g of activated charcoal and admitted to the intensive care unit. The urine drug screen was negative. The use of diphenhydramine to treat muscle rigidity was discussed but ultimately withheld because symptoms seemed to be resolving and there was concern about exacerbating the anticholinergic effects of clozapine. The child improved and was discharged from hospital the next day.

SUGGESTED READINGS

Aks SE, Krantz A, Hryhorczuk DO, et al: Acute accidental lindane ingestion in toddlers. *Ann Emerg Med* 26:647–651, 1995.

Clemessy JL, Favier C, Borron SW, et al: Hypokalaemia related to acute chloroquine ingestion. *Lancet* 346:877–880, 1995.

Collee GG, Samra GS, Hanson GC: Chloroquine poisoning: Ventricular fibrillation following 'trivial' overdose in a child. *Intensive Care Med* 18:170–171, 1992.

Couper RT. Methemoglobinemia secondary to topical lignocain/prilocaine in a circumcised neonate. *J Pediatr Child Health* 36:406, 2000.

Curtis JA, Goel KM: Lomotil poisoning in children. *Arch Dis Child* 54:222–225, 1979.

Cutler EA, Barrett GA, Craven PW, et al: Delayed cardiopulmonary arrest after Lomotil ingestion. *Pediatrics* 65:157–158, 1980.

Dayan PS, Litovitz TL, Crouch BI, et al: Fatal accidental dibucaine poisoning in children. *Ann Emerg Med* 28:442–445, 1996.

Emery D, Singer JI: Highly toxic ingestions for toddlers: When a pill can kill. *Pediatr Emerg Med Reports* 3:111–122, 1998.

Emery DP, Corban JG: Camphor toxicity. *J Paediatr Child Health* 35:105–106, 1993.

Gouin S, Patel H: Unusual cause of seizure. *Pediatr Emerg Care* 12:298, 1996.

Higgins GL, Campbell B, Wallace K, et al: Pediatric poisoning from over-the-counter imidazoline-containing products. *Ann Emerg Med* 20:655–658, 1991.

Holmes JF, Berman DA: Use of naloxone to reverse symptomatic tetrahydrozoline overdose in a child. *Pediatric Emerg Care* 15:193–194, 1999.

Jones DV, Work CE: Volume of a swallow. *Am J Dis Child* 102:427, 1964.

Kelly JC, Wasserman GS, Bernard WD, et al: Chloroquine poisoning in a child. *Ann Emerg Med* 19:47–50, 1990.

Klein-Schwartz W, Gorman R, Oderda GM, et al: Central nervous system depression from ingestion of nonprescription eyedrops. *Am J Emerg Med* 2:217–218, 1984.

Koren G: Medications which can kill a toddler with one tablet or teaspoonful. *Clin Toxicol* 31:407–413, 1993.

Liebelt EL, Shannon MW: Small doses, big problems: A selected review of highly toxic common medications. *Pediatr Emerg Care* 9:292–297, 1993.

McCarron MM, Challoner KR, Thompson GA: Diphenoxylate-atropine (Lomotil) overdose in children: an update (report of eight cases and review of the literature). *Pediatrics* 87:694–700, 1991.

Mady S, Wax P, Wang D, et al: Pediatric clozapine intoxication. *Am J Emerg Med* 14:462–463, 1996.

Mahieu LM, Rooman RP, Goossens E: Imidazoline intoxication in children. *Eur J Pediatr* 152:944–946, 1993.

Phelan WJ: Camphor poisoning: Over-the-counter dangers. *Pediatrics* 57:428–430, 1976.

Potter JL, Hillman JV: Benzocaine-induced methemoglobinemia. *JACEP* 8:26–27, 1979.

Prescott LF, Hamilton AR, Heyworth R: Treatment of quinine overdosage with repeated oral charcoal. *Br J Clin Pharmacol* 27:95–97, 1989.

Riou B, Barriot P, Rimailho A, et al: Treatment of severe chloroquine poisoning. *N Engl J Med* 318:1–6, 1988.

Rumack BH, Temple AR: Lomotil® poisoning. *Pediatrics* 53:495–500, 1974.

Segel E, Wason S: Camphor toxicity. *Pediatr Clin North Am* 33:375–379, 1986.

Smilkstein MJ, Kulig KW, Rumack BH: Acute toxic blindness: Unrecognized quinine poisoning. *Ann Emerg Med* 16:98–101, 1987.

Tobias JD: Central nervous system depression following accidental ingestion of Visine eye drops. *Clin Pediatr* 35:539–540, 1996.

Townes PL, Geertsma MA, White MR: Benzocaine-induced methemoglobinemia. *Am J Dis Child* 131:697–698, 1977.

Wolf LR, Otten EJ, Spadafora MP: Cinchonism: Two case reports and review of acute quinine toxicity and treatment. *J Emerg Med* 10:295–301, 1992.

Wolowich WR, Hadley CM, Kelley MT, et al: Plasma salicylate from methyl salicylate cream compared to oil of wintergreen. *J Toxicol Clin Toxicol* 41:355–358, 2003.

26

Nontoxic Exposures

Sage W. Wiener
Robert S. Hoffman

CASE PRESENTATION

A worried mother calls after her 3-year-old boy is found playing with an open container of glue. The mother says that she can see some of the glue in and around the child's mouth. The boy is alert, playful, interactive, and without complaints. She estimates that less than 1 ounce is missing from the 4-ounce container, and confirms that no other products were found near the child. The mother identifies the product as Elmer's Glue-All. The package states that the product is nontoxic, and was manufactured in 2002 by Elmer's Products, Inc.

INTRODUCTION AND EPIDEMIOLOGY

Paracelsus, the father of toxicology, stated in his *Third Defense*, "What is there that is not poison? All things are poison and nothing [is] without poison. Solely, the dose determines that a thing is not a poison" (see Chapter 1). Although this remains true today, there are many products that are of such low toxicity that all reasonably possible exposures are unlikely to cause significant harm. The ability to identify these exposures can reassure anxious parents and caregivers, prevent unnecessary emergency department visits, and conserve limited health care resources.

Poison Center Data

In 2001, Poison Control Centers in the United States received almost 1.5 million calls for pediatric exposures (age <20 years), representing 66% of all exposures. Almost one quarter of these pediatric cases were not followed up by the poison specialist because the exposure was considered nontoxic. An additional quarter were followed and found to produce no ill effects. About 90% of calls for children under 12 years old were managed on site. This likely reflects the fact that unintentional pediatric exposures tend to involve small ingestions of single products through hand-to-mouth behavior. Thus, although children tend to have more exposures than their adult counterparts, their exposures are more often nontoxic. In one study, 64% of children seen in the emergency department for acute poisoning required no care. Unfortunately, 95% of these patients or their parents had not contacted their local poison center. These cases represent missed opportunities to intervene and prevent unnecessary emergency visits.

CRITERIA FOR NONTOXIC EXPOSURES

In 1984, Mofenson and Greensher proposed a set of criteria for identifying nontoxic ingestions that have been widely adopted with minor modifications. Most sources consider all of the following criteria necessary for an exposure to be considered nontoxic:

1. Identification of the product and its ingredients with absolute certainty
2. Absence of the signal words *caution, warning,* or *DANGER* on the container
3. Unintentional exposure, with no evidence of suicidality, abuse, or neglect
4. Exposure to a single product only
5. A reliable assessment of the dose
6. A reliable assessment of the route of exposure
7. A completely asymptomatic patient
8. Follow-up care must be available and a reliable adult must be available for telephone follow-up

These criteria have never been prospectively validated and were not developed specifically for children, but they represent a reasonable, conservative approach to the nontoxic exposure and have been accepted for 20 years. We now examine each of the criteria in depth, with specific attention to their application to a pediatric population.

IDENTIFICATION

History, POISINDEX, and Poison Centers

Products and their ingredients must be identified with reasonable certainty if an exposure is to be considered nontoxic. This identification must start with a thorough history. Important elements include the brand name of the product including the exact spelling, the ingredients and their quantities, as well as the manufacturer, the date of manufacture, and any telephone contact number listed on the packaging. People sometimes store household products for years, and contact with a manufacturer may reveal a significant change in a product's formulation, making current POISINDEX data not applicable. The

product also must be in its original container for accurate identification. Numerous cases of caustic ingestions are caused by household cleaning products stored in soft drink containers. Although absolute identification is preferable, the intended use of the product may be sufficient if *no* product in this generic category poses any significant risk, such as children's chewable multivitamin tablets without iron.

The regional poison center should be contacted to assist in product identification, rather than relying on history and use of the POISINDEX database alone. Although the POISINDEX database is a valuable resource, the experience of the poison specialist can shed light on otherwise confusing cases. Patients may later develop symptoms in ingestions initially thought to be nontoxic, and early involvement of the poison center can help identify medication errors, misidentification of a product, or patterns of possible product tampering.

Plants

Plants are very commonly implicated in pediatric exposures, and rank sixth in overall frequency reported to poison centers in 2001. Although only 525 of approximately 300,000 identified plants are suspected of being poisonous to humans, identification of these potentially toxic plants is difficult (see Chapter 80). Because most plant exposures result in minimal toxicity, asymptomatic children exposed to unknown plants can be managed at home with close follow-up. For symptomatic children, if parents do not know the common or scientific names of the plant to which the child was exposed, the child should have a medical evaluation and possible gastrointestinal decontamination. Parents should bring the plant, or clippings from it, to the emergency department to aid in identification.

SIGNAL WORDS

The Federal Hazardous Substance Labeling Act of 1960 required labeling of certain products with the signal words *caution, warning,* or *danger*. In 1972, The Consumer Product Safety Act created the Consumer Product Safety Commission, which has instituted the same labeling rules for many household products. Patients who are exposed to products labeled with any of these words have a potentially toxic exposure, and should be evaluated at a health care facility. Absence of these words on a package, although reassuring, does not guarantee the benign nature of its contents.

INTENTION

Pediatric exposures can generally be categorized by the age and developmental stage of the child. Histories that deviate from these categories should raise the suspicion of intentional poisoning or abuse. Any history consistent with a suicide attempt or possible abuse or neglect excludes a nontoxic ingestion because the history is unreliable. These scenarios should prompt a medical evaluation in a health care facility.

Infants

Children under 6 months of age are rarely exposed to poisons, except through medication errors. Without a clear history of this type of exposure, intentional poisoning must be considered, and the ingestion should not be classified as nontoxic.

Toddlers

Toddlers, aged 1 to 3 years, are at the peak age for pediatric poisoning. Children at this stage of development are becoming mobile, have the ability to pick up objects, and are inquisitive about their environment. They tend to explore their environment by putting things in their mouths. All of these factors put them at great risk for toxic exposures. Fortunately, most of these encounters are benign. Among all age groups, these children have the lowest fatality rate and the highest rate of nontoxic exposures.

Children and Adolescents

It is much less common for children above the age of 5 to have unintentional exposures, and adolescent exposures should be assumed to be intentional unless there is a very clear history to the contrary. Whereas 99.4% of exposures in children under 6 years old are unintentional, 45.7% of exposures in adolescents age 13 to 19 are reported as intentional. Intentional exposures may involve experimentation by ingestion or inhalation of household products in attempts to get high or suicide attempts and gestures.

SINGLE PRODUCT

There is a general concern that products that are nontoxic by themselves might cause toxicity when combined, thus exhibiting a synergistic effect. However, ingestion of two clearly nontoxic products does not automatically constitute toxicity. A more important concern in pediatric exposures relates to the intent behind them. Ingestion of multiple agents raises the concern of suicidal intention in an adolescent, and of abuse or neglect in the younger child. For these reasons, these children should be evaluated in a health care facility, even if the exposure is unlikely to cause toxicity, unless there is a reasonable explanation of the circumstances. An example would be a child found chewing on a pencil and a crayon from an open art supply kit.

DOSE

It must be possible to reliably determine the dose of an exposure for it to be considered nontoxic.

Worst-Case Scenario Approach

For some products such as acetaminophen and salicylates, the dose–response curve for toxicity is so well established that potential toxicity may be excluded if the dose can be accurately determined. A safe approach to these cases is to assume a worst-case scenario of the dose. For example, a child is found with an open bottle of liquid medication, some of which is spilled on the face, clothes and floor, and some of which is ingested. The maximal possible dose that the child could have ingested can be estimated from the volume remaining in the bottle. Although this may overestimate the possible dose, if the calculated amount falls below the minimum toxic dose, the chance for toxicity is extremely low, and the ingestion may be considered nontoxic. These determinations should be made in conjunction with the regional poison control center, which can assist with the subtleties of a given case.

Swallowing Volume

Sometimes, children will be observed to take one gulp or one sip of a product before the parent is able to intervene. Although it can be difficult to accurately assess these exposures quantitatively, some estimate a child's swallowing volume as 0.21 mL/kg. It is important to remember that this is only an estimate based on water, and may not apply to fluids with different physical properties, such as high viscosity, or a bad taste. This gross approximation should not be solely relied upon to exclude a toxic exposure and should never replace the worst-case scenario approach.

ROUTE

Some products are relatively innocuous by one route of exposure, but are toxic by a different route. For example, cyanoacrylate ingestion or dermal exposure is relatively benign, whereas exposure to the eyes should prompt medical evaluation. Similarly, many household cleaning products that have minimal toxicity when ingested can be devastating if aspirated. An accurate and detailed history about the route or routes of exposure is essential to clarify these cases.

SYMPTOMS

Because symptoms are clinical manifestations of toxicity, exposures cannot be considered nontoxic when symptoms are present. This may be a semantic distinction in many cases, because there are many *minimally toxic* products that predictably cause minor symptoms. Patients with minor symptoms that are expected from a particular agent can be managed at home despite the fact that they are not technically nontoxic. For example, vomiting and diarrhea would be expected after an ingestion of hand dishwashing soap, but would not necessitate an emergency department visit unless they persisted. This approach is supported by American Association of Poison Control Centers data showing lack of subsequent problems when these cases are managed at home.

FOLLOW-UP

A basic assumption in any decision to manage an exposure at home is the presence of a responsible adult and the ability to contact that adult for follow-up. If there are any doubts about the ability and willingness of the responsible adult to monitor the child's condition, or to comprehend instructions and communicate with the physician or poison center for follow-up, the child should be brought to a health care facility. At follow-up, it should be confirmed that the child has remained asymptomatic or has experienced limited predictable toxicity. Information about what should prompt another call to the physician or poison center should be reinforced. Finally, the responsible adult should be educated about poisoning prevention and safety.

MANAGEMENT

Disposition and Follow-up

When it is determined that a nontoxic or minimally toxic exposure has occurred, there is a responsible adult pres-

ent, and there is no concern of abuse, neglect, or suicidal intent, the patient can be safely managed at home, with follow-up by the physician or poison center. It is important to remember that products initially believed to be nontoxic may sometimes contain toxic contaminants due to manufacturing errors or product tampering, and errors in identification occur. Furthermore, products generally considered nontoxic may later be discovered to cause unrecognized toxicity. Follow-up of these cases permits prompt identification of these problems and public health intervention when appropriate.

Prevention

Up to 30% of children who have one episode of ingestion will subsequently repeat this behavior. The most important intervention for the patient with a nontoxic or minimally toxic exposure is to educate parents about poisoning prevention. Parents should also be encouraged to ask the child's primary care physician for poisoning prevention information at the follow-up visit.

CASE OUTCOME

The label does not contain the words *CAUTION, WARNING,* or *DANGER.* The mother is offered reassurance and instructed to continue to observe the child at home, and to bring the child to the emergency department if any symptoms develop. A telephone contact number is obtained for follow-up. The poison control center is contacted to report the exposure.

The poison control center calls the mother to follow up about 1 hour later and finds that the child remains asymptomatic. The mother is educated about poisoning prevention and advised to schedule a follow-up visit for her child with his pediatrician. Because no delayed toxicity is expected, subsequent follow-up calls are not made. A phone sticker with the poison center number is mailed to the home.

SUGGESTED READINGS

Bizovi KE, Smilkstein MJ: Acetaminophen. In: Goldfrank LR, Flomenbaum NE, Lewin NA, et al, eds: *Goldfrank's Toxicologic Emergencies.* 7th ed. New York: McGraw-Hill; 2002:480–501.
Centers for Disease Control: Update: Childhood poisoning—United States. *MMWR* 34:117–118, 1985.
Chafee-Bahamon C, Lovejoy FH: Effectiveness of a regional poison center in reducing excess emergency room visits for children's poisonings. *Pediatrics* 72:164–169, 1983.

Deichmann WB, Henschler D, Holmstedt B, et al: What is there that is not poison? A study of the Third Defense by Paracelsus. *Arch Toxicol* 58:207–213, 1986.

Fine JS: Pediatric principles. In: Goldfrank LR, Flomenbaum NE, Lewin NA, et al, eds: *Goldfrank's Toxicologic Emergencies.* 7th ed. New York: McGraw-Hill; 2002:1629–1639.

Gaudreault P, McCormick MA, Lacouture PG, et al: Poison exposures and use of ipecac in children less than 1 year old. *Ann Emerg Med* 15:808–810, 1986.

Jones DV, Work CE: Volume of a swallow. *Am J Dis Child* 203:427, 1966.

Litovitz TL, Flagler SL, Manoguerra AS, et al: Recurrent poisoning among pediatric poisoning victims. *Med Toxicol Adverse Drug Exp* 4:381–386, 1989.

Litovitz TL, Klein-Schwartz W, Rogers GC, et al: 2001 annual report of the American Association of Poison Control Centers Toxic Exposure Surveillance System. *Am J Emerg Med* 20:391–453, 2002.

Mofenson HC, Greensher J, Caraccio TR: Ingestions considered nontoxic. *Emerg Med Clin North Am* 2:159–174, 1984.

Mofenson HC, Greensher J, Caraccio TR: Ingestions considered nontoxic. *Clin Lab Med* 4:587–602, 1984.

Mofenson HC, Greensher J: The nontoxic ingestion. *Pediatr Clin North Am* 17:583–590, 1970.

Peterson RG, Rumack BH: Toxicity of acetaminophen overdose. *JACEP* 7:202–205, 1978.

U.S. Consumer Product Safety Commission Homepage. Available from URL: http://www.cpsc.gov. Accessed March 9, 2003.

Weisman R: Principles and techniques to identify the nontoxic exposure. In: Goldfrank LR, Flomenbaum NE, Lewin NA, et al, eds: *Goldfrank's Toxicologic Emergencies.* 7th ed. New York: McGraw-Hill; 2002:40–43.

27
Over-the-Counter Medications

Stacey Bangh

HIGH-YIELD FACTS

- Toxicity can occur with regular use of an OTC medication if administered in the wrong dose, or if combination products containing the same ingredients are given over an extended period of time.

- Cold medications, vitamins, acetaminophen, ibuprofen, and diaper rash products account for the majority of OTC medication exposures in children <6 years old.

- Intertional abuse of OTC cold medications by adolescents has been increasing over the last few years, especially in substances containing dextromethorphan.

- Some of the medications with the most potential to cause toxicity are found in topical preparations, such as wart removers, muscle rubs, teething gels, and chest rubifacients.

Over-the-counter (OTC) medications are widely available and often used in children. An estimated 50% of American children are given an OTC medication each month. Although it is commonly thought that OTC medications are nontoxic because they do not require a prescription, in reality OTC medications can be toxic under a variety of circumstances. A child gaining access to a bottle and ingesting the medication inside is the most common scenario resulting in toxicity. Toxicity can also occur with regular use of an OTC medication if administered in the wrong dose, or if combination products containing the same ingredient are given, over an extended period of time.

The Poison Prevention Packaging Act of 1970 (PPPA) was enacted to prevent young children from accidentally ingesting hazardous substances, including OTC medications, by requiring that these substances be packaged in such as way that it would be difficult for children less than 5 years to open them. This child-resistant packaging is not child proof, and children can still gain access to the product. There is also an exemption to the PPPA, which allows manufacturers the option of marketing one size of their product in non–child-resistant packaging.

EPIDEMIOLOGY

Cold medications, vitamins, acetaminophen, ibuprofen and diaper rash products account for the majority of OTC medication exposures in children less than 6 years old. The majority of these cases are handled outside of a health care facility, and very few actually result in substantial toxicity (Table 27–1).

DEVELOPMENTAL CONSIDERATIONS

Most medications intended for children are colored and flavored. Grape-, cherry-, orange-, and bubble gum-flavored medications are common. Parents may persuade children to take medication by calling it *candy,* which can lead to inadvertent ingestion of a potentially toxic substance. Last, children may ingest medication to imitate adult behavior.

MOST COMMON TOXINS

The five most common categories of OTC medications ingested by children less than 6 years old in 2001 were

Table 27–1. Common OTC Medication Ingestions in Children <6 Years Old

Medication	Exposures (*n*)	Treated in HCF (%)	Major Effects (%)[a]
Cold medications	64,781	14	0.01
Vitamins	39,396	7	0.00
Acetaminophen	37,132	15	0.03
Ibuprofen	31,802	7	0.00
Diaper rash products	27,646	1	0.00
Antacids	17,800	2	0.01
Diphenhydramine (OTC)	9,524	18	0.02
Methyl salicylate	7,556	9	0.00
Camphor	6,987	11	0.07
Aspirin	3,837	12	0.05
Wart preparations	1,038	10	0.00

[a]Major effects include symptoms that were life threatening or resulted in significant residual disability or disfigurement, such as repeated seizures, cardiovascular instability, and patients who required intubation and mechanical ventilation

Abbreviations: HCF, health care facility; OTC, over the counter.

cold medications, diaper rash ointment, ibuprofen, vitamins, and acetaminophen.

Cold Medications

Cold medications often contain a combination of ingredients. Ingestion by children can cause various symptoms, depending on the ingredients (Table 27–2). Intentional abuse of OTC cold medications by adolescents has been increasing over the last few years, especially in substances containing dextromethorphan. Teens taking dextromethorphan for its psychotropic effects may not realize they are at risk for toxicity from other ingredients.

Diaper Rash Ointment

Although it is not inherently toxic, ingestion of diaper rash ointment is very common; there are over 40,000 exposures per year. Most products contain either zinc oxide or vitamin A or D in an ointment base. Large ingestions of these products may produce gastrointestinal (GI) upset, but serious toxicity is not likely. Many of the calls to poison control centers are prompted by the warning on the back of the tube which states, "In case of accidental ingestion contact poison control immediately," which may lead parents to believe that serious toxicity will occur. No treatment is generally necessary for these exposures.

Ibuprofen

There are many formulations of ibuprofen available, including adult and pediatric formulations. Fortunately, it takes a relatively large amount ingested before toxicity occurs (>200 mg/kg) and the most common effects are GI upset. Severe effects such as apnea, metabolic acidosis, and acute renal failure are rare but may occur in very large ingestions (see Chapter 31).

Table 27–2. Common Ingredients in OTC Cold Medications and Clinical Effects Associated With Overdose

Category	Drug	Clinical Effects
Analgesic	Acetaminophen	Nausea, vomiting, hepatotoxicity
	Ibuprofen	Abdominal pain, nausea, vomiting
Cough suppressant	Dextromethorphan	Drowsiness, ataxia, hyperexcitability, toxic psychosis
Antihistamine	Diphenhydramine	Drowsiness, anticholinergic effects, nausea, vomiting
	Chlorpheniramine	
	Brompheniramine	
Decongestant	Pseudoephedrine	Tachycardia, hypertension, agitation, tremor, vomiting

Abbreviation: OTC, over the counter.

Vitamins

Over 30,000 children ingest multivitamins each year; the majority ingesting pediatric formulations. The primary concern in an acute ingestion is the iron; most children's multivitamins contain between 3 and 18 mg whereas adult preparations may contain up to 65 mg, especially prenatal vitamins. In chronic overdose, vitamins A and D cause the most severe toxicity (see Chapter 33).

Acetaminophen

Despite the very low incidence of toxic effects, acetaminophen toxicity remains a concern because of its wide use in children. Cases of hepatotoxicity owing to acetaminophen are more often associated with dosing errors than a child merely getting into a container and ingesting the medication themselves. In one study, children younger than 10 were at greatest risk of acetaminophen overdose owing to incorrect measuring device or concentration of product used. Adolescents, on the other hand, tend to underestimate the potential toxicity of many OTC medications, including acetaminophen. Risk factors contributing to toxicity include multiple overdoses, delayed referral and therapy, as well as concomitant ingestion of enzyme-inducing drugs, which increase the toxic acetaminophen metabolite (see Chapter 28).

MOST DANGEROUS TOXINS

Topical Medications

Some of the medications with the most potential to cause toxicity are found in topical preparations. These include wart removers, muscle rubs, teething gels, and chest rubifacients. Wart removers and muscle rubs contain potent forms of salicylate, salicylic acid and methyl salicylate respectively. A teaspoon of either of these products has the potential to cause salicylate toxicity in a small child (see Chapter 30).

Teething gels contain benzocaine. Although children with accidental exposure to OTC benzocaine-containing products rarely develop significant toxicity, methemoglobinemia has occurred with oral or rectal administra-tion of as low as 100 mg (¼ teaspoonful of 7.5% gel) in infants under 1 year, and with ½ teaspoonful in older children (see Chapter 74).

Chest rubs for colds such as Vicks Vaporub contain camphor. Camphor is a volatile, aromatic compound that is rapidly absorbed following ingestions and is highly toxic. Death can occur from respiratory depression or complications of seizures, although acute camphor poisoning secondary to ingestion of a "taste" or small amount is unlikely (see Chapter 50).

SUGGESTED READINGS

Baker SD, Borys DJ: A possible trend suggesting increased abuse from coricidin exposures reported to the Texas Poison Network: Comparing 1998 to 1999. *Vet Human Toxicol* 44:169–171, 2002.

Banerji S, Anderson IB: Abuse of Coricidin HBP Cough & Cold tablets: Episodes recorded by a poison center. *Am J Health Sys Pharm* 58:1811–1814, 2001.

Chan TY: Medicated oils and severe salicylate poisoning: Quantifying the risk based on methyl salicylate content and bottle size. *Vet Human Toxicol* 38:133–134, 1996.

Gunn VL, Taha SH, Liebelt EL, et al: Toxicity of over-the-counter cold medications. *Pediatrics* 108:e52–62, 2001.

Heubi JE, Barbacci MB, Zimmerman HJ: Therapeutic misadventures with acetaminophen: Hepatotoxicity after multiple doses in children. *J Pediatr* 132:22–27, 1998.

Huott MA, Storrow AB: A survey of adolescents' knowledge regarding toxicity of over-the-counter medications. *Acad Emerg Med* 4:214–218, 1997.

Litovitz TL, Klein-Schwartz W, Rodgers GC, et al: 2001 annual report of the American Association of Poison Control Centers Toxic Exposure Surveillance System. *Am J Emerg Med* 20:391–452, 2002.

Litovitz TL, Klein-Schwartz W, Caravati EM, et al: 1998 pediatric exposures. Report extracted from the 1998 Annual Report of the American Association of Poison Control Centers Toxic Exposure Surveillance System. *Am J Emerg Med* 17:435–487, 1999.

Rivera-Penera T, Gugid R, Davis J, et al: Outcome of acetaminophen overdose in pediatric patients and factors contributing to hepatotoxicity. *J Pediatr* 130:300–304, 1997.

Wolowich WR, Hadley CM, Kelley MT, et al: Plasma salicylate from methyl salicylate cream compared to oil of wintergreen. *J Clin Toxicol* 41:355–358, 2003.

28

Acetaminophen

Leon Gussow
Kenneth Bizovi

HIGH-YIELD FACTS

- Owing to wide availability in both prescription and OTC preparations, acetaminophen is a leading cause of pediatric poisoning.

- Acetaminophen toxicity is a potentially preventable cause of hepatic failure.

- *N*-acetylcysteine (NAC) is the antidote for acetaminophen overdose.

- NAC should be utilized in any case of acetaminophen-induced hepatotoxicity, regardless of the time elapsed since ingestion.

- Starting therapy with NAC does not absolutely commit the patient to a full course of 17 doses.

CASE PRESENTATION

A 15-year-old girl is brought to the hospital by her parents 6 hours after ingesting forty 500-mg acetaminophen tablets (Figure 28–1). She vomited once shortly before arrival. On questioning, the patient says that she had just broken up with her boyfriend but did not really know why she ingested the medicine. She denies suicidal ideation or any other ingestion. Her medical history is negative. Physical examination is unremarkable except for slight epigastric tenderness. Serum electrolytes, liver enzymes, and complete blood count are all normal. A urine drug screen and a pregnancy test are negative. A serum acetaminophen level is sent, but the results will not be back for 8 hours. The patient is given an oral load-ing dose of NAC, 140 mg/kg mixed with juice, but promptly vomits. The dose is repeated and retained after treatment with metoclopramide, 10 mg intravenously (IV), as an anti-emetic. She is admitted to the pediatric service with suicide precautions. Psychiatric consultation is ordered for the next day.

EPIDEMIOLOGY

In 2002, 62,881 cases of acetaminophen ingestion in patients younger than 19 years of age were reported to poison control centers in the United States. Despite the large number of reports, only five deaths occurred, all in adolescents, the majority of whom also ingested other drugs. Although *N*-acetylcysteine (NAC) is a very effective antidote for acetaminophen overdose if given early, initial signs and symptoms of toxicity are nonspecific, and the therapeutic window in which treatment is completely effective may be missed unless acetaminophen levels are routinely obtained when any drug ingestion is suspected. Delayed presentation and delayed treatment increase the risk for hepatocellular injury. Factors associated with acetaminophen overdose in children include parental misunderstanding of dosing and measurement instructions, concomitant use of multiple products containing acetaminophen, and use of adult or extended-release preparations instead of pediatric products. Young children are more likely to be administered liquid acetaminophen preparations, which are absorbed more rapidly than pills, or rectal suppositories, which have prolonged and unpredictable absorption. Adolescents often are not aware that acetaminophen ingestion can be lethal, and may unknowingly take a life-threatening amount as a suicidal gesture.

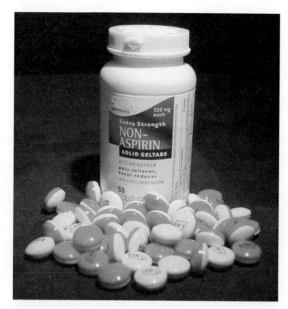

Fig. 28–1. Generic acetaminophen is widely available in many over the counter products including pain relievers, fever reducers, as well as cough and cold medications.

AGE AND DEVELOPMENTAL CONSIDERATIONS

Young children have a low incidence of hepatotoxocity after acetaminophen exposure, a phenomenon that may be due to early presentation after ingestion, an increased rate of spontaneous vomiting, or differences in drug metabolism compared to adults. In a 1984 study of 417 cases of acetaminophen overdose in children 5 years of age or younger, Rumack found that the rate of hepatotoxicity (serum glutamic-oxaloacetic transaminases [SGOT] >1000 IU/L) in patients with acetaminophen levels in the probably hepatic toxicity range on the Rumack-Matthew nomogram was more than five times less than that of adolescents and adults with similar levels (5.5% versus 29%). In 1994, Bond and associates were able to find only one reported death resulting from acute (single-dose) ingestion of acetaminophen in a child 6 years of age or less. The metabolism of acetaminophen in children changes as they age, with the major hepatic conjugation pathway switching from sulfonation to glucuronidation at some point between the ages of 9 and 12 years. The clinical implication of this change has not yet been determined. Laboratory studies have shown that young animals synthesize glutathione at a much higher rate than do older animals. Because glutathione is the primary detoxifier of *n*-acetyl-*p*-benzoquinoneimine (NAPQI, the metabolite of acetaminophen that causes liver damage), this observation may partially explain the young child's relative resistance to acetaminophen-induced hepatotoxicity.

PHARMACOLOGY AND TOXOKINETICS

Acetaminophen (also called APAP or paracetamol) is a synthetic analgesic and antipyretic that lacks the anti-inflammatory effects found in salicylates and nonsteroidal agents. Clinical effects are most likely mediated by inhibition of prostaglandin synthesis.

The therapeutic dose of APAP in children is 15 mg/kg given every 4 to 6 hours, with a maximum recommended daily dose of 75 mg/kg (or five doses). Therapeutic serum levels are 5 to 20 μg/mL. Acetaminophen is well absorbed after an oral therapeutic dose, with peak levels generally occurring at 30 to 60 minutes. However, after overdose the peak level may be delayed for up to 4 hours. Absorption of liquid elixir is more rapid than that of tablets or caplets. Following gastrointestinal absorption, APAP is taken up by the liver, where tissue concentrations are high. Serum half-life is 1 to 3 hours after a therapeutic dose, but may be prolonged significantly following hepatotoxic ingestion.

Volume of distribution is 1 L/kg, with plasma protein binding approximately 50%. Acetaminophen is eliminated primarily by hepatic pathways. After a therapeutic dose, 90% of the drug is metabolized to inactive sulfate and glucuronide conjugates. In young children, unlike in adults and adolescents, the sulfate conjugate predominates. Less than 5% is excreted unchanged in the urine. Two to 4% is metabolized by the cytochrome-P450–mixed-function-oxidase (MFO) system to the toxic intermediate NAPQI. In the presence of adequate hepatic stores of glutathione, NAPQI is rapidly converted to nontoxic mercapturic acid and cysteine conjugates. In the overdose setting, the sulfate and glucuronide pathways become saturated, and increased amounts of acetaminophen are shunted through the P450–MFO system. Glutathione becomes depleted and free NAPQI forms covalent bonds with structures on the hepatocytes. Necrosis ensues, distributed in a centrilobular fashion corresponding to the area of greatest MFO activity.

Acetaminophen can be toxic to organs other than the liver. Local metabolism to a toxic metabolite in the kidney can rarely cause proximal tubular necrosis and renal failure, even if the liver is relatively unaffected. Pancreatitis can also occur, particularly when severe hepatic necrosis is present. Such nonhepatic manifestations, however, are virtually never seen in children. Susceptibility to acetaminophen-induced hepatotoxicity may vary significantly among individuals, but the approach outlined for acute acetaminophen exposure has a margin of safety that is adequate to compensate for this variability. Acute ingestion of more than 140 mg/kg of acetaminophen establishes potential risk for acetaminophen-induced hepatic injury and requires emergent evaluation.

It is important to remember that acetaminophen is found in many combination products. For example, if a patient comes in comatose after taking a codeine–acetaminophen preparation, the clinician should not neglect to measure an acetaminophen level, and begin treatment if indicated. It is essential not to overlook this aspect of the case while dealing with the more evident and dramatic opioid effects.

CLINICAL PRESENTATION: THE FOUR STATES OF ACETAMINOPHEN TOXICITY

Stage 1 (0 to 24 hours): Gastrointestinal Irritation

Patients may be asymptomatic, but young children frequently vomit after acetaminophen overdose. In massive overdose or in children on chronic therapy with medications that induce specific cytochrone P450 enzymes, an anion gap metabolic acidosis can rarely occur within hours of ingestion. Enzyme-inducing medications include isoniazid, rifampin, and carbamazepine.

Stage 2 (24 to 48 hours): Latent Period

As nausea and vomiting resolve, patients appear to improve, but rising transaminase levels reveal evidence of hepatic necrosis. On physical examination, hepatic tenderness and enlargement may be apparent.

Stage 3 (72 to 96 hours): Hepatic Failure

Severe hepatotoxicity presents with jaundice, hypoglycemia, renewed nausea and vomiting, right upper quadrant pain, coagulopathy, encephalopathy, hyperbilirubinemia, and markedly elevated transaminase levels. In this stage, APAP-induced hepatotoxicity is usually accompanied by an SGOT > 1000 IU/L. In fulminant hepatic failure, the SGOT can rise to levels of 20,000 or 30,000 IU/L. It is very unusual, but not unprecedented, for children younger than 6 to develop fulminant effects from acute APAP ingestion.

Stage 4 (4 to 14 days): Recovery or Death

Patients who ultimately recover show improvement in laboratory parameters of hepatic function starting at about day 5, and eventually recover completely. Follow-up histology is normal. Other patients show progressive encephalopathy, renal failure, bleeding diatheses, and hyperammonemia. They have a high fatality rate unless liver transplant is performed.

LABORATORY AND DIAGNOSTIC TESTING

An acetaminophen level is drawn 4 hours after an acute ingestion, or immediately if more than 4 hours have elapsed since the ingestion. Levels drawn earlier than 4 hours may not represent the peak serum concentration and thus may be misleadingly low. In cases where the acetaminophen level is above the possible toxicity line on the nomogram, additional laboratory tests that influence management or indicate prognosis include liver enzymes, amylase, bilirubin, electrolytes, creatinine, and prothrombin time.

MANAGEMENT

Gastrointestinal Decontamination

Induction of emesis with syrup of ipecac is contraindicated in known or suspected acetaminophen ingestion. Aside from being relatively ineffective as a method of gastric emptying, it delays administration of NAC. Gastric lavage is generally not indicated but can be considered if the patient presents within 1 hour of ingestion *and* has taken a life-threatening overdose of another drug or drugs in addition to acetaminophen. Standard doses of activated charcoal can be given if patients arrive within 1 hour of ingesting acetaminophen alone, or if other toxic substances are also involved.

Antidote

A glutathione precursor, NAC restores the liver's ability to detoxify NAPQI and prevents hepatonecrosis (Figure 28–2). It is most effective if started within 8 hours after an acute overdose. However, there is now good evidence that NAC has some benefit even if started very late, possibly even up to days after ingestion when hepatic failure has already ensued. It should not be withheld on the basis of an arbitrary time limit.

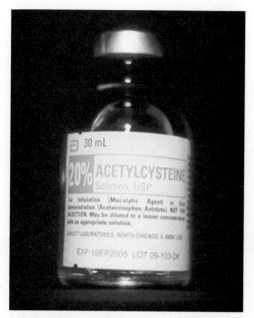

Fig. 28–2. NAC is most effective if started within 8 hours after an acute acetaminophen overdose.

The Rumack-Matthew nomogram indicates which patients require treatment with NAC following an acute ingestion at a known time (Figure 28–3). It was devised using data from a relatively small number of adult patients, but is also applied to children. The original studies indicated that 60% of patients whose levels are above the probable toxicity line after single acute APAP overdose will go on to develop severe hepatotoxicity (serum transaminases > 1000 IU/L). The lower possible toxicity line was added to give a margin of safety. Any patient with a level that falls in the range of possible or probable hepatotoxicity is treated with NAC. Frequent repeat APAP levels are unnecessary, and do not change management. In cases where the patient has not taken a single acute overdose, but rather has taken multiple doses or overdoses of APAP, or has ingested APAP chronically, the nomogram cannot be used to predict hepatotoxicity. Note that the risk line on the nomogram starts at 4 hours. Although after a therapeutic oral dose APAP is rapidly absorbed and achieves peak level within 30 minutes to 1 hour in most patients, the nomogram requires a level drawn at >4 hours, because absorption and time to peak level can be delayed after massive overdose. Recently, based on a computer pharmacokinetic model, Anderson and associates suggested that with children aged 1 to 5

years, a 2-hour level >225 mg/L is a reliable indicator of possible toxicity. The safety and effectiveness of this suggestion has not been tested in a prospective clinical study.

If the time of ingestion is unknown, treatment is started for any detectable level of acetaminophen, or any elevation of aspartate aminotransferase (AST) or alanine aminotransferase (ALT). Patients with normal liver function tests and undetectable acetaminophen levels do not require treatment. Patients chronically on medication that induces the P450 system may be at increased risk for APAP-induced hepatotoxicity. With such patients, the threshold for treatment indicated on the Rumack-Matthew nomogram should be reduced. Some advocate treating with NAC if the acetaminophen level is more than half that on the nomogram indicating possible toxicity.

The oral NAC protocol approved by the United States Food and Drug Administration for treating APAP toxicity is a loading dose of 140 mg/kg followed by 17 additional doses of 70 mg/kg given at 4-hour intervals. The commercial 20% solution (Mucomyst, Mead Johnson & Company) is unpalatable and should be diluted with three parts fruit juice or soda. If vomiting occurs within 1 hour of treatment, the dose is repeated. Persistent vomiting that interferes with therapy can be suppressed with metoclopramide (0.25 mg/kg IV over 5 minutes) or ondansetron (0.15 mg/kg over 5 minutes). If necessary, NAC can be infused slowly through a nasogastric tube. If activated charcoal has been administered, the usual dose of NAC does not need to be increased, but is best given at least 30 to 60 minutes after the charcoal.

In a review of APAP toxicity over the first 35 years of the drug's use, Rumack describes how the NAC treatment regimen was originally derived from theoretical calculations, with individual doses and length of treatment tripled to provide a margin of safety. Rumack states: "The 72-hour oral NAC protocol is probably unnecessary in many cases where the drug has a shorter half-life [than 4 hours] and disappears before the full dosage is completed" (Rumack, 2002). Based on a retrospective chart review of 75 mostly adult patients, Woo and co-workers suggested that, because evidence of APAP-induced hepatotoxicity (increased GOT and/or GPT) is apparent within 36 hours of acute ingestion, treatment could be stopped at that time if liver enzymes were normal and APAP levels undetectable. Some poison centers have adopted this guideline.

Intravenous NAC is commonly used in Europe, and has recently been approved by the U.S. Food and Drug Administration. In cases of significant overdose where oral NAC is either contraindicated or not tolerated despite all efforts mentioned, the IV preparation

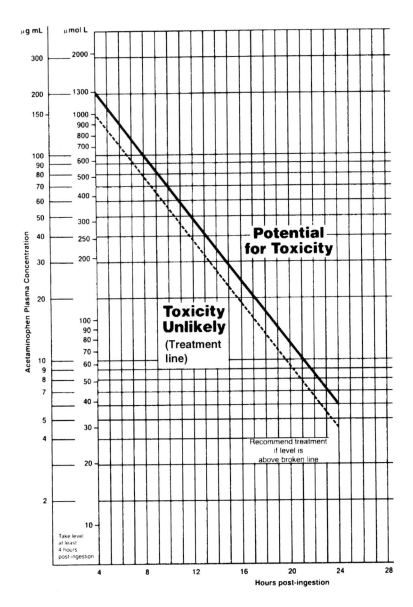

Fig. 28–3. The Rumack-Matthew nomogram indicates which patients will require treatment with NAC following an acute ingestion at a known time.

(Acetadote, Cumberland Pharmaceuticals) can be administered. It differs from the oral form only in that it is certified to be free of pyrogens and bacterial products that can cause a febrile reaction. A recent study by Perry and Shannon of 25 pediatric patients (only 2 of whom were younger than 5 years) found that 52 hours of IV NAC was as effective as the 72-hour oral regimen. In cases where use of IV NAC is considered, a poison control center should be consulted for precise instructions and proper dosing. In young pediatric patients such as neonates and infants, the IV preparation may cause fluid overload if not monitored carefully.

CHRONIC ACETAMINOPHEN POISONING

There have been very rare cases reported in which children appear to have developed severe hepatotoxicity after ingestion of moderately supratherapeutic doses of acetaminophen, administered over several days. The Rumack-Matthew nomogram cannot be used to evaluate these patients; it applies specifically to acute overdose. Doses above 150 mg/kg/d can cause toxicity. Even lower doses may cause hepatic injury in children with such predisposing factors as malnutrition or chronic use of drugs that induce specific cytochrome P450 enzymes (e.g., isoniazid, rifampin, carbamazepine). For patients with these predisposing factors, evaluation for acetaminophen-induced hepatic injury should be considered after ingestion of more than 90 mg/kg/d. Patients with chronic APAP poisoning can present with encephalopathy, vomiting, anorexia, hypoglycemia, coagulopathy, and increased liver enzymes and serum ammonia. Serum APAP levels may be either elevated or nondetectable. Differential diagnosis of acute hepatitis with fulminant hepatic failure includes Reye syndrome, viral hepatitis, septic shock, various metabolic conditions (e.g., Wilson disease), autoimmune liver disease, and other toxin-induced disorders. Toxins that can affect the liver, in addition to APAP, include iron, isoniazid, salicylates, carbon tetrachloride, valproic acid, and amanita mushrooms. Centrilobular necrosis seen on liver biopsy is consistent with drug-induced liver disease. Children with elevated liver enzymes and suspected chronic APAP toxicity should be treated with NAC, in consultation with a poison center. Other possible toxic and nontoxic causes in the differential diagnosis should be ruled out.

Disposition

Use of the Rumack-Matthew nomogram can help to assess risk for hepatotoxicity after a single acute ingestion of APAP. Asymptomatic patients whose APAP level falls below the possible toxicity line can be medically cleared. They should not be discharged home until appropriate interventions have been accomplished. These interventions may include psychiatric assessment in the case of suicidal gesture or attempt, social service consultation for suspected abuse, or counseling of parents or caregivers about the principles of poison prevention. If the APAP level is above the possible toxicity line, the patient should be admitted for treatment with NAC.

Patients with suspected chronic overdose can be medically cleared if liver enzymes are normal and APAP level is undetectable. Asymptomatic or minimally symptomatic patients needing admission can be sent to general pediatric service. Any patient with evidence of fulminant hepatic failure (encephalopathy, hypoglycemia, coagulopathy, acidosis) is admitted to intensive care. All patients whose exposure resulted from an attempt at self-harm need psychiatric evaluation and adequate suicide precautions.

CASE OUTCOME

The patient's 6-hour serum APAP level is 130 μg/mL, above the treatment line on the Rumack-Matthew nomogram. NAC is continued at a dose of 70 mg/kg q4h orally, and is well tolerated. The patient does not develop any symptoms. A psychiatric consultation determines that the ingestion was a suicidal gesture, but that there is no ongoing suicidal ideation and the patient is not at risk for self-harm. At 36 hours, repeated tests reveal that the liver enzymes have remained normal and APAP level is undetectable. She is discharged to the care of her parents with outpatient psychiatric visits scheduled.

SUGGESTED READINGS

Alander SW, Down MD, Bratton SL, et al: Pediatric acetaminophen overdose: Risk factors associated with hepatocellular injury. *Arch Pediatr Adolesc Med* 154:346, 2000.

American Academy of Pediatrics—Committee on Drugs: Acetaminophen toxicity in children. *Pediatrics* 108:1020, 2001.

Anderson BJ, Holford NHG, Armishaw JC: Predicting concentrations in children presenting with acetaminophen overdose. *J Pediatr* 135:290, 1999.

Anker A: Acetaminophen. In: Ford MD, Delaney KA, Ling LJ, et al, eds: *Clinical Toxicology.* Philadelphia: Saunders; 2001: 265–274.

Bond GR, Krenzelok EP, Normann SA, et al: Acetaminophen ingestion in childhood—Cost and relative risk of alternative referral strategies. *Clin Toxicol* 32:513, 1994.

Day A, Abbott GD: Chronic paracetamol poisoning in children: A warning to health professionals. *Aust N Z Med J* 107:201, 1994.

Heubi JE, Bien JP: Acetaminophen use in children: More is *not* better. *J Pediatr* 130:175, 1997.

Huott MA, Storrow AB: A survey of adolescents' knowledge regarding toxicity of over-the-counter medications. *Acad Emerg Med* 4:214, 1997.

James LP, Wells E, Beard RH, et al: Predictors of outcome after acetaminophen poisoning in children and adolescents. *J Pediatr* 140:522, 2002.

Kearns GL, Leeder JS, Wasserman GS: Acetaminophen intoxication during treatment: What you don't know *can* hurt you. *Clin Pediatr* 39:133, 2000.

Kearns GL: Acetaminophen poisoning in children: Treat early and long enough. *J Pediatr* 140:495, 2002.

Keays R, Harrison PM, Wendon JA, et al: Intravenous acetylcysteine in paracetamol induced fulminant hepatic failure: a prospective controlled trial. *BMJ* 303:1026, 1991.

Kociancic T, Reed MD: Acetaminophen intoxication and length of treatment: How long is long enough? *Pharmacotherapy* 23:1052, 2003.

Kozer E, Koren G: Management of paracetamol overdose. *Drug Safety* 24:503, 2001.

Lavalette JH, Tucker JR, Wiley JF: Inherited metabolic disease masquerading as chronic acetaminophen toxicity (abstract). *Clin Toxicol* 36:443, 1998.

Longford JS, Sheikh S: An adolescent case of sulfhemoglobinemia associated with high-dose metoclopramide and *N*-acetylcysteine. *Ann Emerg Med* 34:538, 1999.

Perry HE, Shannon MW: Efficacy of oral versus intravenous *N*-acetylcysteine in acetaminophen overdose: Results of an open-label clinical trial. *J Pediatr* 132:149, 1998.

Peterson RG, Rumack BH: Age as a variable in acetaminophen overdose. *Arch Intern Med* 141:390, 1981.

Rivera-Penera T, Gugig R, Davis J, et al: Outcome of acetaminophen overdose in pediatric patients and factors contributing to hepatotoxicity. *J Pediatr* 130:300, 1997.

Rumack BH: Acetaminophen overdose in young children: Treatment and effects of alcohol and other additional ingestants in 417 cases. *Am J D is Child* 138:428, 1984.

Rumack BH: Acetaminophen overdose in children and adolescents. *Pediatr Clin North Am* 33:691, 1986.

Rumack BH: Acetaminophen overdose? A quick answer. *J Pediatr* 135:269, 1999.

Rumack BH: Acetaminophen hepatotoxicity: The first 35 years. *Clin Toxicol* 40:3, 2002.

Tucker JR: Late-presenting acute acetaminophen toxicity and the role of *N*-acetylcysteine. *Pediatr Emerg Care* 14:424, 1998.

Watson WA, Litoviz TL, Rodgers GC, et al: 2002 Annual Report of the American Association of Poison Centers Toxic Exposure Surveillance System. *Am J Emerg Med* 21:353, 2002.

Woo OF, Mueller PD, Olson KR, et al: Shorter duration of oral *N*-acetylcysteine therapy for acute acetaminophen overdose. *Ann Emerg Med* 35:363, 2000.

29

Anticholinergic Poisoning

Mark Su

HIGH-YIELD FACTS

- Anticholinergic poisoning is manifested by a constellation of both peripheral and central signs and symptoms. Central anticholinergic toxicity is characterized by delirium, hallucinations, and seizures. Peripheral anticholinergic toxicity is characterized by tachycardia, dry skin and mucous membranes, urinary retention, decreased bowel sounds, and hyperthermia.

- Many drugs and various plant species contain anticholinergic properties.

- In most cases of anticholinergic toxicity, supportive care, activated charcoal for gastric decontamination, and benzodiazepines for agitation are adequate therapies.

- Physostigmine can be used as an antidote for severe central anticholinergic toxicity. The usual dose is 0.02 mg/kg (maximum 0.5 mg) infused over at least 5 minutes. Redosing may be necessary.

- Cyclic antidepressant toxicity should be excluded by history and electrocardiogram prior to the administration of physostigmine.

CASE PRESENTATION

A 16-year-old boy presents to the emergency department with altered mental status and ataxia after ingesting an unknown quantity of diphenhydramine. He is speaking incoherently and is very agitated. He has no significant past medical history, is not taking any medications, and has no known allergies.

On physical examination, he has a blood pressure of 150/102 mmHg; pulse of 150 bpm; respiratory rate of 22 breaths per minutes; and a rectal temperature of 101°F. His pupils are dilated and minimally reactive; mucous membranes are dry. Cardiac examination is unremarkable except for tachycardia. His lungs are clear to auscultation bilaterally. The abdominal examination reveals decreased bowel sounds. There are no localizing findings on the neurologic examination.

Laboratory studies, including a serum chemistry and complete blood count are unremarkable. Serum acetaminophen, salicylate, and ethanol concentrations are all negative. An arterial blood gas on room air reveals a pH of 7.41, PCO_2 of 35 mmHg and PO_2 of 94 mmHg. An electrocardiogram demonstrates sinus tachycardia at a rate of 140 bpm with a narrow complex QRS, and normal QT_c duration. The patient is treated orally with a single 50-g dose of activated charcoal and has one episode of vomiting. The same dose of activated charcoal is repeated and tolerated by the patient.

INTRODUCTION AND EPIDEMIOLOGY

Anticholinergic toxicity is quite common and may result from both pharmaceutical preparations, as well as various plant species. According to American Association of Poison Control Center (AAPCC) data, from 1997 to 2001, there were 25,730 exposures to anticholinergic drugs, with 696 major outcomes and 26 deaths. Specific examples of anticholinergic agents are seen in Table 29–1.

Table 29–1. Anticholinergic Agents

Pharmaceuticals	Plants
Atropine	*Atropa belladonna* (deadly nightshade)
Astemizole (removed from market)	*Datura stramonium* (jimson weed)
Cyproheptadine	*Hyosycamus niger* (black henbane)
Diphenhydramine	*Lantana camara* (red sage)
Dimhydrinate (diphenhydramine/ chlorotheophylline)	*Mandragora officinarum* (mandrake)
Doxylamine	*Solanum dulcamara* (bittersweet)
Hyoscyamine	
Other classes of drugs	
Antiparkinsonian agents	
Antispasmodics	
Antipsychotics	
Cyclic antidepressants	

DEVELOPMENTAL CONSIDERATIONS

Anticholinergic toxicity in toddlers and young children is likely to be due to unintentional excessive administration of medication by caretakers. This might occur when a child has an upper respiratory tract infection and is administered a cold medicine for several consecutive days. The child is then brought to health care because of persistent fever and/or an alteration in mental status owing to anticholinergic toxicity. Older children, especially adolescents, may ingest parts of the jimson weed plant for its hallucinatory effects. Significant quantities of atropine, hyoscyamine, and scopolamine are distributed throughout both the plant and its seeds, and anticholinergic poisoning can be severe when this plant is ingested.

PHARMACOLOGY AND PATHOPHYSIOLOGY

Anticholinergic agents act by inhibiting the normal physiologic response to the neurotransmitter acetylcholine (Ach) at muscarinic receptors. Muscarinic receptors are found throughout the central nervous system (CNS) and sympathetic and parasympathetic ganglia. Ach is also an agonist at nicotinic receptors located at the neuromuscular junction of skeletal muscle. The anticholinergic agents do not antagonize the effects at nicotinic receptors, and therefore may be thought of as antimuscarinic agents.

Anticholinergic toxicity, or antimuscarinic toxicity, may be divided into central and peripheral effects. *Central effects* include alteration in mental status including delirium, hallucinations, agitation, and seizures. *Peripheral effects* include mydriasis, tachycardia, flushing, dry skin and mucous membranes, urinary retention, and decreased gastrointestinal (GI) motility. The onset of anticholinergic toxicity varies depending on the particular toxin, but usually occurs within several hours except in cases of diphenoxylate-atropine (Lomotil) poisoning, in which delayed toxicity can occur. Although central and peripheral anticholinergic effects are commonly seen simultaneously, the central effects may occasionally persist after the peripheral effects have resolved.

CLINICAL FINDINGS

An often-used mnemonic to remember the clinical manifestations of anticholinergic toxicity is

Hot as a hare

Blind as a bat

Dry as a bone

Red as a beet

Mad as a hatter

The most concerning and serious form of anticholinergic toxicity is due to blockade of muscarinic receptors in the brain. The excessive CNS excitation that results clinically manifests as agitation, anxiety, delirium, lethargy, drowsiness, coma, and occasionally seizures. Peripheral blockade of muscarinic receptors leads to cardiovascular effects such as tachycardia from antagonism of vagal tone, mydriasis with the inability to accommodate, decreased activity of sweat glands, hyperthermia, urinary retention, and reduced gut motility.

LABORATORY AND DIAGNOSTIC TESTING

The diagnosis of anitcholinergic toxicity is generally based on recognition of the signs and symptoms characteristic of the toxidrome. However, basic screening tests such as an electrocardiogram and serum electrolytes should be obtained. An electrocardiogram is very important because cyclic antidepressants, certain phenothiazines, and diphenhydramine have Type IA antidysrhythmic properties in addition to anticholinergic effects. A prolonged QRS interval duration with subsequent prolonged QT_c duration may result, and severe cardiac dysrhythmias can occur. Astemizole, a drug no longer marketed in the United States because of its cardiotoxicity, was reported to cause torsades de pointes. Serum drug concentrations are neither readily available nor helpful in the clinical setting. In suicide attempts, a screening acetaminophen level is indicated, because products containing a combination of acetaminophen and antihistamine are common. Patients with severe psychomotor agitation and seizures should have a serum creatine kinase checked because of the possibility of rhabdomyolysis. Additionally, patients who ingest the antihistamine doxylamine are reported to have delayed rhabdomyolysis. Doxylamine is an over-the-counter sleep-inducing agent that has been associated with massive elevations in serum creatine phosphokinase in the absence of trauma. Injury is likely due to direct drug injury to striated muscle.

MANAGEMENT

Patients with anticholinergic poisoning should have immediate stabilization of the airway, breathing, and circulation. Continuous cardiac monitoring and pulse oximetry are essential. Depending on the particular substance and the route of exposure, decontamination should be performed. Although most anticholinergic toxicity results from ingestion, systemic anticholinergic toxicity has been reported from cutaneous absorption and from ocular exposure. If a significant quantity of cyclic antidepressants is believed to have been recently ingested, GI lavage is indicated. If the patient presents beyond 1 hour postingestion, because of decreased GI motility, lavage may be theoretically effective at drug removal. For most other cases, as long as mental status is not severely impaired, activated charcoal (1 g/kg) should suffice as initial therapy. Syrup of ipecac is contraindicated.

In most cases of anticholinergic toxicity, supportive care (i.e., benzodiazepines to treat agitation or seizures; cooling for hyperthermia) is adequate therapy. Other associated complications, such as rhabdomyolysis from doxylamine, are also usually treated supportively with good outcome. Following an overdose of doxylamine, however, renal failure and subsequent need for hemodialysis is reported. Wide complex cardiac dysrhythmias from cyclic antidepressants and diphenhydramine should be treated with boluses (1 to 2 mEq/kg) of IV sodium bicarbonate to reverse the local anesthetic properties of these drugs (as described in Chapter 43).

For patients demonstrating severe central anticholinergic toxicity (delirium, hallucinations, tachydysrhythmias, or seizures), not responsive to traditional doses of benzodiazepines, physostigmine may be used as antidotal therapy (Figure 29–1). Physostigmine is an anticholinesterase drug that antagonizes the effects of anticholinergic agents and is sufficiently lipophilic to cross the blood–brain barrier. It is therefore able to counteract both the peripheral and central effects of anticholinergic toxicity. The usual dose in children is 0.02 mg/kg (maximum 0.5 mg) and in adults 1 to 2 mg infused IV over at least 5 minutes. The onset of action of physostigmine is usually within several minutes. The half-life of the drug is approximately 15 minutes. For agents that have a

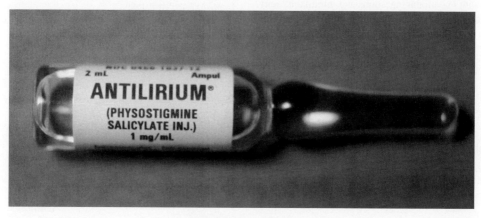

Fig. 29–1. Physostigmine.

prolonged anticholinergic effect on the CNS such as scopolamine, redosing may be necessary.

It should be noted that prior to the administration of physostigmine, anticholinergic agents with potential cardiotoxicity such as cyclic antidepressants or phenothiazines should be excluded historically, or by electrocardiogram. If the QRS and QT$_c$ intervals are normal, these agents are unlikely to be the cause of anticholinergic toxicity. In the past, physostigmine was routinely used as an analeptic agent to reverse toxins with CNS depressant properties. Several deaths are associated with the administration of physostigmine in cases of cyclic antidepressant toxicity, and it is no longer advocated for this purpose. Other adverse effects of physostigmine, especially with rapid administration, include inducing a cholinergic crisis with increased bronchial secretions, bradycardia, and seizures. When administering physostigmine, it is therefore imperative to closely monitor the patient and be prepared for cholinergic toxicity with oral and laryngeal suction, endotracheal intubation, and atropine as needed.

DISPOSITION

Patients who have significant anticholinergic toxicity (and are treated with physostigmine) should be admitted to an intensive care setting for observation. Patients exposed to anticholinergic agents with additional toxicity, such as cyclic antidepressants and phenothiazines should also be closely observed for cardiac dysrhythmias. Children with unintentional ingestions or minimal anticholinergic toxicity should be given activated charcoal and observed in the emergency department for a minimum of 6 hours. For all other hemodynamically stable patients with intentional ingestions and minimal toxicity, a psychiatric evaluation is necessary prior to disposition.

CASE OUTCOME

The patient was treated with 1 mg of physostigmine IV and his delirium quickly resolved. He disclosed that he intentionally ingested the diphenhydramine tablets as an experiment. He was admitted to the pediatric intensive care unit for observation where he remained hemodynamically stable and developed no further evidence of CNS anticholinergic toxicity. He was transferred to the psychiatry service the following day.

SUGGESTED READINGS

Asthana S, Greig NH, Hegedus L, et al: Clinical pharmacokinetics of physostigmine in patients with Alzheimer's disease. *Clin Pharmacol Ther* 58:299–309, 1995.

Bernhardt DT: Topical diphenhydramine toxicity. *Wisc Med J* 90:469–471, 1991.

Clark RF, Vance MV: Massive diphenhydramine poisoning resulting in a wide-complex tachycardia: Successful treatment with sodium bicarbonate. *Ann Emerg Med* 21:318–321, 1992.

Farrell M, Heinrichs M, Tilelli JA: Response of life threatening dimenhydrinate intoxication to sodium bicarbonate administration. *J Toxicol Clin Toxicol* 29:527–535, 1991.

Frankel D, Dolgin J, Murray BM: Non-traumatic rhabdomyolysis complicating antihistamine overdose. *J Toxicol Clin Toxicol* 31:493–496 1993.

Holzgrafe RE, Vondrell JJ, Mintz SM: Reversal of postoperative reactions to scopolamine with physostigmine. *Anesth Analg* 52:921–925, 1973.

Koppel C, Ibe K, Oberdisse U: Rhabdomyolysis in doxylamine overdose. *Lancet* 21:442–443, 1987.

Leybishkis B, Fasseas P, Ryan KF: Doxylamine overdose as a potential cause of rhabdomyolysis. *Am J Med Sci* 322:48–49, 2001.

Litovitz TL, Klein-Schwartz W, Rodgers GC Jr, et al: 2001 Annual report of the American Association of Poison Control Centers Toxic Exposure Surveillance System. *Am J Emerg Med* 20:391–452, 2002.

Litovitz TL, Klein-Schwartz W, White S, et al: 2000 Annual report of the American Association of Poison Control Centers Toxic Exposure Surveillance System. *Am J Emerg Med* 19:337–395, 2001.

Litovitz TL, Klein-Schwartz W, White S, et al: 1999 annual report of the American Association of Poison Control Centers Toxic Exposure Surveillance System. *Am J Emerg Med* 18:517–574, 2000.

Litovitz TL, Klein-Schwartz W, Caravati EM, et al: 1998 annual report of the American Association of Poison Control Centers Toxic Exposure Surveillance System. *Am J Emerg Med* 17:435–487, 1999.

Litovitz TL, Klein-Schwartz W, Dyer KS, et al: 1997 annual report of the American Association of Poison Control Centers Toxic Exposure Surveillance System. *Am J Emerg Med* 16:443–497, 1998.

McCarron MM, Challoner KR, Thompson GA: Diphenoxylate-atropine (Lomotil) overdose in children: An update (report of eight cases and review of the literature) *Pediatrics* 87:694–700, 1991.

Mendoza FS, Atiba JO, Krensky AM, et al: Rhabdomyolysis complicating doxylamine overdose. *Clin Pediatr* 26:595–597, 1987.

Pentel P, Peterson CD: Asystole complicating physostigmine treatment of tricyclic antidepressant overdose. *Ann Emerg Med* 9:588–590, 1980.

Shervette RE 3rd, Schydlower M, Lampe RM, et al: Jimson "loco" weed abuse in adolescents. *Pediatrics* 63:520–523, 1979.

Soto LF, Miller CH, Ognibere AJ: Severe rhabdomyolysis after doxylamine overdose. *Postgrad Med* 93:227–229, 232, 1993.

Reilly JF Jr, Weisse ME: Topically induced diphenhydramine toxicity. *J Emerg Med* 8:59–61, 1990.

Thompson HS: Cornpicker's pupil: Jimson weed mydriasis. *J Iowa Med Soc* 61:575–578, 1971.

Wiley JF 2nd, Gelber ML, Henretig FM, et al: Cardiotoxic effects of astemizole overdose in children. *J Pediatr* 120:799–802, 1992.

30

Aspirin

Michele Zell-Kanter

HIGH-YIELD FACTS

- Salicylate poisoning may result from oral and/or topical exposure.
- Unlike adults, children do not typically display respiratory alkalosis after acute aspirin ingestion.
- Metabolic acidosis may be the presenting sign.
- Pediatric patients are managed primarily with supportive care, activated charcoal, and alkalinization of the urine.
- Hemodialysis is reserved for severely intoxicated patients and patients with altered mental status, seizures, renal failure, pulmonary edema, and acidosis that does not correct with standard therapy.

CASE PRESENTATION

A 22-month-old girl ingested 30 children's aspirin several hours ago. The mother noticed that the child was tachypneic, and brought the patient to the Emergency Department. Her past medical history was noncontributory, she was on no medications, and had no known allergies.

On physical examination, the patient appeared lethargic and dehydrated, with a pulse of 140 bpm and respiratory rate of 48 breaths per minute. The temperature was 100.0°F and blood pressure was measured at 70/40 mmHg. Pupils were equal and reactive to light. Auscultation of the heart and lungs was normal. Abdominal examination revealed mild epigastric tenderness. Stool testing was negative for occult blood.

INTRODUCTION

Salicylates were used by the Greeks more than 2400 years ago to treat pain and gout. Salicylic acid is derived from the extract of willow bark. The acetylated form of salicylic acid was synthesized in 1853, resulting in present-day aspirin.

One fourth of all aspirin exposures reported to the American Association of Poison Control Centers in 2002 occurred in patients less than 6 years of age. Thirty-two percent of the reported exposures were in patients 6 to 19 years old. Aspirin use in children has decreased since its association with Reye syndrome. However, children's aspirin tablets may be more commonly found in homes now, because adults are using this dosage form for the prevention of stroke and myocardial infarction (Figure 30–1). Salicylates are available in many cough and cold preparations. Topical preparations containing salicylic acid are routinely available. Oil of wintergreen and Pepto-Bismol also contain salicylic acid. Many herbal remedies advertised for their analgesic effects contain derivatives of white willow, and therefore some derivative of salicylic acid.

DEVELOPMENTAL CONSIDERATIONS

Children with Kawasaki disease require unusually high doses of aspirin (up to 180 mg/kg/d) to maintain therapeutic salicylate levels during the acute febrile period of this disease. Aspirin absorption is thought to be impaired during this period of time. Levels should be closely monitored. The aspirin dose must be reduced once the fever has resolved. Juvenile rheumatoid arthritis patients typically require aspirin doses that approach toxic levels. Doses must be closely titrated and monitored to avoid toxicity.

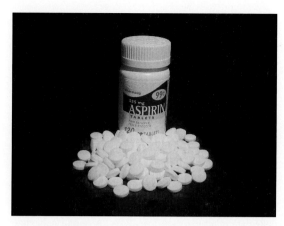

Fig. 30–1. OTC generic aspirin product.

No fetal or neonatal toxicity has been observed when aspirin has been used in doses of 40 to 150 mg/d to prevent pregnancy-induced hypertension, preeclampsia, eclampsia, and the fetal risks associated with intrauterine growth retardation. It is theorized that only maternal and not fetal cyclooxygenase is inhibited at this dose. Aspirin use in late pregnancy, especially within 1 week of delivery, may have an effect on the neonate's coagulation status and may cause premature closure of the ductus arteriosus. Adolescents who intentionally ingest aspirin in a suicide attempt may present with serious toxicity because larger doses of aspirin have been ingested.

PHARMACOLOGY AND TOXICOKINETICS

Salicylates inhibit cyclooxygenase and thereby inhibit prostaglandin synthesis. This imparts analgesic, anti-inflammatory, and antipyretic effects. Ingestions of less than 150 mg/kg are considered nontoxic. Patients who ingest 150 to 300 mg/kg exhibit mild to moderate toxicity, and ingestions of greater than 500 mg/kg are considered potentially lethal.

Aspirin is rapidly absorbed from the small intestine at normal doses. Concretions may form in overdose settings, thus delaying absorption. Aspirin has a narrow therapeutic range. When used as an anti-inflammatory, serum salicylate concentrations approach toxic levels. Salicylates are highly bound to plasma proteins, and have a small volume of distribution (0.1 to 0.2 L/kg). The volume of distribution increases in overdose. Aspirin is rapidly hydrolyzed to salicylic acid in the intestinal wall, liver, and red blood cells. Glycine and glucuronide-conjugated metabolites are produced by the liver and kidneys. The pharmacokinetics of aspirin changes from first-order to enzyme saturable zero-order when serum levels reach the upper limit of therapeutic. This means that as the dose is being titrated up, patients may develop toxicity because their enzymes have been saturated and they can no longer metabolize the aspirin as quickly. Excretion of both the glycine and glucuronide conjugates is diminished in toxicity and there is an increase in salicylic acid excretion. Aspirin's half-life may increase from 4 hours with therapeutic doses to 10 to 45 hours in overdose. Peak serum salicylate levels may be delayed after multiple tablet ingestion because of concretion formation. Ingestion of enteric-coated or sustained-release products may delay peak levels for up to 12 hours.

Aspirin has a pK_a of 3.0 and is ionized in an alkalotic environment. In its ionized state, aspirin cannot cross cell membranes and diffuse into critical organs such as the brain. The goal in managing overdose patients is to maintain serum pH between 7.4 and 7.5 to limit toxicity and prevent salicylate diffusion.

Salicylate products vary widely in concentration. It is critical to be certain of the concentration of a specific product so that a patient's serum level can be estimated. Oil of wintergreen contains 100% methylsalicylate. As little as 4 mL of oil of wintergreen may be fatal in a child. An aspirin-equivalent dose can be calculated using aspirin conversion factors to estimate toxicity when using non–aspirin containing salicylates.

PATHOPHYSIOLOGY

Salicylates irritate the gastric mucosa and stimulate the chemoreceptor trigger zone, causing nausea and vomiting. Tinnitus and impaired hearing results from vasoconstriction of the auditory microvasculature. Respiratory alkalosis results for direct stimulation of the respiratory center, which causes tachypnea.

Unlike adults, aspirin toxic children may not exhibit a respiratory alkalosis prior to developing metabolic acidosis.

Several metabolic pathways are affected by salicylate overdose. Metabolic acidosis is a consequence of (1) Krebs cycle inhibition resulting in accumulation of pyruvic and lactic acids, (2) uncoupling of oxidative phosphorylation, resulting in depletion of high-energy phosphates, increased oxygen consumption, increased carbon dioxide production, and increased heat production, and (3) increased tissue glycolysis causing gluconeogenesis, lipolysis, and increased ketone production. Accumulation of organic acids causes an increased anion-gap metabolic acidosis. The kidney excretes bicarbonate, sodium, and potassium as a compensatory response to the metabolic acidosis. Dehydration ensues because of increased sodium and potassium excretion, as well as increased insensible losses and vomiting.

Noncardiogenic pulmonary edema or acute lung injury can result from salicylate toxicity to the pulmonary endothelium. This causes increased pulmonary vascular permeability to fluids and proteins. Salicylates inhibit platelet aggregation, inhibit factor VII, and decrease prothrombin.

CLINICAL PRESENTATION

Acute aspirin toxicity is much more common in children than chronic toxicity. Chronic toxicity occurs at lower salicylate levels (30 to ≤60 mg/dL) than acute toxicity (40 to ≥100 mg/dL). Symptoms of acute toxicity in children occur more rapidly and are generally more severe than in adults. This occurs in part because of enhanced distribution of salicylate to the brain, kidney, and liver in the pediatric patient. The earliest symptoms are gastrointestinal, and patients may complain of nausea, vomiting, and epigastric pain. Hematemesis and hyperventilation may be present. Patients may also complain of tinnitus and/or deafness. Children often develop fever. With increasing levels, neurologic toxicity including delerium, seizures, and coma may develop as toxicity worsens and acidemia increases. Rhabdomyolysis may result in oliguric renal failure. Hypotension and noncardiogenic pulmonary edema may ensue.

Severe fluid and electrolyte disturbances may occur. Patients become dehydrated and develop hypokalemia. Younger children are particularly vulnerable to dehydration. Hypoglycemia can occur in the pediatric patient because of increased peripheral glucose demand, increased rate of tissue glycolysis, and an impaired rate of glucose synthesis from non-carbohydrate sources. In some patients hyperglycemia occurs.

LABORATORY AND DIAGNOSTIC TESTING

The therapeutic range for salicylates is 15 to 25 mg/dL. Anti-inflammatory effects occur in the high-therapeutic range. Special attention must be given to the units of measurement which are typically listed in mg/dL, but also may be listed as mg/L. Serum salicylate levels should be measured serially in the overdose setting until declining concen-

trations have been documented. There is increased morbidity and mortality when patients on chronic salicylate therapy develop toxic levels. In this setting, clinical findings are more indicative of toxicity than are serum levels.

The ferric chloride test is a rapid bedside determination for the qualitative presence of salicylates. Two to three drops of ferric chloride are added to 1 mL of urine. A purple color results if salicylates are present, and a positive result should occur 30 minutes after salicylate ingestion. Both acetoacetic acid and phenylpyruvic acid will cause the ferric chloride test to turn purple. Phenistix will turn brownish-purple in the presence of salicylate.

Other laboratory tests should include arterial or venous blood gases, serum electrolytes, glucose, creatinine, coagulation profile, and urinalysis. A serum salicylate level should be considered in all suspected overdoses because of the morbidity and mortality associated with toxicity and delayed diagnosis. A nomogram to interpret serum salicylate levels was described by Done in 1960, but has very limited utility in the overdose setting.

MANAGEMENT

The goals of treatment of salicylate toxicity include preventing its further absorption, enhancing its elimination, and correcting fluid and electrolyte abnormalities. In ventilated patients, maintaining a slight respiratory alkalosis will potentially reduce salicylate distribution into the CNS. Most salicylate toxic patients are severely dehydrated, and require aggressive fluid resuscitation with isotonic crystalloids. Hypokalemic patients require potassium replacement once urine flow is established.

Gastric decontamination should be instituted in ingestions of >150 mg/kg or when the amount ingested is not known. If given soon after ingestion, activated charcoal may prevent further absorption of salicylates. An initial dose of activated charcoal at 1 g/kg is generally recommended. Multiple doses of activated charcoal may enhance salicylate elimination. The theoretical benefits for using multiple-dose activated charcoal (MDAC) in salicylate poisoning are that (1) charcoal acts as a form of peritoneal or gut dialysis leaching salicylate from a higher concentration in the plasma to a lower concentration in the gut and (2) MDAC will adsorb any salicylate that may desorb from the initial charcoal dose. The dose of MDAC is 0.5 g/kg every 2 to 4 hours.

Whole bowel irrigation with polyethylene glycol solution may be considered if a sustained-release preparation has been recently ingested or if there is suspicion of a gastric concretion.

Urinary alkalinization is used to enhance salicylate excretion. The goal is to maintain the urine pH between 7 and 8 and a urine output between 1 and 2 mL/kg/h. When the urine pH is 8, a large concentration gradient exists between the nonionized salicylate in the blood/peritubular fluid, and the tubular luminal fluid. The nonionized salicylate passes from the peritubular fluid into the urine. If patients become hypokalemic, it will be very difficult to achieve alkaline urine because the kidney preferentially reabsorbs potassium in exchange for hydrogen. Use caution to avoid overalkalinization, hypernatremia, and fluid overload.

Hemodialysis effectively removes salicylate and corrects electrolyte and acid–base disturbances. Indications for hemodialysis include neurologic depression, seizures, renal failure, noncardiogenic pulmonary edema, and severe acid–base disorder. An absolute salicylate level should not be used as the sole criteria for instituting hemodialysis. Guidelines for instituting hemodialysis in an acute ingestion are a level >100 mg/dL, and >50 mg/dL in a patient with chronic salicylate poisoning.

DISPOSITION

Poison control center guidelines for assessing the accidental ingestion of salicylates are: (1) Ingestion of <150 mg/kg is considered nontoxic and can be generally treated at home with fluids and telephone follow-up. This recommendation must be cautiously interpreted because the history of the amount ingested can be intentionally or unintentionally incorrect. (2) Ingestion of 150 to 300 mg/kg may result in mild to moderate toxicity. (3) Ingestion of >500 mg/kg should be considered a potentially lethal ingestion.

In toxic patients, serial levels must be obtained before disposition can be made. Asymptomatic patients with normal acid/base status and who have two consecutive serum levels drawn at least 2 hours apart that are less than 30 mg/dL may be discharged. Children with serious toxicity, seizures, acid–base disturbances, and those requiring hemodialysis should be admitted to a pediatric intensive care unit.

CASE OUTCOME

The following laboratory studies were determined: Arterial blood gas pH 7.46, P_{CO_2} 20, P_{O_2} 115, O_2 saturation 99%, base excess 14. A metabolic profile revealed a sodium of 141 mEq/L, potassium 3.3 mEq/L, chloride 103 mEq/L, bicarbonate 15 mEq/L, BUN 18 mEq/L, creatinine 0.8 mEq/L, and glucose 97 mg/dL. The anion gap was 23 and the serum salicylate level was 60 mg/dL. The patient was treated with activated charcoal, IV sodium bicarbonate for urinary alkalinization, and IV potassium supplementation. Repeat serum salicylate levels were ordered every 2 hours until the level began to decline.

The patient's repeat salicylate level 5 hours later was 43 mg/dL, and the urine pH was greater than 7.5. The serum salicylate level was 10 mg/dL 22 hours after therapy was begun, and the patient was discharged home.

SUGGESTED READINGS

Briggs GG, Freeman RK, Yaffe SJ: *Drugs in Pregnancy and Lactation.* Philadelphia: Lippincott Williams & Wilkins; 1998.

Boldy D, Vale JA: Treatment of salicylate poisoning with repeated oral charcoal. *Br Med J* 292:136, 1986.

Done AK: Salicylate intoxication: Significance of measurements of salicylate in blood and cases of acute ingestion. *Pediatrics* 26:800–807, 1960.

Koren G, MacLeod SM: Difficulty in achieving therapeutic serum concentrations of salicylate in Kawasaki disease. *J Pediatr* 105:991–995, 1984.

Kozer E, Nikfar S, Costie A, et al: Aspirin consumption during the first trimester of pregnancy and congenital anomalies: A meta-analysis. *Am J Obstet Gynecol* 187:1623–1630, 2002.

Manikian A, Stone S, Hamilton R, et al: Exchange transfusion in severe infant salicylism. *Vet Human Toxicol* 44:224–227, 2002.

Mayer AL, Sitar DS, Tenenbein M: Multiple-dose charcoal and whole-bowel irrigation do not increase clearance of absorbed salicylate. *Arch Intern Med* 152:393–396, 1992.

Notarianni L: A reassessment of the treatment of salicylate poisoning. *Drug Safety* 7:292–303, 1992.

Perneger TV, Whelton PK, Klag MJ: Risk of kidney failure associated with the use of acetaminophen, aspirin, and non-steroidal anti-inflammatory drugs. *N Engl J Med* 331:1675–1712, 1994.

Riordan M, Rylance G, Berry K: Poisoning in children 2: painkillers. *Arch Dis Child* 87:397–400, 2002.

Watson JE, Tagupa ET: Suicide attempt by means of aspirin enema. *Ann Pharmacother* 28:467–469, 1994.

Watson WA, Litovitz TL, Rodgers GC, et al: 2002 annual report of the American association of poison control centers toxic exposure surveillance system. *Am J Emerg Med* 21:353–421, 2003.

Yip L, Dart RC, Gabow PA: Concepts and controversies in salicylate toxicity. *Emerg Med Clin North Am* 12:351–363, 1994.

31

Nonsteroidal Anti-Inflammatory Drugs

Michele Zell-Kanter

CASE PRESENTATION

A 3-year-old, 14-kg girl is brought to the emergency department (ED) after ingesting an unknown quantity of children's liquid ibuprofen. The bottle initially contained 16 ounces, and 4 ounces remained. The concentration of the liquid was 100 mg/5 mL, the maximum amount potentially ingested was 72 g. The patient had one episode of spontaneous emesis at home, and another episode in the ED. On physical examination, the patient appeared lethargic. Vital signs were temperature of 97.9°F, pulse 80 bpm, respiratory rate of 24 breaths per minute, and a blood pressure of 90/60 mmHg. The cardiopulmonary examination was normal. The rest of the physical examination was unremarkable.

INTRODUCTION AND EPIDEMIOLOGY

Many NSAIDs are currently available, with several more awaiting approval. Both ibuprofen and naproxen are available without prescription (Figure 31–1). A second generation of NSAIDs known as the cyclooxygenase 2 (COX-2) inhibitors, or *coxibs,* was introduced in the late 1990s. They were touted to cause less GI and renal toxicity with chronic use, as well as having platelet-sparing effects when compared to traditional NSAIDs.

More than 51,000 ibuprofen exposures in children younger than 19 years were reported to the American Association of Poison Control Centers in 2002. There were more than 9000 exposures secondary to all other traditional NSAIDs in this same age group. Now that there are three coxibs available, accidental childhood exposures to the coxibs has increased by 50% in 1 year, to more than 3000. No NSAID-related pediatric deaths were reported during this time period.

Adult deaths related to chronic NSAID use in patients with rheumatoid arthritis and osteoarthritis in the United States has been conservatively estimated at 16,500 in 1997, and was similar in magnitude to the number of AIDS-related deaths for that year. Over-the-counter NSAID-related deaths were not included in this statistic.

DEVELOPMENTAL CONSIDERATIONS

There are published case reports of neonates who developed oligohydramnios and renal failure associated with maternal high-dose indomethacin or ibuprofen therapy used early in gestation and for prolonged periods. In these cases, NSAIDs were used as tocolytics or in the management of polyhydramnios. There have been reports describing persistent neonatal pulmonary hyper-

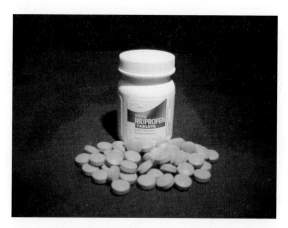

Fig 31–1. OTC generic ibuprofen product.

din synthesis involve two major organs, the gut, and kidney. Gastric irritation and bleeding occur when synthesis of the cytoprotective prostaglandins I_2 and E_2 is inhibited. These prostaglandins are also involved in maintaining fluid and electrolyte balance, renin release leading to aldosterone regulation, potassium loss, blood pressure control, and renal blood flow, especially in states when renal perfusion is decreased.

Celecoxib, rofecoxib, and valdecoxib are the coxibs that are currently available in the United States. By specifically blocking COX-2, these agents have reduced GI toxicity and bleeding, complications of traditional NSAIDs. They are generally well tolerated by patients who are well hydrated and who have normal renal function. These agents should be avoided in patients with preexisting renal impairment.

tension associated with NSAIDs used to treat patent ductus arteriosus in the third trimester. Early indomethacin use for patent ductus arteriosus in extremely premature infants has been associated with neonatal necrotizing enterocolitis. Other therapeutic misadventures associated with NSAIDs in pediatric patients include necrotizing fasciitis and facial scarring.

PHARMACOLOGY AND TOXICOKINETICS

The NSAIDs are classified according to their chemical structures, and the toxicokinetics are specific for individual agents. The specific characteristics of ibuprofen will be presented here, because ibuprofen is available over the counter, and it is the NSAID that is most commonly reported to poison control centers. Ibuprofen is rapidly absorbed in therapeutic doses, and maximum blood levels are reached in 1 to 2 hours. Its volume of distribution is 0.1 L/kg in adults, but is increased in patients between 3 months and 2.5 years of age. Ibuprofen is 95% bound to plasma proteins, and has a half-life of 2 hours. Liver metabolites are mostly conjugated with glucuronic acid and excreted by the kidney.

A few NSAIDs have prolonged half-lives (24 hours or greater) because of enterohepatic recirculation. These include nabumetone, oxaprozin, phenylbutazone, and piroxicam. Celecoxib has the largest volume of distribution (about 400 L) of the currently available coxibs.

PATHOPHYSIOLOGY

Traditional NSAIDs act by inhibiting both COX-1 and -2, and thus inhibiting synthesis of prostaglandins from arachidonic acid. Toxicities associated with prostaglan-

CLINICAL PRESENTATION

Patients who ingest NSAIDs typically exhibit GI toxicity, including nausea, vomiting, and epigastric pain. Ulceration and bleeding are associated with chronic use. Patients may exhibit CNS toxicity with larger overdoses. Symptoms include drowsiness, dizziness, and lethargy. Rarely, patients may develop hypotension and tachycardia, probably secondary to hypovolemia.

The traditional NSAIDs have been associated with renal failure from both acute and chronic use, especially in high-risk individuals such as diabetics and patients with hypertension. Acute interstitial nephritis/proteinuria may develop at any time, but typically develops after months to years of NSAID therapy, and is reversible upon discontinuation of therapy. NSAID-induced papillary necrosis is the least common renal toxicity and is irreversible.

An anion gap metabolic acidosis is associated with NSAID abuse, usually from massive ingestions such as adolescent suicidal ingestions of more than 20 to 25 g. Idiosyncratic findings associated with NSAID use include aseptic meningitis, aplastic anemia, hemolytic anemia, and decreased platelet aggregation.

LABORATORY AND DIAGNOSTIC TESTING

Laboratory tests that should be performed in symptomatic patients include serum electrolytes, a complete blood count, serum blood urea nitrogen, and creatinine. Assays for determining ibuprofen levels are available; however, there is no clinical correlation between levels and toxicity.

Arterial blood gases should be obtained if acidosis is suspected. Serum salicylate and acetaminophen levels should be obtained to rule out analgesic coingestants, particularly in patients who have deliberately overdosed.

MANAGEMENT

Patients are managed with supportive care. Gastric decontamination with activated charcoal is indicated for recent ingestions. There are no antidotes for the NSAIDs. Extracorporeal methods and multiple-dose activated charcoal are ineffective for NSAID removal because of their high degree of plasma protein binding and short half-lives. Enhanced elimination techniques have not been studied in NSAIDs with prolonged half-lives.

DISPOSITION

Children who unintentionally ingest <150 mg/kg of ibuprofen can be observed at home. Observation may be considered with ibuprofen ingestions of 150 to 199 mg/kg. All ingestions of ibuprofen 200 mg/kg or greater and all intentional ingestions should be referred to a health care facility. Patients can be monitored for 4 to 6 hours, and if they are asymptomatic, can be discharged. Any patient with altered mental status, unstable vital signs, and/or metabolic acidosis should be monitored in an intensive care setting.

CASE OUTCOME

Laboratory findings revealed ABG: pH 7.37, P_{CO_2} 37, P_{O_2} 108, and O_2 sat 97%. Electrolytes were normal, an-

ion gap was 14. The complete blood count revealed a white blood cell count of 12.1, hemoglobin of 10.6, and platelet count of 240,000. Serum salicylate and acetaminophen levels were below detectable limits. The child was given one dose of activated charcoal. The patient did well with no adverse effects. The parents were educated regarding poison prevention in the home.

SUGGESTED READINGS

Diaz Jara M, Perez Montero A, Gracia Bara MT, et al: Allergic reactions due to ibuprofen in children. *Pediatric Dermatol* 18:66–67, 2001.

Fujii AM, Brown E, Mirochnick M, et al: Neonatal necrotizing enterocolitis with intestinal perforation in extremely premature infants receiving early indomethacin treatment for patent ductus arteriosus. *J Perinatol* 22:535–540, 2002.

Hall AH, Smolinske SC, Conrad FL, et al: Ibuprofen overdose: 126 cases. *Ann Emerg Med* 15:1308, 1986.

Hall AH, Smolinske SC, Stover B, et al: Ibuprofen overdose in adults. *Clin Toxicol* 30:23, 1992.

Litalien C, Jacqz-Aigrain E: Risks and benefits of nonsteroidal anti-inflammatory drugs in children: A comparison with paracetamol. *Paediatr Drugs* 3:817–858, 2001.

Martinez R, Smith DW, Frankel LR: Severe metabolic acidosis after acute naproxen sodium ingestion. *Ann Emerg Med* 18: 1102, 1989.

Smolinske SC, Hall AH, Vandenburg SA, et al: Toxic effects of nonsteroidal anti-inflammatory drugs in overdose. *Drug Safety* 5:252–274, 1990.

Watson WA, Litovitz TL, Rodgers GC, et al: 2002 Annual report of the American association of poison control centers toxic exposure surveillance system. *Am J Emerg Med* 21: 353–421, 2003.

32

Caffeine

Carson R. Harris

HIGH-YIELD FACTS

- Caffeine is present in many beverages, over-the-counter products, and prescription medications.
- Caffeine is a stimulant that can be easily abused by teens and may lead to seizures, tachydysrhythmias, and psychomotor agitation.
- Treatment is generally supportive. With severe toxicity, hemodialysis and charcoal hemoperfusion enhance elimination of caffeine.

CASE PRESENTATION

A 3-year-old child is brought to the emergency department (ED) at 3:00 AM for being hyperactive, with a history of multiple diarrheal stools the previous evening. The child's mother states that he will not go to bed, and has been very active since leaving the pediatric clinic earlier in the afternoon. The patient was seen for flu syndrome. The mother has not given the child any medications and she does not believe he has ingested any other medications at home.

On physical examination, the child is very active and will not sit still in the room. He jumps on and off the examination table and attempts to play with the chair pushing it around the examination room and making car noises. He appears diaphoretic. The nurse estimated the child's pulse to be 180 bpm and blood pressure (BP) 130/78 mmHg. The tympanic temperature is 99.9°F. The pupils are 4 to 5 mm and reactive to light, mucus membranes moist, and tympanic membranes are clear. The neck is supple. Heart examination reveals tachycardia. The child does not appear to be tender in the abdomen. The skin reveals no bruising or abnormal rash.

INTRODUCTION AND EPIDEMIOLOGY

Caffeine is widely consumed throughout the world, and is probably the most frequently ingested pharmacologically active substance. It is commonly found in beverages, chocolates, and in prescription and over-the-counter (OTC) medications. The caffeine content of various beverages and medications are listed in Tables 32–1, 32–2, and 32–3.

DEVELOPMENTAL CONSIDERATIONS

Caffeine is a source of energy for many people who seek increased stamina to maintain their rigorous schedules. Many are unaware of the dangers associated with too much caffeine, especially for chronic users. Diet aids are a multibillion dollar business marketed across all ages, including to preteens and adolescents. Many of these products contain caffeine or guarana, a natural caffeine-like substance.

Parents may administer a child caffeinated beverages during the course of an acute illness; if the intake is not closely monitored, the child may become caffeine toxic. Adolescents are attuned to the effects of certain beverages, and advertisers tend to target this population, increasing their vulnerability to the effects of excess use of caffeine.

Table 32–1. Caffeine Content of Beverages

Beverage	Caffeine Content
Coffee	
Regular drip	106–164 mg/5 oz
Regular percolated	93–134 mg/5 oz
Regular instant	7–68 mg/5 oz
Decaffeinated	2–5 mg/5 oz
Tea	
1-min brew	21–33 mg/5 oz
3-min brew	35–46 mg/5 oz
5-min brew	39–50 mg/5 oz
Canned iced tea	22–36 mg/5 oz
Cocoa and chocolate	
Cocoa beverage (mix)	2–8 mg/6 oz
Milk chocolate	6 mg/oz
Sweet chocolate	20 mg/oz
Baking chocolate	35 mg/oz
Hot cocoa	14 mg
Chocolate milk	2–7 mg/8 oz

Source: From: Cheesebrow D: Caffeine. In: Harris CR, ed: *Emergency Management of Selected Drugs of Abuse.* Dallas: ACEP; 2000.

PHARMACOLOGY AND TOXICOKINETICS

Caffeine is rapidly absorbed after oral administration. The presence of food in the stomach does not alter its absorption. It is freely and equally distributed throughout body water, and has a volume of distribution of 0.5 L/kg. The plasma half-life is approximately 3.5 hours. Once absorbed, caffeine is metabolized by the liver into the inactive metabolites of methyluric acid and methylxanthine. The major active metabolite of caffeine is theophylline.

Doses greater than 2.6 mg/kg/d can lead to adverse effects in children. Definite toxicity can be expected with greater than 6 mg/kg/d, including CNS and cardiovascular symptoms. Ventricular dysrhythmia, seizures, pulmonary edema, and severe metabolic acidosis have been associated with intake of 200 to 300 mg/kg.

PATHOPHYSIOLOGY

Caffeine is an analeptic or psychostimulant that is a derivative of methylxanthine. It increases the permeability of the sarcoplasmic reticulum to calcium, thus leading to increased contractility of cardiac and skeletal muscles. Caffeine antagonizes adenosine receptors, specifically A_1, which increases sympathomimetic effects. Inhibition of phosphodiesterase increases cyclic adenosine monophosphate, and there is inhibition of smooth muscle contraction. Caffeine causes an increase in gastric secretions and has moderate diuretic properties. Excess doses of caffeine result in increased levels of norepinephrine, dopamine, and serotonin in the brain. These neurotransmitters can cause the common clinical effects noted with caffeine use and toxicity.

Table 32–2. Caffeine Content in Soft Drinks

Soft Drink	Average Caffeine Content (mg)	Soft Drink	Average Caffeine Content (mg)
Krank20 (bottled water)	71 mg/12 oz	Sugar-free Mr. Pibb	58
Surge	53	Mountain Dew	55
Water Joe	45 mg/12oz	Mello-Yello	53
Kick	58	Coca-Cola Classic	47
Red Bull (8.3 oz)	80	Diet Coke	47
Jolt	72	Dr. Pepper	40
Josta	58	Sunkist Orange	40
RC Edge	70	Pepsi Cola	38
XTC Power Drink	70	Canada Dry Jamaica Cola	30
Battery Energy Drink	46	Shasta Cherry Cola	44
KMX	53	Tab	47

The U.S. Food & Drug Administration allows a maximum of 72 mg of caffeine per 12-oz serving (6 mg/oz).
Sources: Christian Science Monitor, Prevention, and erowid.org.

Table 32–3. Caffeine Content of OTC and Prescription Medications

Medication	Caffeine Content
Stimulants	
No-doz	100
Vivarin	200
Pain relievers	
Anacin	32
Excedrin	65
Excedrin PM	0
Midol (for cramps)	32
Midol (PMS)	0
Vanquish	33
Dexatrim	200
Prescription	
Cafergot	100
Darvon compound-65	32.4
Fioricet/Fiorinol	40
Migralam	100

Source: Information on caffeine content and standard dosages obtained from *Physician's Desk Reference* (2002) and *Physician's Desk Reference for Non-prescription Drugs* (2002).

CLINICAL PRESENTATION

In children, acute oral doses of 80 to 100 mg/kg of caffeine have produced severe symptoms. Stimulation of the myocardium causing tachycardia, dysrhythmias, and extrasystoles can occur. Hypertension secondary to vasoconstriction is common. Patients may appear agitated and anxious, with increased psychomotor activity. A hyperadrenergic state is seen in most children with acute caffeine toxicity; manifestations include excitement, insomnia, flushed face, gastrointestinal (GI) complaints, rambling thoughts and speech, periods of inexhaustibility, and psychomotor agitation. Seizures can occur in significant overdoses. Hyperglycemia can result from catecholamine-induced increase in gluconeogenesis, lipolysis, and glycogenolysis. Potassium can be shifted intracellularly through a catecholamine-induced mechanism leading to hypokalemia. Rhabdomyolysis has been reported after caffeine overdose.

Other manifestations of caffeine use/abuse fall into several typical presentations. The anxiety presentation in children and adolescents mimics hyperactivity. Symptoms include diuresis, restlessness, tremulousness, hyperactivity, irritability, dry mouth, dysesthesias, tinnitus, ocular dyskinesias, and scotomata. In a hypochondriasis-like presentation, the patient complains of vague, nonspecific complaints such as generalized discomfort, tremor, and myalgias. The insomnia and/or headache presentation is characterized by difficulty sleeping, or increased motility during sleep. Withdrawal headaches with nausea and vomiting can occur in moderate or sporadic users of caffeine products. Other withdrawal symptoms include nausea, yawning, drowsiness or lethargy, rhinorrhea, irritability, nervousness, and poor attention in school. The depressive presentation is seen in heavy users of caffeine products (>750 mg/d). Patients generally present with a depressed mood and affect.

LABORATORY AND DIAGNOSTIC TESTING

The diagnosis of caffeine toxicity is made by a detailed history and exclusion of other organic etiologies. A comprehensive urine toxicology screen may detect caffeine. In selected cases evaluation of serum electrolytes may be indicated to assess serum potassium. An electrocardiogram is indicated in patients with severe toxicity and associated tachycardia or dysrhythmias.

MANAGEMENT

In the majority of cases, caffeine overuse in children is due to beverages and activated charcoal has no value. If, however, the child has ingested a significant amount of a caffeine-containing medication and presents to the ED within 1 hour, activated charcoal can be administered at a dose of 1 g/kg.

Supraventricular tachydysrhythmias can be treated with esmolol 500 μg/kg over 2 minutes, then a 200-μg/kg/min infusion. Ventricular dysrhythmias should be managed according to standard protocol. Seizures can be treated with benzodiazepines or phenobarbital. Hemodialysis and charcoal hemoperfusion have been safely used to remove caffeine in severe intoxications. There is no specific antidote for caffeine overdose.

DISPOSITION

Children presenting with severe intoxication such as dehydration, dysrhythmia, or seizures should be monitored as inpatients. Cardiac monitoring and seizure precautions are necessary. Generally, mild and moderate toxicity can be monitored in the ED or observation unit for 6 to 10 hours and the patient can be discharged if stable.

CASE OUTCOME

The mother is given instructions to push fluids upon leaving the pediatrician's office. The only fluid she could get the child to drink was Mountain Dew, which contains 54 mg of caffeine for every 12 ounces of fluid. The patient was admitted to the pediatric ward and monitored for 12 hours. He was treated with intravenous fluids and gradually returned to normal activity and vital signs at discharge. The parents were educated on caffeine content of popular beverages at discharge.

SUGGESTED READINGS

Benowitz NL, Osterloh J, Goldschlager N, et al: Massive catecholamine release from caffeine poisoning. *JAMA* 248:1097–1098, 1982.

Cheesebrow D: Caffeine. In: Harris CR, ed: *Emergency Management of Selected Drugs of Abuse*. Dallas: ACEP; 2000.

Christian MS, Brent RL: Teratogen update: evaluation of the reproductive and developmental risks of caffeine. *Teratology* 64:51–78, 2001.

Ford RPK, Schluter PJ, Mitchell EA, et al: Heavy caffeine intake in pregnancy and sudden infant death syndrome. *Arch Dis Child* 78:9–13, 1998.

Field AS, Laurienti PJ, Yen YF, et al: Dietary caffeine consumption and withdrawal: Confounding variables in quantitative cerebral perfusion studies? *Radiology* 227:129–135, 2003.

Hurlbut, KM, Hall AH, Kuffner E, et al: Caffeine. In: *Thomson POISINDEX*. Micromedex Healthcare Series, Vol. 115, expires 3/2003.

Nawrot P, Jordan S, Eastwood J, et al: Effects of caffeine on human health. *Food Addit Contam* 20:1–30, 2003.

33

Vitamins

Deborah L. Anderson

HIGH-YIELD FACTS

- Acute toxicity is unlikely following ingestion of vitamin products that do not contain iron or fluoride.

- Chronic use of vitamins A and D can cause toxicity.

- An excessive amount of vitamin A can cause increased intracranial pressure.

- Acute ingestion of niacin can cause dermal flushing and pruritis.

- The diagnosis of vitamin overdose is usually based on the history of ingestion.

CASE PRESENTATION

A mother calls after finding her 5-year-old son feeding her 2-year-old, 12-kg daughter an unknown number of children's chewable multivitamins. She reports finding a 100-count bottle with the child-resistant top removed and vitamins in her daughter's mouth. The child is asymptomatic.

INTRODUCTION AND EPIDEMIOLOGY

Vitamins are one of the top ten substances involved in pediatric poisoning exposures, with 42,150 exposures in children younger than 6 years reported to U.S. poison centers in 2001. In addition, there were 4739 ingestions in children ages 6 to 19 years of age. A variety of vitamin products account for these exposures, including multiple vitamins in pediatric and adult formulations, products with or without iron and/or fluoride, tablet and liquid preparations, and single-ingredient formulations. The single most important factor leading to overdose is simply the accessibility of multiple vitamin preparations. Given the wide use of vitamins, the scarcity of reported adverse effects suggests that these products as a group are fairly safe. Ingestion of vitamin products that do not contain iron or fluoride are unlikely to cause acute toxicity, but chronic use of vitamins A and D certainly may.

DEVELOPMENTAL CONSIDERATIONS

Vitamin overdose is common among toddlers. Parental concern over children's eating patterns results in routine vitamin supplementation to ensure adequate nutrition. The candy-like appearance, the sweet fruity flavors, and the animal or cartoon character shapes make these products attractive to children (Figure 33–1). Child-resistant containers may slow children down, but do not remove the threat of poisoning. Dean and Krenzelok determined that the child's own dietary supplement was implicated in 93% of reported vitamin exposures. In 18.2% of these cases, more than one child was involved in the poisoning incident. Adolescents may take megavitamin therapy for their advertised health benefits, or with the belief that more is better. In addition, with the widespread availability of vitamin supplements, suicidal adolescents will have access to a variety of these products right in their own homes.

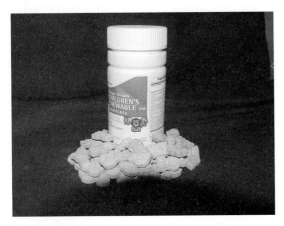

Fig. 33–1. Generic children's chewable multivitamins.

PHARMACOLOGY, TOXICOKINETICS, AND PATHOPHYSIOLOGY

Vitamin A

Vitamin A is a fat-soluble vitamin that when absorbed is transported by retinol-binding protein to its primary storage site, the liver. Hypervitaminosis A occurs when the retinal-binding protein carrying system and the liver become saturated from excessive intake of vitamin A (Table 33–1). The free vitamin A in plasma binds with lipoprotein membranes, causing increased permeability and decreased stability, and is responsible for dermatologic abnormalities and bone malformations. Excessive deposition of vitamin A in liver cells leads to hepatoxicity. The mechanism by which vitamin A causes increased intracranial pressure is unknown. Acute ingestions of 300,000 IU of vitamin A in children can cause toxicity, with signs and symptoms developing within 4 to 8 hours postingestion. Chronic hypervitaminosis A has occurred with repeated ingestion of 25,000 IU/d for 2 or more weeks.

Vitamin B$_6$

Vitamin B$_6$, or pyridoxine, is a water-soluble vitamin that when taken acutely elicits no ill effects. Chronic low-dose therapy of as little as 200 mg/d can produce a sensory neuropathy in some individuals; the mechanism by which this occurs is unknown.

Vitamin C

Vitamin C, or ascorbic acid, is a water-soluble vitamin that is metabolized to oxalic acid. Excessive doses may increase oxalate excretion and produce nephrolithiasis. Unexplained hemolysis has occurred in patients deficient in glucose 6-phosphate. Premature neonates may be susceptible to hemolytic anemia associated with vitamin C supplementation.

Vitamin D

Vitamin D is a fat-soluble vitamin synthesized in the skin from a combination of cholesterol and exposure to sunlight. Toxic effects are usually due to over-supplementation; acute ingestion rarely causes toxicity. Chronic ingestion of more than 2000 IU/d from supplements, fortified dairy products, or infant formulas causes an increase in calcium levels by facilitating calcium absorption and mobilizing calcium from bone.

Niacin

Niacin, or vitamin B$_3$, is a water-soluble vitamin that commonly produces an acute vasodilatory syndrome that is prostaglandin mediated. Intense cutaneous flushing can last up to 2 to 3 hours; there is no other known toxicity. Chronic use of sustained-release preparations has caused hepatoxicity by an unknown mechanism.

CLINICAL FINDINGS

Most acute overdoses of multivitamins are associated with nausea, vomiting, and diarrhea.

Vitamin A

Acute exposure may produce significant increases in intracranial pressure. This may result in anorexia, vomiting, irritability, lethargy, and, in infants, bulging fontanelles. With chronic use of vitamin A, it is common to see alopecia, skin desquamation and erythema, fissuring at lip corners, pruritis, photophobia, headache, hepatomegaly, joint pain, bone pain and tenderness, and premature epiphyseal closure. As with acute toxicity, increased intracranial pressure can also occur.

Vitamin B$_6$

Sensory neuropathy is the primary manifestation of chronic exposure. Muscular incoordination, decreased or absent deep tendon reflexes, and decreased sensation to touch, pain, and temperature in a stocking-glove distribution are common. Muscle strength is preserved. With

Table 33–1. Signs and Symptoms of Pediatric Vitamin Toxicity

	Acute	Chronic
Vitamin A	Anorexia Bulging fontanelles Increased intracranial pressure Irritability Lethargy Vomiting	Alopecia Anorexia Bone pain and tenderness Bulging fontanelles Fissuring at lip corners Headache Hepatomegaly Increased intracranial pressure (pseudotumor cerebri) Irritability Joint pain Lethargy Photophobia Premature epiphyseal closure Pruritis Skin desquamation Skin erythema Vomiting
Vitamin B_1 (thiamine)	Gastrointestinal irritation	
Vitamin B_2 (riboflavin)	Turns the urine bright yellow	
Vitamin B_3 (niacin)	Gastrointestinal irritation Cutaneous flushing Headache Pruritis Vasodilation	Hepatotoxicity

Vitamin B_6 (pyridoxine)	Gastrointestinal irritation	Sensory neuropathy
		  – Muscular incoordination
		  – Diminished deep tendon reflexes
		  – Decreased sensation to touch,
		    pain, temperature

Vitamin B_{12} (cyanocobalamin)	Gastrointestinal irritation	

Vitamin C	Gastrointestinal irritation
	Large ingestions
	  – Acute renal failure
	  – Anemia
	  – Hemoglobinuria
	  – Hemolysis
	  – Nephrolithiasis	

Vitamin E	Gastrointestinal irritation	
Folic acid	Gastrointestinal irritation	

time, most patients recover fully, although permanent deficits can result.

Vitamin C

Self-limited gastrointestinal (GI) symptoms such as nausea and vomiting are common with overdose. Nephrolithiasis, acute renal failure, hemolysis, anemia, and hemoglobinuria can rarely occur.

Vitamin D

Symptoms seen with chronic excessive intake of vitamin D are similar to those of hypercalcemia: GI upset, headache, irritability, weakness, hypertension, renal tubular injury, and occasionally cardiac arrhythmias. Some infants may present simply with failure to thrive.

Niacin

Acute ingestion of regular release formulations of niacin commonly causes cutaneous flushing, vasodilation, headache, and pruritis. Niacin-induced hepatoxicity is uncommon, but when it occurs it is generally dose related and associated with sustained-release products.

LABORATORY AND DIAGNOSTIC TESTING

Diagnosis of vitamin overdose is most commonly made based on history of ingestion. When assessing the potential for toxicity it is important to identify the specific ingredients in the preparation, especially to ensure that the product does not contain iron or fluoride. It is also useful to calculate the quantity of vitamins A and D ingested, and to determine if the exposure is acute or chronic.

A plasma vitamin A level is useful in confirming a suspected diagnosis after chronic exposure, but is not clinically useful in determining prognosis or treatment. In patients with symptomatic chronic hypervitaminosis A, elevated levels of aminotransferases, alkaline phosphatase, and bilirubin and increased INR are commonly seen. Hypercalcemia and an elevated erythrocyte sedimentation rate are common. Increased intracranial pressure can be confirmed via computed tomography of the head or higher entry pressures on lumbar puncture. Bone radiography may reveal osteopenia and periosteal new bone growth in children.

Measuring other vitamin concentrations is not useful. With chronic vitamin D exposure, monitor calcium and phosphate levels as well as renal function tests to rule out damage from hypercalciuria. With large ingestions of vitamin C, consider obtaining a urinalysis to rule out uricosuria. Radiographs for visualization of the vitamin supplement are not useful for products that do not contain iron.

MANAGEMENT

Exposure to the vitamin preparation should be discontinued. There are no specific antidotes for vitamin toxicity. Gastric decontamination is generally unnecessary, except with acute vitamin A exposures exceeding 300,000 IU in children. Fluid loss caused by vomiting and diarrhea should be treated with oral or intravenous fluids. Antiemetics or antidiarrheals are helpful for prolonged or severe vomiting and diarrhea.

Increased intracranial pressure from acute and chronic hypervitaminosis A commonly improves upon discontinuation of vitamin A. Rarely, more aggressive therapy with mannitol, steroids, and hyperventilation may be necessary.

Patients with hypercalcemia from vitamin D toxicity should be placed on a low calcium diet. In severe cases hydration, loop diuretics, steroids, calcitonin, sodium EDTA, or mithramycin may be considered.

DISPOSITION

The majority of vitamin ingestions can be managed over the telephone, and advised that an emergency department visit is unnecessary. Children who develop more than mild GI symptoms should be referred to a health care facility for evaluation. In most cases, symptoms begin to resolve within days of discontinuation of vitamin use, and patients can be monitored on an outpatient basis. Hospital admission is necessary for patients with significant hypercalcemia, hemolysis, renal or hepatic failure, or cardiac dysrhythmias.

CASE OUTCOME

The caller is prompted to read the label and determines that there is no iron or fluoride in the multivitamin product. A tablet count is performed to help estimate the maximum number of tablets the child could have ingested. The child could have ingested 43 tablets by estimation, each containing 2,500 IU of vitamin A. The total amount of vitamin A ingested is calculated to be 107,500 IU, a quantity well below the threshold for causing acute toxicity. After explaining that the child may experience some minor GI irritation and a bright yellow discoloration of the urine, dilution to decrease the gastrointestinal irritability is recommended, along with observation at home.

SUGGESTED READINGS

Ballin A, Brown EJ, Koren G, et al: Vitamin C-induced erythrocyte damage in premature infants. *J Pediatr* 113: 114–120, 1988.

Chesney RW: Vitamin D: Can an upper limit be defined? *J Nutr* 119:1825–1828, 1989.

Dean BS, Krenzelok EP: Multiple vitamins and vitamins with iron: accidental poisoning in children. *Vet Hum Toxicol* 30:23–24, 1988.

Hathcock JN, Hattan DG, Jenkins MY, et al: Evaluation of vitamin A toxicity. *Am J Clin Nutr* 52:183–202, 1990.

Jacobus CH, Holick MF, Shoa Q, et al: Hypervitaminosis D associated with drinking milk. *N Engl J Med* 326:1173–1177, 1992.

Litovitz, TL, Klein-Schwartz W, Rodgers GC, et al: 2001 annual report of the American Association of Poison Control Centers Toxic Exposure Surveillance System. *Am J Emerg Med* 20:391–452, 2002.

Menna VJ: Index of suspicion. Case 2. Diagnosis: Niacin overdose. *Pediatr Rev* 14:433–435, 1993.

Meyers DG, Maloley PA, Weeks D: Safety of antioxidant vitamins. *Arch Intern Med* 156:925–935, 1996.

Pasquariello PS, Schut L, Borns P: Benign increased intracranial hypertension due to chronic vitamin A overdosage in a 26-month-old child. *Clin Pediatr* 16:379–382, 1977.

Pundzien B, Dobilien D, Surkus J: Severe vitamin D overdose in two infants (abstract). *J Toxicol Clin Toxicol* 39:310, 2001.

Schaumburg H, Kaplan J, Windebank A, et al: Sensory neuropathy from pyridoxine abuse: A new megavitamin syndrome. *N Engl J Med* 309:445–448, 1983.

34

Prescription Drugs

Frank P. Paloucek

HIGH-YIELD FACTS

- Prescription drug products have been a significant source of serious and fatal pediatric poisonings.

- Comparing recent findings to data from 10 years previously, it can be noted that there have been some changes in pediatric poisoning epidemiology from medicinal agents and prescription drugs.

- Most prescription drug-related pediatric fatalities over the past 5 years have resulted from opioids, antidepressants, cardiovasculars, sedative-hypnotics, and anticonvulsant toxicity.

- Ferrous sulfate is no longer the most common cause of unintentional pediatric poisoning deaths as compared to 10 years ago.

- Opioid agents such as methadone have become the leading a cause of unintentional pediatric deaths from prescription drugs over the past 5 years.

- Interventions targeted at preventing pediatric opioid poisoning may reduce pediatric mortality secondary to unintentional exposures.

Prescription drug products have long been a significant source of serious and fatal pediatric poisonings. Surveillance of the epidemiology of pediatric poisonings has led to packaging innovations and legal limits to total doses that have had a profound impact on pediatric poisoning mortality. This is most classically illustrated with children's aspirin, but can also be noted with recent packaging initiatives for ferrous sulfate.

The most important epidemiologic database for identifying common agents, most lethal agents, and emerging trends in pediatric poisonings is the Toxic Exposure Surveillance System (TESS) of the American Association of Poison Control Centers. This report, published annually since 1984, summarizes all calls to participating certified poison control centers in the United States for the previous year. Beginning with all calls for 1983 and through the recent summary for 2002, the cumulative database represents 33.8 million human exposures. Although this is an impressive cumulative total, it must be balanced with the inherent flaws of the data collection method, which probably under represents the true frequency and mortality of poisonings. All annual TESS data summaries since 1984 are also available at www.aapcc.org/poison1.htm. This database has been analyzed for pediatric poisoning epidemiology twice. First, all pediatric exposures reported from 1985 to 1989, a total of 3.8 million exposures, were analyzed to generate a hazard factor rating and to list the most common causes of pediatric fatalities from pharmaceutical and nonpharmaceutical ingestions. Second, all pediatric exposures for 1998 were extracted from the cumulative 1998 database. The purpose of this chapter is to review the cumulative TESS data for the 5-year period of 1997 through 2001, focusing on pharmaceutical agent exposures in pediatric patients (Table 34–1).

From 1997 to 2001, TESS recorded 11,070,553 toxic exposures; 5,799,010 occurred in patients 19 years or less in age. The overall incidence of pediatric exposures is consistently about 60%. Most exposures occurred in the under 6 age group. Despite representing a majority of

Table 34–1. Cumulative Total and Pediatric Exposures in the TESS, 1997 to 2001

	1997	1998	1999	2000	2001	5-Year Total
Total calls	2,192,088	2,241,082	2,201,156	2,168,248	2,267,979	11,070,553
Pediatric calls						
<6 y	115,0931	1,181,006	1,154,799	1,142,796	1,169,478	5,799,010
6–12 y	152,988	158,351	154,606	151,221	156,612	773,778
13–19 y	160,707	158,518	157,993	160,505	165,657	803,380
Total deaths	786	775	873	920	1,074	4,428
<6 y	25	16	24	20	26	111
6–12 y	4	5	8	6	12	35
13–19 y	48	46	53	66	77	290

exposures, pediatric exposures account for only about 10% of reported fatalities. It is important to note the increased trends in the 13- to 19-year-old age group for pediatric deaths compared to the 6 to 12 year olds. This is mostly likely due to an increase in intentional overdose as well as drug abuse and misuse.

Of the 436 pediatric toxic exposure deaths listed in Table 34–1, 418 occurred in patients less 18 years old or younger. In this population, the most common cause of death was prescription medications. When over-the-counter medications were added, medicinal substances contributed to 52% of pediatric deaths. Street drugs (13%) and nonpharmaceutical substances (33%) represented the remainder of reported causes of death. It is interesting to note that the nonpharmaceutical substances category also included the volatile hydrocarbons. Intentional abuse of these chemical substances was implicated to be the cause of death in 48 of the 140 deaths in this category (Table 34–2).

The five most common categories of substances involved in toxic exposure deaths for all ages has remained unchanged over the 1997 to 2001 period, although there has been some changes in the order (Table 34–2). These five categories typically account for 70% to 75% of all deaths reported in TESS. Regarding medicinal substances involved in pediatric deaths, that there is little change from the overall data. Analgesics, antidepressants, cardiovasculars, sedative-hypnotics/antipsychotics, and anticonvulsants constitute the five most common substances implicated. However, these five categories only account for 40% of pediatric deaths. This is most likely explained by the overrepresentation of nonmedicinals as a cause of death in pediatrics versus adults, owing to intentional abuse of volatile substances.

One of the most significant findings in the death data is the relative absence of iron as a cause of pediatric mortality (Table 34–3). In the review of TESS data from 1985 to 1989, iron caused 11 unintentional pediatric deaths. Over the 1997 to 2001 data, there were only three reported iron deaths; two were unintentional. This strongly suggests federally mandated packaging require-

Table 34–2. Categories With Largest Numbers of Deaths (All Ages) in the TESS From 1997 to 2001

Rank	1997	1998	1999	2000	2001
1	Analgesics	Analgesics	Analgesics	Analgesics	Analgesics
2	Antidepressants	Antidepressants	Antidepressants	Antidepressants	Sedative/antipsychotics
3	Sedative/ antipsychotics	Stimulants/ street drugs	Cardiovasculars	Sedative/ antipsychotics	Antidepressants
4	Stimulants/ street drugs	Cardiovasculars	Stimulants/ street drugs	Stimulants/ street drugs	Stimulants/street drugs
5	Alcohols	Sedative/ antipsychotics	Sedative/ antipsychotics	Cardiovasculars	Cardiovasculars

Table 34–3. Pediatric Deaths From Medicinal Products (Intentional and Unintentional) Reported by TESS for 1997 Through 2001

Deaths Category	(% of pediatric deaths)
Analgesics	88 (21)
Acetaminophen	33
Opioids	31
Methadone	11
Oxycodone	8
Morphine	6
Hydrocodone	3
Others	3
Aspirin	24
Antidepressants	41 (9.8)
TCAs	28
SSRIs	13
Cardiovasculars	13 (3.1)
Calcium channel blockers	5
Digoxin	2
Others	6
Sedative-hypnotics/antipsychotics	11 (2.6)
Anticonvulsants	8 (2)
Carbamazepine	5
Valproic acid	3
Fosphenytoin	2
Others	27

Abbreviations: SSRIs, selective serotonin reuptake inhibitors; TCAs, tricyclic antidepressants.

ments instituted for iron in 1997 are direct cause for the reduction in mortality. This represents the second significant success in reducing pediatric mortality from toxic exposures, after child-resistant caps and package tablet count limits were mandated for children's aspirin. It is noteworthy that methadone is the most frequent opioid responsible for pediatric deaths (11 cases). These findings were not duplicated in the adult population. This may be explained by the fact that methadone is commonly dispensed as in a liquid formulation, mixed with juice, and dosed for patients with significant tolerance to opioid activity. This suggests a need for patient and caretaker education, and potentially an intervention in packaging or formulation. Also noteworthy is the large number of oxycodone deaths (eight cases). This may represent the introduction and significant prescribing of new, intensely marketed oxycodone products.

Table 34–4. Medicinal Substances Involved in Pediatric Deaths Associated With Therapeutic Errors Reported by TESS, 1997 to 2001

Medicinal substances	Number of Deaths
Acetaminophen	4
Digoxin	2
Fosphenytoin	2
Others	12

Fourteen of the pediatric deaths involved adverse reactions; no medicinal substance was listed more than once. There were 20 deaths, 12 in children younger than 2, involving therapeutic errors. These are summarized in Table 34–4.

Significant is the three specific agents listed. All four acetaminophen deaths occurred in children 2 years of age or younger. Three were chronic overmedications cases and one involved acute acetaminophen use with ecstasy exposure. Over the 5-year period for all age groups, digoxin has been the most commonly involved medicinal substance, accounting for approximately 70% of all cases. This agent is clearly underrepresented in pediatrics. The two reported pediatric fosphenytoin deaths over the entire period were in children between the ages of 1 and 2 years.

For unintentional general exposures, an analysis of pediatric toxic exposures deaths reported by TESS from 1983 to 1990 identified 97 total deaths from unintentional exposure, 53 from medicinal substances. In descending order, the four most common causes of unintentional death were ferrous sulfate ($n = 16$), antidepressants ($n = 10$), salicylates ($n = 6$; 4 due to methyl salicylate), and calcium channel blockers ($n = 4$).

Table 34–5. A Comparison of the Most Common Medicinals Associated With Unintentional Pediatric Deaths Reported by TESS 1983 to 1990 Versus 1997 to 2001

Rank	1983 to 1990 (deaths, n)	1997 to 2001 (deaths, n)
1	Ferrous sulfate (16)	Opioids (6)
2	Antidepressants (10)	Salicylates (3)
3	Cardiovascular (7)	Antidepressants (2)
4	Salicylates (6)	Ferrous sulfate (2)
5	Anticonvulsants (3)	Cardiovascular (2)

The data from 1997 to 2001 revealed only 54 total deaths, with 21 from medicinal substances (Table 34–5). Opioids caused six deaths with methadone responsible for half of these fatalities. Salicylates caused three deaths, none of which were due to methyl salicylate. Antidepressants and ferrous sulfate each caused two deaths. No other agent or category was implicated in more than one death.

CONCLUSION

The TESS data provide an opportunity to adapt clinical toxicology and poison prevention education or interventions on the basis of a very large database. Comparing recent findings to data from 10 years previously, it can be noted that there have been some changes in pediatric poisoning epidemiology from medicinal agents. Ferrous sulfate being diminished in incidence and mortality is one of the most significant changes. Medicinals do remain significantly associated both with pediatric exposures in general, and with pediatric mortality secondary to toxic exposure. Analgesics, antidepressants, cardiovasculars, sedative-hypnotics/antipsychotics, and anticonvulsants remain agents requiring education, intervention, and research. Toxic opioid exposure from agents like methadone appears to require focused attention with the intent that this overrepresented pediatric cause of mortality be reduced.

Chapters 35 through 45 discuss individual prescription drugs that can lead to significant toxicity in the pediatric patient. Each chapter discusses the epidemiology, toxicologic profile, diagnosis, and management of each specific pharmacologic agent.

SUGGESTED READINGS

Litovitz TL, Klein-Schwartz W, Dyer KS, et al: 1997 annual report of the American Association of Poison Control Centers Toxic Exposure Surveillance System. *Am J Emerg Med* 16:443–497, 1998.

Litovitz TL, Klein-Schwartz W, Caravati EM, et al: 1998 annual report of the American Association of Poison Control Centers Toxic Exposure Surveillance System. *Am J Emerg Med* 17:435–487, 1999.

Litovitz TL, Klein-Schwartz W, White S, et al: 1999 annual report of the American Association of Poison Control Centers Toxic Exposure Surveillance System. *Am J Emerg Med* 18:517–574, 2000.

Litovitz TL, Klein-Schwartz W, White S, et al: 2000 annual report of the American Association of Poison Control Centers Toxic Exposure Surveillance System. *Am J Emerg Med* 19:337–395, 2001.

Litovitz TL, Klein-Schwartz W, Rodgers GC, et al: 2001 annual report of the American Association of Poison Control Centers Toxic Exposure Surveillance System. *Am J Emerg Med* 20:391–452, 2002.

Litovitz TL, Manoguerra A: Comparison of pediatric poisoning hazards: An analysis of 3.8 million exposure incidents. *Pediatrics* 89:999–1006, 1992.

35

Antihypertensives, β-Blockers, and Calcium Antagonists

Kenneth Bizovi

HIGH-YIELD FACTS

- β-Blockers are made in both immediate-release and sustained-release formulations. The formulation of the drug affects the onset of symptoms and the length of observation after exposure.

- Cardiovascular manifestations of β-blocker toxicity include hypotension, bradycardia, heart block, and congestive heart failure.

- In patients with symptomatic bradycardia and hypotension from β-blocker toxicity, glucagon is often used to reverse the toxic effects.

- Additional treatment of β-blocker toxicity includes aggressive fluid resuscitation and adrenergic agonists. Epinephrine is the adrenergic agonist of choice.

- Different pharmacologic profiles of calcium channel blockers cause various presentations, but in all cases, the cardiovascular effects predominate. Verapamil and diltiazem typically cause bradycardia and hypotension.

- In calcium channel blocker overdose with hypotension, fluid administration, calcium salts, glucagon, and therapy with adrenergic agonists is indicated.

- High-dose insulin and dextrose therapy has been shown to be effective in the management of calcium channel blocker overdose.

- Clonidine-induced bradycardia is treated with atropine if it is associated with hypotension.

- Naloxone may reverse the opiate-like side effects of clonidine on mental status and respiration.

CASE PRESENTATION

The patient is a 3-year-old child who presents after getting into his grandfather's blood pressure medications 2 hours prior to presentation to the emergency department (ED). Presenting vital signs demonstrate a heart rate of 60 bpm, blood pressure of 70/40 mmHg, respiratory rate of 16 breaths per minute, and a temperature of 97°F. The child is sleepy, but easily awakened with an intact airway. The lungs are clear to auscultation and the heart examination reveals a bradycardic, regular rate and rhythm. The abdomen is soft and nontender with normoactive bowel sounds. Examination of the child's extremities reveals thready peripheral pulses without cyanosis. The parents bring in an empty pill bottle of atenolol 50 mg (#30) that was filled 2 weeks prior.

β-ADRENERGIC BLOCKING AGENTS

β-Blockers are a diverse category of drugs that are used in the treatment of hypertension, thyrotoxicosis, dysrhythmias, angina, migraine headaches, withdrawal states, and glaucoma. In 2002, the American Academy of Poison Control Centers (AAPCC) reported 14,113 β-blocker exposures. There were 3501 (24%) in children younger than 6 years of age, and 1056 (7.5%) in children ages 6 to

19 years. There were a total of 39 deaths, with one pediatric death after metoprolol exposure. The rate of mortality after exposure for β-blocker overdose is much lower than that of overdose from calcium channel antagonists or digoxin, but it is still 10 times higher than the mortality rate for all other exposures.

Pharmacology

β-Blocker properties that determine the drug's effect are β_1-antagonist activity, β_2-antagonist activity, intrinsic sympathomimetic activity, and membrane-stabilizing activity. Labetalol is the only β-blocker that has α-antagonist activity. β_1-Antagonist activity causes decreased cardiac contractility and conduction. β_2-Antagonist activity causes increased smooth muscle tone, which manifests as bronchospasm, increased peripheral vascular tone, and increased gut motility. Although many β-blockers are β_1-selective at therapeutic doses, these drugs have both β_1 and β_2 effects in overdose.

The intrinsic sympathomimetic property of some β-blockers causes an agonist–antagonist activity, which may lead to paradoxical effects of hypertension and tachycardia in overdose. The membrane-stabilizing activity of β-blockers causes a quinidine-like effect, leading to decreased contractility. This effect is additive to the β_1 toxic effects. Membrane-stabilizing activity also causes central nervous system (CNS) depression. Lipophilic β-blockers with membrane-stabilizing activity, such as propranolol, acebutolol, and oxprenolol, have markedly increased mortality in overdose—up to 5 times greater than β-blockers without this characteristic. The α-antagonist activity of labetalol causes decreased peripheral vascular resistance. Sotalol is a β-blocker with class III antiarrhythmic properties. In overdose, this drug can cause prolongation of the QT interval and ventricular arrhythmias, including torsades de pointes. Each different β-blocker preparation may have only some of the described activities, and clinical manifestations may vary. By being aware of all of the possible effects, the clinician will be prepared to monitor the patient and address them as they occur.

Pharmacokinetics

The absorption, distribution, and elimination of β-blockers vary with the preparation. β-Blockers are available in both immediate and extended-release preparations. As with all extended-release preparations, the onset of toxic effects may be delayed. β-Blockers are rapidly absorbed, with a 30% to 90% bioavailability. The elimination half-life

varies from 2 to 24 hours, depending on the drug. In many cases, the half-life is significantly increased in overdose.

Pathophysiology

Suppression of the cardiovascular system is the hallmark of β-blocker overdose. β_1-Blockade leads to negative inotropic and chronotropic effects. Membrane-stabilizing activity further exacerbates cardiotoxicity. Deaths from β-blockers toxicity are associated with bradydysrhythmias and asystole. Ventricular arrhythmias are less common. Respiratory compromise during β-blocker overdose can result from cardiogenic shock, decreased respiratory drive, or β_2-antagonist effects. β_2-Blockade causes bronchospasm and usually affects patients with previously diagnosed bronchospastic disease. Hypoglycemia may occur secondary to β_2-mediated decrease in glycogenolysis and gluconeogenesis. CNS depression may be caused by direct toxicity, hypoxia, hypoglycemia, or shock. Drugs with membrane-stabilizing properties cause direct CNS depression.

Clinical Presentation

Owing to the rapid absorption of many β-blockers, the onset of symptoms may be as soon as 30 minutes after ingestion, but it most commonly occurs within 1 to 2 hours. The cardiovascular manifestations include hypotension, bradycardia, heart block, and congestive heart failure.

Aside from atrioventricular (AV) block, electrocardiographic (ECG) manifestations of toxicity include prolongation of the PR interval, QRS complex, and QT interval, as well as bundle branch block. Respiratory toxicity includes noncardiogenic pulmonary edema, pulmonary edema, exacerbation of asthma, and decreased respiratory drive. Patients may also present with CNS depression or seizures.

Laboratory Evaluation

Laboratory tests for blood levels of β-blockers are available from reference laboratories. These are helpful only in confirming the exposure, and are rarely clinically useful. Serum electrolytes are obtained and abnormalities addressed. Serum glucose may be low. Arterial blood gas measurement may be useful in the patient with respiratory signs or symptoms. Chest radiograph is obtained for patients who are admitted or have respiratory signs or symptoms.

All patients with a history of β-blocker ingestion are placed on a cardiac monitor and receive an ECG. ECG findings related to β-blockers exposure include first-degree heart block, QRS prolongation, QTc prolongation, and bradycardia. In one case series the majority of symptomatic patients (69%) had heart rates above 60 bpm, but systolic blood pressures below 90 mmHg.

Management

The patient with a history of β-blocker ingestion is placed on a cardiac monitor and intravenous (IV) access is established. Gastric emptying and administration of activated charcoal can decrease absorption. If the ingestion occurred less than 1 hour prior to presentation and the dose is potentially lethal, gastric emptying should be considered. Ipecac is contraindicated because rapid CNS depression may occur, leading to aspiration. In cases that present early, lavage is the preferred method of gastric decontamination. The airway should be protected in patients with altered mental status. Activated charcoal is administered after lavage. Charcoal alone is used for patients who present late after ingestion.

The patient with respiratory compromise is evaluated for the presence of pulmonary edema or bronchospasm. The patient with pulmonary edema is supported with oxygen and, if necessary, endotracheal intubation.

Patients with symptomatic bradycardia and hypotension owing to β-blocker toxicity may respond to glucagon. It is a positive inotrope that appears to work by increasing cyclic adenosine monophosphate (cAMP). In adults and older adolescents, an initial bolus of glucagon is administered IV at a dose of 3 to 5 mg over 1 minute. If symptoms recur, a repeat bolus is given. If symptoms persist, an infusion may be started at 1 to 5 mg/h. Pediatric doses of 0.05 to 0.10 mg/kg are administered IV, followed by a continuous infusion at 0.07 mg/kg/h. If glucagon is administered multiple times or as an infusion, it is mixed in normal saline or sterile water (Figure 35–1). Patients who do not respond to glucagon are treated with aggressive fluid resuscitation and sympathomimetics.

Epinephrine can be given as a continuous infusion, starting at a rate of 0.1 μg/kg/min, titrated to perfusion parameters. Dopamine, dobutamine, or the β-agonist isoproterenol may also be beneficial. It is reasonable to try atropine for patients with bradycardia, but it is frequently ineffective. For patients with bradycardia and hypotension refractory to pharmacologic intervention, temporary pacing is an option, but it too may not reverse the cardiac depression of severe β-blocker overdose.

Interventions such as intra-aortic balloon pump, extracorporeal membrane oxygenation, or cardiac bypass are considerations for patients with toxicity refractory to all other therapy. Hemodialysis and hemoperfusion are rarely useful in the setting of β-blocker overdose. Most β-blockers have a large volume of distribution and are highly protein bound, making drug removal by hemodialysis impractical. A few drugs, such as nadolol, sotalol, atenolol, and acebutolol, can be dialyzed, but information is limited to case reports. Hemodialysis can be considered for renal failure and hemodynamic instability in a drug with a low volume of distribution and low protein binding. Unstable patients often cannot tolerate the procedure, making their care difficult.

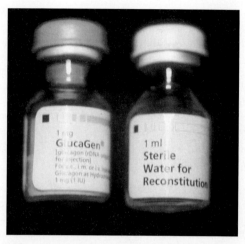

Fig. 35–1. Glucagon is the antidote of choice for β-blocker overdose.

Disposition

A patient with a history of immediate-release β-blocker ingestion is observed on a cardiac monitor for 6 hours after ingestion. Patients who have signs of cardiovascular, respiratory, or CNS toxicity are admitted to a monitored bed. Patients with a history of ingestion of extended-release preparations are admitted and monitored for 24 hours. A patient who ingested a β-blocker can be discharged home after the observation period if there are no signs of toxicity found by clinical examination, ECG, or cardiac monitoring.

CALCIUM CHANNEL BLOCKERS

Calcium channel blockers are used to treat hypertension, coronary artery disease, atrial fibrillation, and to prevent cerebral vasospasm. They decrease peripheral and coronary vascular tone, and to slow AV node conduction.

In 2002, the AAPCC reported 9585 calcium channel antagonist exposures. There were 2770 (29%) exposures in children, with 2256 (24%) in children younger 6 years old, and 514 (5.4%) in children ages 6 to 19 years. There were a total of 68 deaths (0.7%). There were four pediatric deaths reported, one after nifedipine exposure and three after verapamil exposure.

Pharmacology

Calcium channel blockers decrease contraction of vascular muscle and myocardium by inhibiting the influx of calcium into the cell. This action decreases activity of the calcium-dependent actin-myosin ATPase. The three calcium channel blockers, verapamil, diltiazem, and nifedipine, are structurally different. Each drug affects a different subset of calcium channels, leading to a unique set of physiologic effects. Verapamil affects both the myocardium and the peripheral arterioles, causing decreased contractility, AV node conduction, and peripheral vascular resistance. Diltiazem has less effect on peripheral vasodilatation and myocardial contractility than verapamil. Diltiazem slows AV node conduction and causes coronary artery dilatation. Nifedipine has the greatest effect on peripheral vascular resistance, and also decreases contractility, with minimal effect on AV node conduction (Figure 35–2).

The unique properties of each drug define their therapeutic and toxic effects; however, in overdose, any of these drugs can cause peripheral vasodilatation, decreased AV conduction, and decreased myocardial contractility.

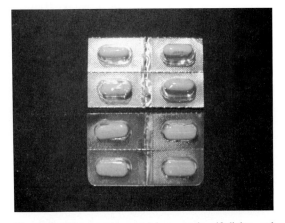

Fig. 35–2. Blister packs containing generic nifedipine and diltiazem.

Pharmacokinetics

The various calcium channel blockers have slightly different pharmacokinetic properties. They are 90% absorbed, with a significant first-pass metabolism. The onset of action is 30 minutes. All three drugs have a large volume of distribution, are highly protein bound, and metabolized in the liver. The half-life of calcium channel blockers varies from 3 to 7 hours, but can be greatly increased in the setting of overdose. It is extremely important to be aware that sustained-release preparations can have a delayed onset of life-threatening effects owing to their prolonged absorption time. Patients need to be monitored for 24 hours after significant ingestion prior to medical clearance.

Pathophysiology

In overdose, the pharmacologic effects of calcium channel blockers may lead to life-threatening physiologic sequelae. Slowing of the sinus node causes bradycardia. Slowing of conduction can cause heart blocks or asystole. Decreased contractility can cause heart failure and shock. Lowered peripheral vascular resistance leads to hypotension, which may exacerbate the hypotension associated with bradycardia, bradyarrhythmias, and heart failure. Patients with cardiac disease and those on other medications that suppress heart rate and contractility may develop severe toxic effects after mild overdose, or even at therapeutic doses.

Clinical Presentation

The different pharmacologic profile of calcium channel blockers causes various presentations; however, in all cases, cardiovascular effects predominate. Verapamil and diltiazem typically cause bradycardia and hypotension.

Hypotension may be due to sinoatrial node depression, atrioventricular node depression leading to AV blocks, negative inotropic effects, or decreased peripheral vascular resistance. Nifedipine primarily affects the arterioles, causing decreased peripheral vascular resistance, which leads to hypotension and reflex tachycardia. Neurologic and respiratory findings are usually secondary to cardiovascular toxicity and shock. Respiratory effects include decreased respiratory drive, pulmonary edema, and acute respiratory distress syndrome (ARDS). Neurologic sequelae include depressed sensorium, cerebral infarction, and seizures.

Nausea, vomiting, and constipation can occur. The most important gastrointestinal (GI) consequence to recognize is a concretion of sustained-release capsules. In addition to causing a bowel obstruction, the concretion can be a source of continued toxicity. Evacuation of sustained-release capsules from the GI tract may decrease morbidity and mortality.

Laboratory

Metabolic abnormalities may occur; decreased insulin release can lead to hyperglycemia. Hypoperfusion may lead to profound lactic acidosis. Hypocalcemia is the most frequent electrolyte abnormality. Hypokalemia and hyperkalemia have also been reported.

Drug levels for calcium channel blockers are available by reference laboratories. These levels are generally not available in a time frame that is useful for patient management, but they can be used to confirm the presence of a suspected agent.

An ECG and cardiac monitoring is obtained for any patient with a history of calcium channel blocker overdose and is assessed for blocks, bradycardia, and ischemic changes. Electrolytes are evaluated, specifically Na^+, Ca^{2+}, Mg^{2+}, and K^+. Arterial blood gas can be useful in evaluating oxygenation and acid–base status. Chest radiographs are obtained for patients with respiratory signs or symptoms. Sustained-release tablets may be radiopaque. An abdominal radiograph may be useful for patients with signs of obstruction or history of recently ingesting sustained-release tablets.

Management

In the unstable patient, supportive care and antidotal therapy are instituted immediately. The patient is placed on a cardiac monitor, IV access is established, and fluid resuscitation with crystalloid is initiated in hypotensive patients. In the patient with altered mental status, bedside evaluation of oxygen and capillary blood glucose is obtained. Intubation may be necessary for airway protection or for patients with respiratory failure secondary to pulmonary edema or ARDS.

If the patient is stable, he or she is monitored for signs of toxicity and measures are taken to decrease absorption. Ipecac is contraindicated because rapid CNS depression may occur, leading to aspiration. If the ingestion occurred less than 1 hour prior to presentation and a potentially lethal dose is suspected, gastric emptying with lavage can be considered. Charcoal is administered after lavage. Charcoal alone is used for patients who present late in their clinical course.

For patients who have ingested sustained-release preparations, whole bowel irrigation can potentially be helpful. The goal of whole bowel irrigation is to move the pills through the entire GI tract prior to their being absorbed. Whole bowel irrigation is accomplished by administering polyethylene glycol solution at a rate of 25 mL/kg/h by mouth or nasogastric tube until the rectal effluent is clear. A dose of charcoal is administered prior to initiating whole bowel irrigation, because it can adsorb drug that is released while the pills remain in the GI tract.

Although there are multiple antidotes for calcium antagonist overdose, there is little evidence available to guide their use. The clinician should be prepared to use an agent up to its maximum dose and add a subsequent agent if the adverse effects of the overdose are not adequately controlled.

Calcium is one antidote available for calcium channel antagonist. Increasing extracellular calcium increases the influx of calcium into the cell, thus augmenting the calcium reserve of the sarcoplasmic reticulum. This reserve makes calcium available to the calcium-dependent ATPase, increasing contractility. Calcium is indicated for patients with hypotension, bradycardia, or heart blocks.

Two calcium salts are available: calcium gluconate and calcium chloride (Figure 35–3) Both of these are supplied in 10% solutions, but each contains a different quantity of calcium. Calcium chloride contains 1.30 mEq/mL of calcium and calcium gluconate contains 0.45 mEq/mL of calcium. The recommended pediatric doses are 0.1 to 0.2 mL/kg of 10% calcium chloride or 0.2 to 0.3 mL/kg of 10% calcium gluconate by slow IV push. The dose is repeated in 10 to 15 minutes for patients with persistent hypotension or bradycardia. Calcium chloride can contribute to acidosis; therefore, calcium gluconate is preferred for patients with acidosis.

The calcium salts primarily reverse hypotension due to vasodilation, and may have little or no effect on heart rate or conduction. There have been several cases in which calcium salts failed to reverse toxic effects. For patients with symptomatic bradycardia or heart block, atropine administered at 0.02 mg/kg may be helpful. However, hypotension is often related to peripheral vasodilation and does not respond to an increase in heart rate. Conversely, in a patient with stable blood pressure despite bradycardia, atropine will be of no benefit.

Adrenergic agents are useful antidotes include for calcium channel blocker overdose. Dopamine is a reasonable first-line option. If it is ineffective, therapy with epinephrine, norepinephrine, or dobutamine may be helpful.

Glucagon is another antidote for calcium channel blocker toxicity. It stimulates adenylate cyclase, which increases the formation of cAMP and promotes intracellular calcium influx. The adult dose is 3 to 5 mg slow IV

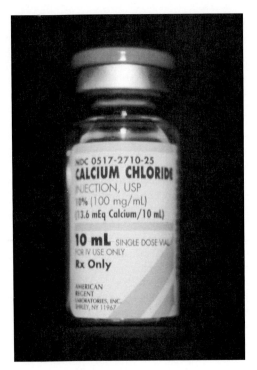

Fig. 35–3. Calcium chloride.

push over 1 minute. It can be infused at a rate of 1 to 5 mg/h. Pediatric doses of 0.05 to 0.10 mg/kg are administered IV, followed by a continuous infusion at 0.07 mg/kg/h. If glucagon is administered multiple times or as an infusion it can be mixed in normal saline or D_5W. Nausea and vomiting are frequent side effects of glucagon administration that should be considered when using this agent.

High-dose insulin has been used in the management of calcium channel blocker overdose in patients refractory to calcium and glucagon therapy. Insulin improves myocardial contractility by improving myocardial carbohydrate utilization. Insulin can be administered as a bolus of regular insulin, 0.5 to 1.0 U/kg along with 0.5 to 1.0 g/kg of dextrose. This is followed by an infusion of 0.5 U/kg/h. Serum glucose must be monitored at least hourly during the infusion and dextrose administered to maintain euglycemia. Glucose infusion can be initiated at 0.5 g/kg/h and adjusted based on the results of blood glucose levels. A decrease in serum potassium is anticipated owing to an intracellular shift of potassium. Serum potassium should be monitored and replaced to maintain serum potassium levels at 2.8 to 3.2 mEq/L.

Inamrinone, a phosphodiesterase inhibitor used in treating congestive heart failure, has been reported in both case reports and animal models to be effective in reversing hypotension secondary to calcium channel blocker overdose. Inamrinone can be given as an initial bolus of 0.75 mg/kg over 2 to 3 minutes, followed by an infusion of 5 to 10 μg/kg/min. Currently, clinical experience with inamrinone is in pediatric cases is limited.

Hemodialysis and hemoperfusion are very rarely indicated in the setting of calcium channel blocker overdose. The calcium channel blockers have a large volume of distribution and are highly protein bound, making elimination of the drug not feasible. Dialysis could be considered in a patient who has renal failure. There has been one case of clinical improvement after hemoperfusion in a patient with combined diltiazem and metoprolol ingestion.

Disposition

Children who have signs of cardiovascular, respiratory, or CNS compromise are admitted to an intensive care unit. Children with a history of sustained-release ingestion are observed with cardiac monitoring for at least 24 hours. Those patients with no signs of toxicity, no history of sustained-release ingestion, and no ECG abnormalities can be observed for 6 to 8 hours after the time of ingestion. If they do not develop any signs of toxicity or ECG abnormalities during this period, they may be discharged.

CLONIDINE

Clonidine is widely used as an antihypertensive agent, a treatment for opiate withdrawal, and a treatment for attention deficit hyperactivity disorder (ADHD). Especially in young children, even small doses of clonidine can cause serious toxicity. The frequency of therapeutic use in the pediatrics for ADHD has increased markedly since the 1990s. Unlike other antihypertensive medications, many of pediatric clonidine exposures involve the child's own medication. Although accidental exposure is most common in children younger than 12 years old, exposures related to self-harm are the most common etiology in children ages 12 to 19 years old.

Clonidine is available in tablets and sustained-release patches. Children have been reported to ingest both preparations. There are accidental cases of toxicity related to clonidine patches. These exposures have occurred owing to a patch mistakenly applied as a band-aid, and inadvertent manipulation of patches that led to increased delivery. Clonidine has also been reported in pediatric cases of Munchausen syndrome by proxy.

In 2002, the AAPCC reported 5222 clonidine exposures. There were 3370 (65%) exposures in children, with 1638 (31%) in children younger than 6 years old and 1732 (33%) in children aged 6 to 19 years. There were a total of six deaths (0.1%). There were 2.5 times as many clonidine exposures in children in 1999 as in 1993.

Pathophysiology

Clonidine is an α_2-agonist that functions at the level of the brain stem by blocking sympathetic flow. It decreases heart rate, cardiac output, and peripheral vascular resistance. Clonidine also functions as a CNS depressant by depressing noradrenergic activity. At high doses, it can stimulate peripheral α_1-receptors and actually cause hypertension, although this effect is transitory, and is usually followed by hypotension.

Clonidine is rapidly absorbed from the GI tract, with a decrease in blood pressure noted 30 to 60 minutes after ingestion. Hypotensive effects can last up to 24 hours. Severe toxicity has been reported after a pediatric ingestion of as little as 0.1 mg.

The effects of an overdose of clonidine vary, but largely reflect CNS toxicity. They include altered mental status, somnolence, respiratory depression, and, especially in children, recurrent apnea. CNS depression can last for 24 hours. Miosis can occur, which, in combination with altered mental status and depressed respiratory drive, can appear similar to opioid toxicity. In addition to miosis, the neurologic examination may reveal ataxia, hypotonia, and decreased reflexes. Seizures are rare. Some patients may develop hypothermia.

Bradycardia and hypotension are the predominant cardiovascular manifestations, although patients can initially be hypertensive. Cardiac arrhythmias can occur. The cardiovascular effects can develop hours after the onset of mental status changes; thus, initially normal vital signs do not exclude the possibility that cardiovascular instability will ensue.

Management

The initial management of clonidine overdose focuses on stabilizing the airway. Respiratory depression may require ventilatory support. A trial of naloxone prior to intubation is appropriate. This is important given the difficulty in distinguishing clonidine ingestion from an opioid overdose. In addition, naloxone may reverse the effects of a clonidine overdose.

After the airway is stabilized, GI decontamination is indicated. Ipecac-induced emesis should be avoided owing to the potential for aspiration. Gastric lavage is the preferred method given the tendency of clonidine to cause CNS depression and seizures. In this setting, the airway should be protected to avoid aspiration. Following lavage, activated charcoal is administered. For patients who are asymptomatic or exhibit mild toxicity, activated charcoal alone is adequate.

Clonidine-induced bradycardia is treated with atropine if it is associated with hypotension. Hypotension is treated with aggressive fluid resuscitation. For hypotension that does not respond to fluids, moderate-dose dopamine may be useful. Dopamine may also ameliorate bradycardia. For patients with hypertension, it is important to realize that this side effect is transient and should be treated only if there is evidence of end-organ compromise. A short-acting agent, such as nitroprusside, is used to avoid precipitating profound hypotension, which can occur if a longer-acting agent is administered.

As mentioned, there may be a role for naloxone in reversing the opioid-like side effects of clonidine on mental status and respiration and there is some indication that it can reverse clonidine-mediated hypotension. However, data on this subject are conflicting and naloxone cannot be considered a specific antidote for clonidine overdose. Although there are no contraindications to its use, the administration of naloxone in the setting of clonidine overdose has been associated with hypertension, and blood pressure monitoring is necessary during its administration.

Tolazoline is an α-antagonist agent that has been reported to reverse clonidine-mediated hypotension. However, it is not the specific antidote for clonidine. Data on its use are conflicting. It can cause profound hypotension, and its use should be restricted to the most refractory cases.

Disposition

Children who have signs of respiratory, CNS, or cardiovascular compromise secondary to clonidine toxicity are admitted to an intensive care unit. Those patients with no signs of toxicity can be observed for 6 to 8 hours after the time of ingestion. If they do not develop any signs of toxicity during this period, they may be discharged.

CASE OUTCOME

The child is placed on a cardiac monitor and pulse oximeter in the ED. IV access is established, and a 20-cc/kg normal saline bolus is administered. The patient is given 25 g of activated charcoal via a nasogastric tube. With no change in the child's blood pressure and pulse following the initial fluid bolus, it is elected to give IV glucagon at 0.1 mg/kg. The child's blood pressure responds, increasing to 85/60 mmHg; the pulse increases to 110 bpm. The child is admitted to the pediatric intensive care unit where a continuous glucagon infusion is started at 0.07 mg/kg/h. The patient requires one additional IV bolus of glucagon at 0.1 mg/kg during the night, and recovers uneventfully 24 hours after admission.

SUGGESTED READINGS

β-Blockers

Brimacombe JR: Use of calcium chloride for propranolol overdose. *Anaesthesia* 47:907, 1992.

Litovitz TL, Manoguerra A: Comparison of pediatric poisoning hazards: An analysis of 3.8 million exposure incidents: A report from the American Association of Poison Control Centers. *Pediatrics* 88:999, 1992.

Love JN, Enlow B, Howell JM, et al: Electrocardiographic changes associated with β-blocker toxicity. *Ann Emerg Med* 40:603–610, 2002.

Love JN, Litovitz TL, Howell JM, et al: Characterization of fatal beta-blocker ingestion: A review of the American Association of Poison Control Center's data from 1985–1995. *J Toxicol Clin Toxicol* 35:353–359, 1997.

Love JN, Tandy TK: Beta-adrenoreceptor antagonist toxicity: A survey of glucagon availability. *Ann Emerg Med* 22:267, 1993.

Reith DM, Dawson AH, Epid D, et al: Relative toxicity of beta blockers in overdose. *J Toxicol Clin Toxicol* 34:273–278, 1996.

Calcium Channel Blockers

Cimpello LB, Craig S, Lawrence E, et al: A calcium channel blocker and ibuprofen overdose. *Curr Opin Pediatr* 10:303–307, 1998.

Kerns JA: Calcium channel antagonists. In: Ford MD, Delaney KA, Ling LJ, et al, eds: *Clinical Toxicology.* Philadelphia: Saunders; 2001:370–378.

Kline JA, Raymond RM, Schroeder JD, et al: The diabetogenic effects of acute verapamil poisoning. *Toxicol Appl Pharmacol* 145:357–362, 1997.

Kline JA, Tomaszewski CA, Schroeder JD, et al: Insulin is a superior antidote for cardiovascular toxicity induced by verapamil in the anesthetized canine. *J Pharmacol Exp Ther* 267:744–750, 1993.

Kozlowski JH, Kozlowski JA, Schuller D: Poisoning with sustained release verapamil. *Am J Med* 85:127, 1996.

Litovitz TL, Klein–Schwartz W, White S, et al: 1999 annual report of the American Association of Poison Control Centers Toxic Exposure Surveillance System. *Am J Emerg Med* 18:517–574, 2000.

Yuan TH, Kerns WP, Tomaszewski CA, et al: Insulin-glucose as adjunctive therapy for severe calcium channel antagonist poisoning. *J Toxicol Clin Toxicol* 37:463–474, 1999.

Clonidine

Broderick-Cantwell JJ: Case study: Accidental clonidine patch overdose in attention-deficit/hyperactivity disorder patients. *J Am Acad Child Adolesc Psychiatr* 38:95–98, 1999.

Killian CA, Roberge RJ, Krenzelok EP, et al: "Cloniderm" toxicity: Another manifestation of clonidine overdose. *Pediatr Emerg Care* 13:340–341, 1997.

Klein-Schwartz W: Trends and toxic effects from pediatric clonidine exposures. *Arch Pediatr Adolesc Med* 156:392–396, 2002.

Lustof KJ, Lameijer W, Zweipfenning PG: Use of clonidine for chemical submission. *J Toxicol Clin Toxicol* 38:329–332, 2000.

Maloney MJ, Schwam JS: Clonidine and sudden death. *Pediatrics* 96:1176–1177, 1995.

Tessa C, Mascalchi M, Matteucci L, et al: Permanent brain damage following acute clonidine poisoning in Munchausen by proxy. *Neuropediatrics* 32:90–92, 2001.

36

Colchicine

Yaron Finkelstein

HIGH-YIELD FACTS

- Pediatric colchicine overdose is uncommon but potentially life threatening, with a high mortality rate.

- Onset of gastrointestinal symptoms within 10 to 24 hours suggests severe intoxication. Death occurs secondary to rapidly progressive multiorgan failure.

- Colchicine has a narrow therapeutic-toxic index, with no clear-cut line between nontoxic, toxic, and lethal doses.

- Although a specific treatment for colchicine overdose (colchicine-specific Fab fragments) exists, it is not commercially available.

- Extreme caution is necessary when prescribing colchicine, and parents should be alerted to its potential toxicity in children.

CASE PRESENTATION

A 3-year-old girl presents to the emergency department (ED) after ingesting an unknown amount of her grandfather's gout medication several hours prior to presentation. The child vomited three times prior to arrival with some streaks of blood noted by her parents. Vital signs on presentation are as follows: pulse, 150 bpm; respiratory rate, 28 breaths per minute; blood pressure 70/40 mmHg; and temperature of 99°F. In the ED, the child is noted to be lethargic with an intact airway.

INTRODUCTION AND EPIDEMIOLOGY

Colchicine is a neutral lipophilic alkaloid with weak anti-inflammatory activity. It is extracted from two plants: *Colchicum automnale* (meadow saffron) and *gloriosa superba* (glory lily). The drug's name is derived from the name of the ancient district of Colchis on the eastern shore of the Black Sea, where these plants were indigenous. It has been used for centuries for the treatment of acute gouty arthritis because of its anti-inflammatory action and prophylactic effect against recurrences. It has been proven effective in children for treatment of familial Mediterranean fever (FMF) and preventing amyloidosis and recurrent pericarditis, and may also play a role in the treatment of scleroderma, Behçet syndrome, and Sweet syndrome. The use of colchicine is limited by its toxicity. Acute pediatric colchicine poisoning is uncommon, but associated with a very high mortality rate. The youngest reported patient with a colchicine overdose is a 3-year-old girl. A fatal case of a colchicine overdose was reported in a 13-year-old boy.

DEVELOPMENTAL TOXICOLOGY

Studies of colchicine administration during pregnancy reported small amounts of the drug in cord blood samples, suggesting that it may cross the placenta. However, a few small series failed to demonstrate any effect on rate of fetal abnormalities, birth weight, duration of pregnancy, or miscarriage rate. Most current policies recommend continuing colchicine therapy during pregnancy with amniocentesis performed in the fourth or fifth month.

Colchicine is present in breast milk. Most authors do not recommend breastfeeding for mothers receiving colchicine therapy. Nevertheless, the estimated daily amount of colchicine ingested by the nursing infant is less than one-tenth the therapeutic dose. This finding, together with the favorable outcome of more than 50 infants breast fed by colchicine-treated mothers, has led to a reconsideration of the guidelines by some authors.

Prolonged use of colchicine in children raises some concerns of chronic toxicity to various organs. Sperm motility, which depends on microtubular function, may theoretically be affected, although in vivo studies show that for this to occur, serum concentration needs to be 3000 times higher than achieved with appropriate dosing. There is no convincing evidence of a negative effect of colchicine treatment on female fertility. By controlling attacks in pregnant women with FMF, colchicine may reduce peritoneal adhesions and mechanical infertility.

The potential effect of colchicine on childhood growth is also of concern, because the latter results from cell division. However, one study found that growth was within the normal percentiles even in children treated with colchicine (0.5 to 1.0 mg/d) for long periods.

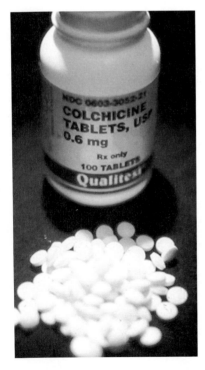

Fig. 36–1. Colchicine tablets.

TOXICOKINETICS AND PHARMACOKINETICS

Colchicine can be administered orally in 0.5- or 0.6-mg tablets (Figure 36–1) or as an intravenous (IV) 0.5 mg/mL solution. It is rapidly absorbed from the gastrointestinal (GI) tract; levels peak at 0.5 to 3.0 hours after ingestion. Absorption is not significantly delayed with overdose. The drug undergoes extensive hepatic first-pass metabolism, which accounts for its relatively low bioavailability of 25% to 50%. After absorption, colchicine is rapidly distributed from plasma to all tissues. In therapeutic doses, the mean half-life of oral colchicine is 9 to 16 hours and its volume of distribution 4.3 ± 2.9 L/kg. In intoxicated patients, the mean half-life may reach 11 to 32 hours and the volume of distribution 21 L/kg. Colchicine is highly protein-bound (30% to 50%).

IV colchicine is occasionally prescribed as a substitute for the oral form when a rapid response is desired. The risk of severe systemic toxicity with IV administration of the drug is significantly increased, partly owing to lack of early GI symptoms. Toxicity in these cases depends on the total cumulative dose given in a course, which should not exceed 2 to 4 mg in adults. No colchicine, by any route, should be given for 7 days thereafter. The failure to follow these guidelines led to severe toxicity and death at 1 to 40 days after IV drug administration in 20 adults between 1983 and 2000. The dose should be further reduced in patients with organ failure.

Colchicine is eliminated primarily by hepatic metabolism by the CYP 3A4 isoform of cytochrome P450. Its metabolites undergo significant enterohepatic recirculation before excretion in bile and feces. This high exposure time to intestinal mucosa explains the vulnerability of the GI tract to colchicine's side effects. Renal clearance accounts for 20% to 30% of colchicine elimination. Colchicine clearance is significantly impaired in children with kidney or liver failure.

Interaction of colchicine with other drugs or compounds that are metabolized by the same enzyme interrupts its metabolic pathway and may lead to increased drug levels and toxicity. The main specific inhibitors of CYP 3A4 in children are erythromycin, ketoconazole, and natural grapefruit juice. Drugs that have a general inhibitory effect on the cytochrome system, such as cimetidine, may also increase colchicine levels when administered concomitantly.

PATHOPHYSIOLOGY

Colchicine has a potent reversible binding capacity to intracellular tubuli. Impairment of microtubular-dependent neutrophil chemotaxis and phagocytosis results in a re-duced inflammatory response, which is the main thera-peutic mechanism of action. The systems with the high-est turnover rate, including bone marrow, GI tract, and hair follicles, are the most affected. Colchicine may also have a direct toxic action on myocardial cells.

The inhibition of other important microtubular func-tions may also be involved in the devastating processes leading to multiorgan failure in cases of drug overdose. Several recent studies of colchicine toxicity have focused on the role of P-glycoprotein (P-gp). P-gp is an integral membrane ATPase efflux pump that serves as an energy-dependent transporter of several drugs, including col-chicine. It acts in such manner that ATP hydrolysis coun-teracts the effects of colchicine.

In general, the risk of colchicine toxicity is dose depen-dent, with a high fatality rate when ingestion exceeds 0.5 mg/kg in acute cases. Some studies demonstrated only GI and coagulation disorders in doses less than 0.5 mg/kg, bone marrow aplasia, and a 10% mortality rate in patients ingesting 0.5 to 0.8 mg/kg, and cardiovascular collapse followed by death in doses exceeding 0.8 mg/kg in acute ingestions. Colchicine exhibits a great variation in the dose required to cause significant morbidity or mortality.

Adult patients have survived ingestion of more than 60 mg; lethal outcome was reported after an ingestion of only 7.5 and 26 mg. Severe pediatric intoxications have been reported even with chronic prophylactic oral doses of 1 to 2 mg/d. There is no clear-cut line between non-toxic, toxic, and lethal doses of colchicine in either adults or children.

CLINICAL MANIFESTATIONS

The clinical course of colchicine toxicity is well de-scribed. It may be divided into three sequential and usu-ally overlapping phases (Table 36–1). The *GI phase* oc-curs within a few to 24 hours after ingestion. Possible symptoms are severe nausea, vomiting, abdominal pain, and diarrhea, which may be hemorrhagic, reflecting GI mucosal damage. A cholera-like syndrome of severe fluid loss, electrolyte imbalance, and hypovolemic shock may develop. The *second phase* may occur between 24 hours and 7 days after ingestion. It is characterized by multiorgan failure, which may include respiratory dis-tress syndrome, cardiac arrhythmias, congestive heart failure, and cardiovascular collapse. Renal failure, liver

Table 36–1. Clinical Stages of Significant Colchicine Toxicity

Stage	Time of Onset	Features
1. GI phase	2–24 h postingestion	Nausea, vomiting, diarrhea, abdominal discomfort
		Hypovolemia
		Leukocytosis
2. Multiorgan failure phase	1–7 days postingestion	Respiratory distress syndrome
		Cardiac arrhythmias, failure, arrest
		Encephalopathy, brain edema
		Convulsions
		Renal failure
		Liver failure
		Disseminated intravascular coagulation
		Bone marrow suppression
		Pancytopenia
		Hemolysis
		Metabolic derangements: metabolic acidosis, hypokalemia, hyponatremia, hypocalcemia, hypoglycemia, hypophosphatemia
		Myopathy
		Secondary sepsis
3. Recovery phase	7–21 days postingestion	Resolution of organ system derangements
		Rebound leukocytosis
		Alopecia

failure, and bone marrow suppression, which reaches a nadir within 4 to 8 days of ingestion, have also been described. Hemolytic anemia, disseminated intravascular coagulation, and central nervous system disorders such as convulsions, encephalopathy, cerebral edema, and coma have also been reported. Metabolic derangements such as hyponatremia, hyperglycemia or hypoglycemia, hypocalcemia, hypokalemia, and metabolic acidosis are common in severe toxicity. Myopathies and neuropathies have been reported as isolated reversible manifestations of chronic colchicine treatment in children.

Death from acute oral colchicine overdose is usually due to hemodynamic collapse and cardiac arrhythmias, infectious, or hematologic complications. Patients with early hemodynamic collapse have a particularly poor prognosis. If the patient survives, the *third phase* of colchicine toxicity develops 7 or more days after ingestion. It is characterized by recovery of bone marrow with rebound leukocytosis, resolution of organ failure, and development of transient alopecia, followed by complete recovery.

LABORATORY STUDIES

Baseline laboratory studies indicated in a child with colchicine overdose include complete blood count (CBC), glucose, electrolytes, renal and hepatic function tests, coagulation studies, creatine phosphokinase level, chest radiograph, urinalysis, and electrocardiogram. Pregnancy test is recommended in female patients of childbearing age. Serial CBCs are monitored to detect possible hematologic toxicity. Specific colchicine plasma levels are neither readily available in the clinical setting, nor useful for the management of acute intoxication.

MANAGEMENT

The mainstays of treatment of colchicines toxicity consist of early GI decontamination and aggressive supportive care. In children presenting within 1 hour of ingestion, gastric lavage may be beneficial. Activated charcoal is indicated following ingestion of colchicine pills or colchicine-containing plant parts. Repeated doses of activated charcoal administration may be efficacious, because colchicine undergoes enterohepatic recirculation.

Treatment is basically supportive. Cardiac monitoring is indicated, because sudden malignant arrhythmias have been reported. If clinical signs of toxicity develop, pediatric intensive care modalities may be required, including mechanical ventilation, vasopressor drugs, blood products, granulocyte colony-stimulating factor, and broad-spectrum antibiotics.

Effective experimental treatment with colchicine-specific Fab fragments for severe colchicine toxicity in an adult has been reported. Colchicine-specific Fab fragments consist of the light chain and variable region of the heavy chain of antibodies derived from goats immunized with a conjugate of colchicine and serum albumin. Their mechanism of action in the clinical setting is similar to that of digoxin-specific Fab fragments. Binding to the target drug allows redistribution into the extracellular space and intravascular compartment, and thus the removal of substantial amounts from peripheral tissues. The high affinity of the Fab fragments for colchicine prevents the drug from returning to the peripheral binding sites.

Because of the large volume of distribution and 30% to 50% binding rate to plasma proteins, hemodialysis and hemoperfusion are ineffective in the treatment of acute overdose.

DISPOSITION

Any child with a known or suspected colchicine overdose is admitted for observation for 24 hours. If no symptoms develop, the child may be discharged. In cases of IV colchicine overdose, GI symptoms may not appear, and a higher index of suspicion regarding potential toxicity is necessary. Follow-up blood counts may be necessary to exclude bone marrow toxicity.

CASE OUTCOME

The child experiences several more episodes of vomiting and bloody diarrhea in the emergency department. The child is given an IV fluid bolus and admitted to the pediatric intensive care unit. Initial CBC demonstrates a mild leukocytosis with a normal hemoglobin and platelet count. Within 24 hours, the child develops fever, neutropenia, anemia, and renal insufficiency. IV antibiotics are initiated. No colchicine-specific Fab fragments are available. The child recovers after 7 days of supportive care in the ICU with normalization of CBC and renal function.

SUGGESTED READINGS

Achtert G, Scherrmann JM, Christen MO: Pharmacokinetic bioavailability of colchicine in healthy male volunteers. *Eur J Drug Metab Pharm* 14: 317–322, 1989.

Altiparmak MR, Pamuk ON, Pamuk GE, et al. Colchicine neuromyopathy: A report of six cases. *Clin Exp Rheumatol* 20:S13–16, 2002.

Baud FJ, Sabouraud A, Vicaut E, et al: Brief report: Treatment of severe colchicine overdose with colchicine-specific Fab fragments. *N Engl J Med* 332:642–645, 1995.

Ben-Chetrit E, Backenroth R, Levy M: Colchicine clearance by high-flux polysulfone dialyzers. *Arthritis Rheum* 41:749–750, 1998.

Ben-Chetrit E, Levy M. Colchicine: 1998 update. *Semin Arth Rheum* 28:48–59, 1998.

Ben-Chetrit E, Levy M. Does the lack of the P-glycoprotein efflux pump in neutrophils explain the efficacy of colchicine in familial Mediterranean fever and other inflammatory diseases? *Medical Hypotheses* 51:377–380, 1998.

Bonnel RA, Villalba ML, Karwoski CB, et al: Deaths associated with inappropriate intravenous colchicine administration. *J Emerg Med* 22:385–387, 2002.

Borron SW, Scherrmann JM, Baud FJ: Markedly altered colchicine kinetics in a fatal intoxication: Examination of contributing factors. *Hum Exp Toxicol* 15:885–890, 1996.

Briggs GG, Freeman RK, Yaffe RS: *Drugs in Pregnancy and Lactation*. 4th ed. Baltimore: Williams & Wilkins; 1994.

Ehrenfeld M, Bzezinski A, Levy M, et al: Fertility and obstetric history in patients with familial Mediterranean fever on long-term colchicine therapy. *Br J Obstet Gynecol* 94:1186–1191, 1987.

Elwood MG, Robb GH: Self poisoning with colchicine. *Postgrad Med J* 65:752–755, 1989.

Ferron GM, Rochdi M, Jusko WJ, et al: Oral absorption characteristics and pharmacokinetics of colchicine in healthy volunteers after single and multiple doses. *J Clin Pharmacol* 36:874–883, 1996.

Finkelstein Y, Aks S, Erickson T: Colchicine toxicity: Back to the roots. *Pediatrics* (in press).

Goldbart A, Press J, Sofer S, et al: Near fatal acute colchicine intoxication in a child. A case report. *Eur J Pediatr* 159:895–897, 2000.

Guven AG, Bahat E, Akman S, et al: Late diagnosis of severe colchicine intoxication. *Pediatrics* 109:971–973, 2002.

Harel L, Mukamel M, Amir J, et al: Colchicine-induced myoneuropathy in childhood. *Eur J Pediar* 157:853–855, 1998.

Hunter AL, Klaassen CD: Biliary excretion of colchicine. *J Pharmacol Exp Ther* 192:605–617, 1974.

Jarvie D, Park J, Stewart MJ: Estimation of colchicine in a poisoned patient by using high performance liquid chromatography. *Clin Toxicol* 14:375–381, 1979.

Jones GR, Singer PP, Bannach BB: Application of LC-MS analysis to a colchicine fatality. *J Anal Toxicol* 26:365–369, 2002.

Maxwell MJ, Muthu P, Pritty PE: Accidental colchicine overdose. A case report and literature review. *Emerg Med J* 19:265–267, 2002.

Putterman C, Ben-Chetrit E, Caraco Y, et al: Colchicine intoxication, clinical pharmacology, risk factors, features and management. *Semin Arthritis Rheum* 21:143–155, 1991.

Roberts WN, Liang MH, Stern SH: Colchicine in acute gout: Reassessment of risks and benefits. *JAMA* 257:1920–1922, 1987.

Rochdi M, Sabouraud A, Baud FJ, et al: Toxicokinetics of colchicine in humans: Analysis of tissue, plasma and urine data in ten cases. *Hum Exp Toxicol* 11:510–516, 1992.

Sarica K, Suzer O, Gurler A, et al: Urological evaluation of Behçet patients and the effect of colchicine on fertility. *Eur J Mol* 22:39–42, 1995.

Stahl N, Weinberger A, Benjamin D, et al: Fatal colchicine poisoning in a boy with familial Mediterranean fever. *Am J Med Sci* 278:77–81, 1979.

Stapczynski JS, Rothstein RJ, Gaye WA, et al: Colchicine overdose: Report of two cases and review of the literature. *Ann Emerg Med* 10:364–369, 1981.

Tateiski T, Soucek S, Caraco Y, et al: Colchicine biotransformation by human liver microsomes: Identification of CYP 3A4 as a major isoform responsible for colchicine demethylation. *Biochem Pharmacol* 10:111–116, 1997.

Thomas G, Girre C, Scherrmann JM, et al: Zero-order absorption and linear disposition of oral colchicine in healthy volunteers. *Eur J Clin Pharmacol* 37:79–84, 1989.

Valenzuela P, Paris E, Oberpauer B, et al: Overdose of colchicine in a three-year-old child. *Vet Human Toxicol* 37:366–367, 1995.

Wallace SL, Ertel NH: Plasma levels of colchicine after administration of a single dose. *Metabolism* 22:749–753, 1973.

Wallace SL, Omokoku B, Ertel NH: Colchicine plasma levels: Implications as to pharmacology and mechanism of action. *Am J Med* 48:443–448, 1970.

Zahir A, Scherrmann SM, Wechsler B, et al: Transplacental passage of colchicine in familial Mediterranean fever. *J Rheumatol* 21:383, 1994.

Zemer D, Livneh A, Danon YL, et al: Long-term colchicine treatment in children with familial Mediterranean fever. *Arth Rheum* 34:973–977, 1991.

37

Digoxin

Jerrold B. Leikin
Steven E. Aks

HIGH-YIELD FACTS

- Toxic oral dose of digoxin is over 0.05 mg/kg.
- Serum digoxin concentration must be used in conjunction with clinical symptoms and electrocardiogram to confirm diagnosis of digoxin intoxication.
- Usual symptoms associated with acute poisoning include vomiting, atrioventricular block, bradycardia, hyperkalemia, and mental status changes.
- Digoxin-immune Fab fragments is the specific antidote for digoxin poisonings.

CASE PRESENTATION

A 1-week-old boy discharged from the newborn nursery on digoxin elixir for paroxysmal supraventricular tachycardia presents to the emergency department (ED) with a 1-day history of emesis and decreased formula intake.

Prior to delivery, fetal tachycardia was noted on prenatal ultrasound, and the mother was digitalized 4 days prior to delivery. The patient was delivered vaginally, with APGAR scores of 7 at 1 minute, and 9 at 5 minutes. His initial evaluation included a total digoxin level of 0.6 ng/mL on day 1 of life; an echocardiogram on day 2 revealed occasional irregular beats, a small left-to-right atrial shunt, and a small patent ductus arteriosus. A 24-hour Holter monitor revealed several episodes of nonsustained paroxysmal supraventricular tachycardia, ranging from 3 to 11 seconds to 3 minutes, with spontaneous resolution.

The patient was discharged from the newborn nursery at 4 days of age in stable condition, on a prescribed maintenance digoxin elixir (Lanoxin Elixir Pediatric, 50 μg/ mL) of 7 μg/kg/d (0.2 mL PO bid). The prescription directions were improperly labeled by a community pharmacy as 2.0 mL PO bid of digoxin elixir (50 μg/mL). The patient received approximately 60 μg/kg/d for 3.5 days.

The patient presents to the ED 1.5 hours after receiving the last dose of digoxin, and is alert but extremely irritable. Initial vital signs are as follows: blood pressure 76/52 mmHg, apical pulse 100/min and irregular, respiratory rate 32 breaths per minute, and axillary temperature 96.6°F. The patient appears mildly to moderately dehydrated. Fluid resuscitation is initiated with isotonic saline, and cardiac rhythm strips are obtained, which reveal a heart rate between 80 and 90 bpm, with a high degree of atrioventricular (AV) block, frequent preventricular contractions (PVCs), and occasional bigeminy.

INTRODUCTION AND EPIDEMIOLOGY

Digoxin is used today for the treatment of congestive heart failure and supraventricular dysrhythmias. There are great risks for children who accidentally ingest this potentially life-threatening substance. There have been numerous case reports documenting severe toxicity occurring in children associated with life-threatening dysrhythmias. There were no fatalities in children younger than 6 years of age reported to the American Association of Poison Centers Toxic Exposure Surveillance System in 2002. However, there were two deaths in 2001. One fatality was in a 1 month old, and another in a 2 year old. Both were due to therapeutic error.

There are several plants that contain cardiac glycoside or digoxin-like substances including foxglove, oleander, lily of the valley, and red squill, which are discussed Chapter 80. Recently, the use of digoxin-specific Fab fragments has been shown to be effective in children. Mortality rates of 68% for tachycardia and 100% for ventricular fibrillation were noted prior to the development of digoxin-immune Fab fragments.

DEVELOPMENTAL CONSIDERATIONS

Although there are some serious digoxin overdoses that are accidental, many of the fatalities represent dosing errors. It is essential for clinicians and caretakers to be especially vigilant in dosing digoxin in infants and neonates. The other major consideration in neonates and children is the change in the pharmacokinetics over age ranges (Table 37–1). In neonates, the volume of distribution is 7.5 to 10 L/kg. It increases to 16 L/kg in children, and decreases to 7 L/kg in adults. Also, the elimination of digoxin fluctuates across age ranges. The elimination half-life in premature infants ranges from 61 to 170

hours; in infants it decreases to 18 to 25 hours, and increases to about 35 hours in children and adults. Consideration of the kinetics with respect to age is essential to avoid toxicity.

PHARMACOLOGY AND PATHOPHYSIOLOGY

Digoxin functions as a positive inotrope, and increases the force and velocity of myocardial contraction. In the failing heart it can increase cardiac output, and decrease elevated ventricular end-diastolic pressures. Digoxin enhances both the efficiency of the heart and the work it can perform.

On the cellular level it is felt that digoxin functions by binding to and inactivating the Na^+–K^+ ATPase in the heart. This blockade results in an increased intracellular sodium concentration. Additionally, enhanced contractility depends on intracellular ionized calcium concentrations during systole. At toxic concentrations, it is felt that

Table 37–1. Digoxin Pharmacokinetics

Pharmacodynamics	Pharmacokinetics
Onset of action	Distribution
Oral: 0.5–2.0 h	Distribution phase: 6–8 h
IV: 5–30 min	V_d (L/kg)
Maximum effect:	Neonates, full-term: 7.5–10
Oral: 2–8 h	Children: 16
IV: 1–4 h	Adults: 7
Duration (adults): 3–4 d	Renal disease: decreased V_d
	Protein Binding: 20–25%
	Bioavailability (%)
	Capsules: 90–100
	Elixir: 70–85
	Tablets: 60–80
	Half-life, elimination (dependent upon age, renal and cardiac function)
	Premature: 61–170 h
	Neonates, full-term: 35–45 h
	Infants: 18–25 h
	Children: 35 h
	Adults: 38–48 h
	Anephric adults: >45 d
	Anuric adults: 3.5–5 d
	Elimination: 50–70% excreted unchanged in urine
	Dialysis: Nondialyzable (0–5%)

calcium concentrations are increased, and that the membrane potential is unstable. This may lead to dysrhythmias. Furthermore, there is a decrease in conduction through the sinoatrial and AV nodes at toxic concentrations of digoxin.

The absorption of oral digoxin is approximately 75%. Malabsorption syndromes and decreased gut motility slow absorption. Digoxin is approximately 25% protein bound. The half-life is approximately 1.6 days. Most digoxin is excreted renally, with limited hepatic metabolism. There is only a small amount of enterohepatic recirculation of digoxin in contrast to the large recirculation of digitoxin. Pharmacokinetic data are listed in Table 37–1.

There are numerous factors that predispose the patient to digoxin toxicity. Both hypokalemia and hyperkalemia increase the chance of developing digoxin toxicity. Hypokalemia reduces the rate of Na$^+$–K$^+$ ATPase pump turnover.

Patients on concurrent diuretic therapy are at risk of developing hypokalemia and chronic digoxin toxicity. Hyperkalemia can cause further depolarization, and may lead to clinically significant conduction delays. Hypomagnesemia, hypercalcemia, renal insufficiency, and underlying heart disease are all known causes predisposing to digoxin toxicity. There are also numerous drugs that interact with digoxin elimination, which can result in toxicity (Table 37–2).

CLINICAL PRESENTATION

The presentation of digitalis toxicity in the pediatric setting varies. It is important for the clinician to distinguish between the acute and chronic forms of toxicity. Acute toxicity generally responds well to supportive therapy, whereas chronic toxicity is more refractory to treatment. Chronic toxicity is more commonly seen among the elderly when patients are treated with both digitalis and diuretics. They may be on other medications that may alter the clearance of digoxin. However, many children are also on chronic digoxin therapy, and with those underlying heart disease will similarly be at high risk for toxicity. Children can also be at risk for ingesting a family member's digitalis preparation.

Early signs and symptoms of digitalis may be very subtle. Anorexia, nausea, vomiting, and diarrhea are clues to toxicity. Other symptoms that may be present in children include visual disturbances such as photophobia and altered red–green color perception. Other symptoms consistent with toxicity are fatigue, malaise, weakness, headache, rashes, altered mental status, and paresthesias. Bradycardia, hyperkalemia, and vomiting are the most predictive symptoms in patients with acute digoxin intoxication.

Cardiovascular toxicity is clearly the most important factor in determining morbidity and mortality. Symptoms reflecting cardiovascular toxicity include palpitations and dizziness usually secondary to hypotension. There are a myriad of abnormal rhythms that can be seen with digoxin toxicity. There is no pathognomonic rhythm. Dysrhythmias can be supraventricular, nodal, and ventricular in nature. Commonly occurring rhythms include ventricular premature beats, junctional escape beats, and rhythms (especially accelerated junctional rhythms), paroxysmal atrial tachycardia with block, and AV block of varying degrees (Table 37–3). The most common electrocardiographic manifestation of digitalis toxicity is the presence of ventricular premature beats of any morphology. Sinus bradycardia or first-degree AV block are also commonly noted in pediatric patients.

Table 37–2. Factors Altering Serum Digoxin Concentration

	Drugs That Interact With Digoxin	
Increases Risk of Digoxin Toxicity	**Decreased Elimination**	**Decreased Bioavailability**
Hypokalemia	Indomethacin	Cathartics
Hyperkalemia	Verapamil	Antacids
Hypomagnesemia	Potassium-sparing diuretics	Cholesterol-binding agents
Hypercalcemia	Excessive diuretic use	
Age (elderly)	Quinidine	
Renal insufficiency	Cyclosporine	
Hypothyroidism	Amiodarone	
Antibiotics (erythromycin)		

Table 37–3. Electrocardiographic Changes and Abnormal Rhythms Associated With Digitalis Toxicity

Ventricular premature beats
Sinus bradycardia
Increased PR interval
First-degree AV block
Second-degree AV block
    Mobitz I
    Mobitz II
Third-degree AV block
ST-Segment abnormalities
Sinoatrial pause or arrest
Junctional rhythms
Supraventricular dysrhythmias
Paroxysmal atrial tachycardia with block
Ventricular tachycardia
Ventricular fibrillation
Asystole

Abbreviation: AV, atrioventricular.

The key to correct diagnosis is for the clinician to have a high index of suspicion for digoxin toxicity. A history of the exact amount of digoxin ingested is extremely helpful because an ingested dose of greater than 0.1 mg/kg has been suggested as an indication for the use of digoxin-specific Fab fragments. Additionally, the treating physician must suspect chronic toxicity in children presenting with vague, nonspecific symptoms who are on digoxin. Malaise, headache, fatigue, and mild gastrointestinal symptoms may be all that is presented to the clinician in the setting of digoxin toxicity.

LABORATORY

Appropriate laboratory studies in the setting of digoxin toxicity include a complete blood count, serum electrolytes, magnesium, calcium, blood urea nitrogen, creatinine, and an electrocardiogram. If the condition is severe, arterial blood gases will reveal metabolic acidosis from hypoperfusion. If the ingestant is unknown, it is appropriate to obtain acetaminophen and salicylate levels, as well as a urine toxicology screen.

Digoxin level should be ordered whenever there is clinical suspicion for digoxin toxicity. Therapeutic digoxin levels are usually considered to be between 0.8 to 1.8 ng/mL. Levels are obtained upon admission, and again at 6 hours after ingestion to account for full distribution of the drug. Serum digoxin concentrations obtained between 6 and 12 hours postingestion correlate well with the clinical course of intoxication.

In neonates and newborns, one must consider falsely elevated digoxin levels secondary to digoxin-like immunoreactive substances. These substances have been described with greatest frequency in babies 1 to 2 days after birth. Rarely, these substances can be present in older children. They are thought to be due to a steroid substance that is present in the neonatal period.

Toxicity can be seen with digoxin levels above 2.0 ng/mL, especially in the chronic setting. In children with acute toxicity, a level of 2.6 ng/mL does not correlate with signs and symptoms of digoxin toxicity. Woolf has recently suggested a cutoff level of 5 ng/mL alone as an indication for Fab therapy in acutely toxic patients. However, the clinician must keep in mind that toxicity may not correlate well with levels, and treatment should be guided by the entire clinical picture of the patient rather than simply the level.

The distinction between acute and chronic ingestion is very important. In the acute setting, the patient has more dramatic clinical and laboratory findings than in the chronic setting. In the acute group, the onset of symptoms is more abrupt, with severe nausea and vomiting. In chronic cases, there may be only mild nausea and vomiting. Serum levels are higher in the acute setting. Patients with chronic toxicity are symptomatic and more unstable with lower digoxin serum levels. Finally, the potassium level is higher in the acute group, reflecting the acute action on the Na^+–K^+ ATPase pump. Patients with chronic digoxin toxicity may be on diuretic therapy, and may actually have low or normal potassium concentrations.

MANAGEMENT

It is essential for children with possible digoxin toxicity to be managed aggressively. This is justified by the high potential for morbidity. All patients should have IV access, frequent vital sign assessment, and continuous cardiac monitoring.

Syrup of ipecac is relatively contraindicated in the asymptomatic child because of the potential for hemodynamic instability and alteration in mental status that can predispose to aspiration. It is absolutely contraindicated in any patient who presents with abnormal vital signs or is drowsy. Lavage is appropriate with adequate protection of the airway if the ingestion occurs within 1 hour of presentation. Vagal stimulation owing to tube placement may exacerbate heart block or bradycardia. Activated charcoal can be administered as a single dose. Whole bowl irrigation may be useful in alert patients following large ingestions. Multiple doses of charcoal have been reported to be of value for digitoxin preparations where there is avid enterohepatic recirculation, and may be useful if antidotal therapy is not available.

Digoxin-immune Fab fragments are specific antidigoxin antibodies raised in sheep (Figure 37–1). Only the Fab fragment is used to decrease the risk of immunogenicity. This antidote has been used successfully in adults since 1976; its first use in children was in 1982. The use of the Fab fragments is indicated in cases of severe digitalis intoxication suspected by history, a high level, or a child manifesting significant signs and symptoms of toxicity. An ingestion of more than 0.1 mg/kg is considered to be an indication for Fab fragments. A digoxin level of greater than 5 ng/mL in the acute setting is another suggested indication. The presence of a life-threatening dysrhythmia or conduction delay would be an indication in and of itself. Also, if the patient's condition is deteriorating, Fab fragments are indicated. Again, this may be seen at lower digoxin levels in the case of chronic toxicity.

Because hyperkalemia can potentiate digoxin toxicity, hyperkalemia higher than 5.5 mEq/L is another indication to consider the use of Fab fragments. Standard modalities to treat hyperkalemia may also be used (glucose, insulin, bicarbonate), with the exception of calcium salts. It is felt that the administration of calcium in the face of digoxin toxicity may exacerbate the development of dysrhythmias.

Dosage of Fab fragments is based either on the amount ingested or on the serum level. Guidelines are available in the package insert. Each vial of Fab fragments contains 40 mg of drug, which will bind approximately 0.6 mg of digoxin.

Calculations

$$\text{Dose (\# of vials)} = \frac{\text{Total digitalis body load (mg)}}{0.6 \text{ mg of digitalis bound/vial}}$$

If the digoxin serum level is available the following formula can be used to estimate the dose in adults (Table 37–4):

Dose (# of vials) =

$$\frac{\text{Serum digoxin concentration (ng/mL)} \times \text{Wt (kg)}}{100}$$

Although supporting literature is limited and anecdotal, empiric Fab fragment therapy of 1 to 2 vials for symptomatic children with elevated digoxin levels due to chronic poisoning is also an acceptable approach.

Allergic reactions are rare, but should be anticipated. In cases where Fab fragments have been effective the results can be seen in the range of 30 minutes to 4 hours after the dose. It is important to note that subsequent digoxin levels will be falsely elevated after the administration of Fab fragments, and this will take several days to correct. Radioimmunoassay measures all digoxin, not just free digoxin, therefore giving a falsely elevated result.

Along with administration of Fab fragments, standard treatment of dysrhythmias or blocks is indicated. Atropine or pacing may be necessary to temporize while Fab fragments are taking effect. Phenytoin can improve AV conduction. Magnesium can also be a useful in digoxin-induced ventricular tachydysrhythmias. Hyperkalemia should be treated with standard therapy. Cardioversion and lidocaine are appropriate in case of ventricular dysrhythmias or ventricular tachycardia and ventricular fibrillation.

Extracorporeal methods of hemodialysis and hemoperfusion do not aid in the management of digoxin toxicity. Plasma exchange also is not useful.

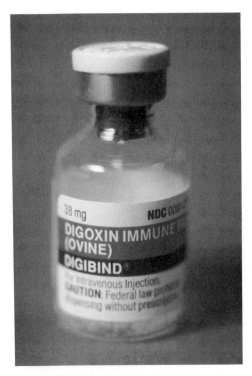

Fig. 37–1. Digoxin immune Fab fragments.

Table 37–4. Dosing for Infants and Small Children: Dose Estimates of Digibind (in mg) from Steady-State Serum Digoxin Concentration

Weight	Serum Digoxin Concentration (ng/mL)						
(kg)	1	2	4	8	12	16	20
1	0.4	1.0	1.5	3.0	5.0	7.0	8.0
3	1.0	3.0	5.0	10.0	15.0	19.0	24.0
5	2.0	4.0	8.0	16.0	24.0	32.0	40.0
10	4.0	8.0	16.0	32.0	48.0	64.0	80.0
20	8.0	16.0	32.0	64.0	96.0	128.0	160.0

Note: For very small doses, the drug should be diluted. A reconstituted vial containing 40 mg can be diluted with 36 mL of sterile isotonic saline to achieve a concentration of 1 mg/mL. The required dose can be administered with a tuberculin syringe.

Reproduced from Burroughs Wellcome dosing for Infant and Small Children Dose Estimates of Digibind (in mg) from Steady-State Serum Digoxin Concentration.

DISPOSITION

Children with trivial ingestions with no evidence of signs or symptoms, dysrhythmias, and no detectable levels of digoxin 4 hours after ingestion may be discharged from the ED after 6 hours of observation.

Any child that has signs and symptoms of digoxin toxicity should be admitted to a monitoring bed. All patients with significant signs and symptoms, and where the use of Fab fragments is being considered, should be admitted to a pediatric intensive care unit (PICU). Consultation with the poison control center, a toxicologist, or a cardiologist familiar with the treatment of these cases is suggested.

CASE OUTCOME

Based on an estimated total digoxin dose of 600 μg since discharge from the newborn nursery, and prior to receiving the results of the digoxin assay, the patient was given Fab digoxin-specific antibodies, 40 mg in 24 mL of normal saline IV over 1 hour and transferred to the PICU. The initial total digoxin level sent from the ED prior to administration of Fab was 25.0 ng/mL, and initial potassium level was 8.6 mEq/L. Another serum potassium 5 hours after admission was 4.3 mEq/L. Seven hours after admission, the total digoxin was greater than 10 ng/mL, with a free digoxin of 0.6 ng/mL. Maintenance potassium

(20 mEq/L) was subsequently added to the IV fluids, and the patient remained hemodynamically stable in sinus rhythm. The potassium level 24 hours after admission was 5.5 mEq/L with a total digoxin level still greater than 10 ng/mL, and a free digoxin level of 3.9 ng/mL.

The patient was started on oral feedings of glucose and electrolyte solution, and rapidly advanced to full formula feedings. Digoxin levels continued to decline throughout the remainder of his hospitalization, and the patient was discharged after 3 days, in normal sinus rhythm with a corrected maintenance digoxin prescription.

SUGGESTED READINGS

Gittleman MA, Stephan M, Perry H: Acute pediatric digoxin ingestion. *Pediatr Emerg Care* 5:359–362, 1999.

Hastreiter AR, van der Horst RL, Chow-Tung E: Digitalis toxicity in infants and children. *Pediatr Cardiol* 5:131–148, 1984.

Hicks JM, Brett EM: Falsely increased digoxin concentrations in samples from neonates and infants. *Ther Drug Monit* 6:461–464, 1984.

Jeager A, Bilbault P, Meziana F, et al: Digoxin antibodies, when? How much? *J Toxicol Clin Toxicol* 414:424–425, 2003.

Kaufman J, Leikin J, Kendzierski D, et al: Use of digoxin Fab immune fragments in a seven-day-old infant. *Pediatr Emerg Care* 6:118–121, 1990.

Kearns GL, Moss M, Clayton BD, et al: Pharmacokinetics and efficacy of digoxin specific Fab fragments in a child following massive digoxin overdose. *J Clin Pharmacol* 29:901–908, 1989.

Keller F, Kreutz G, Vohringer H, et al: Effect of plasma exchange on the steady state kinetics of digoxin and digitoxin. *Clin Pharmacokinet* 10:514–523, 1985.

Leikin J, Vogel S, Graff J, et al: Use of Fab fragments of digoxin-specific antibodies in the therapy of massive digoxin poisoning. *Ann Emerg Med* 14:175–178, 1985.

Litovitz T, Klein-Schwartz W, Rodger GC, et al: 2001 annual report of the American Association of Poison Control Centers Toxic Exposure Surveillance System. *Pediatrics* 20:391–452, 2002.

Ma G, Brady WJ, Pollack M, et al: Electrocardiographic manifestations: Digitalis toxicity. *J Emerg Med* 20:145–152, 2001.

Pap C, Zacher G, Karteszi M: Estimation of the risk of patients with acute digoxin intoxication. *J Toxicol Clin Toxicol* 41:501–502, 2003.

Van Duesen SK, Birkhahn RJ, Gaeta TJ: Treatment of hyperkalemia in a patient with unrecognized digitalis toxicity. *J Toxicol Clin Toxicol* 41:373–376, 2003.

Watson W, Litovitz T, Rodgers GC, et al: 2002 annual report of the American Association of Poison Control Centers Toxic Exposure Surveillance System. *Pediatrics* 21:353–421, 2003.

38

Theophylline

Frank P. Paloucek
Michael Shannon

HIGH-YIELD FACTS

- Compared to most therapeutic agents, theophylline has a narrower therapeutic index and significantly greater morbidity and mortality.

- Age <2 years or >60 years in chronic intoxication, or serum concentration >100 mg/L in acute overdose, are associated with increased morbidity and mortality.

- Status epilepticus secondary to theophylline intoxication has greater morbidity and mortality than from other causes.

- Theophylline poisoning is a well-established indication for the use of multiple doses of oral activated charcoal.

- Extracorporeal removal is highly efficacious and should be started as early as possible if indicated. High-clearance hemodialysis is safer and as effective as hemoperfusion.

CASE PRESENTATION

An 8-day-old neonate (33 weeks' gestational age) in a neonatal intensive care unit (NICU) is noted one morning to have poor feeding, jitteriness, and tachycardia. Nursing staff, experienced with similar cases, recognized the possibility of theophylline toxicity. The neonate had been receiving theophylline 1.1 mg/kg intravenous (IV) bolus every 8 hours for 4 days. A total of 12 doses had been administered, and the morning dose was held pending the results of a stat theophylline concentration. The

serum concentration (8 hours after the last dose) was 57 mg/L. Serum potassium was 3.2 mEq/L. The NICU staff contacted a poison information specialist at the regional poison control center; the specialist discussed the case with the on-call medical toxicologist.

The patient's birth weight was 1.5 kg but had decreased to 1.35 kg over the following 8 days. The specialist determined that a failure to adjust the dose for decreasing weight led to chronic overmedication. Supportive therapy with fluids was started. Because of the infant's prematurity, young age, and the possibility of necrotizing enterocolitis, oral charcoal was not administered. A pediatric nephrology consultant concluded that the patient's size precluded the use of extracorporeal elimination therapies, such as hemodialysis or hemoperfusion, and that the magnitude of the serum concentration was not an indication for such therapies. The staff observed the patient in the NICU and obtained serial measurements of theophylline.

INTRODUCTION AND EPIDEMIOLOGY

There have been several historical clusters of theophylline toxicity since its introduction as a medicinal agent for asthma. The first pediatric events were in the 1950s, with fatalities associated with the use of adult-strength suppositories in children. In the 1980s, the introduction of sustained-release dosage forms led to a significant increase in the incidence of theophylline toxicity, which became one of the top 10 causes of poisoning death nationwide. The introduction of newer agents, dosage forms, and practice guidelines for the treatment of asthma during the 1990s have significantly reduced both the prescribing of theophylline and the incidence of theophylline poisoning. The 1997–2001 American Association of Poison

Control Centers Toxic Exposure and Surveillance System summaries reported a total of 2917 childhood theophylline exposures, which represented 33% of the total for this drug. Although the mean number of exposures was 583 annually, the numbers of cases decreased consistently over the period. Only 2 of the total 63 who died were children, a 15-year-old (intentional suicide) and a 3-year-old (unintentional).

Important factors leading to theophylline morbidity and mortality are its narrow therapeutic index, the proliferation of multiple dosage forms, availability as a nonprescription product (thigh-reducing cream), and multiple drug–drug, drug–disease, and drug–food interactions. Theophylline remains a common cause of fatal adverse drug events in adults.

It is critical to classify theophylline toxicity as acute, acute-on-chronic, or chronic in its development. Unfortunately, there is no consensus on the definitions of these terms. In this discussion, *acute* refers to toxicity that occurs after one or more excessive doses within an 8-hour interval; *acute-on-chronic*, after a single excessive dose in a patient who has been ingesting theophylline for >24 hours; and *chronic*, during maintenance drug therapy (Table 38–1).

DEVELOPMENTAL CONSIDERATIONS

Hepatic metabolism of theophylline in neonates differs from that in older infants, resulting in a comparatively prolonged half-life (24 hours). The cytochrome isoenzymes CYP1A2 (the main enzymatic metabolic pathway), CYP2E1, and CYP3A4 are not fully expressed in neonates. CYP1A2 specifically is not mature until 5 to 6 months of life. Neonates thus rely more heavily on N-methyltransferase pathways and renal elimination than do older babies. However, both CYP1A2 and methyltransferases may become saturated in neonates who have supratherapeutic theophylline concentrations. These de-

Table 38–1. Classification of Theophylline Toxicity

Acute
    One or more excessive doses within an 8-h interval
Acute-on-Chronic
    Single excessive dose after regular dosing >24 h
Chronic
    During maintenance drug therapy

velopmental issues appear to prolong theophylline half-life, increase caffeine formation (via N-methyltransferase), decrease caffeine elimination (owing to impaired CYP2E1 and CYP3A4 activity), and increase concentrations of both theophylline and caffeine. Neonates appear relatively tolerant to supratherapeutic theophylline concentrations. They often fail to demonstrate the life-threatening complications seen in older children, adolescents, and adults despite comparable or higher serum concentrations. The highest reported theophylline concentration associated with survival—330 mg/L—was in a neonate.

PHARMACOLOGY AND TOXICOKINETICS

Theophylline is marketed in parenteral and oral (immediate- and sustained-release) oral dosage forms. It is absorbed readily (80% to 100%) after ingestion. The parenteral dosage form, although primarily intended for older children and adults, is also administered to neonates for the treatment of apnea and bradycardia. This usage requires careful dilution and dosage calculations. Dose miscalculations are a common etiology for medication errors, particularly 10-fold dosing errors. The ingestion of sustained-release theophylline preparations may delay or prolong absorption (or both), and therefore delay manifestations and severity of symptoms following overdose. Food and other drugs may affect theophylline absorption; sustained-release products are also known to form concretions or pharmacobezoars in the overdose setting. In cases of intentional overdose, peak serum theophylline concentrations have occurred as late as 24 to 27 hours after arrival in the emergency department (ED).

The volume of distribution (V_d) of theophylline is fairly consistent for individuals but decreases from 0.6 L/kg in children to 0.5 L/kg in adults. There is no evidence that the V_d changes in the overdose setting. This allows approximation of the peak concentration following an oral overdose. The worst-case peak concentration (mg/L) estimate for most overdoses of parenteral and immediate-release theophylline is twice the exposure dose (mg/kg) for overdoses of sustained-release products, where the peak is equal to the dose.

Theophylline metabolism occurs primarily via the hepatic mixed-function oxidase systems (cytochrome P450), with a mean elimination half-life of 6 to 8 hours in adults. CYP1A2 accounts for the majority of metabolism, demethylating theophylline to 1-methylxanthine and 3-methylxanthine, and forming 1,3-dimethyluric acid. CYP2E1 and CYP3A4 also account for a portion of theophylline metabolism. Multiple factors such as disease, drugs, age, gender, and diet may either enhance or impair theophylline metabolism. Common factors contributing to chronic overmedication include decreased metabolism at extremes of age (<2 or >60 years), symptomatic congestive heart failure, hepatic disease, acute viral infections, and concomitant treatment with erythromycin, cimetidine, fluoroquinolones, and allopurinol. Other etiologies for chronic toxicity include the recent discontinuation of elimination-enhancing factors without concomitant theophylline dosage adjustment, such as smoking, barbiturates, carbamazepine, phenytoin, or rifampin.

PATHOPHYSIOLOGY

The exact mechanism of theophylline toxicity is unknown. The majority of its effects appear to reflect direct adenosine-receptor antagonist activity. It is known to exert a number of pharmacodynamic effects, summarized in Table 38–2. Many of these effects, and theophylline-induced cellular shifts in electrolytes, are mediated via stimulation of β_2-adrenergic receptors. Manifestations of theophylline toxicity are direct extensions of some of these properties.

CLINICAL FINDINGS

Acute, acute-on-chronic, and chronic theophylline toxicity generally lead to similar clinical findings, although there are some variations in laboratory findings and unique manifestations that distinguish them.

The primary clinical manifestations of acute theophylline toxicity are in the gastrointestinal (GI), cardiovascular, and neurologic systems. Disturbances in serum electrolytes (potassium, bicarbonate, and glucose), have

Table 38–2. Pharmacodynamic Effects of Theophylline

CNS stimulation
Stimulation of the medullary vomiting center
Positive cardiac inotropy and chronotropy
Reduction of peripheral arteriolar resistance
Increase in renal blood flow and GFR
Stimulation of secretion of gastric acid and pepsin

Abbreviations: CNS, central nervous system; GFR, glomerular filtration rate.

Table 38–3. Clinical Manifestations of Theophylline Toxicity

Gastrointestinal
    Nausea
    Severe and refractory vomiting
    Hemorrhage
Cardiovascular
    Tachyarrhythmias (especially multifocal atrial tachycardia)
    Hypotension
    Cardiac arrest
Neurologic
    Mental status changes
    Tremor
    Seizures
    Coma
Electrolyte disturbances
    Hypokalemia
    Hypophosphatemia
    Hypercalcemia
Miscellaneous
    Diuresis
    Rhabdomyolysis
    Tachypnea
    Hyperglycemia

been observed as well. These manifestations are summarized in Table 38–3.

GI findings include nausea, severe and refractory vomiting, and GI bleeding. Nausea and vomiting are nonspecific and may occur with therapeutic use. Vomiting may be severe enough to limit the use of activated charcoal. GI bleeding has been reported in acute childhood overdoses of the oral form. There are no reports of clinically significant blood loss, and the bleeding probably represents mild esophageal or gastric erosions.

Cardiovascular findings include tachyarrhythmias, hypotension, and cardiac arrest. Sinus and supraventricular tachycardias are the most common presentations of theophylline toxicity, regardless of etiology. They are also the findings most likely to reveal previously unrecognized intoxication in the neonatal patient. These are not generally life threatening in the absence of other underlying cardiac disease. Specific to acute or chronic toxicity, although not pathognomonic, are multifocal atrial tachycardias. Ventricular ectopy is reasonably common, but significant or life-threatening ventricular arrhythmias are very rare. Peripheral β_2-receptor–stimulated vasodilation is responsible for the hypotension that is unique to acute theophylline overdoses and is associated with serum concentrations >100 mg/L.

Neurologic manifestations include mental status changes, tremor, seizures, and coma. Seizures, typically generalized tonic–clonic, are a grave sign. Status epilepticus may occur and is associated with greater morbidity and mortality than other causes of status epilepticus in children. A serum theophylline concentration >100 mg/L predisposes to seizures. Literature reviews suggest that 20% of patients with reported theophylline-induced seizures die. Death may be a direct consequence of seizures, but is more commonly due to secondary complications, particularly after cardiac events. Postictal coma, probably an indirect consequence, has also been reported.

Electrolyte disturbances, fairly typical in the acutely intoxicated patient, include hypokalemia, hypophosphatemia, and hypercalcemia. These concentration-dependent changes reflect transient cellular shifts associated with β_2-adrenergic stimulation, and are not associated with any significant pathology if theophylline alone is the cause. Specifically, there is an inverse linear relationship between potassium concentration and theophylline concentration when the latter exceeds 35 mg/L. All forms of acid–base disorders have been reported with theophylline poisoning, mostly related to underlying diseases and coingestants. Theophylline-induced lactic acidosis has been reported very rarely in severe acute toxicity.

Miscellaneous manifestations of theophylline toxicity include diuresis (related to transient increase in renal blood flow that follows acute exposure), rhabdomyolysis, and tachypnea. Hyperglycemia may also occur, presumably as an acute stress response.

LABORATORY AND DIAGNOSTIC TESTING

The single most important laboratory evaluation for suspected theophylline toxicity is a serum theophylline concentration. The normal adult range is 10 to 20 mg/L; the toxic range is >20 mg/L, although symptoms of toxicity may occur at concentrations of 10 to 20 mg/L. Significant toxicity is likely with concentrations >100 mg/L for acute overdoses. Ingestion of ≥50 mg/kg or ≥100 mg/kg sustained-release tablets can potentially produce a theophylline concentration of ≥100 mg/L. Increased mortality is associated with age <2 years or serum theophylline concentration >100 mg/L in acute pediatric overdoses.

Depending on the laboratory methodology used, significant cross-reaction in the presence of caffeine, uremia, or hyperbilirubinemia may produce false reports of elevated theophylline concentrations. It is critical, especially in known sustained-release overdoses, that serial concentrations be measured every 1 to 2 hours, until two consecutive theophylline concentrations establish a decreasing trend. This allows for appropriate monitoring of the absorption phase of these products, as well as identification of concretions or pharmacobezoars. Serum concentration monitoring should continue until theophylline is undetectable. If a sustained-release dosage form has been ingested, three consecutive decreasing concentrations should be obtained, at least one of which should more be than 24 hours after the ingestion. Concretions or bezoars should be suspected with essentially unchanged or markedly prolonged increases in serum concentrations over a period greater than 24 hours.

Additional initial laboratory testing includes fingerstick glucose, serum electrolytes, arterial blood gas, and 12-lead electrocardiogram. An acetaminophen concentration is indicated in the overdose patient to rule out a concomitant ingestion.

MANAGEMENT

Patients presenting with acute theophylline toxicity are managed with conventional supportive care and individualized treatment of specific complications (Table 38–4). There is no specific antidote for theophylline toxicity.

Options for GI decontamination are limited for acute and acute-on-chronic presentations. Syrup of ipecac is contraindicated owing to potential seizure activity associated with theophylline toxicity. Gastric lavage should be considered if it can be performed within 1 hour after a large, life-threatening ingestion. However, a lavage tube sufficiently large to accommodate most sustained-release theophylline products may not be practical, especially in a small child.

Activated charcoal is the gastric decontamination treatment of choice. The ideal decontamination dose should be calculated to deliver 10 g of charcoal for every gram of ingested theophylline. The use of weight-based dosing, 1 g/kg, is unlikely to provide an adequate amount of charcoal for decontamination, given the amounts found in conventional theophylline products. The initial dose of activated charcoal should be 50 to 100 g of charcoal in adolescents, and 15 to 25 g in children. This represents ideal decontamination of 1.5 g (or five 300 mg tablets) of theophylline. It is important to note that achieving a 10:1

Table 38–4. Management of Theophylline Toxicity

Conventional supportive care
Specific antidote: None
GI decontamination
    Activated charcoal
Elimination enhancement
    Multiple-dose activated charcoal (bolus or
        continuous nasogastric infusion)
    Hemodialysis (or charcoal hemoperfusion)
    Continuous renal replacement modalities
    Exchange transfusion
    Plasmapheresis
Treatment of complications
    Seizures
        First line: benzodiazepines
        Second line: barbiturates (consider paralysis)
    Arrhythmias
        Short-acting β_2-receptor antagonists (esmolol)
        Calcium channel antagonists (avoid verapamil)
    Hypotension
        Short-acting β_2-receptor antagonists (esmolol)
    Persistent vomiting
        Slow charcoal administration
        Metoclopramide (up to 0.5 mg/kg)
    Electrolyte disturbances
        Avoid overcorrection (often resolve
          spontaneously)

ratio ultimately may require multiple doses, best accomplished with aliquots of 12.5 to 25.0 g hourly. In the absence of a known or even estimable amount ingested, a reasonable approach would be to use serial theophylline concentrations following the administration of the initial dose to assess the apparent severity of the ingestion. A very small number of neonates, including premature infants who received inadvertent parenteral overdoses, have tolerated serial doses of oral activated charcoal when extracorporeal methods for elimination enhancement were unavailable.

Elimination enhancement is an important component of the management of severe theophylline toxicity. Potential modalities include multiple-dose oral activated charcoal, hemodialysis, charcoal hemoperfusion, other continuous renal replacement modalities, exchange transfusions, and plasmapheresis. For any significant ingestion, oral activated charcoal 12.5 to 25.0 g every 1 to 2 hours should be initiated and continued until concentrations are <20 mg/L. These may be administered as boluses or a continuous nasogastric infusion.

Hemodialysis and charcoal hemoperfusion are indicated prophylactically in patients with theophylline concentration >100 mg/L, or when charcoal therapy is contraindicated or poorly tolerated. Withholding these modalities until toxicity occurs is undesirable; severe toxicity may cause hypotension, seizures, and tachyarrhythmias, which may preclude initiation of these procedures. Hemoperfusion was once preferred to hemodialysis because it achieves higher clearance rates; however, newer hemodialysis machines achieve clearances comparable to those of hemoperfusion. For adequate hemoperfusion, the charcoal cartridge should be exchanged every 2 hours to avoid saturation and loss of efficacy. Both hemodialysis and charcoal hemoperfusion have been used simultaneously, although there is no comparative clinical data to suggest that the practice improves outcome.

Although limited, there is some experience to indicate that exchange transfusion or plasmapheresis may benefit the intoxicated neonate or infant, and should be considered when hemodialysis is not feasible.

The treatment of choice for seizures is benzodiazepine administration. Barbiturates should be second-line therapy. Phenytoin is contraindicated in the absence of any known prior indications; in vitro studies show that it lowers seizure threshold in theophylline intoxication and is clinically ineffective. The development of repetitive seizures or status epilepticus is an indication for barbiturate coma, with or without paralysis. Isolated seizure activity does not require long-term maintenance anticonvulsant therapy.

Arrhythmias are treated with β-receptor or calcium channel blockade. Short-acting β-receptor antagonists such as esmolol are preferred; verapamil should be avoided, because it may inhibit theophylline metabolism. Ventricular arrhythmias and cardiac arrests should be managed conventionally. Hypotension refractory to conventional support may be β_2-mediated, and therefore may respond to β-receptor blockade.

Persistent vomiting may respond to several interventions, none of which has proven superior. Slow charcoal administration over 15 to 20 minutes or infusion via GI feeding tube systems may be effective. Metoclopramide, 10 mg IV, has been proven effective in approximately 50% of theophylline poisonings that require ICU admission. Larger doses may be necessary in severe cases (up to 0.5 mg/kg). Alternatively, the patient may be treated with odansatron for intractable vomiting.

Electrolyte disturbances that are the result of acute theophylline overdose do not require acute correction and often resolve spontaneously. The cellular shifts of electrolytes are transient, resolving within 2 to 3 hours, and are nonpathologic. In cases of extreme values (e.g., K^+ <3.0 mEq/L), a single conventional replacement dose of the appropriate salt is indicated. Symptomatic overcorrection has occurred in patients with serial replacement doses without interval reassessment. Lactic acidosis should be managed conventionally.

Acute-on-Chronic Theophylline Toxicity

Patients with acute-on-chronic theophylline toxicity present with the same clinical manifestations as those with acute toxicity, but signs develop at lower theophylline concentrations. Historical details or the presence of multifocal atrial tachycardias, hypotension, or hypokalemia may provide clues to the diagnosis of acute-on-chronic toxicity. An elevated theophylline concentration confirms the diagnosis. Seizures occur with the same frequency as in acute presentations, but may occur at concentrations as low as 30 mg/L. Significant toxicity is likely with concentrations >60 mg/L in acute-on-chronic and chronic presentations, as opposed to >100 mg/L in acute overdose. Worst-case estimates for acute toxicity should be made with the conservative addition of 20 mg/L to the serum level to represent the chronic maintenance concentration.

Management is similar to the acute toxic overdose. The only variation occurs with the use of elimination-enhancing treatment. The endpoint of multiple-dose activated charcoal is 30 mg/L, not 20 mg/L, if theophylline therapy remains indicated. Hemodialysis and charcoal hemoperfusion are indicated prophylactically in patients with theophylline concentrations >100 mg/L in an acute or acute-on-chronic overdose.

Chronic Theophylline Toxicity

Chronic theophylline toxicity does not cause GI bleeding, hypotension, or hypokalemia. These findings in a patient on chronic theophylline therapy imply another etiology. All other toxic manifestations of theophylline occur in chronic patients, but at much lower serum levels. Severe toxic symptoms are often the presenting complaint.

Seizures in chronic patients present typically as either a few (1 to 3) partial-complex or generalized tonic–clonic seizures; there are no known predisposing factors for seizures in chronic toxicity. Seizures have been re-ported in chronic patients with theophylline concentrations >20 mg/L; and the incidence increases significantly with serum concentrations >60 mg/L. Age greater than 60 years is the best-documented poor prognostic factor for patients with chronic toxicity. Although there is no definitive data to support the observation, serum theophylline concentrations >60 mg/L in a chronic scenario appear to be associated with an increased incidence of significant morbidity and mortality. Increased morbidity and mortality are more likely when the intoxication is due to drug-underlying disease-state etiologies than drug–drug or drug–diet interactions. Status epilepticus is also associated with significant morbidity and mortality.

GI decontamination is not indicated for the chronic patient, although there is a role for elimination enhancement. For theophylline concentrations >30 mg/L, oral activated charcoal, 25 g every 2 hours, should be initiated and continued until concentrations are <30 mg/L or GI complications occur. Either hemodialysis or charcoal hemoperfusion is indicated in the chronic patient over 60 years of age, especially when the concentration is greater than 60 mg/L, although there is less support for this recommendation than for acute ingestions with concentrations >100 mg/L. Electrolyte disturbances are treated conventionally in the chronic overdose patient.

DISPOSITION

Patients who have ingested sustained-release preparations and have elevated or rising serum concentrations should be admitted to an intensive care unit. Patients who are asymptomatic (or have symptoms that resolve readily) and have concentrations that do not exceed 30 mg/L should be managed in the ED. Neonates suffering medication errors should be admitted to, or remain in, the NICU until symptoms resolve and concentrations are in an acceptable therapeutic range. Patients with histories of massive ingestion and rapidly rising concentrations should be considered for transfer to another institution if extracorporeal removal methods are not readily available at the presenting institution, even if they are asymptomatic or mildly symptomatic.

CASE OUTCOME

The patient did well over the day, and her heart rate and jitteriness improved significantly by the night shift; urinary output doubled. Analysis of three declining serum concentrations allowed calculation of a theophylline half-life of 25.5 hours, consistent with normal neonatal metabolism. Caffeine concentrations were not obtained. Toxicokinetic analysis of the first concentration suggested that even the simultaneous IV administration of all 12 doses 1 hour earlier could not have led to a concentration of 57 mg/L. In addition, chronic intoxication could not have realistically explained the elevation. The only likely explanation is that theophylline in excess of the history had to have been provided; a 10-fold dilution error in dosage calculation or drug preparation had most likely occurred.

Careful chart review revealed that a temporarily assigned health care provider was responsible for a 10-fold dosing admixture error on the last day (Day #4) of therapy, affecting last three doses. Staff education was instituted to improve awareness of this preventable error.

SUGGESTED READINGS

Cooling DS: Theophylline toxicity. *J Emerg Med* 11:415–425, 1993.

Henderson A, Wright DM, Pond SM: Management of theophylline overdose patients in an intensive care unit. *Aneasth Inten Care* 20:56–62, 1992.

Jain R, Tholl DA: Activated charcoal for theophylline toxicity in a premature infant on the second day of life. *Dev Pharmacol Ther* 19:106–110, 1992.

Lowry JA, Jarrett RV, Wasserman G, et al.: Theophylline toxicokinetics in premature newborns. *Arch Pediatr Adolesc Med* 155:934–939, 2001.

Osborn HH, Henry G, Wax P, Hoffman R, Howland MA: Theophylline toxicity in a premature neonate—elimination kinetics of exchange transfusion. *J Toxicol Clin Toxicol* 4:639–644, 1993.

Paloucek FP: Theophylline toxicokinetics. *J Pharm Pract* 6:57–62, 1993.

Paloucek FP, Rodvold KA: Evaluation of theophylline overdoses and toxicities. *Ann Emerg Med* 17:135–144, 1988.

Powell EC, Reynolds SL, Rubenstein JS: Theophylline toxicity in children: A retrospective review. *Pediatr Emerg Care* 9:129–133, 1993.

Sessler CN: Theophylline toxicity and overdose: Predisposing factors, clinical features, and outcome of 116 consecutive cases. *Am J Med* 88:567–576, 1990.

Shannon M, Amitai Y, Lovejoy F: Multiple dose activated charcoal for theophylline poisoning patients. *Pediatrics* 80:368–370, 1987.

Shannon M: Effect of acute versus chronic intoxication on clinical features of theophylline poisoning in children. *J Pediatr* 121:125–130, 1992.

Shannon M: Predictors of major toxicity after theophylline overdose. *Ann Intern Med* 119:1161–1167, 1993.

Skinner MH: Adverse reactions and interaction with theophylline. *Drug Safety* 5:275–285, 1990.

Woo OF, Pond SM, Benowitz NL, et al: Benefit of hemoperfusion in acute theophylline intoxication. *J Toxicol Clin Toxicol* 22:411–424, 1984.

39

Sedative-Hypnotics

Timothy B. Erickson
Donna Seger

CASE PRESENTATION

A 2-year-old girl presents to the emergency department (ED) 2 to 3 hours after ingesting several of her grandmother's lorazepam when the grandmother fell asleep while babysitting the child. The patient is otherwise healthy. The child arrives in the ED lethargic with a pulse of 80 bpm; blood pressure of 80/50 mmHg; respiratory rate of 8/min; a temperature of 97°F; and a pulse oximetry of 88%. The child's pupils are 4 mm and sluggishly reactive to light. No gag reflex is appreciated.

INTRODUCTION AND EPIDEMIOLOGY

This chapter focuses on those sedative-hypnotic agents commonly encountered in the pediatric population, including barbiturates, benzodiazepines, chloral hydrate, and γ-hydroxybutyrate (GHB). Other sedative-hypnotic agents such as meprobamate, glutethamide, and ethchlorvynol are much less common in the pediatric patient population and more relevant to adult patients. According to the 2001 American Association of Poison Control Centers (AAPCC) annual report, there were 10,943 exposures to benzodiazepines, 1023 toxic exposures to barbiturates, 81 exposures to chloral hydrate, and 395 cases of GHB in children under 20 years of age. There were two reported deaths in adolescent patients overdosing on benzodiazepines, and one from GHB toxicity.

BENZODIAZEPINES

Benzodiazepines are among the most commonly prescribed drugs in the world, and they constitute the majority of sedative-hypnotic overdoses. They are used for their anxiolytic, muscle relaxant, and anticonvulsant properties. Benzodiazepines produce less CNS and respiratory depression than barbiturates. Flunitrazepam is a potent benzodiazepine that has recently been popularized as a street drug of abuse and has been implicated as a date-rape drug. Flunitrazepam pills are often referred to as *roofies*.

Age and Developmental Considerations

Young children and toddlers are typically involved in accidental exposures and ingest small doses of benzodiazepines. Adolescent patients may ingest larger amounts of drug in the setting of a suicide gesture or attempt, or for recreational use. In addition, teenagers are more likely to exhibit chronic dependence and the potential for withdrawal symptoms.

Pharmacology

Benzodiazepines vary in onset and duration of action depending on lipid solubility and presence of active metabolites. The more lipid soluble the agent, the more rapidly it crosses the blood–brain barrier. The half-life of specific agents varies ranging from 1.5 to 2.5 hours with midazolam, to 30 to 60 hours with diazepam. Benzodiazepines can be administered intravenously, intramuscularly, orally, or rectally.

Pathophysiology

The benzodiazepines act by binding to benzodiazepine receptors on γ-aminobutyric acid (GABA) complexes, which increase the affinity of GABA for its receptor. Substances that increase GABA receptor-complex activity cause CNS depression. Benzodiazepines have anxiolytic, muscle relaxant, sedative-hypnotic, amnestic, and anticonvulsant properties. Pure benzodiazepine overdoses result in a mild to moderate CNS depression. Deep coma requiring assisted ventilation can occur. In severe overdoses, benzodiazepines can induce cardiovascular and pulmonary toxicity, but fatalities resulting from pure benzodiazepine overdoses are rare.

Clinical Presentation

Following an acute overdose, the patient classically presents with sedation, somnolence, ataxia, slurred speech, and lethargy. Profound coma is rare, and its presence should prompt a search for coingestions or reasons for coma. The elderly and very young children are more susceptible to the CNS depression of these drugs.

Benzodiazepines can also induce paradoxical reactions such as anxiety, delirium, combativeness, and hallucinations, particularly in children. Pupils are typically

dilated, and the patient may be hypothermic. As opposed to other sedative-hypnotics, benzodiazepines rarely cause significant cardiovascular manifestations, although bradycardia and hypotension have been reported in severe overdoses.

Laboratory

Quantitative benzodiazepine concentrations correlate poorly with pharmacologic or toxicologic effects, and are poor predictors of clinical outcome. However, qualitative screening for benzodiazepines in the serum or urine can be useful in diagnosing patients with coma of unknown etiology. Many standard urine toxicology screens are insufficiently sensitive to detect low levels of potent benzodiazepines like flunitrazepam.

Treatment

The most critical management intervention is stabilization of the patient's airway and respiratory status. Ipecac is contraindicated owing to the CNS depressant effects of these agents. In older children with a life-threatening ingestion, gastric lavage may be useful in obtunded patients who present within 1 hour of ingestion. Activated charcoal may be considered in significant overdoses. Forced diuresis is not efficacious and, because benzodiazepines are highly bound to plasma proteins, hemodialysis and hemoperfusion are also ineffective.

Flumazenil (Figure 39–1) is an antidotal agent that reduces or terminates benzodiazepine effects by competitive inhibition at the central nervous system GABA sites. According to the 2001 AAPCC database, flumazenil was the fifth most common antidote administered. In comatose children, initial doses of 0.01 mg/kg IV have been recommended. If no response is elicited, this dose can be repeated. In neonates, an IV loading dose of 0.02 mg/kg is suggested, with a maintenance drip of 0.05 mg/kg/h if indicated. The duration of flumazenil is less than 1 hour; thus, repeat doses or continuous infusions may be necessary.

Contraindications to flumazenil administration include seizure disorders, chronic benzodiazepine use, and coingestion of proconvulsant agents such as tricyclic antidepressants, cocaine, or isoniazid. Therefore, flumazenil should not be administered to children with coma of unknown cause. Administration of flumazenil is safe in healthy children with altered mental status caused by acute benzodiazepine overdose. If a coingestion is suspected, a urine drug screen and electrocardiogram should be obtained to rule out concomitant cyclic antidepressant

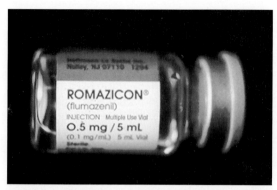

Fig. 39–1. Flumazenil is an antidotal agent that reduces or terminates benzodiazepine effects by competitive inhibition at the CNS GABA sites.

toxicity before flumazenil is administered. In this setting, reversal of benzodiazepine intoxication with flumenazil may be more problematic than providing respiratory support while the patient clears the drug via metabolism.

BARBITURATES

Pharmacology

The barbiturates are classified as either ultrashort acting (thiopental), short acting (pentobarbital), or long acting (phenobarbital). In the overdose setting, however, the duration of action varies with dose, rate of absorption, and rate of distribution and elimination. The shorter-acting agents are highly lipid soluble and rapidly penetrate the CNS. In addition, the shorter-acting barbiturates are more highly protein bound, have a higher pKa, and have larger volumes of distribution. Long-acting agents like phenobarbital are metabolized more slowly in the liver with a greater fraction of unchanged drug excreted in the kidney. These factors help to explain why enhanced renal elimination via alkalinization may be more effective with longer-acting agents. In addition, phenobarbital undergoes enterohepatic recirculation, making repetitive dosing of charcoal potentially advantageous.

Pathophysiology

These agents are primarily used as anticonvulsants in children, and for induction of anesthesia. Barbiturates are primarily CNS depressants that mediate their effect through inhibition of aminobutyric synapses of the brain. The reticular activating system and the cerebellum appear to be most susceptible to the depressant effects of barbiturates. Toxicity can result in suppression of skele-

tal, smooth, and cardiac muscle, leading to depressed myocardial contractility, bradycardia, vasodilation, and hypotension.

Clinical Presentation

In the overdose setting, the pediatric patient presents with CNS depression, often accompanied by respiratory depression. Vital signs may reveal hypotension, bradycardia, and hypothermia. Pupils are constricted early in the clinical course, but can be dilated in later stages of coma. As with most sedative-hypnotic agents, noncardiogenic pulmonary edema has been described in severely toxic patients. After prolonged coma, the patient can develop bullous skin lesions over dependent body parts, but this is rare. Cases of phenobarbital-induced hepatotoxicity have also been described in children.

Laboratory

In addition to baseline laboratory studies, a quantitative serum phenobarbital level is obtained to document the toxicity, but is not mandatory for definitive management. Therapeutic concentrations of phenobarbital range between 15 and 40 mg/L. Patients with levels >50 mg/L will exhibit mild toxicity, and those with levels >100 mg/L are typically unresponsive to pain and suffer from respiratory and cardiac depression.

Treatment

The primary management of barbiturate toxicity is support and stabilization of the airway and circulation. Comatose patients may require intubation. Hypotensive patients are managed with fluid resuscitation, and if necessary, pressor agents. Gastric lavage may be useful in obtunded patients presenting within 1 hour postingestion. Because most barbiturate ingestions cause CNS and respiratory depression, syrup of ipecac is contraindicated. Several investigations have demonstrated that multiple-dose activated charcoal significantly reduces the serum half-life of certain barbiturates such as phenobarbital, which undergoes enterohepatic circulation. Phenobarbital also has the physical characteristics that allows it to undergo gastric dialysis and be pulled from the blood into the gut, and adsorbed by charcoal. An initial dose of activated charcoal of 1 g/kg is recommended, followed by 0.25 g/kg every 4 to 6 hours. Physicians must be aware that some charcoal preparations are premixed with a cathartic. With multidosing regimens of activated charcoal, repeated doses of any cathartic agent are contraindicated to avoid dehydration and electrolyte imbalances. However, a small dose of sorbitol (0.2 to 0.5 g/kg) may be given with the first dose of activated charcoal in older children to prevent constipation. It should be noted that administration of multiple doses of charcoal has not been shown to change overall clinical outcome in phenobarbital toxicity.

Urinary alkalinization with sodium bicarbonate to a pH of 7.5 to 8.0 can hasten the renal excretion of phenobarbital, which is a weak acid and primarily renally excreted. Alkalinization can be accomplished with an initial sodium bicarbonate bolus of 1 mEq/kg, followed by a continuous infusion. This infusion is made by adding 100 to 150 mEq of sodium bicarbonate to 850 mL of dextrose 5% in water, and titrating it to maintain a urine pH of greater than 7.5 with an arterial pH less than 7.5. The rate must be assessed hourly to avoid excessive administration of fluid or bicarbonate, which can cause pulmonary or cerebral edema or electrolyte imbalance. It should be noted that no clinical evidence exists that shows this form of enhanced elimination ultimately improves patient outcome. Alkalinization does not increase excretion of shorter-acting agents, which are hepatically metabolized and are not primarily renally excreted.

In unstable patients not responsive to standard therapeutic measures, or in those with renal failure, hemodialysis is indicated for long-acting barbiturates. Fortunately, extracorporeal elimination is rarely indicated because most barbiturate overdoses do well with supportive care alone. Charcoal hemoperfusion seems more efficacious for shorter-acting agents, which possess greater fat and protein binding.

CHLORAL HYDRATE

Chloral hydrate is frequently used in the pediatric population for sedation prior to procedures or radiologic testing. It is an uncommon cause of overdose.

Pharmacokinetics

Chloral hydrate is rapidly absorbed from the gastrointestinal (GI) tract, with an onset of action within 30 minutes. It is metabolized in the liver by alcohol dehydrogenase. In adults, the parent compound has a half-life of a few minutes. Children metabolize chloral hydrate more slowly. The parent compound can be detected for several hours after administration in neonates and in children up to 2 years of age, and for 28 to 40 hours in preterm infants. The major active metabolites of chloral hydrate are

trichlorethanol (TCE) and trichloroacetic acid. TCE has a half-life of 6 to 12 hours. In pediatric patients, the TCE metabolite may be detected for up to 48 hours. Ethanol enhances the formation of TCE by alcohol dehydrogenase by increasing the availability of NADH. When the two are mixed, a synergistic sedative-depressant effect is rapidly produced. This interaction is the basis for the famous Mickey Finn cocktail or knock-out drops.

Pathophysiology

Chloral hydrate is an effective sedative-hypnotic that produces minimal respiratory and circulatory depression when given in therapeutic doses. Although most authorities recommend regimens of 25 to 50 mg/kg/dose, doses up to 80 to 100 mg/kg have been reported as safe and effective for pediatric sedation. Its structure is similar to that of the general anesthetic agent halothane. The sedative action of TCE is mediated by the $GABA_A$ receptor site, similar to barbiturates and benzodiazepines. In large overdoses, chloral hydrate can depress myocardial contractility and sensitize the myocardium to catecholamines, causing dysrhythmias.

Clinical Presentation

Signs and symptoms of chloral hydrate toxicity are very similar to those seen in barbiturate overdoses, with respiratory and CNS depression and cardiovascular manifestations. Pupils are typically miotic early in the clinical course but dilate in later stages of coma.

Following ingestion a child's breath may have a classic pear-like odor. GI upset with vomiting and abdominal pain is common, and occasionally elevation of hepatic enzymes is seen. Cardiac dysrhythmias can include atrial fibrillation, multifocal premature ventricular contractions, ventricular tachycardia, and ventricular fibrillation, which may progress to torsades de pointes. Inadvertent IV administration has been reported and may irritate the surrounding skin, but seems no more toxic than oral exposure. In severe overdose, the pediatric patient can exhibit hypothermia, hypotension, and noncardiogenic pulmonary edema.

Laboratory

Chloral hydrate levels can assist in documenting the ingestion, but correlate poorly with clinical findings. Trichlorethanol levels may be a more reliable indicator of toxicity, but management is not delayed awaiting their result. If the ingestion is recent, an abdominal radiograph is obtained to confirm the diagnosis, because chloral hydrate may be radiopaque.

Treatment

As with the other sedative-hypnotics, the child's airway is stabilized. Close attention is paid to the cardiovascular status owing to the potential for cardiotoxicity. Gastric decontamination considerations are similar to those of the other sedative-hypnotic agents. Ventricular dysrhythmias have responded to lidocaine, β-blockers, and magnesium administration; however, such cases have been anecdotal. If the patient is unstable, hemodialysis should be considered because this effectively removes the active metabolite trichlorethanol.

γ-Hydroxybutyrate

GHB was synthesized in 1960, and used as an anesthetic agent and for the treatment of sleep disorders because it induces REM sleep. However, its use was halted when the drug was found to induce seizure activity when given as an anesthetic agent. An erroneous study in the 1970s reported that GHB may stimulate growth hormone production; therefore, the drug became popular in the body building community. In addition, owing to its euphoric and mind-altering effects, it has become a very popular drug of abuse with adolescents. Common street names include Liquid Ecstasy, Scoop, Somatomax, Grievous Body Harm, Bioski, Blue Thunder, and Georgia Home Boy. The U.S. Drug Enforcement Agency (DEA) has classified GHB as a federally controlled substance. It has also been allegedly used in date rape owing to its rapid onset and amnestic-inducing properties. Currently, it is under U.S. Food and Drug Administration investigation for use in narcolepsy.

GHB is a colorless, odorless liquid or gel. As a powder, it has a salty taste. It is obtainable on the street, over the Internet, and can be easily produced in the home. With increased federal DEA regulation of GHB, its precursors γ-butyrolactone and 1,4-butandiol have gained recent popularity.

Pharmacology

The time of onset for clinical symptoms begin approximately 15 minutes after ingestion, with a peak effect in 30 to 45 minutes. The duration of action is from 1 to 5 hours. GHB is eliminated via hepatic biotransformation, with a small percentage excreted unchanged in the urine. Blood levels are generally undetectable after 6 hours of exposure.

Pathophysiology

Structurally, GHB is similar to the inhibitory neurotransmitter GABA. GHB crosses the blood–brain barrier and acts as a neurotransmitter affecting $GABA_B$ and dopaminergic receptors, causing CNS and respiratory depression. Theories regarding seizure activity include stimulation of presynaptic $GABA_A$ receptors and release of excitatory amino acids such as glutamine. 1,4 Butandiol is converted to hydroxybutaldehyde by alcohol dehydrogenase and to GHB via aldehyde dehydrogenase.

Clinical Presentation

GHB ingestion results in drowsiness, dizziness, and disorientation. Peak effects occur within 45 minutes of ingestion. The duration of action may be prolonged with coingestion of ethanol. High doses may result in a depressed respiratory drive, bradycardia, anesthesia, and coma. Myoclonic jerking and seizure activity have been well described. The hallmark of GHB toxicity is marked agitation with stimulation despite apnea and hypoxia. Awakening from coma may occur suddenly, with a startle. Deaths associated with GHB generally involve massive overdoses or coingestions.

Laboratory

GHB is eliminated by biotransformation in the liver, with a small percentage excreted in the urine. Urinary levels are best measured using gas chromatography-mass spectrometry or high-performance liquid chromatography. Serum levels may be detected for only 4 to 6 hours postingestion. Coma is generally seen with serum levels of 250 mg/L; at levels of 150 to 250 mg/L the patient may arouseable; at 50 to 150 mg/L some spontaneous movement with eye opening is likely; at levels below 50 mg/L the patient is typically awake.

Management

Treatment involves airway protection and maintenance of ventilation. Atropine may be used for profound bradycardia. Activated charcoal may be considered for gastric decontamination following recent ingestions. There is no proven antidote for GHB, although some anecdotal reports claim physostigmine may reverse the effects of GHB. Currently, this practice is not widely supported in the literature. Patients typically awaken very suddenly.

Disposition

Pediatric patients who are symptomatic with significant CNS or respiratory depression following a sedative-hypnotic overdose should be admitted and monitored for airway and cardiovascular stability.

CASE OUTCOME

The child remains lethargic with a depressed respiratory drive. A rapid bedside serum glucose of 100 mg/dL is measured. There is no response to IV naloxone. Before the child is orally intubated, an IV dose of flumazenil is administered. The child immediately awakens and starts crying. Her pulse oximetry improves to 98% and her respiratory drive increases to 28 breaths per minute. The child receives an additional dose of flumazenil in the ED 1 hour later, and is admitted to the pediatric intensive care unit for monitoring. She receives one more subsequent dose of flumazenil during the night, and recovers uneventfully. She is discharged home 24 hours after admission.

SUGGESTED READINGS

Amitai Y, Degan Y: Treatment of phenobarbital poisoning with multiple dose activated charcoal in an infant. *J Emerg Med* 8:449–450, 1990.

Centers for Disease Control and Prevention: GHB use 1995–1996. *JAMA* 277:1511, 1997.

Frenia ML: Multiple dose activated charcoal compared to urinary alkalinization for the enhancement of phenobarbital elimination. *J Toxicol Clin Toxicol* 34:169–175, 1996.

Grahm SR, Day RO, Lee R, et al: Overdose with chloral hydrate: A pharmacological and therapeutic review. *Med J Aust* 149:686, 1988.

Gueye PN, Hoffman JR, Talboulet P, et al: Empiric use of flumazenil in coma patients: Limited applicability of criteria to define low risk. *Ann Emerg Med* 266:24, 1996.

Jones RD, Lawson AD, Andrew LJ, et al: Antagonism of the hypnotic effect of midazolam in children: A randomized, double-blind study of placebo and flumazenil administered after midazolam-induced anaesthesia. *Br J Anaesth* 66:660–666, 1991.

Lacayo A, Mitra N: Report of a case of phenobarbital-induced dystonia. *Clin Pediatr* 31:252, 1992.

Li J, Stokes SA, Woeckener A: A tale of novel intoxication: Seven cases of GHB overdose. *Ann Emerg Med* 31:723–728, 1998.

Liebelt EL: Sedative Hypnotics. In: Ford M, Delaney K, Ling L, et al, eds: *Clinical Toxicology.* Philadelphia: Saunders; 2001:558–568.

Lindberg MC, Cunningham A, Lindberg NH: Acute phenobarbital intoxication. *South Med J* 85:803–807, 1992.

Litovitz TL, Schwartz-Klein W, Rodgers GC S, et al: 2001 annual report of the AAPCC Toxic Exposure Surveillance System. *Am J Emerg Med* 20:391–452, 2002.

Mason PE, Kern WP: Gamma hydroxybuteric acid: GHB intoxication. *Acad Emerg Med* 9:730–739, 2002.

Nicholson KL, Balster RL: GHB: A new and novel drug of abuse. *Drug Alcohol Depend* 63:1–22, 2001.

Richard P, Auret E, Bardol J, et al: The use of flumazenil in a neonate. *J Toxicol Clin Toxicol* 29:137–140, 1991.

Rosenberg J, Benowitz NL, Pond S: Pharmacokinetics of drug overdose. *Clin Pharmacokinet* 6:161–192, 1991.

Schiebel N, Vicas I: Barbiturates. In Ford M, DeLaney K, Ling L, et al, eds: *Clinical Toxicology.* Philadelphia: Saunders; 2001:569–574.

Shannon M, Quang LS: Gamma-hydroxybutyrate, gamma-butyrolactone, and 1,4-butanediol: A case report and review of the literature. *Pediatr Emerg Care* 16:435–440, 2000.

Sugarman JM, Paul RI: Flumazenil: A review. *Pediatr Emerg Care* 10:37–49, 1994.

Veerman M, Espejo MG, Christopher MA, et al: Use of activated charcoal to reduce elevated serum phenobarbital concentrations in the neonate. *Clin Toxicol* 29:53–58, 1991.

Viera AJ, Yates SW: Toxic ingestion of gamma-hydroxybutyric acid. *South Med J* 92:404–405, 1999.

Waltzman ML: Flunitrazepam: A review of "roofies." *Pediatr Emerg Care* 15:59–60, 1999.

Yates SW, Viera AT: Physostigmine in the treatment of GHB overdose. *Mayo Clinic Proc* 75:401–406, 2000.

40

Hypoglycemic Agents and Insulin

Marianne Ingels

HIGH-YIELD FACTS

- Admission is recommended for any child who has:
  - Overdosed on long-acting insulin.
  - Overdosed on shorter-acting insulin if there is recurrent hypoglycemia within 6 hours of observation.
  - Overdosed on any of the oral agents other than the α-glucosidase inhibitors.
  - Ingested even a single tablet of a sulfonylurea.
  - A hypoglycemic episode suspicious for child abuse.
  - Suicidal behavior.
- Feed the patient as soon as possible after a hypoglycemic episode.
- A patient must maintain euglycemia without being on a glucose infusion to be considered medically clear.
- C-peptide levels are low after administration of exogenous insulin, but are high after administration of a sulfonylurea or a meglitinide.

CASE PRESENTATION

A 13-year-old boy presents to the emergency department (ED) after his mother finds him unresponsive in his bedroom at dinnertime. He has no past medical history. He had spent the afternoon with a friend who is asympto-matic. On physical examination the patient is a well-developed young man who is responsive to pain only. Heart rate is 122 bpm, respiratory rate 18 breaths per minute, blood pressure 126/72 mmHg, and temperature 97.1°F. Pupils are equal, round, and reactive to light at 4 mm. Oropharynx is clear. Neck is supple. Heart sounds are rapid and regular. Lungs clear to auscultation. Abdomen is soft, nondistended, and nontender. Extremities are atraumatic and without cyanosis. Skin is diaphoretic.

INTRODUCTION AND EPIDEMIOLOGY

Type 1 diabetes, also known as juvenile-onset diabetes or insulin-dependent diabetes mellitus (IDDM), is the result of an autoimmune or idiopathic process in which the pancreas ceases insulin production. Treatment of type 1 diabetes requires the use of exogenous insulin. Type 2 diabetes, also known as adult-onset or non–insulin-dependent diabetes mellitus (NIDDM) is caused primarily by decreased sensitivity of insulin receptors to insulin, and also by deficient pancreatic insulin secretion. Type 2 diabetes may be treated by using oral agents and/or insulin. This chapter discusses the toxicity of insulin preparations (Table 40–1) and of the oral agents: sulfonylureas, biguanides, α-glucosidase inhibitors, thiazolidinediones, and meglitinides (Table 40–2).

In 2001, American poison centers reported 118 insulin exposures in children <6 years of age, and 108 exposures in children 6 to 19 years of age. Although the incidence remains rare, these numbers represent 2% and 8% increases over 1999 figures. In 2001, there were 2652 exposures to hypoglycemic agents in children under 6, and 544 in children 6 to 19 years old, representing 24% and 35% increases over 1999. This increase is temporally associated with an increase in the incidence of type 2 diabetes in children.

Table 40–1. Insulin Preparations

Class	Formulation	U.S. Trade Name	Duration (h) at Therapeutic Doses
Rapid acting	Aspart	Novolog	3–5
	Lispro	Humalog	2–5
	Regular	Humulin R, Novolin R	5–8
Intermediate acting	NPH	Humulin N, Novolin N	18–24
	Lente	Humulin L, Novolin L	18–24
Long acting	Ultralente	Humulin U	20–36
	Glargine	Lantus	24–30

Children are always at risk for exposure to medications belonging to the adults in their lives. There is now also increasing risk that children may incur unintentional or intentional exposures to hypoglycemic agents of their own, their siblings, or their peers.

DEVELOPMENTAL CONSIDERATIONS

In the neonatal period, exposures to medications via breast milk must be considered. Insulin is not excreted into breast milk and is therefore safe for use in breast-feeding mothers. Of the first-generation sulfonylureas, tolbutamide is felt to be safest for nursing mothers. Because of the high, nonionic protein binding of the second-generation sulfonylureas, glyburide and glipizide, these agents are also felt to be unlikely to be passed to infants through breast milk, but monitoring the infants for signs of hypoglycemia is still recommended. Little information is available about the other oral agents.

Toddlers are at high risk for ingesting any unattended medication, including oral hypoglycemics, but acciden-

Table 40–2. Oral Hypoglycemic Agents

Class	Formulation	U.S. Trade Name	Duration (h) at Therapeutic Doses
Sulfonylureas			
First generation	Acetohexamide	Dymelor	12–18
	Chlorpropamide	Diabinese	24–72
	Tolazamide	Tolinase	16–24
	Tolbutamide	Orinase	6–12
Second generation	Glimepiride	Amaryl	24
	Glipizide	Glucotrol	16–24
	Glyburide	Diabeta, Glynase, Micronase,	18–24
Biguanides	Metformin	Glucophage	1.5–4.5
	Phenformin	(not available)	6–8
α-Glucosidase inhibitors	Acarbose	Precose	2
	Miglitol	Glyset	2
Thiazolidinediones	Pioglitazone	Actos	16–24
	Rosiglitazone	Avandia	12–24
Meglitinides	Nateglinide	Starlix	2–4
	Repaglinide	Prandin	1–3
Combination drugs	Metformin/glyburide	Glucovance	
	Metformin/rosiglitazone	Avandamet	

tal insulin-induced hypoglycemia in nondiabetic toddlers or infants is very unlikely and should raise the question of child abuse. Adolescents may have difficulty complying with the strict diet and medication regimens of diabetes, and are at risk for accidental hypoglycemia from their own medications. Suicide attempts and risk-taking behavior, including experimentation with prescription drugs, also become more common in this age group, putting adolescents at risk for hypoglycemic episodes from intentional exposures.

PHARMACOLOGY AND TOXICOKINETICS

Insulin

Insulin is administered parenterally, because oral absorption of the active substance is prevented due to its breakdown in the stomach. Insulin's duration of action depends on the product formulation and ranges from fewer than 5 hours to 36 hours. (Table 40–1). Degradation of insulin primarily occurs in the liver, kidney, and muscle. Renal impairment may lead to increased circulating insulin and hypoglycemia at previously therapeutic doses. Insulin receptors are saturable, and so there is not a direct correlation between the amount injected and the degree of hypoglycemia. Massive overdoses may prolong the duration of hypoglycemia owing to a depot effect at the injection site. Delay in absorption may cause prolonged duration of action even in short-acting preparations, perhaps owing to depot effect or hypoglycemia-induced decrease in peripheral perfusion. Hypoglycemia has been reported as late as 18 hours after Lente insulin overdose, and has been persistent for 6 days after Ultralente overdose.

Sulfonylureas

The sulfonylureas are divided into first- and second-generation agents. The first-generation agents (Table 40–2) have active hepatic metabolites and are excreted renally. Impairment of renal function therefore potentiates their hypoglycemic effect. Their duration of action ranges from 6 to 72 hours.

The second-generation agents are fecally eliminated; glimepiride and glyburide also have active hepatic metabolites. The duration of action of these agents ranges from 16 to 24 hours. Overdose on any of the sulfonylureas can cause delayed hypoglycemia, which has been reported as late as 21 to 48 hours following ingestion.

Biguanides

Metformin (Glucophage) is renally eliminated. The risk of developing lactic acidosis appears to be related in part to renal impairment, most likely because of decreased metformin elimination. The manufacturers of metformin recommend that this drug be discontinued for 48 hours after the administration of iodinated contrast material, because of the risk of renal impairment from the contrast. The elevated metformin levels in overdose have also been associated with the development of lactic acidosis. This has been seen as late as 14 hours after metformin overdose.

Meglitinides

The meglitinides have a duration of action of 1 to 4 hours. Nateglinide has active metabolites. Little data on kinetics in overdose are available on these newer agents.

PATHOPHYSIOLOGY

The human body closely regulates glucose homeostasis with a complex array of regulatory and counterregulatory hormones. In normal individuals an increase in blood glucose results in the secretion of insulin into the bloodstream. The binding of insulin to specific receptors then triggers a variety of processes that result in increased storage and decreased breakdown of carbohydrates, lipids, and proteins. In the fasting state, lower blood glucose causes the pancreas to cease insulin secretion and to begin secreting glucagon. This change in hormonal milieu triggers catabolic processes that mobilize fuel sources from the body's reserves. Lipolysis begins and free fatty acids become the primary fuel of virtually all tissues other than the brain, which relies primarily on glucose but may also utilize ketones. An excess of fatty acids in the liver leads to increased ketone formation. Glucagon promotes glycogenolysis and gluconeogenesis to increase blood glucose levels. Hypoglycemia also stimulates the sympathetic nervous system, and epinephrine released by the adrenal gland triggers glycogenolysis in the liver and lipolysis in adipose tissue.

The major toxic effect of drugs used to treat diabetes is hypoglycemia. The insulin preparations act just like endogenous insulin and trigger the same cascade of responses, including a drop in blood glucose levels. Hypoglycemia may be noted with normally therapeutic doses of insulin if there is inadequate caloric intake or an increase in metabolic demands, such as from exercise or illness.

Of the oral agents, the sulfonylureas and the meglitinides also cause severe hypoglycemia. The sulfonylureas (Table 40–2) produce their hypoglycemic effect by stimulating the β cells of the pancreas to secrete insulin. The sulfonylureas also inhibit aldehyde dehydrogenase; therefore, patients taking these drugs may experience a disulfiram-type reaction if they consume ethanol. Chlorpropamide is unique among these agents in that it has also been associated with the development of the syndrome of inappropriate antidiuretic hormone secretion and hyponatremia. The meglitinides (nateglinide, repaglinide) are structurally unrelated to the sulfonylureas, but also cause increased insulin secretion by the pancreas.

The biguanides (metformin, phenformin) decrease glucose by inhibiting gluconeogenesis and by increasing peripheral glucose uptake. These agents have been associated with lactic acidosis, both in therapeutic dosing and on rare occurrences in overdose. Phenformin interferes with cellular aerobic metabolism and causes decreased hepatic lactic acid consumption and uptake. The mechanism of lactic acidosis due to metformin is thought to be similar, although the incidence of lactic acidosis is 20 times lower with metformin than with phenformin. Phenformin was taken off the market in the United States in 1977 due to its association with lactic acidosis, but remains available in other countries. Hypoglycemia is rarely associated with overdose on these agents.

The thiazolidinediones (pioglitazone, rosiglitazone) increase insulin receptor sensitivity in the liver, skeletal muscle, and adipose tissue and also reduce hepatic gluconeogenesis. They have not been associated with hypoglycemia in overdose, but experience with these drugs is limited. Troglitazone, another thiazolidinedione, was removed from the U.S. market by the Food and Drug Administration in 2000 due to its association with acute liver failure at therapeutic doses.

The α-glucosidase inhibitors (acarbose, miglitol) inhibit the activity of α-glucosidase enzymes in the brush border of the small intestine, limiting absorption of glucose from the small bowel. These agents do not cause hypoglycemia in overdose, but may instead cause gastrointestinal symptoms, such as abdominal pain, nausea, diarrhea, and flatulence. Asymptomatic and reversible elevations in hepatic transaminases have been reported.

CLINICAL FINDINGS

The brain's reliance almost exclusively on glucose for fuel makes it the most sensitive organ to hypoglycemia.

Any CNS abnormality including agitation, psychosis, ataxia, seizures, focal neurologic deficits, and coma, should prompt clinicians to rule out hypoglycemia. Other symptoms are caused by hypoglycemia-triggered catecholamine release, and include tremor, pallor, diaphoresis, tachycardia, anxiety, dry mouth, mydriasis, and hypertension. Angina has also been reported, but is unlikely in children. Hypoglycemic patients may also be hypothermic, particularly if there has been exposure to a cool environment.

LABORATORY AND DIAGNOSTIC TESTING

Glucose monitoring is the mainstay of diagnostic testing. This can be done at the bedside using reagent strips or a glucometer, or in the hospital laboratory. Reagent strips are not as accurate as laboratory testing, and clinicians should be aware of the sensitivity of the particular strips they are using for detecting hypoglycemia. It also must be remembered that the blood glucose levels at which patients show clinical signs of hypoglycemia are variable, and are often higher in diabetics than in nondiabetics.

Plasma C-peptide levels can be determined if there is a question of endogenous versus exogenous insulin as the cause of hypoglycemia. Proinsulin is formed in the pancreas and then cleaved to form insulin and the nonreactive C-peptide. Insulin and C-peptide are secreted in equimolar amounts. When insulin is administered to a patient the C-peptide level is low; commercially available forms of insulin contain only the active insulin. When patients are hypoglycemic due to endogenous insulin production, such as secondary to insulinoma or sulfonylurea ingestion, the C-peptide level is high. Reference laboratories can measure sulfonylurea and meglitinide levels.

Lactic acidosis may be noted indirectly by an elevated anion gap, and directly by measuring serum lactate levels. Other useful studies include electrolytes, blood urea nitrogen, creatinine, and liver function tests.

MANAGEMENT

Initial resuscitation of a hypoglycemic patient from any cause includes administration of glucose. This is given intravenously (IV) at a dose of 0.5 to 1.0 g/kg as $D_{50}W$ in older children (Figure 40–1), $D_{25}W$ in younger children (2 to 4 mL/kg), and $D_{10}W$ in neonates. Patients who are alert should be given oral glucose in the form of food or juice as soon as possible, because an IV glucose bolus

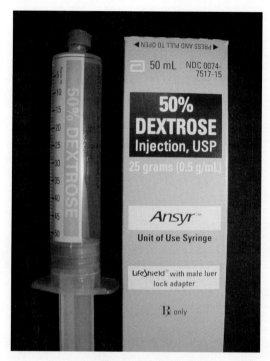

Fig. 40–1. Standard 50% dextrose syringe.

may produce only transient euglycemia. Glucagon should be administered only if IV access is unavailable. This is given at a dose of 0.3 mg/kg intramuscularly (IM) or subcutaneously (SQ) in neonates or 0.025 to 0.100 mg/kg IM/SQ in children, with a maximum dose of 1 mg. Glucagon increases glucose by mobilizing glycogen stores, which may be inadequate in children. Mental status should be monitored closely, and repeat blood glucose measurements should be obtained every 1 to 2 hours. Glucose infusion may be required to maintain euglycemia and is given as either D_5W or $D_{10}W$, titrated as necessary. Patients must maintain euglycemia off glucose infusions before they can be considered medically clear.

Octreotide, a somatostatin analog, may be helpful in the management of hypoglycemia from sulfonylurea or meglitinide ingestion. Somatostatin is secreted by the δ cells of the pancreas and acts to decrease pancreatic insulin secretion. Octreotide decreases insulin secretion by the same mechanism and has a longer half-life than somatostatin. Suggested doses of octreotide are 4 to 5 μg/kg/day (SC or IV), up to 50 μg, divided every 6 hours. Patients should be monitored for 24 hours after discontinuation of octreotide therapy.

Diazoxide is a nondiuretic thiazide that acts as a vasodilator and has been used as an antihypertensive. It also inhibits insulin secretion and has been used to manage hypoglycemia. Its utility is limited because of its hypotensive effects and its tendency to cause sodium retention. Diazoxide is generally recommended only after treatment failure with other agents, including octreotide. It is given as an IV infusion at 0.1 to 2.0 mg/kg/h.

In any overdose, decontamination must be addressed. Unfortunately there is little that can be done in cases of insulin overdose. Excision of insulin injection sites has been reported but is not routinely recommended. For oral agents, syrup of ipecac is not recommended because patients may develop hypoglycemia-related decreased mental status and loss of protective airway reflexes. Activated charcoal has been shown to adsorb sulfonylureas, and is recommended early in patients who have ingested oral agents. There are some data to suggest that patients who have ingested glipizide may benefit from a repeat dose of activated charcoal, given that substance's enterohepatic circulation.

Alkalinization of the urine to a pH of 7 to 8 enhances the elimination of chlorpropamide and decreases its half-life from 49 to 13 hours. Sodium bicarbonate is used to achieve this urine pH, and must be given with great caution to avoid causing hypernatremia and excessive alkalemia. Urinary alkalinization is not effective for other oral agents.

DISPOSITION

It is very important to determine the agent responsible for the hypoglycemia and whether the event was intentional or unintentional. Appropriate interventions must be undertaken for suicidal patients as well as for victims of child abuse or attempted homicide. Patients who have hypoglycemic episodes due to noncompliance or poor understanding of their therapeutic regimen need intensive diabetic education and close follow-up to prevent reoccurrence.

A patient who becomes hypoglycemic due to missing a meal after taking routine insulin doses may be discharged from the hospital after a period of observation. The patient's primary physician should be consulted about possible alteration of the dosing regimen. Patients who have overdosed on long-acting insulin should be admitted, as should patients with overdoses with other formulations of insulin if they develop recurrent hypoglycemia during a 4- to 6-hour observation period without IV glucose administration.

Hospital admission is recommended for children who overdose on sulfonylureas or meglitinides, even if these children are asymptomatic. Management of children with exposure to only 1 tablet of a sulfonylurea is controversial. Hypoglycemia has been reported as late as 16 to 21 hours after ingestion, and so admission with close observation is generally recommended in these patients. Experience with the meglitinides is limited, but because of their shorter half-life, it may be assumed that a child who has ingested one tablet and remains asymptomatic after a 6-hour period of observation may be safely discharged.

Experience with children who have overdosed on metformin or a thiazolidinedione is limited. Because of the rare reports of delayed lactic acidosis and hypoglycemia after metformin overdose, admission of these patients is probably indicated. Until enough clinical experience is generated to determine the incidence of hypoglycemia in thiazolidinedione overdose, admission is also prudent for these patients.

CASE OUTCOME

Bedside glucometer testing reveals a blood glucose of "LOW." The patient is given 50 mL of $D_{50}W$ and becomes alert and oriented. The patient had a recurrence of hypoglycemia and altered mental status 35 minutes after initial administration of $D_{50}W$, but responded to a second dose by again regaining consciousness. At that point he admitted that he had taken one of his friend's mother's "sugar pills" in the hope that it would make him high. The medication was identified as a glyburide 5-mg tablet. He was admitted overnight, given frequent meals, and discharged in good condition the next evening.

SUGGESTED READINGS

Bosse GM: Antidiabetic and hypoglycemic agents. In: Goldfrank LR, Flomenbaum NE, Lewin NA, et al, eds: *Goldfrank's Toxicologic Emergencies.* 7th ed. New York: McGraw-Hill; 2002:593–605.

Brosnan CA, Upchurch S, Schreiner B: Type 2 diabetes in children and adolescents: An emerging disease. *J Pediatr Health Care* 15:187–193, 2001.

Davis SN, Granner DK: Insulin, oral hypoglycemic agents, and the pharmacology of the endocrine pancreas. In: Hardeman, JG, Limbird LE, eds: *Goodman & Gilman's The Pharmacological Basis of Therapeutics.* 10th ed. New York: McGraw-Hill; 2001:1679–1714.

Gerich JE: Novel insulins: Expanding options in diabetes management. *Am J Med* 113:308–316, 2002.

Greger N, Edwin CM: Obesity: A pediatric epidemic. *Pediatr Ann* 30:694–700, 2001.

Harrigan RA, Nathan MS, Beattie P: Oral agents for the treatment of type 2 diabetes mellitus: Pharmacology, toxicity, and treatment. *Ann Emerg Med* 38:68–78, 2001.

Levien TL, Baker DE, White JR, et al: Insulin glargine: A new basal insulin. *Ann Pharmacother* 36:1019–1027, 2002.

Libman I, Arslanian SA: Type II diabetes mellitus: No longer just adults. *Pediatr Ann* 28:589–593, 1999.

Litovitz TL, Klein-Schwartz W, Rodgers GC, et al: 2001 Annual report of poison control centers toxic exposure surveillance system. *Am J Emerg Med* 20:391–452, 2002.

Quadrani DA, Spiller HA, Widder P: Five year retrospective evaluation of sulfonylurea ingestion in children. *Clin Toxicol* 34:267–270, 1996.

Scott PA, Wolf LR, Spadafora MP: Accuracy of reagent strips in detecting hypoglycemia in the emergency department. *Ann Emerg Med* 32:305–309, 1998.

Spencer JP, Gonzalez III LS, Barnhart DJ: Medications in the breast-feeding mother. *Am Fam Phys* 64:119–126, 2001.

Spiller HA, Villalobos D, Krenzelok EP, et al: Prospective multicenter study of sulfonylurea ingestion in children. *J Pediatr* 131:141–146, 1997.

41

Antiepileptic Agents

Fermin Barrueto, Jr.
Lewis S. Nelson

HIGH-YIELD FACTS

- Phenobarbital is a sedative-hypnotic agent commonly used as an antiepileptic in children, which causes central nervous system (CNS) and respiratory depression in the overdose setting.

- Phenytoin toxicity characteristically causes nausea, vomiting, nystagmus, ataxia, and sedation.

- Rapid intravenous (IV) phenytoin can cause hypotension, in part from the diluent (propylene glycol), but when ingested, does not produce hypotension or cardiotoxicity.

- Carbamazepine, structurally similar to the tricyclic antidepressants (TCAs), is one of the more potentially cardiotoxic antiepileptics, but is very well adsorbed by activated charcoal.

- In overdose, valproic acid produces metabolites that both inhibit the urea cycle and cause an increase in serum ammonia with potential hepatotoxicity. L-Carnitine therapy may improve valproic acid-induced hyperammonemia.

- The newer agents gabapentin, vigabatrin, and levetiracetam are the only antiepileptics that are nearly 100% renally eliminated. In overdose, they may cause mild CNS toxicity.

CASE PRESENTATION

A 9-year-old, 35-kg boy presents to the emergency department (ED) after his mother found the child next to an empty bottle of his valproic acid (125-mg sprinkle capsules). The bottle, initially half full, was left on the kitchen table. The patient had an episode of emesis and became increasingly more somnolent over the next 2 hours. The boy has a medical history of epilepsy and mental retardation. He had been taking valproic acid for seizure control and takes no other medications.

The patient has the following vital signs: temperature 99 °F; pulse 105 bpm; blood pressure 105/55 mmHg; respirations 11 breaths/minute; and a pulse oximetry 93% on room air. Physical examination revealed normal pupils and moist oral mucosa. His lungs were clear and the cardiovascular examination was normal. Neurologic exam revealed no focal deficits and no nystagmus. The child was difficult to awaken and mumbled incomprehensible words. There was a good gag reflex; deep tendon reflexes were 2+ bilaterally in upper and lower extremities. Laboratory evaluation revealed a serum ammonia of 225 mmol/L but no other abnormalities. Liver enzymes were within normal limits and the initial serum valproic acid serum concentration was 250 mg/L.

INTRODUCTION AND EPIDEMIOLOGY

A seizure is the result of excessive CNS activity. Epilepsy is commonly defined as two or more unprovoked seizures. Seizures occur in up to 5% of children. True epilepsy is

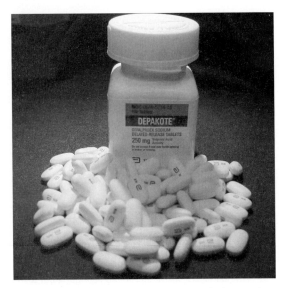

Fig. 41–1. Valproic acid overdoses have greatly increased recently due to this drug's multiple indications.

less common, with a prevalence of 0.5% to 1%. Antiepileptics halt the propagation of action potentials in the CNS and decrease a neuron's ability to fire. There are many new medications that are utilized to control epilepsy, but the four antiepileptics responsible for most reported exposures in children are phenobarbital, phenytoin, carbamazepine, and valproic acid. Valproic acid overdoses have greatly increased over the past several years, probably due to valproic acid's expanded indications, including migraine prophylaxis and bipolar disorder (Figures 41–1 and 41–2).

DEVELOPMENTAL CONSIDERATIONS

Phenobarbital crosses the placenta and enters breast milk. Although no direct causal relationship has been established with congenital malformations, folate deficiency and hypoprothrombinemia have been noted in infants of mothers receiving phenobarbital therapy. Phenytoin use during pregnancy has been associated with the fetal hydantoin syndrome. This is characterized by pre- and postnatal growth insufficiency, microcephaly, and mental retardation. Specific abnormalities include facial hypoplasia, hypertelorism, flattened philtrum, and shortened nasal structure. Human case reports have correlated carbamazepine overdose during the first trimester with potential neural tube defects, but a causal link has not been firmly established. Maternal prenatal valproic acid therapy has been associated with spina bifida.

BARBITURATES

Pharmacology and Pathophysiology

The barbiturates are classified as either ultrashort acting (thiopental), short acting (pentobarbital), or long acting (phenobarbital). These agents are primarily used as anticonvulsants in children and for induction of anesthesia. Barbiturates are primarily CNS depressants that mediate their effect through inhibition of aminobutyric synapses of the brain. Toxicity can result in suppression of skeletal, smooth, and cardiac muscle, leading to depressed myocardial contractility, bradycardia, vasodilation, and hypotension.

Barbiturates increase the duration that the neuronal chloride channel remains open, directly increasing chlo-

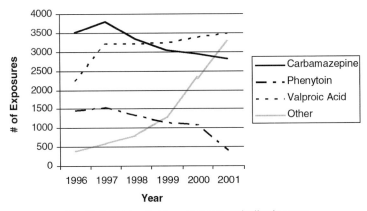

Fig. 41–2. Total pediatric exposures to antiepileptic agents.

ride influx. This augments inhibitory tone, thus preventing seizures. However, because barbiturates produce sedation in therapeutic doses, these agents have been largely supplanted by newer drugs.

Clinical Presentation

In the overdose setting, the pediatric patient presents with altered mental status ranging from sedation to coma, often accompanied by respiratory depression. Vital signs may reveal hypotension, bradycardia, and hypothermia. Pupils are constricted early in the clinical course, but can be dilated in later stages of toxicity. As with most sedative-hypnotic agents, noncardiogenic pulmonary edema has been described in severely toxic patients. After prolonged coma, the patient can develop bullous skin lesions over dependent body parts, but this is rare. Cases of phenobarbital-induced hepatotoxicity have also been described in children.

Laboratory Tests

In addition to baseline laboratory studies, a quantitative serum phenobarbital level is obtained to document the toxicity, but is not mandatory for definitive management. Therapeutic concentrations of phenobarbital range between 15 and 40 mg/L. Patients with levels >50 mg/L exhibit mild toxicity, whereas those with levels >100 mg/L are typically unresponsive to pain, and suffer from respiratory and cardiac depression.

Treatment

The primary management of barbiturate toxicity is support of oxygenation, ventilation, and circulation. Comatose patients may require intubation. Hypotensive patients are managed with fluid resuscitation, and if necessary, pressor agents. Gastric lavage may be useful in patients up to 1 hour postingestion. Syrup of ipecac is not indicated. Several investigations have demonstrated that repeated doses of activated charcoal significantly reduce the serum half-life of phenobarbital, which undergoes enterohepatic circulation. An initial dose of 1 g/kg is recommended, followed by 0.25 g/kg every 4 to 6 hours. When multiple doses of charcoal are used, repeated doses of any cathartic agent premixed with the charcoal product are contraindicated to avoid dehydration and electrolyte imbalances. However, a small dose of sorbitol (0.2 to 0.5 g/kg) may be given with the first dose of activated charcoal in older children to prevent constipation. It should be noted that administration of multiple doses of charcoal has not been shown to significantly change clinical outcome in phenobarbital toxicity.

Urinary alkalinization with sodium bicarbonate to a pH of 7.5 to 8.0 can hasten the renal excretion of phenobarbital, which is a weak acid and primarily renally excreted. This procedure is recommended in severe toxicity. Alkalinization can be accomplished with an initial sodium bicarbonate bolus at 1 mEq/kg followed by a continuous infusion. This infusion is made by adding 100 to 150 mEq of sodium bicarbonate to 850 mL of dextrose 5% in water and titrating it to maintain a urine pH of greater than 7.5. The arterial pH should remain less than 7.5. It should be noted that no clinical evidence exists that shows this form of enhanced elimination ultimately improves patient outcome. Alkalinization does not increase excretion of shorter-acting agents which are hepatically metabolized, and not primarily renally excreted.

In patients who overdose on long-acting barbiturates who remain unstable despite standard therapeutic measures, or in those with renal failure, hemodialysis is indicated. Fortunately, most barbiturate overdoses do well with supportive care alone and dialysis is rarely necessary. Charcoal hemoperfusion seems more efficacious for shorter-acting agents, which possess greater fat and protein binding.

PHENYTOIN

Pharmacology and Pathophysiology

Despite the structural similarity to phenobarbital, at therapeutic doses, phenytoin is nonsedating. It exerts its effects through sodium channel blockade, instead of affecting the chloride ion. Phenytoin also inhibit calcium fluxes, and increases brain GABA levels while potentiating GABA-mediated postsynaptic inhibition. Phenytoin is available as chewable tablets (50 mg) and phenytoin oral suspension (30 mg/5 mL or 125 mg/5mL). For adolescents, 100-mg capsules are available. Even at therapeutic doses, absorption is slow and highly dependent on the formulation. Phenytoin metabolism undergoes Michaelis-Menten kinetics. Supratherapeutic serum concentrations may decrease at a much slower rate owing to saturation of hepatic enzymes, and conversion from first- to zero-order elimination. This partially explains the highly variable elimination half-lives ranging from 7 to 60 hours. Over 90% of phenytoin is protein bound, with a volume of distribution of approximately 0.10 L/kg. Most antiepileptics like phenytoin undergo metabolism by

Table 41–1. Pharmacology of Antiepileptics

Medication	Dose[a] (mg/kg/d)	Therapeutic Serum Levels (mg/L)	Plasma Elimination $t_{1/2}$ (h)	Metabolism	Mechanism of Action
Phenobarbital	4–8	15–40	15–48	Mostly hepatic	Increases neuronal chloride influx
Phenytoin	3–8	10–20	6–60	Mostly hepatic	Na^+ channel blockade
Carbamazepine	5–70	4–12	4.9 – 11.5	Mostly hepatic	Na^+ channel blockade
Valproic acid	15–60	50–120	6–18	β-Oxidation, in overdose more ω-oxidation	Na^+ channel blockade and decrease GABA breakdown
Gabapentin	10–30	1–2	5–7	100% Renal	Multiple, but not primarily GABA
Lamotrigine	5–15	0.5–4.5	14–50	Glucuronidation	Na^+ channel blockade
Vigabatrin	14–57	20–80	4–8	100% Renal	Inhibits GABA transaminase
Ethosuximide	20	N/A	30–50	25% Renal	Blocks Ca^{2+} channels
Levetiracetam	1–3 g/d	10–37	6–10	100% Renal	Unknown, may block Ca^{2+} channels
Topiramate	3–22	14–27	20–30	70% Renal	Unknown, multiple effects

Abbreviation: GABA, γ-aminobutyric acid.
[a]Pediatric doses without the recommended maximal doses, please consult the appropriate reference for precise dosing.

hepatic enzymes such as cytochrome P450 (Table 41–1). This results in the many drug interactions that occur between phenytoin and other medications.

Clinical Presentation

Acute phenytoin toxicity usually results from intentional or accidental oral ingestion. Poisoning may also occur iatrogenically after excessive IV loading doses are administered. In the overdose setting, the patient may develop nystagmus, diploplia, ataxia, and other signs of cerebellar dysfunction. However, the findings of ataxia or nystagmus may be difficult to assess in an infant or preambulatory child. Phenytoin toxicity in this age group may present with lethargy, poor feeding, or hypotonia. With larger overdoses, epileptic children may experience increased frequency of seizures. This phenomenon has been referred to as *paradoxical seizures*. Patients without a history of epilepsy can develop seizure activity in the overdose setting, but this is rare. Seizures in this group of patients should prompt a search for coingestants or other causes of seizures. Gastrointestinal (GI) effects such as nausea and vomiting are common following oral toxicity. Children occasionally have atypical presentations

following overdose, including opisthotonus, chorea, or other movement disorders.

Gingival hyperplasia occurs in 20% of patients on maintenance therapy and is probably the most common presentation of chronic phenytoin toxicity in the pediatric patient. Good oral hygiene can usually minimize this effect; it does not require withdrawal of the medication.

During infusion, propylene glycol, the diluent in IV phenytoin, can cause rate-related hypotension. Fosphenytoin, a water-soluble prodrug form of phenytoin, is converted by serum phosphatases to phenytoin, which takes 5 to 15 minutes. Fosphenytoin was specifically developed to avoid the adverse effects seen with IV phenytoin. Although fosphenytoin can be infused more quickly than phenytoin, it also causes rate-related hypotension, suggesting that the propylene glycol solvent is not fully responsible. The oral preparation is not associated with this adverse effect.

Laboratory Testing

Patients who are chronically on phenytoin should undergo therapeutic drug monitoring, especially when new medications are added or there is a change in dose. Serum phenytoin levels should be obtained in any case of sus-

Table 41–2. Pharmacology of Antiepileptics: Laboratory Testing

	Blood Cell Count	**Electrolytes**	**Hepatic Enzymes**
Phenytoin	Aplastic anemia[a] Megaloblastic anemia Agranulocytosis[a]	Hyperglycemia Hypocalcemia	Hepatotoxic[a]
Carbamazepine	Aplastic anemia[a] Agranulocytosis[a] Thrombocytopenia[a]	Hyponatremia Hypocalcemia	Hepatotoxic[a]
Valproic acid	Aplastic anemia[a] Agranulocytosis[a] Thrombocytopenia[a]	Hypernatremia Anion gap Acidosis	Hepatotoxic[a] Serum Ammonia Lipase[a]

Data derived from AAPCC TESS Reports: http://www.aapcc.org/annual.htm.
[a]Indicates idiosyncratic effects.

pected overdose or in patients on chronic therapy who exhibit signs of toxicity. Factors such as time of ingestion, tolerance to the drug, and protein binding may alter the clinical effects of the drug (see Table 41–1). Signs and symptoms can be present even if the level is therapeutic, and may be absent with elevated serum concentration. Because of the possibility of delayed absorption and slow elimination, serial phenytoin levels are necessary in the acute overdose. Phenytoin, as well as other antiepileptic agents, affects the hematopoietic system, often in an idiosyncratic fashion, and a complete blood cell count may be helpful (Table 41–2). Electrolyte abnormalities are uncommon and usually not clinically significant in the overdose setting.

Management

Management of phenytoin toxicity is supportive with bed rest recommended for ataxic patients. Isolated oral phenytoin exposures do not result in cardiotoxicity, and these patients do not require cardiac monitoring. Reported cases of death are rare, and are usually due to respiratory depression in massive overdoses. In large acute exposures presenting within 1 hour of ingestion, gastric lavage may be beneficial. Activated charcoal is the mainstay of GI decontamination and may be effective hours after ingestion due to the drug's slow absorption properties. The efficacy of multiple dosing of charcoal has not been clearly established. Owing to phenytoin's high protein binding, there is no proven role or benefit from hemodialysis or other extracorporeal drug removal methods in the overdose setting.

CARBAMAZEPINE

Pharmacology and Pathophysiology

Although its mechanism of action is similar to phenytoin, carbamazepine is structurally similar to TCAs like imipramine. It has been used for generalized and partial seizures, trigeminal neuralgia, bipolar disorder, and schizophrenia. It is available as 100-mg chewable tablets, 200-mg tablets, and as a 100 mg/5mL oral suspension. Peak concentrations are reached in 2 to 6 hours in the neonate and 4 to 8 hours in children, but may occur as late as 72 hours after an overdose. Infants and young children often require more frequent dosing and relatively larger daily doses than adults because they have more rapid clearance rates. The volume of distribution ranges from 1.0 to 2.5 L/kg in neonates to 1.2 to 3.5 L/kg in children. Plasma protein binding ranges from 65% in neonates to 75% in older children. Carbamazepine is metabolized in the liver. The primary metabolite is carbamazepine-10,11-epoxide (CBZ-E), which also has anticonvulsant activity. Carbamazepine and CBZ-E limit sustained high frequency repetitive firing of sodium-dependent action potentials and, like phenytoin, block sodium channels at therapeutic doses.

Clinical Presentations

In overdose setting, ataxia, diplopia, nystagmus, and other cerebellar signs are common. Anticholinergic effects, sedation, and CNS and respiratory depression occur with larger overdoses. Myoclonus, dyskinesias, and paradoxical seizures have also been reported. In non-verbal children, symptoms may include lethargy, poor feeding, or behavioral changes. Fatalities are uncommon. Cardiotoxicity manifesting as tachycardia, QRS complex widening, and QT prolongation may occur following overdose, but are far less common than with cyclic antidepressants. It is unknown whether electrocardiographic changes are related to cardiac sodium channel blockade.

Agranulocytosis, thrombocytopenia, and aplastic anemia are rare, and are limited to chronic toxicity. Syndrome of inappropriate diuretic hormone has also been reported with chronic use. Oxcarbazepine is a new antiepileptic agent that is similar to carbamazepine. It is associated with a lower incidence of the anticonvulsant hypersensitivity syndrome and an increased incidence of hyponatremia with chronic use.

Laboratory Testing

Therapeutic carbamazepine levels ranges from 4 to 12 mg/L. The correlation between carbamazepine concentration and clinical symptoms is inconsistent. However, serum levels over 40 mg/L may be associated with respiratory depression, coma, and potential cardiac conduction abnormalities. Serial drug levels are recommended to detect peak plasma concentrations. An electrocardiogram (ECG) should be performed with a significant carbamazepine overdose.

Management

Supportive care is the mainstay for treatment of carbamazepine toxicity. Gastric lavage may be considered with large, recent ingestions. Activated charcoal is indicated for GI decontamination because it adsorbs carbamazepine well. Repeated doses of activated charcoal also decrease the elimination half-life. Because carbamazepine may effect the cardiovascular system, QRS complex widening may be responsive to administration of sodium bicarbonate.

Extracorporeal removal of carbamazepine toxicity is controversial. High protein binding makes conventional hemodialysis ineffective. However, charcoal hemoperfusion may be considered in children with high levels and severe toxicity unresponsive to standard therapy.

VALPROIC ACID

Pharmacology and Pathophysiology

Valproic acid can produce neuronal sodium channel blockade, although it does not appear to effect cardiac sodium channels. It also increases GABA by enhancing glutamate decarboxylase activity and inhibiting GABA transaminase and succinic semialdehyde dehydrogenase (Figure 41–3). Valproic acid has active metabolites which contribute to toxicity. Oral absorption is rapid, with peak serum levels achieved in 1 to 4 hours with therapeutic doses. Peak levels may be delayed up to 18 hours in the overdose setting. The volume of distribution ranges from 0.13 to 0.23 L/kg. Elimination follows first-order kinetics.

Interruption of the carnitine shuttle, which normally transports fatty acids into hepatocytes for metabolism, causes valproic acid to be metabolized through an alternative cytosolic pathway. The resulting metabolites interfere with the urea cycle, causing an elevation of serum ammonia. These same metabolites may contribute to fulminant hepatitis, although depletion of mitochondrial acetyl coenzyme A is probably also a factor. Hyperammonemia, with or without hepatic dysfunction, is well reported and may contribute to sedation. This has been seen both with therapeutic serum concentrations and in overdoses. The hyperammonemia, and perhaps hepatitis, are the result of valproic acid-induced carnitine depletion. In patients with an elevated serum ammonia concentration and no hepatic dysfunction, administration of L-carnitine decreases the production of toxic metabolites.

Clinical Presentation

The indications for valproic acid therapy have been expanded to include bipolar disorder and prevention of migraine headache. As a result, overdose with this agent has become more common. Sedation is the predominant

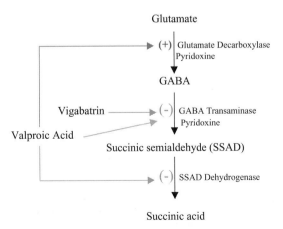

Fig. 41–3. GABA metabolism and antiepileptics.

effect in most overdoses, although there may be ataxia, nausea, vomiting, and anorexia. Pinpoint pupils may be present, mimicking an opioid exposure. Rarely, respiratory depression may occur, particularly with coingestions or massive overdoses. Paradoxical seizures have been rarely reported in patients with underlying seizure disorders. Valproic acid has a variety of idiosyncratic adverse effects such as pancreatitis, alopecia, pancytopenia, metabolic acidosis, and hepatic derangements.

A Reyes-like fulminant hepatitis may occur in approximately 1 in 50,000 patients chronically taking valproic acid. Children younger than 2 years of age and on multiple antiepileptic agents are at an elevated risk for this complication.

Laboratory Testing

Valproic acid is frequently dispensed in a delayed-release formulation that may cause delayed increases in serum concentration. Following oral overdose, serum concentrations of valproic acid should be repeated every 2 to 4 hours until the serum level is reliably decreasing. Elevation in hepatic aminotransferases can occur in an acute overdose and with therapeutic use. A unique laboratory value that may assist with valproic acid exposures is a serum ammonia concentration. Although it may not correlate with the level of sedation, it may guide antidotal therapy with carnitine.

Management

Valproic acid is adsorbed by activated charcoal and may be responsive to multiple dosing. Gastric lavage may be beneficial if performed within 1 hour following a significant, acute ingestion. There is no specific antidote for valproic acid, although there are anecdotal reports of naloxone reversing valproic acid–induced coma and respiratory depression. L-Carnitine is an amino acid that can be administered to patients who develop either hepatotoxicity or hyperammonemia while on valproic acid. Although the dosing of L-carnitine has not been established, and its use is not well defined, there is a trend toward a better clinical outcome in patients with valproic acid–induced hepatitis treated with L-carnitine. Administration of 50 to 100 mg/kg/d, either IV or orally, can be administered in divided doses for valproic acid–induced toxic hepatitis or isolated hyperammonemia. Extracorporeal removal with either hemodialysis or charcoal hemoperfusion has been shown to enhance elimination, and may be beneficial in patients with large overdoses refractory to conventional therapy.

NEWER ANTIEPILEPTIC AGENTS

Pharmacology and Pathophysiology

The newer antiepileptic agents act on voltage-gated calcium channel blockade or inhibition of excitatory neurotransmitters. Only gabapentin, vigabatrin, and levetiracetam are 100% renally eliminated and maintain first-order kinetics following overdose (see Table 41–1). Serum levels of the newer antiepileptics can also be measured, however, not in a clinically relevant or timely fashion. Clinical experience with toxicity from these newer agents in the pediatric patients is limited.

Gabapentin

Gabapentin (Neurontin) is a derivative of GABA that was specifically designed to be a centrally active GABA agonist. Ironically, it was later found to have minimal GABA effects, but to decrease the release of glutamate, an excitatory neurotransmitter, and it has sodium channel blocking effects. The exact mechanism of action is still unclear, and the drug has proved to be more efficacious in neuropathic pain syndromes. There are minimal effects observed after overdose. Lethargy, dizziness, slurred speech, and diplopia have been described. Although data are limited, patients do not appear to suffer life-threatening complications. Sedation and occasional respiratory depression may occur if gabapentin is coingested with other medications. Choereoathatoid movements and facial dyskinesias have been reported during therapy.

Lamotrigine

Although experience with lamotrigine (Lamictal) overdose is limited, a pediatric case report described muscle weakness, ataxia, and an isolated seizure. These symptoms resolved in 24 hours without any sequelae. There are also reports of nystagmus, rash, and blurred vision in adult cases, as well as transient rises in hepatic aminotransferases. No acute respiratory depression has been reported.

Vigabatrin

Vigabatrin, another GABA analog, specifically decreases GABA breakdown by inhibiting GABA transaminase (Figure 41–3). A unique clinical manifestation of this antiepileptic is a reversible psychosis that occurs at therapeutic concentrations and in overdose. Otherwise, sedation is the primary toxic symptom.

Ethosuximide

Used for absence seizures in children, the predominant effects following overdose are GI, including nausea, vomiting, and anorexia. There are also behavioral effects such as anxiety, aggressiveness, and an inability to concentrate. Parkinson-like symptoms and photophobia have been reported.

Levetiracetam

This novel antiepileptic, like many of the newer ones, is more effective treating partial complex epilepsy, and although the mechanism of action is not clear, research indicates that it probably blocks voltage-gated calcium channels. The clinical effects reported in overdose have been minimal, with a predominance of short-lived sedation and respiratory depression.

Topiramate

Although experience with topiramate overdose is limited, adverse effects most often include sedation, lethargy, diplopia, nausea, and anorexia. One adult patient with a large overdose suffered status epilepticus without permanent sequelae. Anorexia has led to weight loss in some patients. A distinctive adverse effect during chronic therapy is the propensity to induce nephrolithiasis from inhibition of carbonic anhydrase.

ANTICONVULSANT HYPERSENSITIVITY SYNDROME

Fever, rash, and internal organ involvement are the constellation of findings that make up the anticonvulsant hypersensitivity syndrome. It typically occurs with the aromatic antiepileptics, like phenytoin, carbamazepine, and barbiturates, but has been described with lamotrigine. This syndrome occurs most often in patients within the first 2 months of initiating therapy, and has a genetic predisposition. Skin manifestations seen with this syndrome can range from a macular erythematous eruption to Stevens–Johnson syndrome or toxic epidermal necrolysis. This rash often spares the mucosal areas, and occurs 1 to 2 weeks into the syndrome. Any organ can be affected, including the liver, cardiac muscle, thyroid, and kidneys. Corticosteroids have been anecdotally reported to be beneficial. Because there appears to be cross-reactivity between phenobarbital, phenytoin, and carbamazepine, these antiepileptic medications should be avoided

in patients who develop the syndrome. Although this has not been proven, it may be prudent to avoid lamotrigine as well.

DISPOSITION

Most patients who overdose on antiepileptic agents recover within 6 to 8 hours. Patients with persistent symptoms are candidates for hospital admission. For patients with respiratory and CNS depression, increasing serum drug levels, or ECG abnormalities, intensive monitoring is necessary. Unless there is an allergic reaction, the ingestion of any single antiepileptic tablet will not result in life-threatening signs or symptoms. The exception to this general rule is respiratory depression associated with adult-strength barbiturates in small children.

CASE OUTCOME

The 9-year-old child became increasingly lethargic, and a repeat valproic acid concentration drawn 4 hours after the first was 409 mg/L. He received 2 g of IV carnitine and his mental status improved over the next 3 hours. He was given a dose of activated charcoal and admitted to the hospital. His subsequent valproic acid level, 12 hours after administration of carnitine, was 205 mg/L and serum ammonia concentration was 85 mmol/L. After 24 hours he was back to his baseline mental status and had normal vital signs. The family was educated on poison prevention in the house and the boy was discharged the next day.

SUGGESTED READINGS

Amitai Y, Degan Y: Treatment of phenobarbital poisoning with multiple dose activated charcoal in an infant. *J Emerg Med* 8:449–450, 1990.

Anderson GO, Ritland S: Life-threatening intoxication with sodium valproate. *J Toxicol Clin Toxicol* 33:279–284, 1995.

Andrews CO, Fischer JH. Gabapentin: A new agent for the management of epilepsy. *Ann Pharmacother* 28:1188–1196, 1994.

Barrueto F Jr., Williams K, Howland MA, et al: Levetiracetam poisoning induces coma: Confirmed by laboratory analysis. *J Toxicol Clin Toxicol* 40:881–884, 2002.

Bohan TP, Helton E, McDonald I, et al: Effect of L-carnitine treatment for valproate-induced hepatotoxicity. *Neurology* 56:1405–1409, 2001.

Briassoulis G, Kalabalikis P, Tamiolaki M: Lamotrigine childhood overdose. *Pediatr Neurol* 19:239–242, 1998.

Brubacher JR, Dahghani P, McKnight D: Delayed toxicity following ingestion of enteric-coated divalproex sodium (Epival). *J Emerg Med* 17:463–467, 1999.

Buckley NA, White IM, Dawson AH: Self-poisoning with lamotrigine. *Lancet* 342:1552–1553, 1993.

Centers for Disease Control and Prevention: GHB use 1995–1996. *JAMA* 277:1511, 1997.

Frenia ML: Multiple dose activated charcoal compared to urinary alkalinization for the enhancement of phenobarbital elimination. *J Toxicol Clin Toxicol* 34:169–175, 1996.

Coulter DL, Allen RJ: Secondary hyperammonemia: A possible mechanism for valproate encephalopathy. *Lancet* 1:1310–1311, 1980.

Davie MB, Cook MJ, Ng C: Vigabatrin overdose [letter]. *Med J Aust* 165:403, 1996.

DeVivo DC, Bohan TP, Coulter DL, et al: L-carnitine supplementation in childhood epilepsy: Current perspectives. *Epilepsia* 39:1216–1225, 1998.

Dreifuss FE, Langer DH, Moline KA, et al: Valproic acid hepatic fatalities. *Neurology* 39:201–207, 1989.

Fischer HJ, Barr AN, Rogers SL, et al: Lack of serious toxicity following gabapentin overdose. *Neurology* 44:982–983, 1994.

Gidal BE, Privitera MD, Sheth RD, et al: A novel therapy for seizure disorders. *Ann Pharmacother* 33:1277–1286, 1999.

Gilman JT. Lamotrigine: An antiepileptic agent for the treatment of partial seizures. *Ann Pharmacother* 29:144–151, 1993.

Hauser WA, Rich SS, Lee J, et al: Risk of recurrent seizures after two unprovoked seizures. *N Engl J Med* 338:429–434, 1998.

Hojer J, Malmlund HO, Berg A: Clinical features in 28 consecutive cases of laboratory confirmed massive poisoning with carbamazepine alone. *J Toxicol Clin Toxicol* 31:449–458, 1993.

Ingels M, Beauchamp J, Clark RF et al: Delayed valproic acid toxicity: A retrospective case series. *Ann Emerg Med* 39:616–621, 2002.

Ishikura H, Matsuo N, Matsubara M, et al: Valproic acid overdose and L-carnitine therapy. *J Anal Toxicol* 20:55–58, 1996.

Knowles SR, Shapiro LE, Shear NH: Anticonvulsant hypersensitivity syndrome: Incidence, prevention and management. *Drug Safety* 21:489–501, 1999.

Lacayo A, Mitra N: Report of a case of phenobarbital-induced dystonia. *Clin Pediatr* 31:252, 1992.

Leiber BL, Snodgrass WR. Cardiac arrest following large intravenous fosphenytoin overdose in an infant [abstract]. *J Toxicol Clin Toxicol* 36:473, 1998.

Levinson DF, Devinsky O: Psychiatric adverse events during vigabatrin therapy. *Neurology* 53:1503–1511, 1999.

Li J, Norwood DL, Li-Feng M, et al: Mitochondrial metabolism of valproic acid. *Biochemistry* 30:388–394, 1991.

Lindberg MC, Cunningham A, Lindberg NH: Acute phenobarbital intoxication. *South Med J* 85:803–807, 1992.

Mauro LS, Mauro V, Brown D, et al: Enhancement of phenytoin elimination by multiple-dose activated charcoal. *Ann Emerg Med* 16:1132–1135, 1987.

McKinney P, Birnbaum K: Carbamazepine and Phenytoin. In: Ford M, DeLaney K, Ling L, et al, eds: *Clinical Toxicology*. Philadelphia: Saunders; 2001:478–992.

Neuvonen PJ, Elonen E: Effect of activated charcoal on absorption and elimination of phenobarbitone, carbamazepine and phenylbutazone in man. *Eur J Clin Pharmacol* 17:51–57, 1980.

Privetera MD. Topiramate: A new antiepileptic drug. *Ann Pharmacother* 31:1164–1173, 1997.

Rogvi-Hansen B, Gram L: Adverse effects of established and new antiepileptic drugs: An attempted comparison. *Pharmacol Ther* 68:425–434, 1993.

Schlienger RG, Knowles SR, Shear NH: Lamotrigine-associated anticonvulsant hypersensitivity syndrome. *Neurology* 51:1172–1175, 1998.

Schiebel N, Vicas I: Barbiturates. In: Ford M, DeLaney K, Ling L, et al, eds: *Clinical Toxicology*. Philadelphia: Saunders, 2001:569–574.

Stremski ES, Brady W, Prasa K, et al: Pediatric carbamazepine intoxication. *Ann Emerg Med* 25:624–630, 1995.

42

Isoniazid

Dominic Chalut

HIGH-YIELD FACTS

- Doses of isoniazid (INH) that cause convulsions are variable and may occur with ingestions of 40 mg/kg or less.

- The clinical triad characteristic of severe acute INH toxicity consists of refractory seizures, profound anion gap metabolic acidosis, and coma.

- Pyridoxine (vitamin B_6) is a specific antidote and usually terminates benzodiazepine-resistant seizures.

- Administer 5 g of pyridoxine intravenously (IV) if the amount of INH ingested is unknown. The pediatric dose is 70 mg/kg, up to 5 g. If the amount of INH ingested is known, the pyridoxine dose in grams is equivalent to the grams of ingested INH.

- Health care facilities often do not have sufficient stocks of pyridoxine, despite its being a very effective and inexpensive antidote.

CASE PRESENTATION

A 15-year-old Native American boy is brought to the emergency department (ED) for convulsions. He was discovered in his room next to an empty bottle of pills, and has been seizing for the last 25 minutes. No other information is available. The patient is brought to the re-suscitation room, where an IV line is inserted, labs are sent, and diazepam is given. The bedside glucose is normal. Despite IV benzodiazepine, the seizure persists.

On physical examination, the seizure is tonic–clonic and generalized. His vital signs are as follows: blood pressure 120/70 mmHg, pulse 130 bpm, and respirations 16 breaths per minute. Pupils are equal, round, and reactive to light. Mucous membranes are moist. The cardiorespiratory assessment is unremarkable. No needle track injuries are visible. Bowel sounds are normal, and there is no urinary incontinence. Laboratory studies reveal a profound metabolic acidosis with increased anion gap.

INTRODUCTION AND EPIDEMIOLOGY

INH, the hydrazide of isonicotinic acid, still remains a first-line antituberculous drug both for treatment and prophylaxis of tuberculosis. When ingested it can produce significant morbidity and mortality. According to the 2001 data from the American Association of Poison Control Centers (AAPCC), there were 426 isoniazid exposures, of which 233 (55%) occurred in patients aged 0 to 19 years. One death was reported in 2001, and 80 patients had an outcome qualified as major in the AAPCC report. Acute INH overdose is a common cause of drug-induced seizures and metabolic acidosis.

INH is readily available and is frequently prescribed to patients who may be at risk of overdose, such as the poor, the homeless, and those lacking social support. However, the rising incidence of AIDS and tuberculosis has meant that people from all socioeconomic strata have increased access to INH. The risk increases in a family where a person is treated or receiving prophylaxis for tuberculosis. According to the 2001 AAPCC report, 50%

of the INH intoxications were intentional and 50% were unintentional. The clinical course of INH may be rapid and devastating, leading to significant morbidity.

DEVELOPMENTAL CONSIDERATIONS

Although INH toxicity is relatively rare, the majority (55%) of overdoses occur in the pediatric population. The 2001 AAPCC report finds that 70% of cases occurred in the 6 to 19 age group, and the remaining 30% were in preschoolers. Children may find the sweet, orange-flavored syrup preparation very attractive.

PHARMACOLOGY AND TOXICOKINETICS

After oral ingestion, 95% of INH is absorbed rapidly from the small intestine. Peak levels are achieved within 2 hours of administration. INH is distributed into all body fluids and tissues, with a volume of distribution estimated at 0.6 L/kg. Only about 10% of INH is protein bound. Seventy-five percent of INH is metabolized via acetylation and dehydralization, and a small amount is excreted unchanged by the kidneys. The rate of acetylation of INH is a major determining factor in the manifestation of toxicity. Persons may be identified as slow or fast acetylators. Approximately 50% of all Caucasian and African Americans are slow acetylators. The vast majority of Asians and Native Americans are fast acetylators. The half-life of INH is 2 to 4 hours in slow acetylators, and 0.7 hours in rapid acetylators. A higher incidence of toxicity might be expected in slow acetylators. Plasma concentrations of rapid INH acetylators are 20% to 50% those of slow

acetylators. INH and its metabolites are excreted by the kidneys, and 75% to 95% of the elimination is completed by 24 hours. INH crosses the blood–brain barrier and the placenta, and is found in breast milk.

PATHOPHYSIOLOGY

INH induces toxicity primarily through its interactions with pyridoxine-5-phosphatase and nicotinamide adenine dinucleotide (NAD) (Figure 42–1). These interactions may explain the complications seen with INH intoxication: seizure and acidosis. INH induces a decrease of the neurotransmitter γ-aminobutyric acid (GABA), which is an inhibitory neurotransmitter in the primary central nervous system (CNS). Lower levels of GABA in the CNS are associated with increased CNS excitability that can result in convulsions.

Acidosis results from increased production of lactate during seizures. However, INH also inhibits NAD, an enzyme that metabolizes lactate to pyruvate, which contributes to an accumulation of lactate.

CLINICAL FINDINGS

Acute Toxicity

The dose of INH that causes convulsions is variable and may occur with ingestion of 40 mg/kg or less. Ingestion of INH between 80 to 150 mg/kg produces severe CNS symptoms. The clinical triad of severe acute INH toxicity consists of refractory seizures, profound anion gap metabolic acidosis (pH 6.8 to 6.9), and coma. Nausea,

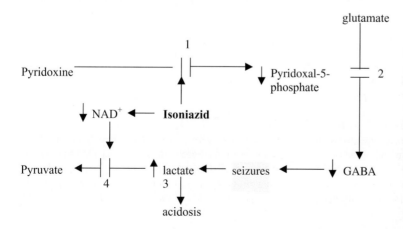

Fig. 42–1. Pathophysiology of INH-induced seizures and acidosis. INH blocks the pyridoxine phosphokinase conversion of pyridoxine to P-5′-P (1), a cofactor necessary for the conversion of glutamate to GABA (2). The decrease in GABA predisposes to seizures. The metabolic acidosis results from lactate produced during the seizures (3) and from INH inhibition of NAD^+ (4), which is required for the conversion of lactate to pyruvate. The result is an accumulation of lactate.

vomiting, dizziness, hyperpyrexia, and hypotension are other abnormalities seen with acute INH toxicity. Patients are usually symptomatic within 30 to 45 minutes of ingestion; however, symptoms may be delayed for up to 2 hours postingestion, when peak serum levels are reached.

Chronic Toxicity

Hepatitis occurs in 0.3% of patients younger than 35 years on INH therapy, but increases to 2.3% in patients older than 50 years. Hepatitis, peripheral neuropathy, optic neuritis, pellagra-like syndrome, hypersensitivity (manifested as hepatitis, fever, rash, joint pain), systemic lupus erythematosus–like syndrome, and rhabdomyolysis have also been reported with the administration of INH.

LABORATORY AND DIAGNOSTIC TESTING

Serum INH concentrations are not commonly available, and therefore are not generally included among routine toxicology screening tests. Serum concentrations, however, are not necessary for treatment of the acutely poisoned patient, and one should initiate specific therapy if clinical suspicion of INH ingestion is high. Other useful laboratory studies include electrolytes, glucose, blood urea nitrogen, creatinine, liver function tests, and blood gases. A patient who presents with seizures following an unknown ingestion may require a chest radiograph if there is concern for aspiration. Radiographic abnormalities suggestive of tuberculosis indicate a potential role of INH in the etiology of seizures.

MANAGEMENT

Aggressive airway management and seizure treatment are the cornerstones of therapy. Maintain the airway and assist ventilation if necessary. Seizures may spontaneously occur early in the course of treatment, so early induction of emesis in a symptomatic patient is not advised. Gastric decontamination of these patients has a limited role, if any, given that INH is absorbed rapidly from the small intestine. Activated charcoal adsorbs INH well. The risk of early seizures must be considered in the decision to administer activated charcoal, because the risk of aspiration increases tremendously in a convulsing patient. If activated charcoal is given, the dose for children is 1 g/kg, up to 50 to 75 g in adult-sized children.

Commonly used anticonvulsants such as benzodiazepines, phenytoin, and phenobarbital, when used alone, may not be effective in controlling INH-induced seizures. Pyridoxine (vitamin B_6), a specific antidote that augments and replaces GABA, usually terminates benzodiazepine-resistant seizures, and should be given as soon as possible. The dose of pyridoxine is equivalent to the amount of INH ingested; administer the pediatric dose of 70 mg/kg, up to 5 g, if the amount of INH is unknown. Pyridoxine may be repeated if the seizures continue or recur. Pyridoxine may also hasten the resolution of metabolic acidosis. If acidosis is not responsive to pyridoxine and seizure control, IV sodium bicarbonate should be considered. If IV pyridoxine is not available, the oral preparation may be crushed and administered via nasogastric tube.

Previous studies have demonstrated that many antidotes, including pyridoxine, are insufficiently stocked in Canadian and U.S. health care facilities. In a 1998 survey mailed to 93 hospital pharmacy directors, only 7% reported having a sufficient quantity of pyridoxine. The standard pyridoxine stock in that study was 1 vial of 10 g, with an acquisition cost of approximately $120. The greatest barrier to adequate pyridoxine supplies is probably a lack of awareness.

With very little protein binding and a low volume of distribution, INH is a good candidate for dialysis, but in view of its short half-life and efficient antagonism with pyridoxine, such procedures may be unnecessary except in the context of renal failure.

DISPOSITION

Asymptomatic patients who have ingested a potentially toxic amount of INH should be observed at least 6 hours because of the possibility of a latent period before toxicity develops. Symptomatic patients with seizure activity or metabolic acidosis should be admitted to an intensive care setting.

CASE OUTCOME

The acute onset of seizures associated with metabolic acidosis prompted the pediatric emergency physician to consider an INH overdose. Five grams of pyridoxine were administered IV, terminating the convulsions. The patient was admitted to the pediatric intensive care unit for close monitoring. He recovered completely and had no neurologic sequelae. He admitted to ingesting his grandmother's tuberculosis medication in a suicide attempt. A psychiatric consultation was obtained.

SUGGESTED READINGS

Bennett WM, Singer I, Golper T, et al: Guidelines for drug therapy in renal failure. *Ann Intern Med* 86:754–783, 1977.

Brown CR: Isoniazid. In: Olson KR, Anderson BA, et al, eds: *Poisoning & Drug Overdose.* 3rd ed. Norwalk, CT: Appleton & Lange; 1999:195–196.

Ellard GA: Variations between individuals and populations in the acetylation of isoniazid and its significance for the treatment of pulmonary tuberculosis. *Clin Pharmacol Ther* 19:610–625, 1976.

Ellenhorn MJ, Schonwald S, Ordog G, et al, eds: Antituberculosis drugs: Isoniazid. In: *Ellenhorn's Medical Toxicology.* 2nd ed. Baltimore: Williams & Wilkins; 1997:240–243.

Gorman SK, Zed PJ, Pursell RA, et al: Antidote stocking in British Columbia hospitals. *Canadian Journal of Emergency Medicine* 5:12–17, 2003.

Henry GC, Haynes S: Isoniazid and other antituberculous drugs: Isoniazid. In: Ford MD, Delaney KA, Ling LJ, et al, eds: *Clinical Toxicology.* Philadelphia: Saunders; 2001:440–444.

Isoniazid (monograph): *Compendium of Pharmaceutical Specialties.* 2003:817–818.

Jeanes CWL, Schaefer O, Eidus L: Inactivation of isoniazid by Canadian Eskimos and Indians. *Can Med Assoc J* 106:331–335, 1972.

Katz GA, Jobin EC: Large doses of pyridoxine in the treatment of massive isoniazid ingestion. *Am Rev Respir Dis* 101:991–992, 1970.

Litovitz T, Klein-Schwartz W, Rodgers GC, et al: 2001 Annual report of the American Association of Poison Control Centers—Toxic Exposure Surveillance System. *Am J Emerg Med* 20:391–452, 2002.

Reilly RH, Killam KF, Jenney EH, et al: Convulsant effects of isoniazid. *JAMA* 152:1317–1321, 1953.

Sievers ML, Herrier RN, Chin L, et al: Treatment of isoniazid overdose. *JAMA* 247:583–584, 1982.

43

Antidepressant Overdose: Tricyclics, Selective Serotonin Reuptake Inhibitors, and Atypical Antidepressants

Gary Lee Geis
G. Randall Bond

HIGH-YIELD FACTS

- Antidepressant use in children is increasing in prevalence, owing to improved diagnosis and increased use of these agents.
- Tricyclic antidepressants (TCAs) taken in overdose can cause conduction delays, dysrhythmias, hypotension, central nervous system (CNS) depression, and seizures.
- Clinical deterioration from TCA overdose can be sudden and unpredictable.
- Serum alkalinization and sodium loading with sodium bicarbonate remains the initial treatment for TCA cardiotoxicity.
- Newer antidepressants, including selective serotonin reuptake inhibitors (SSRIs), have a lower risk of serious toxicity in overdose.

CASE PRESENTATION

A 14-year-old girl is found unresponsive in her bedroom with a suicide note 2 hours following an argument with her mother. She moaned to stimulation at home, but was unresponsive when the rescue squad arrived. During transport to the hospital she developed respiratory arrest requiring intubation. On arrival to the emergency department (ED) she had a self-limited 30-second tonic–clonic seizure. Initial vital signs were significant for heart rate of 140 bpm and blood pressure of 75/40 mmHg. Her electrocardiogram (ECG) revealed a slightly widened QRS interval.

INTRODUCTION AND EPIDEMIOLOGY

Antidepressants continue to represent a large portion of poison center referrals and poisoning fatalities in the United States. From 1991 to 2001, the American Association of Poison Control Centers (AAPCC) reported an increase in poison center calls for antidepressant exposure from 35,871 to 92,675. Per the AAPCC, TCAs were a leading cause of poisoning fatalities until 1993, when only narcotics surpassed TCAs. In recent years, depression has been recognized more frequently in children and adolescents. Because of superior efficacy, a lower adverse side effect profile, and a reduced incidence of serious toxicity, selective SSRIs and atypical antidepressants (Table 43–1) are prescribed more frequently than TCAs. In addition, pediatric uses for antidepressants include neuralgic and chronic pain, migraine headaches, enuresis, attention-deficit hyperactivity disorder, obsessive–compulsive disorder, panic and phobic disorders, and eating disorders. Poisoning center calls parallel these prescribing habits, with SSRIs representing over half of antidepressant exposures in patients younger than 17 years of age in 2001.

PATHOPHYSIOLOGY

In overdose, TCA mainly affect the cardiovascular system, autonomic nervous system, and CNS, leading to conduction delays, dysrhythmias, hypotension, altered mental status, and seizures. The mechanisms involved include inhibition of norepinephrine and serotonin reuptake at central presynaptic terminals, peripheral and central antagonism of muscarinic acetylcholine receptors

Table 43–1. Antidepressants

Generic Name	Trade Name	Antidepressant Class
Amitryptiline	Elavil, Endep	TCA
Amoxapine	Asendin	Dibenzoxapine drug[a]
Bupropion	Wellbutrin	Atypical
Citalopram	Celexa	SSRI[a]
Clomipramine	Anafranil	TCA
Desipramine	Norpramin	TCA
Doxepin	Sinequan	TCA
Fluoxetine	Prozac, Sarafem	SSRI
Fluvoxamine	Luvox	SSRI
Imipramine	Tofranil	TCA
Maprotiline	Ludiomil	Tetracyclic
Mirtazapine	Remeron	Atypical[b]
Nefazadone	Serzone	Atypical
Nortriptyline	Aventyl, Pamelor	TCA
Paroxetine	Paxil	SSRI
Protrityline	Vivactil	TCA
Reboxetine		Atypical
Sertraline	Zoloft	SSRI
Trazadone	Desyrel	Atypical
Trimipramine	Surmontil	TCA
Venlafaxine	Effexor	Atypical

[a]Also considered atypical antidepressants.
[b]Mirtazapine has a tetracyclic structure.
Abbreviations: SSRI, selective serotonin reuptake inhibitors; TCA, tricyclic antidepressant.

(anticholinergic effects), membrane depressant effects on sodium channels of the distal cardiac conduction system, and antagonism of peripheral α_1-adrenergic receptors.

Conduction delays are due to antagonism of the cardiac fast sodium channels. TCAs block the rapid influx of sodium, which slows phase 0 depolarization of the action potential in the His–Purkinje system and ventricular myocardium, manifesting as a prolonged QRS interval. This is referred to as a *quinidine-like effect* because it mirrors the physiology of class Ia anti-arrhythmics. TCAs can also delay ventricular repolarization and phase 4 depolarization causing QT interval prolongation. Although seen more often at therapeutic dosing, this prolonged QT interval can lead to torsades de pointes.

The most common dysrhythmia seen in TCA overdose is sinus tachycardia, owing to the peripheral cholinergic

blockade and inhibition of norepinephrine reuptake. Causes of wide complex tachycardias are multifactorial in origin, including delayed anterograde conduction, nonuniform conduction, and reentry ventricular dysrhythmias. Most wide complexes are probably sinus tachycardia with rate-dependent aberrancy, but risk of ventricular tachycardia exists with associated tissue hypoxia, metabolic acidosis, or use of β_1-adrenergic therapy.

The hypotension found in TCA overdose is multifactorial, including direct myocardial depression, peripheral vasodilation, inhibition of norepinephrine reuptake, and reduced myocardial catecholamine levels. Myocardial depression results from blockade of sodium reentry disrupting coupling of calcium entry into the cells. This decreases myocardial contractility and adds to lowered systemic blood pressures. The peripheral vasodilation is due to direct α-adrenergic blockade by the TCAs.

Altered mental status and CNS depression are due to central anticholinergic effects, but the pathophysiology of lowered seizure threshold is not fully understood. Possible explanations include an increased level of monoamines, antidopaminergic properties, inhibition of neuronal sodium channels, or interaction with the GABA–receptor chloride ionophore complex in the brain.

The toxicity seen following SSRI overdose is an exaggeration of therapeutic pharmacologic activity. These agents specifically inhibit reuptake of serotonin at central presynaptic terminals, thus extending the effects of neuronally released serotonin and altering sensitivities of receptors. They are better tolerated in overdose than TCAs, with a wider therapeutic index and less risk of cardiovascular toxicity. Citalopram is an exception. It has a chemical structure unrelated to that of other SSRIs. It produces antagonism of muscarinic, histaminergic, and adrenergic receptors that has been hypothesized to cause various anticholinergic, sedative, and cardiovascular effects. Citalopram has been shown in dogs to cause seizures, prolonged QT interval, arrhythmias, and torsades de pointes. The atypical antidepressants have various mechanisms of action (Table 43–2), leading to diverse manifestations in acute overdose.

PHARMACOLOGY AND TOXICOKINETICS

There is a higher risk of TCA toxicity in children because TCAs have a small therapeutic index. Taking 10 to 20 mg/kg of most TCAs will cause significant toxicity in most patients. This amounts to only one or two 100-mg

Table 43–2. Pharmacology of Atypical Antidepressants

Antidepressant	Mechanism of Action
Amoxapine	Inhibits norepinephrine reuptake, no effect on serotonin, blocks dopamine receptors.
Bupropion	Unicyclic, mechanism unclear, may inhibit reuptake of biogenic amines (dopamine, norepinephrine, serotonin); moderate anticholinergic activity.
Mirtazapine	Inhibits central α_2-adrenergic receptors, thus increasing neuronal norepinephrine and serotonin; also blocks 5-HT2 and 5-HT3 receptors.
Nefazodone	Inhibits reuptake of serotonin, blocks 5-HT2 receptors.
Reboxetine	Inhibits reuptake of norepinephrine.
Trazadone	Inhibits reuptake of serotonin, some peripheral α-adrenergic blockade.
Venlafaxine	Inhibits reuptake of serotonin, norepinephrine, and dopamine; rapid downregulation of central β-adrenergic receptors.

tablets in an infant or toddler. The small size of pediatric patients means that just one tablet or capsule can cause severe clinical manifestations, including death. Life-threatening exposures in adults are associated with ingestions >1000 mg.

TCAs are rapidly and easily absorbed in the intestine, although in overdose the anticholinergic effects may decrease gut motility, resulting in delayed absorption with prolonged or cyclic symptoms. TCAs and their metabolites are highly lipophilic and extensively protein bound. Despite this protein binding, they each have a large volume of distribution resulting in high tissue:plasma ratios. TCAs have an extensive first pass metabolism in the liver via cytochrome P450 (CYP) oxidative enzymes. Metabolism can be affected by individual differences in CYP enzyme activity (slow metabolizers), other medicines that effect CYP, age, and ethnicity.

SSRIs and atypical antidepressants also have rapid absorption and large volumes of distribution. However,

many atypical agents come in sustained-release preparations. Following overdose, the onset of significant symptoms may be delayed. In addition, their half-lives vary, affecting the persistence of drug actions and side effects. These medications are metabolized by and are inhibitors of P450 (CYP) enzymes, thus can interact with TCAs if taken together.

CLINICAL FINDINGS

TCA poisoning should be suspected in any patient who presents with lethargy, coma, seizures, dysrhythmias, or conduction delay, especially with a past history of depression. Clinical deterioration can be sudden and unpredictable. Most patients demonstrate near maximal symptoms within 4 to 6 hours of presentation. Cardiovascular toxicity manifests as conduction delay, dysrhythmias, and hypotension. Conduction delay is usually identified on ECG as PR, QRS, and QT interval prolongation, with atrioventricular block a rare finding. Dysrhythmias can present as sinus or supraventricular tachycardia, premature ventricular complexes, idioventricular dysrhythmias, or ventricular tachycardia or fibrillation. When severe bradycardia or asystole are seen, they are usually preterminal events.

CNS toxicity manifests as altered mental status, agitation, coma, and seizures. In one study, presenting Glascow Coma Scale (GCS) <8 was a more sensitive predictor of severe complications than QRS interval duration. Seizures are usually generalized, brief, and occur within the first few hours after presentation. Other anticholinergic effects frequently seen are urinary retention, decreased sweating, dry flushed skin, dry mouth, dilated pupils, and hyperthermia. Compared with the classic TCAs, the atypical agents amoxapine and maprotiline have a higher incidence of seizures, but less cardiovascular toxicity. Status epilepticus following amoxapine overdose can be particularly difficult to control, accounting for much of the morbidity and mortality associated with this agent.

Acute SSRI overdose with the most commonly used agents is associated with only nausea, vomiting, dizziness, blurred vision, CNS depression, tremor, sinus tachycardia, and mydriasis. Serotonin syndrome only rarely follows isolated SSRI overdose. A case report of massive sertraline overdose noted QTc prolongation on presentation, followed by development of serotonin syndrome on day 3 of admission. SSRI poisoning should be suspected in any patient with lethargy, coma, or seizures without signs of cardiovascular toxicity.

Table 43–3. Relative Frequency (Not Severity) of Each Finding With Significant
Overdose of Various Antidepressants

	↑HR	↑QRS	↑QTc	↓BP	↓CNS	Sz
TCA	+++	+++	++	++	+++	++
Amoxapine	++	±	±	+	++	++
Citalopram	+	+	+		+	+
Other SSRI	+		±	+	++	±
Trazadone			±	+	++	±
Venlafaxine	+	±	±	+	++	++
Bupropion	++	±	±	±	±	++

Abbreviations: BP, blood pressure; CNS, central nervous system; HR, heart rate; SSRI, selective serotonin reuptake inhibitors; Sz, seizures.

±, reported or rare. Reported experience with nefazodone and mirtazepine overdose are limited.

In contrast with most SSRIs, the course of citalopram overdose may be more severe. A review of acute citalopram overdoses in Sweden showed it to cause prolonged QRS interval and seizures in patients exposed to >600 mg. No deaths were noted in those cases, but six citalopram overdose fatalities were reported in another series.

Serotonin syndrome involves excessive stimulation of 5-HT1 receptors, most commonly following the use of combinations of SSRIs and/or monoamine oxidase inhibitors. Serotonin syndrome involves changes in mental status, autonomic instability, and neuromuscular abnormailities resulting in hyperthermia. For clinical diagnosis, a patient must have three of the following: altered mental status, agitation, myoclonus, hyperreflexia, diaphoresis, tremor, shivering, diarrhea, or incoordination. Serotonin syndrome can result in rhabdomyolysis, acute renal failure, lactic acidosis, hepatic failure, and acute respiratory distress syndrome.

Because atypical antidepressants have varied mechanisms of action (see Table 43–2), their clinical manifestations also vary. Bupropion overdose often manifests with seizures and sinus tachycardia. There are reports of QRS prolongation. The onset of adverse effects can be delayed for hours after presentation and continue up to 48 hours after exposure. Trazadone overdose can cause CNS depression and hypotension, with rare cases of syndrome of inappropriate diuretic hormone and seizures. Bradycardia, heart block, intraventricular conduction delay, prolonged QT, torsades de pointes, and ventricular premature complexes have also been described. There is limited clinical experience with nefazodone overdose, but CNS depression and hypotension similar to trazadone are expected. Venlafaxine overdose has been associated with QRS prolongation and ventricular tachycardia leading to fatalities, as well as hypotension, seizures, and CNS depression. There is a lack of overdose experience with mirtazapine and reboxetine, but pharmacology suggests heart rate, blood pressure, and neurologic status should be closely monitored.

LABORATORY AND DIAGNOSTIC TESTING

Diagnosis of TCA toxicity and risk of serious complications from overdose depends mostly on history, physical examination, close monitoring for changes in clinical condition, and ECG findings. Serum and urine tests are available to assess qualitative presence and quantitative drug levels of TCAs. Positive qualitative drug screens may confirm the presence of TCAs and other coingested medicines, but the results are not readily available at presentation and false or misleading positive results do occur. All patients taking TCAs therapeutically will be positive, so a positive result in an unknown overdose of a patient on TCAs therapeutically does not mean that the patient's symptoms are necessarily related to a TCA overdose. Clinical correlation is required. Diphenhydramine, cyclobenzaprine, cyproheptadine, carbamazepine, and phenothiazines may cause false-positive test results. Serum quantitative levels of TCAs take time to obtain and have not been shown to correlate with clinical toxicity. Serum concentrations of >1000 ng/mL are usually observed in patients with significant toxicity, but seizures have been reported at levels of 571 ng/mL and cardiovascular complications have been reported at levels of 773 ng/mL. Therefore, quantitative TCA levels are of little help in the management of acute overdose.

Sinus tachycardia by itself does not predict complications in TCA overdose. Multiple ECG parameters have been studied for predictive value, including QRS interval duration, terminal 40-millisecond (T40-ms) QRS vector axis, and heights of R-wave and S-wave in lead aVR. Maximal limb lead QRS interval duration has been shown to be a sensitive indicator of toxicity. In one study following TCA ingestion, no patients with a QRS <100 ms had seizures and no patients with a QRS <160 ms had ventricular arrhythmias, whereas patients with QRS >100 ms had a 34% incidence of seizure and a 14% incidence of ventricular arrhythmias. Additionally, there was no statistically significant association between serum drug levels and occurrence of seizures or ventricular arrhythmias when 1000 ng/mL was used as a cutoff.

The T40-ms QRS vector has been shown to be associated with TCA toxicity if it lies between 120 and 270 degrees. One study detailed this association and compared it to the QRS interval duration in detecting TCA overdose. The T40-ms vector had a positive predictive value of 49%, negative predictive value of 90%, and a greater sensitivity than the QRS interval for TCA overdose. However, the T40-ms axis is not readily measured without computer-assisted analysis, thus decreasing its usefulness in the ED. Also, in a retrospective review of pediatric patients with TCA ingestion versus age-matched controls, the T40-ms axis had a large normal variability limiting its usefulness in this age group. In lead aVR, the height of the R-wave and the height ratio of R-wave:S-wave reflect the rightward shift of the terminal QRS axis in TCA toxicity. Comparing R-wave height in aVR and QRS interval duration, having an R-wave height >3 mm in aVR was as sensitive and more specific that QRS >100 ms for TCA toxicity. The clinical utility of these other indicators over CNS depression or QRS widening to mandate more intensive monitoring for severe toxicity is not clear.

No readily available laboratory tests or clinical parameters identify and predict the course of SSRI and atypical antidepressant exposures. Qualitative and quantitative testing do not help in the acute setting. A screening ECG is warranted owing to the risk of coingested medicines, but sinus tachycardia is often the only ECG finding with these overdoses. Because absorption may be significantly delayed with some of these agents, particularly with sustained-release preparations, it is important to monitor patients through the peak of absorption.

MANAGEMENT

The mainstays of therapy for possible TCA overdose are gastrointestinal (GI) decontamination, aggressive supportive care, and close observation. Patients with TCA toxicity can deteriorate rapidly and unexpectedly. For this reason, ipecac-induced emesis is contraindicated. The use of gastric lavage needs to be considered for large ingestions or patients with early presentation (<1 hour) to the ED, but clinical trials do not support its routine use. Activated charcoal, given at a dose of 1 g/kg up to 50 g, is indicated initially, with consideration for a second dose owing to anticholinergic-induced delayed gastric emptying. Owing to TCA's high volume of distribution and high tissue:plasma ratios with TCAs, enhanced elimination with hemodialysis or hemoperfusion is not effective.

Serum alkalinization and sodium loading with intravenous (IV) sodium bicarbonate (Figure 43–1) are the primary therapies for patients with cardiovascular toxicity; however, there are no controlled, prospective trials in the literature. The use of bicarbonate is based on animal studies, case reports, retrospective reviews, and clinical experience. In these studies, alkalinization has been shown to decrease heart rate, narrow QRS intervals, increase blood pressure and reverse dysrhythmias. The exact QRS interval at which to initiate bicarbonate therapy is not clear. It has often been used with QRS >100 to 110 msec, but there is no direct evidence to support prophylactic alkalinization in the absence of life-threatening cardiovascular toxicity. Indications for bicarbonate therapy include hypotension, compromising dysrhythmias, and significantly prolonged QRS interval. This can be

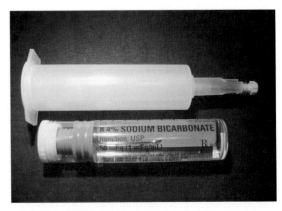

Fig. 43–1. IV sodium bicarbonate.

accomplished by loading doses of 1 to 2 mEq/kg, followed by intermittent dosing or constant infusion. The goal is reversal of cardiovascular toxicity by keeping the serum pH between 7.50 and 7.55.

Hyperventilation of an intubated patient has also been used to achieve serum alkalinization; however, the combined use of IV sodium bicarbonate and hyperventilation can result in profound alkalemia and contribute to death. Capnography to avoid overventilation is important. Serum pH should be monitored. The use of IV hypertonic saline solution (HSS) as a method of sodium loading without alkalinization has theoretical potential. In a randomized, controlled trial using a swine model, HSS was significantly better than sodium bicarbonate or hyperventilation for correcting QRS prolongation and resolving hypotension. Recently, in a case of severe nortriptyline toxicity refractory to optimum serum alkalinization, HSS infusion provided ECG and hemodynamic improvement.

Persistent dysrhythmias or hypotension despite alkalinization require additional therapy. Lidocaine is considered second-line therapy for ventricular dysrhythmias in TCA poisoning. Class Ia, Ic, and III anti-arrhythmics are contraindicated in TCA overdose owing to risk of further sodium channel blockade and prolongation of the QT interval. The use of phenytoin is controversial and not generally recommended owing to its proarrhythmic effects in dogs; however, it has been shown to improve ventricular arrhythmias and conduction abnormalities in human and animal studies. Magnesium sulfate was reported to reverse ventricular tachycardia resistant to lidocaine, bicarbonate and cardioversion in a 20-month-old boy after amitriptyline overdose.

Hypotension should be treated by volume expansion with isotonic saline when indicated. Norepinephrine is second-line therapy for refractory hypotension requiring vasopressors or inotropic support. It offers the advantages of β-agonism for myocardial depression, α-agonism for vasoconstriction, and reversal of depleted norepinephrine stores. Limited clinical data shows it to be more efficacious than dopamine, but at high doses has the risk of exacerbating dysrhythmias. High-dose glucagon was effective in reversing refractory hypotension in a doxepin overdose, but no controlled trials have been performed.

Seizures are usually brief and self-limited, but prolonged seizures can lead to acidosis, hyperthermia, rhabdomyolysis, and hypoxia, all of which can worsen cardiovascular toxicity. Benzodiazepines are first-line treatment, followed by barbiturates. Phenytoin may be effective, but it may also increase the risk of arrhythmogenesis, as discussed.

SSRIs and atypical antidepressants rarely manifest the severe toxicity common with TCAs. Treatment for these includes appropriate use of activated charcoal, supportive care, and close observation. Seizures, hypotension, and conduction disturbances can be managed as for TCA overdose. Serotonin syndrome should be treated with cessation of the offending agent, supportive care, and measures to decrease muscle rigidity.

DISPOSITION

The need for inpatient admission versus close monitoring and discharge to home has been studied for TCA exposure. A summary algorithm has been developed. Patients who at presentation have signs of major toxicity (seizures, coma, dysrhythmia, hypotension, or respiratory depression) or QRS interval >100 msec require admission. Patients who have received appropriate GI decontamination, have no signs of major toxicity, have QRS interval <100 msec, and are observed for 6 hours without change in clinical course or serial ECGs may be medically cleared for discharge home. If overdose was intentional, a psychiatric evaluation is appropriate at this time.

No algorithm for SSRI and atypical antidepressant exposure has been studied or established. Because these agents are generally less toxic, admission is not required in the absence of hypotension or conduction abnormalities. Following overdose of sustained-release products of venlafaxine and bupropion, seizures have occurred many hours after exposure, so admission for observation is indicated if overdose is suspected.

CASE OUTCOME

The 14-year-old patient was presumed to have overdosed on TCAs based on her clinical presentation. She was treated initially with mechanical ventilation, activated charcoal via nasogastric tube, and IV sodium bicarbonate loading. Her QRS interval narrowed after a second 1 mEq/kg bolus of $NaHCO_3$. She also required IV isotonic saline boluses to attain adequate perfusion and blood pressure. A sodium bicarbonate infusion was started and she was admitted to the intensive care unit. No further episodes of seizures occurred and she regained consciousness after 24 hours. At that point she was extubated and later admitted to ingestion of amitriptyline tablets.

SUGGESTED READINGS

Banham NGD: Fatal venlafaxine overdose. *Med J Aust* 169: 445–448, 1998.

Berkovitch M, Matsui D, Fogelman R, et al: Assessment of terminal 40-millisecond QRS vector in children with a history of tricyclic antidepressant ingestion. *Ped Emerg Care* 11:75–77, 1995.

Blackman K, Brown S, Wilkes G: Plasma alkalinization for tricyclic antidepressant toxicity: A systemic review. *Emerg Med* 13:204–210, 2001.

Blythe D, Hackett LP: Cardiovascular and neurological toxicity of venlafaxine. *Hum Exp Toxicol* 18:309–313, 1999.

Boehnert MT, Lovejoy FH: Value of the QRS duration versus the serum drug level in predicting seizures and ventricular arrhythmias after an acute overdose of tricyclic antidepressants. *N Engl J Med* 313:474–479, 1985.

Braithwaite RA, Crome P, Dawling S: Amitryptiline overdose: Plasma concentrations and clinical features. *Br J Clin Pharmacol* 8:388–389, 1979.

Citak A, Soysal DD, Ucsel R, et al: Efficacy of long duration resuscitation and magnesium sulfate treatment in amitryptiline poisoning. *Eur J Emerg Med* 9:63–66, 2002.

Emerman CL, Connors LF, Burnce GM: Level of consciousness as a predictor of complications following tricyclic overdose. *Ann Emerg Med* 16:326–330, 1987.

Glauser J: Tricyclic antidepressant poisoning. *Clev Clinic J Med* 67:704–719, 2000.

Liebelt EL, Francis PD, Woolf AD: ECG lead aVR versus QRS interval in predicting seizures and arrhythmias in acute tricyclic antidepressant toxicity. *Ann Emerg Med* 26:195–201, 1995.

Litovitz TL, Troutman WG: Amoxapine overdose: Seizures and fatalities. *JAMA* 250:1069–1071, 1983.

Malatynska E, Knapp RJ, Ikeda M, et al: Antidepressants and seizure-interactions at the GABA-receptor chloride-ionophore complex. *Life Sci* 43:303–307, 1998.

McCabe JL, Cobaugh DJ, Menegazzi JJ, et al: Experimental tricyclic antidepressant toxicity: A randomized, controlled comparison of hypertonic saline solution, sodium bicarbonate, and hyperventilation. *Ann Emerg Med* 32:329–333, 1998.

McKinney PE, Rasmussen R: Reversal of severe tricyclic antidepressant-induced cardiotoxicity with intravenous hypertonic saline solution. *Ann Emerg Med* 42:20–24, 2003.

Merigian KS, Woodard M, Hedges JR, et al: Prospective evaluation of gastric emptying in the self-poisoned patient. *Am J Emerg Med* 8:479–483, 1990.

Ostrom M, Eriksson A, Thorson J, et al: Fatal overdose with citalopram. *Lancet* 348:339–340, 1996.

Personne M, Sjoberg G, Persson H: Citalopram overdose—Review of cases treated in Swedish hospitals. *Clin Toxicol* 35:237–240, 1997.

Physicians' Desk Reference. 56th ed. 2002:1365.

Pond SM, Lewis-Driver DJ, Williams GM, et al: Gastric emptying in acute overdose: A prospective randomised clinical trial. *Med J Aust* 163:345–349, 1995.

Sensky PR, Olczak SA: High-dose intravenous glucagon in severe tricyclic poisoning. *Postgrad Med J* 75:611–612, 1999.

Shrier M, Diaz JE, Tsarouhas N: Cardiotoxicity associated with bupropion overdose. *Ann Emerg Med* 35:100, 2000.

Sternbach H: The serotonin syndrome. *Am J Psychiatry* 148:705–713, 1991.

Teba L, Schiebel F, Dedhia HV, et al: Beneficial effect of norepinephrine in the treatment of circulatory shock caused by tricyclic antidepressant overdose. *Am J Emerg Med* 6:566–568, 1988.

Tibbles PM, Burns MJ, Spencer FA, et al: Trazodone cardiotoxicity following overdose (abstract). *J Toxicol Clin Toxicol* 35:499, 1997.

Tokarski GF, Young MJ: Criteria for admitting patients with tricyclic antidepressant overdose. *J Emerg Med* 6:121–124, 1998.

Vanpee D, Laloyaux P, Gillet J-B: Seizure and hyponatremia after overdose of trazodone. *Am J Emerg Med* 17:430–431, 1999.

Vohra J, Burrows G, Hunt D, et al: The effect of toxic and therapeutic doses of tricyclic antidepressants drugs on intracardiac conduction. *Eur J Cardiol* 3:219–227, 1975.

Wolfe TR, Caravati EM, Rollins DE: Terminal 40-ms frontal plane QRS axis as a marker for tricyclic antidepressant overdose. *Ann Emerg Med* 18:348–351, 1989.

Wrenn K, Smith BA, Slovis CM: Profound alkalemia during treatment of tricyclic antidepressant overdose. *Am J Emerg Med* 10:553–555, 1992.

44

Lithium

Elisabeth F. Bilden

HIGH-YIELD FACTS

- Serum lithium levels do not correlate well with clinical presentation.

- Factors that may lead to toxicity include those that cause a decrease in lithium elimination such as dehydration, sodium imbalance, and acute or chronic renal failure.

- Lithium does not adsorb well to activated charcoal.

- Peak serum concentration of lithium may be delayed with ingestion of an extended-release formulation.

- Dialysis provides rapid removal of lithium from the body, but the indications for its use remain controversial.

CASE PRESENTATION

A 15-year-old girl with a history of bipolar disorder is brought to the emergency department (ED) by her mother following an ingestion of an unknown amount of Lithobid 300-mg tablets about 20 minutes prior to arrival. Her past medical history is significant for Asperger syndrome, hypothyroidism, and previous self-injurious behaviors. Her other medications include levothyroxine and haloperidol. She has no known drug allergies.

On physical examination, the patient is awake and alert. Her vital signs were BP 112/60 mmHg, pulse 90 bpm, respiratory rate 16 breaths per minute, temperature 36.7°C, and O_2 saturation 98% on room air. Her pupils are equal and reactive to light; extraocular muscles in-

tact, and there is no nystagmus. Her mucous membranes are slightly dry. Cardiac examinations reveals regular rhythm and rate with no rubs, gallops, or murmurs. The are lungs clear to auscultation and the abdomen is nondistended, soft, and nontender. The extremities were normal. The patient is alert and oriented. Cranial nerves are intact, speech clear, and there is no clonus or rigidity.

Laboratory studies reveal a sodium of 133 mEq/L, potassium 3.7 mEq/L, chloride 106 mEq/L, bicarbonate 29 mEq/L, blood urea nitrogen (BUN) 16 mEq/L, creatinine 1.0 mEq/L, and an initial serum lithium level 2.0 mEq/L at 45 minutes postingestion.

INTRODUCTION AND EPIDEMIOLOGY

Lithium is an alkali metal with single valence like sodium and potassium, and has a similar atomic radius to magnesium. In the mid 1800s lithium was used to treat gout and nephrolithiasis. In 1871 lithium bromide was used to treat acute depression (*Melancholia*) and acute mania. In the 1930s, lithium was an additive in antacid lithiated lemon soda (7-Up). In the 1940s it was used as a salt substitute in patients with cardiovascular disease, but this use was discontinued when deaths were attributed to lithium toxicity. The Food and Drug Administration approved lithium for treatment of acute mania in 1970, and for prevention of recurrent mania in 1974. Lithium is currently used for the treatment of bipolar disorder, acute mania, behavior disorders with mood instability, depression, schizoaffective disorders, cluster headaches, and to stimulate white blood cell production in the setting of neutropenia.

Significant toxicity can occur from lithium therapeutic use and misuse. According to the American Association of Poison Control Centers' database, in 2001 no child died from lithium toxicity; however, about 1000 lithium exposures in individuals up to age 19 years old were reported to American poison centers. Of these, 25% involved children less than 6 years old.

DEVELOPMENTAL CONSIDERATIONS

Animal studies have demonstrated a teratogenic risk of lithium, but the effect on humans is uncertain. An increased incidence of Ebstein anomaly, great vessel defects, and other heart defects have been reported in small studies. Lithium toxicity in the neonatal period has been described even when mothers have been on therapeutic doses. Manifestations of toxicity included a depressed neurologic state, hypotonia, cyanosis, cardiovascular abnormalities, and goiter.

In toddlers, a toxic ingestion is most likely accidental, because lithium is rarely used therapeutically in this age group. Lithium is used therapeutically in patients aged 5 to 12 years old, placing these children at risk for toxicity due to chronic use as well as acute exposure. Among adolescents, suicide attempts may lead to toxicity following ingestion of a patient's own or another individual's lithium. In general, children may be less at risk for toxicity than adults, who may have a higher risk of compromised renal function.

PHARMACOLOGY AND TOXICOKINETICS

Lithium has a narrow therapeutic index. In an immediate-release formulation, lithium is absorbed within 1 to 2 hours of ingestion and peak levels occur at 2 to 4 hours postingestion. In a sustained-release formulation, initial absorption may be delayed for 6 to 12 hours, and not completed for an additional 8 hours. Peak absorption may be delayed even longer following overdose.

Lithium is a small ion, is not protein bound, and has a steady-state volume of distribution of 0.6 to 0.9 L/kg. Lithium is initially distributed to extracellular fluid, then accumulates at different rates in various tissues. Lithium enters the liver and kidney quickly and enters muscle, bone, and brain at a much slower rate. This explains the delay between peak serum levels and central nervous system (CNS) effects after an acute overdose. Lithium has an elimination half-life of 20 to 24 hours, which may increase in the setting of chronic use, reduced renal function, or overdose.

Ninety-five percent of lithium is cleared by the kidneys. Between 4% and 5% is secreted in sweat and sali-

vary glands and 1% or less excreted in the feces. A small amount is also excreted in breast milk. Eighty percent of the lithium filtered by the kidneys is reabsorbed and 20% excreted unchanged. Lithium is reabsorbed in the proximal tubules in preference to sodium. The rate of elimination may be altered with compromised renal function, because the rate of clearance is proportional to the glomerular filtration rate (GFR). The rate of lithium clearance is 20 to 30 mL/min, about 25% of the GFR.

Dehydration from any cause may precipitate chronic lithium toxicity secondary to a decreased volume of distribution and increased renal tubular reabsorption. However, lithium toxicity may also lead to dehydration when it causes nausea and vomiting, polyuria, or decreased oral intake owing to mental status changes. It is useful to consider toxic exposure to lithium in three categories:

1. *Acute toxicity* occurs when a patient not currently taking lithium takes an overdose of the drug. This is the most likely ingestion in the pediatric patient.

2. *Acute-on-chronic toxicity* occurs when a patient receiving lithium therapy ingests a toxic dose.

3. *Chronic toxicity* occurs when the use of prescribed lithium becomes toxic without an acute ingestion. Chronic toxicity is more common among adults, particularly in the elderly with renal compromise and patients with chronic psychiatric illness.

Chronic toxicity may be precipitated by dosing errors, dehydration, renal disease, cardiac disease, sodium restriction, or drug interactions with nonsteroidal anti-inflammatory medications (NSAIDs). Angiotensin-converting enzyme inhibitors, haloperidol, diuretics, and selective serotonin reuptake inhibitors have also been implicated.

PATHOPHYSIOLOGY

The mechanisms of action for lithium are complex and not yet fully defined. Lithium enters cells and substitutes for sodium or potassium. It stabilizes cell membranes and interferes with magnesium metabolism. In the CNS, lithium interacts with cyclic adenosine monophosphate (cAMP) and the phosphoinositide second messenger systems. Lithium alters norepinephrine activity via cAMP. It downregulates α- and β-adrenergic function. It interacts with G proteins and with protein kinase C, resulting in a decrease of free brain inositol, which is a mediator of intracellular calcium release. Lithium has regulatory effects on other neurotransmitters. It may prevent upregulation of dopamine$_2$ receptors and it increases γ-aminobutyric acid neurotransmission. Lithium increases the synthesis and turnover of serotonin in presynaptic neurons resulting in a net increase release of serotonin, especially in the hippocampus.

The cardiovascular system may be affected by lithium's inhibition of potassium influx into myocardial cells, causing a decrease in the resting membrane potential of Purkinje fibers. It can cause a decreased velocity of conduction and prolonged depolarization.

Lithium produces nephrogenic diabetes insipidus by blocking the action of antidiuretic hormone–sensitive adenylate cyclase. This can cause dehydration and result in chronic lithium toxicity. Interstitial nephritis and nephrotic syndrome have also been reported.

Lithium causes hypothyroidism. It is concentrated in the thyroid gland, blocks iodine uptake, reduces the release of triiodothyronine (T_3) and thyroxine (T_4), may decrease sensitivity of the gland to thyroid-stimulating hormone (TSH), prevents conversion of T_4 to T_3, and may be responsible for the formation for antithyroid antibodies. Most of these effects with therapeutic use are reversible when lithium is discontinued.

CLINICAL FINDINGS

The severity of symptoms depends on several factors, including type of exposure, serum lithium level, duration of intoxication, and individual tolerance. Signs and symptoms of acute intoxication usually occur within 2 to 4 hours of ingestion.

In the setting of an acute ingestion, lithium toxicity usually presents with gastrointestinal (GI) symptoms including nausea, vomiting, and diarrhea, which result in fluid loss. Lightheadedness and orthostatic hypotension may result. Dehydration further concentrates lithium in the body and exacerbates the toxicity. Neurologic symptoms following an acute ingestion are often delayed. In mild intoxication tremor, weakness, and hyperreflexia can occur. With moderate toxicity, tinnitus, slurred speech, apathy, drowsiness, or agitation may develop. Severe lithium toxicity manifests with confusion, delirium, ataxia, and, potentially, seizures. Extrapyramidal symptoms such as dystonia, lingual and buccal spasm, facial grimacing, opisthotonis, torticollis, and oculogyric palsies can occur. Hyperthermia, encephalopathy, and coma are possible complications. Neuroleptic malignant syndrome has been reported, but only in combination with neuroleptic agents.

Cardiac toxicity produces nonspecific electrocardiogram changes, including T-wave depression, T-wave inversion, prolonged QT interval, preventricular contractions, atrioventricular block, bradycardia, symptomatic sinus node dysfunction, and sinus node arrest. However, dysrhythmias are unusual except in patients with pre-existing cardiac disease or rhythm abnormalities. Cardiogenic shock has also been observed.

With chronic use, a high total body burden of lithium already exists. In toxic patients, there are often no GI symptoms, and neurologic findings often predominate. They are similar to those seen with acute lithium exposure. Long-term neurologic sequelae have been described, such as Parkinson disease, peripheral neuropathy, ataxia, psychosis, memory deficits, personality changes, and idiopathic intracranial hypertension.

Cardiovascular abnormalities may be seen and are similar to those with acute ingestion. Myocarditis and cardiovascular collapse have also been reported. In newborns of mothers on lithium, bradycardia, myocardial depression, cyanosis, and dystonia have been described.

Hypothyroidism occurs with therapeutic use of lithium. Myxedema goiter with increased TSH and decreased T_4 has been reported. Hyperparathyroidism has been described in association with lithium therapy and the resultant hypercalcemia may cause an osmotic diuresis.

Nephrogenic diabetes insipidus is common. Interstitial nephritis and renal failure have been reported, although no evidence exists to show that lithium has a direct nephrotoxic effect. It can induce water and electrolyte disturbances, which may impair renal function, and therefore decreases lithium elimination by the kidney. Lithium may have dermatologic effects such as dermatitis, skin ulcers, and localized edema.

With acute-on-chronic exposure, individuals can present with symptoms of either chronic, acute, or both types of exposure. Symptoms may be more severe or prolonged with this type of exposure and can quickly result in toxicity.

LABORATORY AND DIAGNOSTIC TESTING

The therapeutic serum level for lithium is 0.6 to 1.2 mEq/L. A dose of 1 mEq/kg (40 mg/kg) produces a serum level of approximately 1.2 mEq/L. In acute ingestion, a serum level may be markedly elevated with few or no symptoms if the lithium has not distributed fully from the extracellular space to tissues. With time, the serum level falls but the lithium increasingly distributes into the brain, causing neurologic symptoms that lag behind serum levels. With chronic toxicity, the serum level may be only slightly elevated or even therapeutic, but prominent symptoms of toxicity can be present. Cerebral spinal fluid levels have been reported to be 40% to 80% of that in serum, but do not correlate with symptoms.

In the setting of potential or actual toxicity, serum lithium concentration should be checked on presentation, and then at intervals to assess ongoing absorption and response to therapy. A level of 1.5 to 2.5 mEq/L 12 hours after an acute ingestion is thought to be a mild to moderate elevation. A level of 2.5 to 3.5 mEq/L 12 hours after ingestion is described as severe, and a level greater than 3.5 mEq/L at 12 hours may be life threatening. Other laboratory studies which assist in management include serum electrolytes, BUN, and creatinine. If the clinical picture is consistent with diabetes insipidus, serum and urinary osmolality may offer confirmation.

MANAGEMENT

The lithium-toxic patient should have intravenous (IV) access established and cardiac monitoring instituted. Gastric lavage may be helpful if performed within 1 hour of ingestion. Whole bowel irrigation with a polyethylene glycol electrolyte solution at 20 cc/kg/h has been used to decontaminate the GI tract, and should be considered especially if a sustained-release preparation is ingested. Activated charcoal does not bind well to lithium and should only be considered if coingestants are suspected. There is evidence that sodium polystyrene sulfonate (Kayexalate), an exchange resin usually used to treat hyperkalemia, binds lithium and may lower elevated serum levels. If administered, it is necessary to monitor patients for potential hypokalemia. However, there is no experience with the use of sodium polystyrene sulfonate in the treatment of lithium toxicity among children.

Evidence does not support forced diuresis with diuretics and large amounts of IV fluid. Urine output should be monitored to assess renal function and observe for diabetes insipidus.

Close follow-up of the lithium level, electrolytes, BUN, and creatinine is useful. In chronic toxicity with initial levels less than or equal to 2.5 mEq/L, a goal to achieve a lithium level lower than 1 mEq/L within 30 hours from the start of treatment in stable patients has been suggested.

Hemodialysis is the treatment of choice for rapid removal of lithium in cases of severe toxicity. The goal of treatment is the prevention of neurologic complications. Well-defined guidelines for dialysis in lithium-intoxicated patients have not been established or validated.

However, accepted indications for its use include significant neurologic dysfunction or toxicity, such as decreased level of consciousness, seizures, or altered mental status. Dialysis should also be considered in the setting of renal failure and edematous states such as congestive heart failure and anasarca, in which patients are unable to tolerate volume repletion. Other considerations for hemodialysis include ongoing GI absorption, progressive clinical decline despite conventional therapy, or patient instability.

In an acute exposure, most sources suggest dialysis is indicated for a level ≥4 mEq/L in a patient with neurologic symptoms such as altered mental status and seizures. Asymptomatic patients with elevated lithium levels may be managed with conventional therapy and IV fluids, preferably in an intensive care setting. In chronic exposure, dialysis is indicated in patients with a level of at least 2.5 mEq/L exhibiting neurologic toxicity. A usual course of dialysis is 4 to 6 hours and may be repeated until lithium level remains below 1 mEq/L. Lithium levels should be checked following dialysis and 6 hours later. Lithium levels typically undergo a rebound effect after dialysis owing to continuing equilibration of the intra- and extracellular compartments. If the postdialysis level is high or neurologic symptoms persist, further dialysis may be indicated. Peritoneal dialysis is not any more effective than endogenous lithium clearance by the kidneys. Continuous venous or arterial hemofiltration has been used, but requires a longer duration of treatment than hemodialysis. Although the rate of clearance is decreased, the rebound effect is less pronounced. Hemofiltration requires close monitoring and has been used effectively in children.

DISPOSITION

All intentional ingestions, those in children less than 2 years old, and any symptomatic child regardless of age should be referred to a health care facility. Because lithium is a dangerous toxicant, a worst-case scenario is assumed. At the health care facility, an initial lithium level may document a potentially toxic exposure. A repeat level should be obtained. Patients with lithium levels that are not above the therapeutic range (0.6 to 1.2 mEq/L), are not increasing at 6 hours postingestion, and who remain asymptomatic can be discharged home. Admission is recommended for symptomatic patients, patients with increasing or supratherapeutic serum levels, patients with conditions that may decrease the elimination of lithium, and patients who are suicidal.

CASE OUTCOME

Gastric lavage was performed, and the patient admitted to the intensive care unit. On arrival to the intensive care unit, the patient vomits three times. She is treated with odansatron for the nausea, and whole bowel irrigation started at 500 cc/h. Her lithium levels and electrolytes are followed every 2 hours and the nephrology service is consulted for possible hemodialysis. About 4 hours postingestion, she develops a mild resting tremor and thigh fasciculations. Her speech remains clear and gait is not ataxic. After approximately 6 hours, rectal effluent is clear. Lithium level peaks at 3.8 mEq/L at 6 hours postingestion. At 12 hours after the ingestion level is 2.0 mEq/L. The tremor and fasciculations resolve. The final level is 1.2 mEq/L at 22 hours postingestion. The patient is transferred to the adolescent mental health care unit.

SUGGESTED READINGS

Aita JF, Aita JA, Aita VA: 7-Up anti-acid lithiated lemon soda or early medicinal use of lithium. *Nebr Med J* 75:277–279, 1990.

Alessi N, Naylor MW, Ghaziuddin M: Update on lithium carbonate therapy in children and adolescents. *J Am Acad Child Adolesc Psychiatry* 35:291–305, 1994.

Bailey B, McGuigan M: Comparison of patients hemodialyzed for lithium poisoning and those for whom dialysis was recommended but not done: What lessons can we learn? *Clin Nephrol* 54:388–392, 2000.

Bailey B, McGuigan M: Lithium poisoning from a poison control center perspective. *Ther Drug Monit* 22:650–655, 2000.

Baraban JM, Worley PF, Snyder SH: Second messenger systems and psychoactive drug action: Focus on the phosphoinositide system and lithium. *Am J Psychiatry* 146:1251–1260, 1989.

Filtenborg JA: Persistent pulmonary hypertension after lithium intoxication in the newborn. *Eur J Pediatr* 138:321–323, 1982.

FitzSimons RB, Keane S: Severe lithium intoxication in a child. *Eur J Pediatr* 137:353–354, 1981.

Goetting MG. Acute lithium poisoning in a child with dystonia. *Pediatrics* 76:978–980, 1985.

Groleau G: Lithium toxicity. *Emerg Med Clin North Am* 12:511–531, 1994.

Hansen HK, Amdisen A: Lithium intoxication. *Q J Med* 186:1 23–144, 1978.

Henry GC: Lithium. In: Goldfrank L, Flomenbaum N, Lewin N, eds: *Goldfrank's Toxicologic Emergencies.* 7th ed. New York: McGraw-Hill; 2002:894–900.

Jaeger A, Sauder P, Kopferschmitt J: When should dialysis be performed in lithium poisoning? A kinetic study in 14 cases of lithium poisoning. *J Toxicol Clin Toxicol* 31:429–447, 1993.

Juul-Jensen P: Permanent brain damage after lithium intoxication. *BMJ* 4:673, 1973.

Litovitz, TB, Klein-Schwartz W, Caravati, EM, et al: 1998 annual report of the American association of poison control centers toxic exposures surveillance system. *Am J Emerg Med* 17:435–487, 1999.

Litovitz TB, Klein-Schwartz W, Rodgers GC Jr, et al: 2001 annual report of the American association of poison control centers toxic exposures surveillance system. *Am J Emerg Med* 20:391–452, 2002.

Manji HK, Hsiao JK, Risby ED, et al: The mechanism of action of lithium. I. Effects on serotoninergic and noradrenergic systems in normal subjects. *Arch Gen Psychiatry* 48:505–512, 1991.

Meyer RJ, Flynn JT, Brophy PD, et al: Hemodialysis followed by continuous hemofiltration for the treatment of lithium intoxication in children. *Am J Kidney Dis* 37:1044–1047, 2001.

Moltedo JM, Porter GA, State MW, et al: Sinus node dysfunction associated with lithium therapy in a child. *Tex Heart Inst J* 29:200–202, 2002.

Oakley PW, Whyte IM, Carter GL: Lithium toxicity: An iatrogenic problem in susceptible individuals. *Aust N Z J Psychiatry* 35:833–840, 2001.

Okusa MD, Crystal LJ: Clinical manifestations and management of acute lithium intoxication. *Am J Med* 97:383–389, 1994.

Price LH, Heninger GR: Lithium in the treatment of mood disorders. *N Engl J Med* 331:591–598, 1994.

Scharman EJ: Methods used to decrease lithium absorption or enhance elimination. *Clin Toxicol* 35:601–608, 1997.

Smith SW, Ling LJ, Halstenson CE: Whole-bowel irrigation as treatment for acute lithium overdose. *Ann Emerg Med* 20:536–539, 1991.

Strayhorn JM Jr, Nash JL: Severe neurotoxicity despite "therapeutic" serum lithium levels. *Dis Nerv Syst* 38:107–111, 1977.

Thürmann PA, Steioff A: Drug treatment in pregnancy. *Int J Clin Pharmacol Ther* 39:185–191, 2001.

Tilkian AG, Schroeder JS, Kao JJ, et al: The cardiovascular effects of lithium in man. A review of the literature. *Am J Med* 61:665–670, 1976.

Tunnessen WW Jr, Hertz CG: Toxic effects of lithium in newborn infants: A commentary. *J Pediatr* 81:804–807, 1972.

Weinstein MR, Goldfield MD: Cardiovascular malformations with lithium use during pregnancy. *Am J Psychiatry* 132529–531, 1975.

Weinstein MR, Goldfield MD: Wanted: Reports of lithium babies. *Pediatrics* 48:161–162, 1971.

Woody JN, London WL, Wilbanks GD Jr: Lithium toxicity in a newborn. *Pediatrics* 47:94–96, 1971.

45

Neuroleptic and Antipsychotic Drugs

Anthony M. Burda
Jack W. Lipscomb

HIGH-YIELD FACTS

- Depending on chemical class, neuroleptics cause varying degrees of central nervous system (CNS) depression, anticholinergic symptoms, cardiac toxicity, and movement abnormalities.

- Movement disturbances, known as *extrapyramidal symptoms* (EPS), include acute dystonic reactions, Parkinson dyskinesias, akathisia, and tardive dyskinesia. Many EPS reactions respond to administration of an anticholinergic agent such as diphenhydramine or benztropine mesylate.

- Cardiac conduction disturbances, most notably a prolonged QT interval, are significant complications associated with piperidine phenothiazines (thioridazine) and butyrophenones (haloperidol).

- Neuroleptic malignant syndrome (NMS) is a life-threatening reaction associated with chronic medication therapy and acute drug overdose. Signs and symptoms include hyperthermia, altered mental status, and rigidity.

- Critical interventions with NMS include discontinuation of the offending agent, hydration, rapid cooling, benzodiazepines, and consideration of bromocriptine and/or dantrolene.

- Newer atypical neuroleptics offer therapeutic advantages of lowered incidences of EPS and NMS. Toxicity from these agents may include blood dyscrasias (clozapine), CNS and respiratory depression (clozapine, olanzapine), and hypotension and reflex tachycardia (quetiapine, ziprasidone).

CASE PRESENTATION

A parent brings her 18-month-old, 15-kg son to the emergency department (ED) after observing unusual facial and oral movements. He presents with involuntary tongue wobbling and protrusion, noticeable drooling, and occasional facial grimacing. The child's medical history is unremarkable; he is currently on no medications, and has no known allergies. The parent stated that these symptoms began several hours earlier. She denied that the child had access to any home medications, cleaning products, or plants. He appears slightly drowsy but in no acute distress. His vital signs show a pulse of 120 bpm; respiratory rate of 32 breaths per minute; blood pressure of 82/40 mmHg; a temperature of 99°F; and a pulse oximetry reading of 98% on room air.

On physical examination the patient's pupils are equal and reactive, with no nystagmus noted. His head is noted to be slightly cocked to the right. The child is drooling, but no oral burns, swelling, dysphagia or stridor are observed. The patient's cardiovascular and pulmonary status is normal, and the abdomen is soft and nontender. Extremities have a full range of motion, without rigidity, diaphoresis, or tremors. There is no evidence of trauma or injury. Results of a complete metabolic panel and complete blood count are pending.

INTRODUCTION AND EPIDEMIOLOGY

Neuroleptic is synonymous with *antipsychotic,* and has replaced older nomenclature such as *major tranquilizer,* which refers to agents often prescribed for a wide variety of psychiatric conditions. Previously, *neuroleptic* encompassed all agents possessing antipsychotic properties, along with extrapyramidal effects. The relatively new *atypical neuroleptics* lack these Parkinsonian effects, but still are referred to as neuroleptics.

Since the introduction of chlorpromazine in 1950, neuroleptics have become known for their efficacy in reducing the symptoms of psychosis. They also have antiemetic properties owing to their suppression of the chemoreceptor trigger zone. Promethazine is an example of an agent demonstrating H-1 antagonism, and is prescribed for its antihistaminic properties. Other indications for neuroleptic drugs have included hiccups, migraine headaches, involuntary motor disorders, autism, acute mania, and severe agitation. On occasion, children have been reported to ingest acepromazine, a commonly prescribed veterinary tranquilizer.

Between 1992 and 2001, the Toxic Exposure Surveillance System (TESS) compiled by the American Association of Poison Control Centers reported a total of 32,722 cases of pediatric and adolescent poisoning involving neuroleptic agents. Of those, 45% occurred in children under 6; the remaining 55% occurred in patients age 6 to 18. Fatal outcomes from neuroleptic poisoning

are uncommon. Between 1992 and 2001 only seven pediatric and adolescent deaths were documented in TESS reports. These cases are summarized in Table 45–1.

In a retrospective study involving 86 cases of children and adolescents ingesting phenothiazines or butyrophenones, 70% were under 6 years of age. Most ingestions occurred in the patient's or a relative's home. Depressed levels of consciousness and dystonia were the most common presenting signs. The median length of hospitalization was 2 days; there were no deaths.

DEVELOPMENTAL CONSIDERATIONS

Neonates born to mothers undergoing neuroleptic therapy during pregnancy have been reported to experience CNS depression and extrapyramidal sysmptoms (EPS). Many neuroleptics are rated Pregnancy Category C, and therefore should only be used when the potential therapeutic benefit to the mother outweighs the potential side effects on the fetus.

Breastfed infants may be exposed to phenothiazines and their metabolites excreted in breast milk. Authors of a study of infants whose mothers were treated with chlorpromazine, haloperidol, or trifluoperazine caution that it would be prudent for mothers prescribed these drugs at the upper end of the recommended dose range not to breast feed. Also, breast feeding is generally not recommended during drug treatment with the atypical neuroleptics. Phenothiazine administration has been implicated as a contributing factor in sudden infant death syndrome.

Toddlers are primarily at risk for unintentional poisoning from a family member's medication. Some atypical neuroleptics, such as risperidone, are increasingly being

Table 45–1. Seven Neuroleptic Fatalities Reported in TESS, 1992–2001

Patient Age (y)	Substance	Chronicity	Route	Reason
18	Thioridazine	Chronic	Ingestion	Adverse reaction
16	Quetiapine/valproic acid/ bupropion	Acute on Chronic	Ingestion	Intentional suicide
17	Quetiapine/fluoxetine	Acute	Ingestion	Intentional suicide
7 mo	Promethazine	Acute	Ingestion	Therapeutic error
16	Haloperidol	Chronic	Parenteral	Adverse reaction
12	Trimethobenzamide	Chronic	Other (PR)	Adverse reaction
2	Clozapine	Acute	Ingestion	Unintentional general

prescribed for children and adolescents, although these drugs have yet to be approved by the U.S. Food and Drug Administration (FDA) for this patient population. Adolescents are at risk of neuroleptic toxicity as a result of adverse reactions to therapeutic doses, intentional overdose, or drug abuse.

PHARMACOLOGY AND TOXICOKINETICS

Individual neuroleptic agents are selected for patients based on factors such as their degree of antipsychotic potency, the need for a sedating drug verses a minimally sedating drug, or the potential to cause untoward reactions. Preparations are available in liquid, tablet, capsule, and sustained-release oral formulations. Products are also available for intravenous (IV) and intramuscular (IM) use. Risperidone liquid, rapidly disintegrating olanzapine tablets, and quetiapine sachet packets may facilitate drug administration in certain circumstances.

Specific neuroleptic agents demonstrate a wide variability in oral absorption, because some agents undergo extensive first-pass hepatic metabolism. Most neuroleptics are very lipophilic, highly bound to tissue proteins, and have large volumes of distribution. Neuroleptics undergo complex hepatic metabolism yielding both active and inactive metabolites. The clearance half-life for most agents is long. Typically, there is poor correlation of dose and blood levels with clinical efficacy. After hepatic biotransformation, neuroleptics are eliminated as metabolites in the urine and feces. Therapeutic effects of some depot IM preparations can persist for weeks.

PATHOPHYSIOLOGY

It is believed that excessive dopaminergic activity in the mesolimbic area of the CNS is responsible for disorders such as schizophrenia. Dopamine receptors have been divided into six subtypes: D_1, D_{2A}, D_{2B}, D_3, D_4, and D_5. Neuroleptics have a high affinity for D_2, which is thought to account for their antipsychotic efficacy. The clinical significance of blockade of receptor sites other than D_2 is obscure. Neuroleptics also block dopamine receptors in other areas of the brain. For instance, D_2 antagonism in the mesocortical and nigrostriatal tracts in the basal ganglia results in the array of idiosyncratic movement of the EPS. NMS may represent an extreme form of EPS. Excessive D_2 antagonism in the hypothalamus results in impaired temperature regulation. In addition to their D_2 antagonism in the limbic system, the newer atypical neuroleptics also inhibit serotonin $5HT_{2A}$ and $5HT_{2C}$ receptors. These newer agents possess less affinity for D_2 receptors in the striatum, and thus cause fewer EPS.

Depending on the individual agent, neuroleptics block a variety of other receptors, including α-adrenergic,

Table 45–2. Common Typical Neuroleptics

Chemical Class	Generic Name	Proprietary Name
Phenothiazines		
Aliphatics	Chlorpromazine	Thorazine
	Promethazine	Phenergan
	Acepromazine (veterinary)	Aceprotabs
Piperazines	Prochlorperazine	Compazine
	Trifluoperazine	Stelazine
	Fluphenazine	Prolixin
	Perphenazine	Trilafon
Piperidines	Mesoridazine	Serentil
	Thioridazine	Mellaril
Butyrophenones	Droperidol	Inapsine
	Haloperidol	Haldol
Thioxanthenes	Thiothixene	Navane
Indoles	Molindone	Mobane
Dibenzoxazepines	Loxapine	Loxitane
Diphenylbutylpiperidines	Pimozide	Orap

Table 45–3. Atypical Neuroleptic Agents

Chemical Class	Generic Name	Proprietary Name
Unclassified	Aripiprazole	Abilify
Dibenzodiazepines	Clozapine	Clozaril
	Olanzapine	Zyprexa
Dibenzothiazepines	Quetiapine	Seroquel
Benzisoxazoles	Risperidone	Risperdal
Benzisothiazoyl	Ziprasidone	Geodone
3-[[(Aryloxy)alkyl]piperidinyl]	Iloperidone	Zomaril
-1,2-benzisoxazoles	(investigational)	

muscarinic, histaminic (H_1), and myocardial sodium and potassium channels. These pharmacologic actions explain the myriad of undesirable side effects during drug treatment, and much of the toxicity following intentional overdose.

Neuroleptics include broadly diverse chemical classes. These entities differ in their relative potency as D_2 antagonists, and the degree to which they cause anticholinergic, cardiovascular or EPS reactions (Tables 45–2 and 45–3).

Although they are not used as neuroleptics, trimethobenzamide (Tigan) and metoclopramide (Reglan) are commonly prescribed for pediatric patients for the treatment of nausea and vomiting. Similar to neuroleptics, they exhibit a spectrum of toxic effects including sedation, hypotension, cardiac irregularities, and EPS. Acute dystonia is especially common in children. Metoclopromide may cause NMS and may act as a methemoglobin inducer in infants.

CLINICAL FINDINGS

The clinical manifestations of neuroleptic toxicity can be broadly divided into cardiovascular, neurologic, and motor signs and symptoms. The extent to which any given complication occurs depends on the chemical class from which the drug is derived, the amount ingested, and the presence of coingestants.

Cardiovascular

α_1-Receptor blockade, along with direct myocardial depression, may cause significant hypotension following overdose. Patients may also have orthostatic hypotension owing to α-receptor antagonism while receiving therapy

at standard doses. Sinus tachycardia is the most common dysrhythmia associated with neuroleptic toxicity; however, supraventricular and ventricular tachydysrhythmias can occur. Many agents, most notably the piperidine phenothiazines and the butyrophenones, possess quinidine-like effects on the myocardium. Sodium channel blockade can result in a widened QRS complex, and potassium channel blockade can result a prolonged QTc interval. These conduction aberrations may be accompanied by prolonged PR interval and T-wave inversion. Life-threatening dysrhythmias, including polymorphic ventricular tachycardia (torsades de pointes), may be delayed up to 10 hours. Sudden death may occur. The potential for cardiac toxicity prompted the FDA in late 2001 to issue a new boxed warning mandating an electrocardiogram (ECG) prior to administration of droperidol. Olanzapine does not cause demonstrable effects on the QT interval.

Neurologic

Neuroleptic toxicity can cause varying degrees of CNS toxicity. Altered mental status can range from light sedation to coma. Respiratory depression may occur, especially in infants, or if alcohol or other sedative-hypnotics have been coingested. Neuroleptics are known to lower the seizure threshold. Seizures can occur in an overdose; they are more likely to occur with agents such as loxapine and clozapine.

Other

The anticholinergic and antihistaminic properties of neuroleptics can result in tachycardia, dry skin and mucous membranes, gastrointestinal (GI) hypomotility, and urinary retention. Mydriasis may occur; however, miosis is common, owing to α-adrenergic blockade. Examples of agents exhibiting a significant degree of anticholinergic effect are chlorpromazine, thioridazine, clozapine, and olanzapine. Excessive sialorrhea is noted in clozapine intoxication. Neuroleptic agents also can alter the body's temperature regulation. Hypothalamic dysfunction may induce hypothermia or hyperthermia, which is exacerbated by anticholinergic symptomatology.

Clozapine is well known for its potential to precipitate clinically significant agranulocytosis during chronic therapy and following acute overdose. The Clozaril National Registry reported 1800 patients with a white blood cell count of <2000/mm³ out of 170,000 patients exposed to clozapine. Nineteen patients died as result of agranulocytosis.

Movement Disorders

Perhaps the most distressing adverse reactions experienced by patients treated with neuroleptics are the movement disorders, commonly grouped together as EPS. EPS may occur after overdose or may be observed during chronic drug therapy. The most recognized EPS are acute dystonias, akathisia, Parkinson bradykinesia, and tardive dyskinesia. EPS are more likely to occur with neuroleptics that have high affinity for dopamine receptors in the nigrostriatum but that have minimal anticholinergic activity. Examples of these are the piperazine phenothiazines and the butyrophenones. The newer atypical neuroleptics demonstrate lower incidences of EPS. In one study, 50% of patients with neuroleptic-treated childhood-onset schizophrenia were noted to have withdrawal dyskinesia or tardive dyskinesia. The majority of these abnormal movements were not severe and generally improved over time. Table 45–4 characterizes the four EPS and management strategies.

Neuroleptic Malignant Syndrome

NMS is a rare but potentially life-threatening idiosyncratic reaction with an estimated incidence of 0.02% to 3.2% of treated patients. The overall fatality rate was 11% in one case series of 115 adolescent and adult patients. NMS may occur during chronic drug therapy, especially with high initial doses and rapidly escalating dosages. It also may occur following discontinuation of Parkinson agents or dopaminergic agonists such as L-dopa. It is more commonly associated with neuroleptics with high D$_2$ receptor antagonism. The newer atypical neuroleptics, with a lower affinity for D$_2$ receptors, have a lower potential for precipitating NMS.

The exact incidence of NMS in children is unclear. One review of the literature between 1966 and 1998 revealed 77 cases of NMS in patients ranging from 11 months to 18 years of age. In seven pediatric and young adult cases of NMS, haloperidol alone or in combination with other dopamine antagonists was noted to be a causative agent in 6 of the patients. All patients recovered following intensive supportive care. Risk factors for the development of NMS include prior episodes of NMS, agitation, dehydration, high doses of neuroleptic medication, rapid increase in dosage, and IM administration. Patients with NMS present with a constellation of clinical manifestations including features from each of the following symptom groups:

- *Temperature dysregulation:* fever, which may be life threatening.
- *Altered mental status:* agitation, confusion and delirium, which may be insidious in onset, and ultimately lead to lethargy, obtundation, and coma.
- *Autonomic instability:* fluctuating vital signs, including tachycardia and hypotension or hypertension.
- *Musculoskeletal:* generalized "lead pipe" rigidity, myoclonus, and tremors.
- *Other:* diaphoresis, dehydration, tachypnea, respiratory failure, rhabdomyolysis, and renal failure.

NMS is a diagnosis of exclusion. Important clues are a recent increase in neuroleptic dose or addition of other dopamine antagonists. The toxicologic differential diagnosis includes the serotonin syndrome, monoamine oxidase inhibitor toxicity or interactions with contraindicated foods or medications, and toxicity from anticholinergics or antihistamines. Other possibilities are lithium overdose, sedative-hypnotic or alcohol withdrawal, toxicity from a sympathomimetic such as ecstasy or cocaine, and hallucinogen abuse. The documented causes of death from NMS are cardiorespiratory arrest, pneumonia, pulmonary embolism, sepsis, disseminated intravascular coagulation, profound hyperthermia, or hepatorenal failure.

LABORATORY AND DIAGNOSTIC TESTS

Blood levels for specific neuroleptic agents are not readily available and generally correlate poorly with therapeutic effects or toxicity. Therapy is best guided by the clinical status of the patient.

Some phenothiazines may appear radiopaque on an abdominal radiograph if it is obtained soon after ingestion; however, this is neither sensitive nor specific for

Table 45–4. Neuroleptic-Induced EPS

EPS	Onset	Characteristic Manifestations	Management
Acute dystonia	1–5 d	Oculogyric crisis; torticollis; retrocollis; tortipelvis; jaw, tongue, lip and throat spasms; trismus opisthotonos; facial grimacing; potentially fatal laryngeal dystonia; rare hyperthermia. *Risk factors:* Young age, male gender, high-potency agent, primary psychotic disorder and previous dystonic reaction.	Anticholinergic, benzodiazepines
Akathisia	5–60 d	Irresistible urge to move, restlessness (unable to sit still); repetitive, purposeless movements; may be mistaken for worsening psychosis or agitation. Severity increases with age, usually noted when dose of neuroleptic is increased. Estimated to occur in as many as 75% of patients receiving typical agents.	Reduce neuroleptic dose, switch to lower-potency agent, anticholinergic, benzodiazepines, propranolol (adult dose 20–100 mg/d)
Parkinsonism bradykinesia	5–30 d	Shuffling gait; resting tremor; cog-wheel rigidity; masked facies; rabbit syndrome (perioral tremor); sialorrhea. Most common of the EPS. Affects primarily elderly women.	Reduce neuroleptic dose, anticholinergics
TD/WD	*TD:* Months to years *WD:* D/C drug	Involuntary buccolinguomasticatory movements (persistent lip smacking, rhythmic tongue, and chewing movements) and choreoathetoid movements. Most serious of the EPS. Incidence of TD in children 6%; WD 14%. Less common with atypical neuroleptics. Truncal movements are more common in young adults. Greater risk of TD associated with depot IM agents. Usually noted following reduction of neuroleptic dosage. TD may be permanent or show minimal improvement. Anticholinergics may facilitate the development of TD. TD may be prevented by using low-potency or atypical neuroleptics.	Treatment of TD is often unsatisfactory. Options include discontinuation of causative agent, replacement with another neuroleptic, increase neuroleptic dose, administer cholinergic agent (e.g., choline, lecithin, donepezil), vitamin E, reserpine, calcium channel blockers. WD generally requires no therapy and remits spontaneously.

Abbreviations: EPS, extrapyramidal symptoms; IM, intramuscular; TD, tardive dyskinesia; WD, withdrawal dyskinesia.

313

neuroleptic ingestion and does not modify patient management.

Some phenothiazines may visibly darken the urine. Although rarely performed, some colorimetric tests using ferric chloride reagent or Phenistix may qualitatively detect phenothiazines in the urine. Phenothiazines have been reported to trigger a positive response for tricyclic antidepressants by various qualitative assays.

An ECG is indicated to exclude QRS widening and a prolonged Q–Tc interval. If the patient is obtunded or comatose, pulse oximetry and/or arterial blood gases will help assess the level of respiratory depression. Creatine kinase assays should be performed to rule out rhabdomyolysis in patients experiencing prolonged coma, seizures, severe EPS, hyperthermia, or NMS. Monitor urine for myoglobin. In patients with suspected NMS, monitor electrolytes and liver function tests (LFTs).

Patients with olanzapine overdose should have LFTs ordered to screen for evidence of hepatotoxicity. Monitor serum sodium and potassium in patients intoxicated with risperidone to rule out hyponatremia and hypokalemia. Obtain a baseline leukocyte count with differential for any patient with a history of acute or chronic overdose of clozapine. Follow-up with leukocyte and granulocyte counts once or twice weekly for several weeks.

MANAGEMENT

Although fatalities in pediatric and adolescent patients resulting from neuroleptic poisonings are rare, prompt symptomatic and supportive care is necessary. All patients evaluated in the ED require close monitoring of vital signs, oxygen saturation, and cardiac rhythm. Ventilatory support may be necessary in those patients experiencing marked CNS or respiratory depression. There is no specific antidote for neuroleptic agents. Hyperthermic patients are aggressively cooled, and hypothermic patients are warmed.

Gastrointestinal Decontamination

Ipecac-induced emesis should never be initiated in the prehospital or hospital setting because the onset of CNS depression, dystonia, or seizures places the patient at risk of aspiration pneumonia. Most patients presenting to the ED can be administered aqueous activated charcoal. Oro-gastric lavage is rarely necessary and should be reserved for patients who have ingested life-threatening amounts of medications and present within 1 hour of ingestion.

Hypotension

Most cases of hypotension respond to administration of isotonic fluids. For refractory hypotension, vasopressors may be necessary. In theory, mixed α-/β-adrenergic agents such as dopamine and epinephrine may worsen hypotension owing to unopposed β vasodilation; however, convincing evidence is lacking. A pure α-agonist such as norepinephrine or phenylephrine may be preferred for agents with high α$_1$-blockade, such as chlorpromazine or thioridazine.

Cardiac Toxicity

Cardiac toxicity manifested by a widened QRS complex (greater than 100 msec) is treated by alkalinizing the serum with sodium bicarbonate; the goal is a pH of 7.45 to 7.55. Excessive alkalemia should be avoided. Ventricular tachydysrhythmias may be managed with lidocaine, cardioversion, or defibrillation. All class 1A and 1C antidysrhythmic agents are contraindicated. The use of amiordarone in the setting of neuroleptic-induced cardiac dysrhythmias has not been studied. Torsades de pointes may respond to magnesium sulfate, isoproterenol, or overdrive pacing. Hypokalemia, hypomagnesemia, or hypocalcemia are corrected.

Seizures can be managed with standard anticonvulsant drugs such as the benzodiazepines lorazepam, or diazepam and phenobarbital. Although physostigmine salicylate may reverse central and peripheral signs and symptoms of neuroleptic-induced anticholinergic toxicity, this antidote should be avoided because these symptoms are rarely life threatening and it may aggravate cardiac conduction abnormalities.

Enhanced Drug Elimination

Neuroleptics are highly bound to tissue proteins and possess large volumes of distribution. Therefore, techniques to increase total body clearance, such as multiple-dose activated charcoal or extracorporeal removal methods such as hemodialysis or charcoal hemoperfusion, are not effective.

Acute Dystonic Reactions

Acute dystonic reactions may be effectively treated with an anticholinergic medication such as diphenhydramine or benztropine. The initial dose may be given IM or IV; the IV route is preferable if there is any sign of airway

Table 45–5. Anticholinergic/Antiparkinson Medication Therapy for EPS

Agent	Pediatric Dose	Adult Dose
Diphenhydramine HCl (Benadryl)	PO, IM, or IV (over 2 min) 1.25 mg/kg/dose (37.5 mg/m^2) q6h; max daily dose 300 mg	PO, IM, or IV (over 2 min) 25–50 mg q4h; max dose 100 mg; max daily dose 400 mg
Benztropine mesylate (Cogentin)	PO, IM, or IV Children >3 y. 0.02–0.05 mg/kg/dose 1–2 times daily Use in children <3 y is reserved for life-threatening emergencies.	IM or IV: 1–2 mg for acute dystonia IM or PO: 1–4 mg/dose 1–2 times daily Max daily dose 6 mg
Trihexyphenidyl HCl (Artane)	No established pediatric dose.	PO: 5–15 mg/d in 3–4 divided doses

Abbreviations: EPS, extrapyramidal symptoms; IM, intramuscularly; IV, intravenously; max, maximum; PO, orally.

compromise. If concomitant significant anticholinergic findings are present, such as fever and dry skin and mucous membranes, a benzodiazepine is preferred. After initial resolution is achieved the patient should be prescribed an oral preparation for 2 to 3 days to prevent reoccurrence of dystonia symptoms. Table 45–5 summarizes anticholinergic/antiparkinsonian medication regimens used in the management of neuroleptic-induced extrapyramidal symptoms.

Neuroleptic Malignant Syndrome

Once the diagnosis of NMS has been established, intensive supportive measures are instituted promptly. The offending neuroleptic agent is immediately discontinued. Hyperthermic patients are rapidly cooled using standard measures. Antipyretic agents are ineffective. Anticholinergic agents, which impair heat dissipation, are avoided. Dehydration is corrected with IV crystalloid; large volumes may be required. Benzodiazepines are administered in sufficient doses to control agitation and achieve muscle relaxation, which helps prevent heat generation. Patients with severe muscle rigidity may require paralysis and mechanical ventilation. Nondepolarizing neuromuscular blocking agents should be utilized; succinylcholine is to be avoided.

Bromocriptine mesylate (Parlodel), a central dopamine agonist, has been used in NMS, but supporting evidence is anecdotal. Onset of symptom improvement may be delayed 1 to several days. The adult dose is 5 mg three

times daily orally; this may be increased to a maximum of 20 mg four times daily. Therapy is continued for 10 days. The efficacy and safety of bromocriptine in children under 15 years of age have not been established. Endocrinology references report the use of bromocriptine for prolactin-secreting tumors in children and adolescents in oral doses of 2.5 to 20 mg/d.

Dantrolene sodium (Dantrium; see Chapter 22) has been used for NMS, but supporting evidence has been anecdotal. Dantrolene relieves muscle rigidity by acting in the muscle sarcoplasmic reticulum to inhibit the release of calcium. Dantrolene should not be considered as first-line therapy for NMS because this condition is caused by biochemical derangements in the CNS, rather than at the motor end plate as in malignant hyperthermia. The IV loading dose is 1 to 2 mg/kg to a maximum of 10 mg/kg. IV maintenance dose is 2.5 mg/kg every 6 hours. An alternative oral dose is 1 mg/kg q12h up to 50 mg/dose.

The usual course of therapy of NMS ranges from 5 to 10 days. Neuroleptic drug therapy should be discontinued for 1 to 2 weeks after complete resolution of NMS. At that time, another agent with fewer EPS such as a newer atypical neuroleptic may be initiated.

DISPOSITION

Despite the low incidence of fatalities with neuroleptics, significant effects can result from inadvertent exposure and overdoses. However, clinical effects experienced by

Table 45–6. Case Report/Case Series

Drug	Outcomes
Typical Neuroleptics	
Chlorpromazine	Deaths have been reported in children with ingestions of 20–74 mg/kg. A 350-mg dose was reported to be fatal in a 4-year-old child.
Haloperidol	Two children experienced acute dystonic reactions, changes in mental status, and other EPS after ingestions of 0.26 mg/kg and 0.1 mg/kg over 24 hours.
Promethazine	A 2-year-old boy died after ingesting 200 mg of promethazine. A 5-year-old child who ingested 500 mg and a 6-year-old child who ingested 600 mg both experienced significant neurologic toxicity with recovery.
Atypical Neuroleptics	
Aripiprazole	During clinical trials, one case of an 18-month-old child ingesting 15 mg of aripiprazole and 2 mg of Ativan was reported to be uneventful.
Clozapine	Case reports of as little as 50 mg in children, ranging in age from 21 months to 4 years, have resulted in CNS depression, ataxia, and tachycardia. Death was reported in a 15 year old following an intentional overdose of an unknown amount of clozapine.
Olanzapine	Case reports of 10- to 100-mg ingestions in children have resulted in agitation, CNS depression, EPS, and hypersalivation. A 15 year old required intubation following ingestion of 115 mg of olanzapine along with carbamazepine. In one report, onset of symptoms did not occur until 10 hours postingestion.
Quetiapine	A single case report of a 1300-mg ingestion in an 11 year old resulted only in mental status changes.
Risperidone	Several published series and case reports of pediatric risperidone ingestions, in doses ranging from 1–110 mg, revealed somnolence, agitation, hypotension, tachycardia, and EPS to be the most common symptoms of overdose.
Ziprasidone	During premarketing trials, there were 10 accidental or intentional poisonings, with the highest dose reported as 3240 mg. That patient only experienced mild sedation, slurred speech, and transient hypertension.

Abbreviations: CNS, central nervous system; EPS, extrapyramidal symptoms.

any given patient do not correlate well with specific ingested amounts. All symptomatic patients, intentional overdoses, and ingestions of indeterminate amounts should be transported to the nearest ED as quickly as possible.

Patients who remain asymptomatic for a minimum of 6 hours may be discharged. All symptomatic patients should be admitted with continuous cardiac monitoring. Pediatric patients exhibiting acute dystonic reactions without other evidence of toxicity may be discharged with a 2- to 3-day supply of oral diphenhydramine. Table 45–6 provides some outcomes reported for pediatric/adolescent exposure to typical and atypical neuroleptics.

CASE OUTCOME

An acute dystonic reaction is suspected and a trial of IM diphenhydramine HCl, 1.25 mg/kg, is ordered. A family member is dispatched to retrieve all medications at the residence. Within 30 minutes of administration of IM diphenhydramine, all of the patient's symptoms resolve. All laboratories were reported in the normal range. A family member returns with a variety of medications, one of which was haloperidol 1 mg tablets. They belonged to a visiting grandparent with a history of dementia who admitted to "dropping a few" that morning. A 12 lead ECG was obtained that revealed a normal sinus rhythm with narrow complexes. The child was observed in the ED with no other evidence of neuroleptic toxicity and was discharged. A bottle of diphenhydramine liquid, 12.5 mg/5 mL, was dispensed with instructions to give 11/2 teaspoons four times a day for 3 days.

SUGGESTED READINGS

Andersson C, Chakos M, Mailman R, et al: Emerging roles for novel antipsychotic medications in the treatment of schizophrenia. *Schizophrenia* 21:151, 1998.

Baldessarini RJ, Tarazi FI: Psychosis and mania. In: Hardman JG, Hardman JG, Limbird LE, et al, eds: *Goodman and Gilman's The Pharmacological Basis of Therapeutics.* 10th ed. New York: McGraw-Hill; 2001:485.

Carbone JR: The neuroleptic malignant and serotonin syndromes. *Emerg Med Clin North Am* 18:317, 2000.

Caroff SN, Campbell EC, Havey J, et al: Treatment of tardive dyskinesia with donepezil: A pilot study. *Clin Psychiatry* 62:772–775, 2001.

Catalano G, Catalano MC, Nunez CY, et al: Atypical antipsychotic overdose in the pediatric population. *J Child Adolesc Psychopharmacol* 11:425, 2001.

Dyer KS, Woolf AD: Use of phenothiazines as sedatives in children: What are the risks? *Drug Safety* 21:81, 1999.

Ereshefsky L: Pharmacokinetics and drug interactions: Update of new antipsychotics. *J Clin Psychiatry* 57:12, 1996.

James LP, Abel K, Wilkinson J, et al: Phenothiazine, butyrophenone, and other psychotropic medication poisonings in children and adolescents. *Clin Toxicol* 38:615, 2000.

Kelleher JP, Centorrino F, Alber MJ, et al: Advances in atypical antipsychotics for the treatment of schizophrenia. *CNS Drugs* 16:249, 2002.

Kumra S, Jacobsen LK, Lenae M, et al: Case series: Spectrum of neuroleptic-induced movement disorders and extrapyramidal side effects in childhood-onset schizophrenia. *J Am Acad Child Adolesc Psychiatry* 37:221, 1998.

LoVecchio F, Lewin NA: Antipsychotics. In Goldfrank L, Flomenbaum N, Lewin N, et al, eds: *Goldfrank's Toxicologic Emergencies.* 7th ed. New York: McGraw-Hill; 2002:875.

McDermid SA, Hood J, Bockus S, et al: Adolescents on neuroleptic medications: Is this population at risk for tardive dyskinesia? *Canadian J Psychiatry* 43:629, 1998.

Joshi PT, Capozzoli JA, Coyle JT: Neuroleptic malignant syndrome: Life-threatening complication of neuroleptic treatment in adolescents with affective disorder. *Pediatrics* 87:235, 1991.

Rodnitzky RL: Drug-induced movement disorders in children. *Semin Pediatr Neurol* 10:80, 2003.

Susman VL: Clinical management of neuroleptic malignant syndrome. *Psychiatric Q* 72:325, 2001.

Taketomo CK, Hodding JH, Kraus DM, eds: *Pediatric Dosage Handbook: Including Neonatal Dosing, Drug Administration & Extemporaneous Preparations.* 9th ed. Hudson, OH: Lexi-Comp; 2002.

Tenenbein M: The neuroleptic malignant syndrome: Occurrence in a 15-year-old boy and recovery with bromocriptine therapy. *Pediatr Neurosci* 12:161, 1985–1986.

Toren P, Laor N, Weizmen A: Use of atypical neuroleptics in child and adolescent psychiatry. *J Clin Psychiatry* 59:644, 1998.

Ty EB, Rothner AD: Neuroleptic malignant syndrome in children and adolescents. *J Child Neurol* 16:157, 2001.

Welch R, Chue P: Antipsychotic agents and QT changes. *J Psychiatry Neurosci* 25:154, 2000.

Yoshida K, Smith B, Craggs M, et al: Neuroleptic drugs in breast milk: A study of pharmacokinetics and of possible adverse effects in breast-fed infants. *Psych Med* 28:81, 1998.

46

Household Poisons

Matthew D. Sztajnkrycer

HIGH-YIELD FACTS

- Most household products either have low intrinsic toxicity or are packaged in amounts or concentrations that are nontoxic at doses commonly ingested by children.

- Three hazard levels exist for identified substances, each with a specific signal word. *Danger* is used for substances which are either extremely flammable, corrosive, or highly toxic. *Warning* is used for substances that are moderately toxic, and *caution* applies to substances that are slightly toxic. *Poison* is also used for substances determined to be highly toxic.

- The Poison Prevention Packaging Act of 1970 requires regulated substances to be packaged in child-resistant containers. This packaging must prevent rapid access to substances by individuals under 5 years of age, while not interfering with the ability of normal adults to access the contents.

- The majority of exposures in toddlers are unintentional, nonsuicidal events, occurring as a result of developmental exploration of the environment. Children may be attracted to the color or appearance of the agent, incorrectly identifying it as candy or a beverage.

- Adolescent exposure patterns differ from preschool-aged children, and appear more similar to adult patterns. These exposures may reflect deliberate misuse of a substance, such as abuse of volatile hydrocarbons, or the increased frequency of suicide attempts in this group.

- The five most common categories of household poisons ingested by children over the past 5 years are cosmetics, household cleaning agents, pesticides, arts and crafts supplies, and hydrocarbons. Household cleaning agents typically are either caustic or alcohol containing.

- The most common household products causing pediatric fatalities are hydrocarbons, household cleaning agents, cosmetics, pesticides, and alcohols.

Household products are a diverse group of nonpharmaceutical substances commonly found and utilized during routine activities around the home (Table 46–1). These agents include adhesives and glues, alcohols, automotive products, hydrocarbons, pesticides, and household cleaning agents.

Most of these products either have low intrinsic toxicity or are packaged in amounts or concentrations that are nontoxic at doses commonly ingested by children. Examples of substances considered nontoxic include air fresheners, antiperspirants, charcoal, cosmetics, and sunscreen products. These products may still be hazardous to children, even if they are nontoxic. For example, ingestion of nontoxic cat litter has resulted in aspiration, asphyxiation, and death.

Certain classes of products may be toxic even in small doses, especially to small children. The Federal Hazardous

Table 46–1. Common Household Poison Categories and Representative Products

Adhesives	Deodorizers
Cyanoacrylates	Air fresheners
Epoxy	Toilet bowl deodorizers
Alcohols	**Dyes**
Isopropanol	Fabric
Methanol	Food
Rubbing alcohol	
Arts and crafts supplies	**Hydrocarbons**
Chalk	Benzene
Clay	Gasoline
Crayons	Halogenated hydrocarbons
Glazes	Kerosene
Inks	Lighter fluid
Paints	Toluene or xylene
Typewriter correction fluid	Turpentine
Automotive products	**Paints**
Ethylene glycol	Oil based
Hydrocarbons	Stains
Methanol	Stripping agents
	Varnishes
	Water based
	Wood preservatives
Cleaning products	**Pesticides**
Automatic dishwasher detergents	Fungicides
Bleaches	Herbicides
Carpet and upholstery cleaners	Insecticides
Disinfectants	Moth repellants
Drain cleaners	Rodenticides
Fabric softeners	
Glass cleaners	
Laundry detergents	
Oven cleaners	
Rust removers	
Toilet bowl cleaners	
Wall/floor/tile cleaners	
Cosmetics	**Miscellaneous**
Creams and lotions	Bubble blowing solutions
Dental care products	Charcoal
Deodorants	Desiccants
Eye products	Holiday ornaments
Hair care products	Thermometers
Mouthwash	
Nail care products	
Perfumes	
Suntan products	

Substances Act of 1960 (FHSA), administered by the U.S. Consumer Products Safety Commission, requires that certain household products, defined as *hazardous substances*, be labeled to warn consumers about potential hazards. Hazardous substances are defined under the act as

> **any product that is toxic, corrosive, flammable or combustible, an irritant, a strong sensitizer, or that generates pressure through decomposition, or if the product may cause substantial personal injury or substantial illness during or as a proximate result of any customary or reasonable foreseeable handling or use, including reasonable foreseeable ingestion by children.**

The FHSA does not apply to pesticides foods, drugs, and cosmetics regulated under their respective acts, to substances intended for use as fuels when stored in appropriate containers, or to tobacco products.

Three hazard levels exist for identified substances, each with a specific signal word. *Danger* is used for substances that are either extremely flammable, corrosive, or highly toxic. *Warning* is used for substances that are moderately toxic, and *caution* applies to substances that are slightly toxic. *Poison* is also used for substances determined to be highly toxic.

The Poison Prevention Packaging Act of 1970 requires substances regulated under the FHSA to be packaged in child-resistant containers. This packaging must prevent rapid access to substances by individuals under 5 years of age, while not interfering with the ability of normal adults to access the contents. Since the PPPA, there has been a remarkable decline in pediatric poisoning deaths from toxic household products, including medications.

EPIDEMIOLOGY

According to 2001 data from the American Association of Poison Control Centers (AAPCC), 90% of all exposures occurred in a residential setting, with another 1.6% occurring at school and 2.4% occurring in the workplace. Although pharmaceutical products accounted for 47% of exposures, 36% of all calls to poison control centers involved household products.

Children, defined as victims less than 20 years old, were the subject of 73% of calls involving household products, with children aged 5 years or less accounting for 84% of pediatric exposures. Household products are the most frequently implicated exposure in children.

In 1998, only 8.5% of cases involving children 5 years of age or younger required evaluation and treatment at a health care facility (Table 46–2). In nearly one third of cases, no symptoms were observed following exposure. This reflects both the nontoxic nature of many household products, as well as differences between perceived exposure and actual ingestion, inhalation, or dermal absorption. Moderate toxicity occurred in 0.7%. Severe toxicity and death occurred at a rate of 0.04% and 0.001% respectively (Table 46–2).

Deaths related to household products over the past 5 years are listed in Table 46–3. A total of 33 deaths involving household products were reported to the AAPCC for patients 5 years or younger. All but one case involved a single agent. That case, a 12-month-old exposed to isopropanol and boric acid-containing roach powder, was deemed malicious in nature.

DEVELOPMENTAL CONSIDERATIONS

Children are exposed to potential toxins more than any other age group, with the incidence of both peak poisoning and hospitalization occurring between 1 and 3 years of age. The majority of exposures in toddlers are unintentional, nonsuicidal events, occurring as a result of developmental exploration of the environment. Children may be attracted to the color or appearance of the agent, incorrectly identifying it as candy or a beverage. Younger children are more accepting and more willing to taste

disgusting or dangerous substances than older children. Videotape analysis of exploration behaviors by toddlers has noted an average hand–mouth frequency rate of 9.5 contacts per hour. The amount of agents to which children are exposed is typically small, in contrast to larger exposures associated with deliberate ingestion.

Substances ingested by preschool-aged children are typically nontoxic. In 2001, cosmetics and personal care products accounted for only 4.7% of adult exposures, yet were the leading category of exposure in children less than 6 years of age, accounting for 13.2% of all reported exposures. In half of all accidental poisonings, the product was either in use or had recently been moved from the previous typical storage site.

Adolescent exposure patterns differ from preschool-aged children, and appear more similar to adult patterns. Only 50% of exposures in the adolescent age group are accidental; 46% are intentional. These exposures may reflect deliberate misuse of a substance, such as abuse of volatile hydrocarbons, or the increased frequency of suicide attempts in this group.

MOST COMMON TOXINS

The five most common categories of household poisons ingested by children over the past 5 years are cosmetics, household cleaning agents, pesticides, arts and crafts

Table 46–2. Pediatric (Age ≤5) Household Poison Exposures, 1998: Evaluation by HCF and Outcome

Category	Total	Seen in HCF	No Effect	Moderate Effect	Major Effect	Death
Adhesives	8,701	980	2,345	75	3	0
Alcohols	13,719	1,433	5,865	50	4	1[a]
Art and craft supplies	29,898	572	6,955	23	0	0
Automotive supplies	4,478	1,145	2,216	64	6	0
Batteries	3,771	1,138	1,501	63	9	0
Cleaning agents	126,602	12,131	42,962	1,325	55	0
Cosmetics	157,550	7,013	49,582	687	28	1
Deodorizers	15,467	867	5,077	58	1	0
Dyes	2,178	85	693	2	0	0
Fertilizers	7,377	191	2,347	10	2	0
Hydrocarbons	26,018	5,059	10,318	755	71	4
Paints	13,571	819	3,811	43	4	0
Pesticides	53,199	9,885	21,446	301	38	1[a]
Polishes	5,901	461	2,630	40	2	0
Miscellaneous products	42,119	1,493	9,054	27	0	0

[a] Single patient with exposure to two agents; see text for details.
Abbreviation: HCF, health care facility.

supplies, and hydrocarbons (Table 46–4). Household cleaning agents typically are either caustic in nature or contain alcohols.

The initial approach to the symptomatic patient involves supportive care and correct product identification. Most significant cosmetic ingestions involve alcohols, caustic agents, or hydrocarbons. Several household poisons deserve specific attention, and are discussed below.

Cosmetics

Cosmetics include creams and lotions, dental care products, deodorants, hair care products, mouthwash, and nail

Table 46–3. Pediatric (Age ≤5) Fatalities Related to Household Product Exposure, 1997–2001

Category	Substance	Child's Age
Alcohols	Isopropanol	12 mo
	Methanol	2 d
	Methanol	3 mo
Batteries	AA battery	2 mo
Cleaning Substances	Cleaner	8 mo
	Cleaner in water	11 mo
	Condensed coil cleaner (HF/HCl)	18 mo
	Degreaser (HCl, ABF)	12 mo
	Drain opener (H_2SO_4)	3 y
	Pine oil cleaner	12 mo
	Tire cleaner (HF or ABF)	18 mo
	Wheel cleaner (ABF)	3 y
Cosmetics	Baby oil	15 mo
	Hair oil (safflower/mineral oil)	12 mo
	Hair oil (isoparafin/butyl ether)	9 mo
	Mouthwash (ethanol)	4 y
	Nail polish remover (acetone)	4 y
Deodorizers	Air freshener (propylene glycol, ethoxylate)	5 y
Hydrocarbons	Chlorodifluoromethane	4 y
	Gasoline	19 mo
	Kerosine	12 mo
	Lamp oil	12 mo
	Lamp oil	14 mo
	Lighter fluid	3 mo
	Lighter fluid	15 mo
	Lighter fluid	2 y
	Motor oil	15 mo
	Paint thinner (mineral spirits)	11 mo
Pesticides	Aluminum phosphide	16 mo
	Aluminum phosphide	5 y
	Endosulfan	2 y
	Paraquat	18 mo
	Roach powder (boric acid)	12 mo
Miscellaneous	Cat litter	4 y

Abbreviations: HF, hydrofluoric acid; HCl, hydrochloric acid; ABF, ammonium bifluoride; H_2SO_4, sulfuric acid.

Table 46–4. Pediatric (Age <19) Household Product Exposures per 100,000 Poison Control Center Contacts, 1997–2001

Category	Exposures
Adhesives	383.9
Alcohols	600.4
Art and craft supplies	1366.3
Automotive supplies	193.8
Batteries	170.2
Cleaning agents	5500.9
Cosmetics	6897.8
Deodorizers	674.4
Dyes	98.4
Fertilizers	323.8
Hydrocarbons	1106.1
Paints	586.6
Pesticides	2244.7
Polishes	258.2
Miscellaneous	2023.7

care products (see Table 46–1). These agents are regulated by the Food and Drug Administration, under the Food, Drug and Cosmetic Act of 1919, amended 1997. All agents classified as cosmetics must be nonpoisonous when used according to labeling information. Cosmetics must also conform to the packaging requirements of the PPPA.

Hair Care Products

Hair care products include hair colorants, hair lighteners, hair waving agents, and hair straighteners. Permanent hair colorants require that the dye, typically para-phenylenediamine, be oxidized to a reactive amine intermediate. Additional couplers convert the reactive amine intermediate to an indo dye, which maintains the dye within the hair follicles. The most common oxidizing agent is hydrogen peroxide, typically at a concentration of 6%, but on occasion up to 12%. Semipermanent and temporary hair colorants do not utilize an oxidizing agent, and are less noxious.

Hair bleaches contain 20% to 30% hydrogen peroxide. Additionally, these agents may contain ammonia or sodium persulfate. The pH of these solutions may range between 9.5 and 11.5. Significant accidental exposures are rare owing to the noxious taste and odor associated with these agents.

Hair waving agents consist of a thioglycolate compound and a neutralizing compound. Most noncommer-

cial products use a cold permanent process, involving the chemical ammonium thioglycolate. Waving involves first softening the hair, followed by shaping to the desired appearance, and hardening. Thioglycolates soften the hair by reducing cysteine cross-links in keratin, while neutralizing compounds, typically weak acids and neutralizing agents, reoxidize the cysteine bonds, hardening the reshaped hair. Thioglycolic acids are moderately toxic caustic agents. Bromate-containing neutralizers are especially toxic, and ingestions have resulted in ototoxicity and death, typically from acute renal failure. Ingestion of 5 to 10 cc (1.5 to 3.0 g) of bromate-containing neutralizing agents causes severe toxicity in toddlers.

Hair straighteners are extremely toxic, owing to the alkaline nature of the products (pH 13) and ingestions should be treated as alkaline caustic exposures.

Dental Care Products

Concentrated mouthwashes contain up to 70% ethyl alcohol. Nonconcentrated formulations contain 10% to 25% ethyl alcohol. Alcohol is a CNS depressant, causing altered mental status ranging from emotional lability to coma. Ethanol induced changes in NADH/NAD ratios may cause hypoglycemia, especially in young children.

Fluoride is a general cellular toxin that alters calcium and potassium homeostasis, and affects intracellular enzymatic processes. After ingestion, fluoride interacts with gastric acid to produce hydrofluoric acid, with caustic gastrointestinal (GI) effects. With severe poisoning, hypocalcemia and hyperkalemia may result in cardiac dysrhythmias, respiratory failure and death. GI symptoms occur with ingestion of 3 to 5 mg/kg fluoride, toxicity with 5 to 10 mg/kg fluoride, and death after 16 mg/kg fluoride.

Fluoride-containing toothpaste typically contains sodium monofluorophosphate 0.76%, stannous fluoride 0.4%, or sodium fluoride 0.24%. Accidental pediatric ingestion is typically not associated with significant toxicity, especially if the amount ingested is less than 5 mg/kg. Fluoride-containing toothpaste typically contains 1 mg of fluoride ion per gram, or 28.35 mg per ounce. The maximum amount of fluoride allowed per tube of toothpaste is 260 mg. Children who ingest less than 8 mg/kg fluoride can be given milk and observed at home.

MOST DANGEROUS TOXINS

From 1997 to 2001, 33 deaths related to household products were reported to poison centers. The most common products causing pediatric fatalities were hydrocarbons, household cleaning agents, cosmetics, pesticides, and alcohols (see Table 46–3). Deaths due to cosmetics were from hydrocarbon aspiration or toxic effects of alcohols. Lighter fluid and lamp oil accounted for half of all reported hydrocarbon deaths. Ingestion of traditionally nontoxic agents, including a dry cell battery and cat litter, accounted for two deaths. A propylene glycol/ethoxylate-containing air freshener was responsible for one death.

Ammonium Bifluoride

Hydrofluoric acid or ammonium bifluoride-containing products accounts for half of the household cleaning agent deaths reported over 5 years. As with fluoride-containing toothpaste, ammonium bifluoride reacts with gastric acid to release hydrogen fluoride and fluoride ions. Unlike toothpastes, the concentration of fluoride ions available in ammonium bifluoride-containing products is substantial. Approximately 66.6% of ammonium bifluoride is fluoride ion. One ounce (30 cc) of a 1% solution of ammonium bifluoride contains approximately 200 mg fluoride ion. In a 10-kg toddler, ingestion of one ounce of 1% ammonium bifluoride represents a potentially lethal 20 mg/kg fluoride ion ingestion. Prior to 1997, aluminum wheel cleaners contained as much as 10% ammonium bifluoride and 30% to 50% ammonium fluoride.

Nail Care Products

Nail polish removers typically contain acetone or ethanol. Artificial nail removers are of more concern, historically, because they contain acetonitrile. Acetonitrile is metabolized through hepatic cytochrome P450 systems to an intermediate cyanohydrin, which is metabolized to cyanide and aldehydes. Toxicity is similar to cyanide poisoning, but is delayed 3 to 24 hours owing to the metabolic conversion of the parent compound to the toxic metabolite. Delayed toxicity provides the opportunity to intervene with specific antidotal therapy, but also may lead to misdiagnosis of toxicity.

Unintentional pediatric poisoning and death due to acetonitrile-containing products was first reported in 1988. Since 1992 artificial nail remover products have shifted away from acetonitrile. Many of these products contain either acetone, γ-butyrolactone (GBL), or a combination of both. Acetone, an aliphatic ketone, has a distinctive odor and is a strong mucous membrane irritant. Toxicity is most commonly associated with CNS depression, although hemorrhagic gastritis, tachycardia, and

hypotension have been reported. Urinary ketones are a typical finding. GBL, an industrial solvent, is a precursor of γ-hydroxybutyrate, a γ-aminobutyric acid analog associated with CNS depression. Concentrations of GBL may range from 4.75% to 100%, and acetone concentrations may range from 81.2% to 100.0%.

Ethylene Glycol Monobutyl Ether

An ingredient of many glass cleaners, ethylene glycol monobutyl ether (EGBE) is a common accidental pediatric ingestion. Animal studies have suggested that the toxicity of EGBE is equivalent to or greater than ethylene glycol. Older product formulations, especially those marketed as *concentrated*, contained as much as 25% EGBE, often with isopropyl alcohol added as an antistreaking agent. Current products designed for household use contain much lower concentrations of both EGBE (1% to 3%) and isopropyl alcohol (3% to 6%).

Intentional adult human poisonings have the potential for coma, hypotension, metabolic acidosis, renal injury, and hemolysis. CNS depression is the most common finding, with onset of coma from 1 to 12 hours. These reports involve more concentrated EGBE formulations, large ingested volumes (250 to 500 cc), or both.

Toxicity is unlikely after unintentional ingestion of small amounts by children. Unlike ethylene glycol, which has a sweet taste, EGBE has a very bitter taste, limiting the amount ingested. A retrospective study of 24 pediatric exposures demonstrated no significant toxicity after the ingestion of less than 10 cc of nonconcentrated (less than 10%) EGBE. EGBE does not contribute sufficiently to the osmolal gap to allow prediction of toxicity, and serum EGBE levels are not readily available. As such, treatment decisions are made on clinical grounds.

In the setting of significant ingestion or evidence of toxicity, management is similar to that of the toxic alcohols, with both alcohol dehydrogenase blockade and hemodialysis advocated in the literature.

SUGGESTED READINGS

Augenstein WL, Spoerke DG, Kulig KW, et al: Fluoride ingestion in children: A review of 87 Cases. *Pediatrics* 88:907–912, 1991.

Browning RG, Curry SC: Clinical toxicology of ethylene glycol monoalkyl ethers. *Hum Exp Toxicol* 13:325–335, 1994

Centers for Disease Control: Unintentional poisoning among young children—United States. *MMWR* 32:529–531, 1983

Dean BS, Krenzelok EP: Clinical evaluation of pediatric ethylene glycol monobutyl ether poisonings. *Clin Toxicol* 30:557–563, 1992.

Doyon S. Hairdressers and cosmetologists. In: Greenberg MI, Hamilton RJ, Phillips SD, eds: *Occupational, Industrial, and Environmental Toxicology*. St. Louis: Mosby; 1997:147–152.

Draelos ZK. Hair cosmetics. *Dermatol Clin* 9:19–27, 1991.

Federal Hazardous Substances Act (Codified at 15 U.S.C. 1261-1278) (Public Law 86-613; 74 Stat. 372, July 12, 1960, as amended).

Garrettson LK, Bush JP, Gates RS, et al: Physical change, time of day, and child characteristics as factors in poison injury. *Vet Hum Toxicol* 32:139–141, 1990.

Geller RJ, Elkins BR, Iknoian RC: Cyanide toxicity from acetonitrile-containing false nail remover. *Am J Emerg Med* 9:271–272, 1991.

Hurlburt KM, Rumack BH, Petrie AF, et al: Fluoride. In: *POISINDEX*. MICROMEDEX Healthcare Series, Vol 115, expires 3/2003.

Hymes LC, Bruner BS, Rauber AP: Bromate poisoning from hair permanent preparations. *Pediatrics* 76:975–977, 1985.

Klasner AE, Scalzo AJ, Blume C, et al: Marked hypocalcemia and ventricular fibrillation in two pediatric patients exposed to a fluoride-containing wheel cleaner. Ammonium bifluoride causes another pediatric death. *Ann Emerg Med* 28:713–718, 1996.

Litovitz TL, Klein-Schwartz W, Rodgers GC, et al: 2001 annual report of the American Association of Poison Control Centers Toxic Exposure Surveillance System. *Am J Emerg Med* 20: 391–452, 2002.

Lucas JK: Cosmetics and toilet articles. In: Haddad LM, Shannon MW, Winchester JF, eds: *Clinical Management of Poisoning and Drug Overdose*. 3rd ed. Philadelphia: Saunders; 1998:1169–1174.

Phillips S, Burkhart K, Hartman P, et al: Can dental fluoride exposure less than or equal to 8 mg/kg be managed at home? *Vet Human Toxicol* 34:334, 1992.

Poison Prevention Packaging Act (Codified at 15 U.S.C. 1471-1476) (Public Law 91-601, 84 Stat. 1670, December 30, 1970, as amended).

Rambourg-Schepens MO, Buffet M, Bertault R, et al: Severe ethylene glycol butyl ether poisoning. Kinetics and metabolic pattern. *Human Toxicol* 7:187–189, 1988.

Rambourg-Schepens MO, Buffet M, Durak C, et al: Gamma butyrolactone poisoning and its similarities to gamma hydroxybutyric acid: Two case reports. *Vet Hum Toxicol* 39:234–235, 1997.

Ramu A, Rosenbaum J, Blaschke TF. Disposition of acetone following acute acetone intoxication. *West J Med* 129:429–432, 1978.

Reed KJ, Jimenez M, Freeman NC, et al: Quantification of children's hand and mouthing activities through a videotaping methodology. *J Expo Anal Environ Epidemiol* 9:513–520, 1999.

Rozin P, Hammer L, Oster H, et al:. The child's conception of food: Differentiation of categories of rejected substances in the 16 months to 5 year age range. *Appetite* 7:141–151, 1986.

Trinkoff AM, Baker SP: Poisoning hospitalizations and deaths from solids and liquids among children and teenagers. *Am J Public Health* 76:657–660, 1986.

Wasserman GS: The nontoxic ingestion. *Pediatr Ann* 25:39–46, 1996.

Wolfle J, Kowalewski S: Epidemiology of ingestions in a regional poison control center over twenty years. *Vet Human Toxicol* 37:367–368, 1995.

47

Toxic Alcohols

Timothy B. Erickson
Jeffrey Brent

HIGH-YIELD FACTS

- Ethanol overdose in children may result in hypoglycemia.

- Methanol ingestion is associated with visual disturbance, metabolic acidosis, and possibly multi-organ system failure.

- Ethylene glycol poisoning is associated with metabolic acidosis, renal failure, and possibly death.

- Isopropanol may cause central nervous system (CNS) depression but does not usually cause metabolic acidosis.

- All of the toxic alcohols can produce an osmolal gap.

- Fomepizole, which has been recently approved by the U.S. Food and Drug Administration (FDA), is the antidote for ethylene glycol and methanol toxicity.

- Hemodialysis is indicated in severe toxic alcohol ingestions not responsive to conventional medical therapy, with evidence of end-organ damage, or with severe acidosis.

CASE PRESENTATION

A 2-year-old presents to the emergency department (ED) after drinking an unknown amount of mouthwash from the household bathroom approximately 2 hours prior. The child is lethargic in the ED with a pulse of 120 bpm, a respiratory rate of 16 breaths per minute, and temperature of 95°F. The patient's lungs are clear, and the neurologic examination is nonfocal.

ETHANOL

According to the American Association of Poison Control Centers (AAPCC), there were over 9000 exposures to ethanol in children under 20 years of age in 2001, accounting for 2.5% of all reported exposures. Children under 6 years of age accounted for one third of these cases. There was one documented fatality. Over 6000 additional pediatric ingestions of mouthwash containing ethanol were also reported. The number of total ethanol exposures in the adolescent patient population may be underrepresented in this database.

Sources

In addition to alcohol-containing beverages such as beer, wine, and hard liquors, children have access to mouthwashes that can contain up to 75% ethanol, colognes and perfumes (40% to 60% ethanol), and over 700 ethanol-containing medicinal preparations.

Pharmacokinetics and Pathophysiology

Ethanol undergoes hepatic metabolism via two metabolic pathways: alcohol dehydrogenase and the microsomal ethanol-oxidizing system. The alcohol dehydrogenase pathway is the major metabolic pathway and the rate-limiting step in converting ethanol to acetaldehyde. In general, nontolerant individuals metabolize ethanol at 10 to 25 mg/dL/h and alcoholics metabolize up to 30 mg/dL/h. Children may ingest large amounts of ethanol in relation to their body weight, resulting in rapid development of high blood alcohol concentrations. In children under 5 years of age, the ability to metabolize ethanol is diminished owing to immature hepatic dehydrogenase activity.

Clinical Presentation

Ethanol is a selective CNS depressant at low concentrations, and a generalized depressant at high concentrations. Initially, ethanol produces exhilaration and loss of inhibition, which progresses to lack of coordination, ataxia, slurred speech, gait disturbances, drowsiness, and, ultimately, stupor and coma. The intoxicated child may demonstrate a flushed face, dilated pupils, excessive sweating, gastrointestinal (GI) distress, hypoventilation, hypothermia, and hypotension. Death from respiratory depression may occur at serum ethanol concentrations >500 mg/dL. Convulsions and death have been reported in children with acute ethanol intoxication owing to alcohol-induced hypoglycemia. Hypoglycemia results from inhibition of hepatic gluconeogenesis and is most common in children under 5 years of age. It does not appear to be directly related to the quantity of alcohol ingested.

Laboratory

In symptomatic pediatric patients who have suspected ethanol intoxication, the most critical laboratory tests are the serum ethanol and glucose concentrations. Although blood ethanol concentrations roughly correlate with clinical signs, the physician must treat patients based on the clinical presentation, not the absolute level. If the ethanol level does not correlate with the clinical picture, coingestants or other causes of altered mental status should be considered. If children have experienced fluid losses, serum electrolytes are monitored.

Management

The majority of children with accidental acute ingestions of ethanol respond to supportive care. Attention is directed toward management of the patient's airway, circulation, and glucose status. Obtunded patients should receive 2 to 4 mL/kg of $D_{25}W$ (1 amp of $D_{50}W$ in older children and adolescents), after a specimen for blood glucose level is drawn. Alternatively, a bedside finger stick blood glucose determination can be immediately obtained and dextrose administered if hypoglycemia is documented. If children respond to glucose administration, serial glucose levels are followed to detect recurrent

hypoglycemia. If no response is elicited, or if the patient is not hypoglycemic, administration of naloxone 2 mg intravenous (IV) push is indicated to rule out opioid toxicity.

Unless children are comatose, or coingestion of another drug is suspected, gastric decontamination with a nasogastric tube is unnecessary. Activated charcoal can be administered but is probably not efficacious in isolated ethanol ingestions. Because hemodialysis increases ethanol clearance by 3 to 4 times, it may be considered in massive ethanol ingestions in which patients do no respond to conventional therapy.

Disposition

Any infant with significantly altered mental status following acute ethanol ingestion is admitted for observation of respiratory status, fluid resuscitation, and glucose monitoring. Asymptomatic patients may be discharged home with reliable caretakers. Adolescent patients should be referred for counseling in an alcohol addiction program if a recurrent pattern of ethanol abuse has been reported.

Case Outcome

The child's laboratory studies show a serum glucose concentration of 30 mg/dL and an ethanol level of 80 mg/dL. Acetaminophen and aspirin levels are negative. The patient responds well to an ampule of $D_{25}W$ and an IV dextrose drip. The child is monitored overnight and discharged in stable condition the following morning.

METHANOL

In 2001, there were 387 exposures to methanol reported to the AAPCC in patients younger than 20 years of age. Sixty percent of exposures were reported in children under 6 years of age, with one reported fatality in an infant born to a 28-year-old mother who ingested methanol in a suicide attempt. The infant's methanol level on autopsy was 61 mg/dL.

Sources

Methanol is present in a variety of substances found around the home and workplace, including paint solvents, gasohol, gasoline additives, canned heat products, windshield washer fluid, and duplicating chemicals.

Pharmacokinetics and Pathophysiology

Methanol is rapidly absorbed following ingestion. Peak serum levels can be reached as early as 30 to 90 minutes postingestion. As with ethanol, methanol is primarily metabolized by hepatic alcohol dehydrogenase. The half-life of methanol may be as long as 24 hours, but in the presence of ethanol or fomepizole, it can be longer. Methanol itself is harmless; however, its main metabolite, formic acid, is extremely toxic. Fatalities have been reported after ingestion of as little as 15 mL of a 40% methanol solution, although 30 mL is generally considered a minimal lethal dose. Ingestion of only 10 mL can lead to blindness. Adults have survived ingestions of 500 mL.

Clinical Presentation

The onset of symptoms following methanol ingestion varies from 1 to 72 hours. Patients may have the classic triad consisting of visual complaints, abdominal pain, and metabolic acidosis. Eye signs and symptoms are generally delayed, and include blurring of vision, photophobia, constricted visual fields, snowfield vision, and hyperemia of the optic disk. Although blindness is usually permanent, recovery has been reported.

Patients also typically complain of nausea and vomiting, and can experience GI bleeding and acute pancreatitis. Unlike with the other alcohols, these patients often lack the odor of ethanol on their breath, and typically have a clear sensorium.

Laboratory Testing

Baseline laboratory data include a complete blood cell (CBC) count, serum electrolytes and blood glucose, amylase, blood urea nitrogen (BUN) and serum creatinine, a urinalysis, and an arterial blood gas. Classically, methanol-intoxicated patients develop an elevated anion gap metabolic acidosis, although this may not be present if the patient presents before a significant quantity of formic acid has been generated. The anion gap should be calculated using the equation:

$$(Na) + (Cl - HCO_3).$$

The normal anion gap is 8 to 12 mEq/L. Another valuable clue in establishing the diagnosis is the presence of an elevated osmolal gap, which is the difference between measured and calculated serum osmolarity. An elevated osmolal gap indicates that a highly osmotic compound not normally found in the serum is present in a signifi-

cant quantity. The most accurate determination of the measured osmolality is made using a freezing point depression method, because the standard vapor pressure analysis volatizes alcohols and can produce erroneous results. The formula for calculating serum osmolality is:

$$2(NA) + glucose/18 + BUN/2.8 + ETOH/4.6$$

Normally the difference between the measured serum osmolality and the calculated serum osmolality is less than 10 mOsm. Other toxicologic causes of elevated osmolal gaps include ethylene glycol, ethanol, and isopropanol poisoning, all of which are highly osmotically active compounds. Although the osmolal gap is a useful clue, cases of significant methanol and ethylene glycol overdoses have been reported with normal osmolal gaps.

Measurement of methanol and ethanol levels is critical in diagnosing these poisonings. Generally, levels <20 mg/dL result in no effects. It is generally stated, but undocumented, that CNS effects appear with levels >20 mg/dL and peak levels >50 mg/dL indicate serious toxicity. Ocular effects occur at levels >100 mg/dL, and fatalities have been reported in untreated victims with levels >150 mg/dL. One problem in interpreting levels is the time of ingestion versus the time of patient presentation and serum level assessment. Patients with low serum methanol concentrations may still be significantly poisoned and acidotic when presenting late in their clinical course.

Management

GI decontamination may be efficacious for patients presenting within 1 hour of ingestion, although this is unlikely, particularly with a rapidly absorbed agent such as methanol. Although the utility of activated charcoal and cathartics in preventing absorption of the toxic alcohols has not been well established, 1 g/kg can be administered, particularly if a coingestion is suspected.

If a significant ingestion of methanol is likely, empiric treatment with the IV alcohol dehydrogenase inhibitor fomepizole is recommended, even if laboratory tests are unavailable. Fomepizole (Figure 47–1) competitively binds hepatic alcohol dehydrogenase 500 to 1000 times more avidly than methanol, and prevents the formation of the toxic metabolite formic acid. Other indications for fomepizole therapy include serum methanol levels >20 mg/dL, or acidemia (pH <7.20). A fomepizole loading dose of 15 mg/kg should be administered, followed by doses 10 mg/kg every 12 hours for four doses, until methanol levels are 20 mg/dL. Fomepizole is the only FDA approved antidote for methanol poisoning.

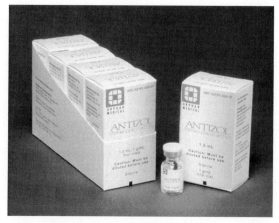

Fig. 47–1. Fomepizole or 4-MP (Antizole).

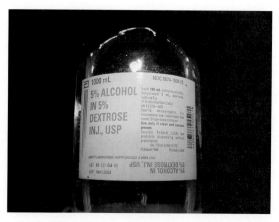

Fig. 47–2. Five percent alcohol solution.

If fomepizole is unavailable, ethanol may be administered in an attempt to block alcohol dehydrogenase (Figure 47–2). To inhibit toxic metabolite formation, ethanol levels are maintained between 100 and 150 mg/dL. An IV solution of 10% ethanol in D_5W is optimal, with a loading dose of 0.6 g/kg. A simplified approximation of the loading dose is 1 mL/kg of 10% diluted absolute ethanol. It is important to note that some hospitals only stock a 5% alcohol solution and the dose should be adjusted accordingly. Using a 5% solution in very young patients can cause fluid overload with excess free water and should be avoided. Close monitoring of the ethanol level every 1 to 2 hours is necessary to adjust the maintenance infusion rate for each individual patient. If IV ethanol preparations are unavailable, oral ethanol therapy can be instituted. Because hypoglycemia is a complication of toxic ethanol levels in young children, serum glucose levels are closely monitored.

Continued therapy with fomepizole or ethanol is recommended until methanol levels fall below 20 mg/dL. Although there is no clinical outcome data confirming the superiority of either of these antidotes, there are significant disadvantages with ethanol therapy. These include difficulties in maintaining therapeutic concentrations, induced hypoglycemia, and CNS depression that may require endotracheal intubation, particularly in children. Unlike ethanol, fomepizole lacks CNS depressant and hypoglycemia effects. According to the 2001 AAPCC data system, fomepizole was the ninth most commonly administered antidote (given 546 times), surpassing ethanol therapy (542) for the first time. Fomepizole has a higher cost than does ethanol therapy.

However, in pediatric cases, the benefits, minimal side effects, and the potential avoidance of hemodialysis make it preferable. A formal economic comparison between fomepizole and ethanol treatment has not been done.

Additional therapies for methanol poisonings may include bicarbonate if the serum pH falls below 7.20 and folic acid. Folate, the active form of folic acid, is a coenzyme in the metabolic step converting the toxic metabolite formate to CO_2 and H_2O, and is indicated in the methanol poisoned patient. Up to 50 mg of folate can be given IV every 4 hours, until the acidosis is corrected and methanol levels fall below 20 mg/dL.

Hemodialysis effectively removes methanol and formic acid. Indications for dialysis include visual impairment, metabolic acidosis not corrected with bicarbonate administration, renal failure, and methanol levels >50 mg/dL (with or without clinical signs or symptoms). It is important to note that ethanol and fomepizole are readily dialyzed, so the rate of IV administration may have to be increased during dialysis. For fomepizole, the recommendation is increasing the frequency of dosing to every 4 hours during hemodialysis.

Disposition

Any patients who are comatose and have abnormal vital signs, visual complaints, metabolic acidosis, or high methanol levels need admission to a pediatric intensive care unit. Asymptomatic patients without evidence of acidosis and with levels <10 mg/dL may be discharged from the ED.

ETHYLENE GLYCOL

In 2001, there were 1400 exposures to ethylene glycol reported to the AAPCC in individuals under 20 years of age, with three reported deaths. Half of the reported cases involved children younger than 6 years of age. Ethylene glycol is an odorless, sweet-tasting compound that is found in antifreeze products, coolants, preservatives, and glycerin substitutes.

Case Presentation

A 17-year-old boy ingested an unknown amount of antifreeze approximately 12 hours prior to presentation to the ED. He was transported by ambulance obtunded with Kussmaul respirations. He had a blood pressure of 150/90 mmHg and a heart rate of 100 bpm. An initial arterial blood gas showed pH 6.93; P_{CO_2} 17 mmHg; and P_{O_2} 76 mmHg. Wood's lamp–induced urine fluorescence was noted in the ED.

Pharmacokinetics and Pathophysiology

Ethylene glycol undergoes rapid absorption from the GI tract, and initial signs of intoxication may occur as early as 30 minutes postingestion. As with the other alcohols, it undergoes hepatic metabolism via alcohol dehydrogenase to form various toxic metabolites, glycolaldehyde, glycolic acid, and ultimately oxalate, which is excreted through the kidney. The hallmark of ethylene glycol toxicity is a severe anion gap metabolic acidosis owing to accumulation of glycolic acid, hypocalcemia, and renal failure, which results from the precipitation of calcium oxalate crystals in the kidney.

Clinical Presentation

The clinical effects of ethylene glycol toxicity can be divided into three stages:

- *Stage I* occurs within the first 12 hours of ingestion, with CNS symptoms similar to that experienced with ethanol. This stage is characterized by slurred speech, nystagmus, ataxia, vomiting, lethargy, and coma. Patients may suffer convulsions, myoclonic jerks, and tetanic contractions owing to hypocalcemia. As with methanol toxicity, patients can demonstrate an anion gap acidosis with an elevated osmol gap. In approximately one third of cases, calcium oxalate crystals are found in the urine, a finding considered strongly suggestive of ethylene glycol poisoning. These types of crystals are also found in the urine of patients ingesting certain vegetable diets.
- *Stage II* occurs within 12 to 36 hours after ingestion and is characterized by rapidly progressive tachypnea, cyanosis, pulmonary edema, adult respiratory distress syndrome, and cardiomegaly. Death is most common during this stage.
- *Stage III* occurs 2 to 3 days postingestion and is heralded by flank pain, oliguria, proteinuria, anuria, and renal failure.

Ethylene glycol poisoning is possible in any inebriated patient lacking an odor of ethanol who has severe acidosis, oxalate crystalluria, hematuria, or renal failure.

Laboratory Testing

Indicated laboratory studies include CBC count, serum electrolytes, blood glucose, calcium, creatine kinase, serum ethanol and ethylene glycol, an arterial blood gas, BUN and serum creatinine, serum osmolarity, and urine for crystals, protein, and blood. Both anion and osmolal gaps are calculated. Because of the potential for severe cardiopulmonary effects in stage II, a chest radiograph and an electrocardiogram are recommended. Because fluorescein is present in many antifreeze products, fluorescence of the patient's urine, gastric aspirate, or perioral area when exposed to light from a Wood's lamp may be a valuable diagnostic clue, although the clinical efficacy and practicality of this test has been challenged in the recent literature.

Management

Gastric lavage may be useful in patients presenting within 1 hour of ingestion. Syrup of ipecac is contraindicated in all significant poisonings. Activated charcoal can be administered, although there are no studies documenting its effectiveness in ethylene glycol toxicity. Patients who develop seizures are treated with standard doses of benzodiazepines and phenobarbital.

The alcohol dehydrogenase inhibitor fomepizole has been FDA approved for treatment of ethylene glycol poisoning, as it has for methanol toxicity. Indications include a metabolic acidosis (pH under 7.20 of unknown cause) or an ethylene glycol level >20 mg/dL. In cases where a significant ingestion is suspected, therapy should not be delayed pending an ethylene glycol level.

Ethanol competitively binds alcohol dehydrogenase with an affinity 100 times greater than ethylene glycol and slows the accumulation of toxic metabolites; it is an alternative to therapy with fomepizole. If an IV preparation of ethanol is unavailable, patients can be loaded orally to achieve an ethanol level of 100 to 150 mg/dL. Because toxic ethanol levels result in profound hypoglycemia in small children, serial glucose measurements are monitored.

Bicarbonate administration is recommended for patients with pH <7.20. Serum calcium levels are monitored and hypocalcemia is treated with 10% calcium gluconate if the patient has clinical signs of hypocalcemia. Calcium replacement is not indicated for hypocalcemia alone, because this encourages the formation of calcium oxalate crystals. Additionally, thiamine (50 to 100 mg IM or IV q6h) and pyridoxine (vitamin B_6, 50 mg IM or IV q6h) are recommended in ethylene glycol poisonings to shunt or reroute the metabolism of ethylene glycol toward less toxic metabolites (Table 47–1).

Hemodialysis effectively removes ethylene glycol, as well as its major circulating toxic metabolite, glycolic acid. It is indicated in the setting of metabolic acidosis not responsive to bicarbonate administration, pulmonary edema, and renal failure. Serum ethylene glycol levels >50 mg/dL, regardless of clinical signs, is an indication of hemodialysis in patients treated with ethanol. Whether pretreatment with fomepizole would obviate the need for hemodialysis in patients with comparable ethylene glycol levels remains to be determined.

Case Outcome

A renal consult was obtained and the 17-year-old patient was admitted to the intensive care unit. Fomepizole, sodium bicarbonate, thiamine, and pyridoxine were administered IV. The patient's ethylene glycol on admission was 62 mg/dL. He underwent emergent hemodialysis for 4 hours with a postdialysis ethylene glycol level of 17 mg/dL. The patient developed ventricular tachycardia 16 hours after admission, which responded to amiodarone and epinephrine infusions. Computed tomography of the head demonstrated massive cerebral edema and herniation. Brain death was confirmed and life support was withdrawn 48 hours after admission.

ISOPROPANOL

In 2001, there were 5800 cases of isopropanol exposure reported to the AAPCC in individuals under 20 years of age. Of note, 90% of exposures occurred in children under 6 years of age. Isopropanol is a common solvent and disinfectant with CNS depressant properties similar to ethanol. Exposure from isopropyl alcohol occurs more frequently in children under 6 years old than ethanol, methanol, or ethylene glycol ingestions. Toxicity results from both accidental and intentional ingestions, as well as inhalation and dermal exposures in young children given rubbing alcohol sponge baths for fever.

Pharmacokinetics and Pathophysiology

Isopropanol is rapidly absorbed across the gastric mucosa, with acute intoxication occurring within 30 minutes of ingestion. It is metabolized by alcohol dehydrogenase, but, unlike the other alcohols, is not metabolized to an acidic end product. Rather, isopropanol is converted to the CNS depressant acetone. Respiratory elimination of the acetone causes a fruity-acetone odor on the patient's breath similar to diabetic ketoacidosis. Because 70% isopropanol is a potent inebriant that is about twice as intoxicating as ethanol, a level of 50 mg/dL is comparable to an ethanol level of 100 mg/dL.

Table 47–1. Toxic Alcohol Antidotes

Methanol	Ethylene Glycol
Fomepizole	Fomepizole
Folate	Thiamine
Ethanol	Pyridoxine
	Ethanol

Table 47–2. Comparisons of Toxic Alcohols

Parameter	Methanol	Ethylene Glycol	Isopropanol
Anion gap Acidosis	+	+	−
Osmolal gap	+	+	+
CNS depression	+	+	+
Eye findings	+	−	−
Renal failure	−	+	−
Ketones	−	−	+
Oxalate crystals	−	+	−

Abbreviation: CNS, central nervous system.

Clinical Presentation

Isopropanol-intoxicated patients are classically lethargic or comatose, hypotensive, and tachycardic, with the characteristic breath odor of rubbing alcohol or acetone. Coma develops at levels >100 mg/dL. Hypotension results from peripheral vasodilation and cardiac depression. GI irritation with acute abdominal pain and hematemesis can also occur. With isopropanol, unlike the other toxic alcohols, acidosis, ophthalmologic changes, and renal failure are absent. However, like ethanol, methanol, and ethylene glycol, isopropanol can produce a significant osmolal gap (Table 47–2).

Laboratory Testing

Patients are tested for the presence of acetonemia and acetonuria. Unlike diabetic ketoacidosis, the acetone is typically found in the absence of glucosuria, hyperglycemia, or acidemia. Indicated laboratory studies include a CBC, serum electrolytes, an arterial blood gas, and blood glucose, serum ethanol, and isopropanol levels, serum osmolarity, and BUN and creatinine. Isopropanol levels >400 mg/dL correspond to severe, life-threatening toxicity.

Management

Patients are managed with particular attention paid to the integrity of the airway. Hypotension is treated with IV crystalloid. Because isopropanol is so rapidly absorbed from the GI tract, gastric decontamination with a nasogastric tube is unlikely to be of any benefit. The efficacy of activated charcoal for isopropanol poisoning alone is questionable. Activated charcoal may be administered if there is a coingestion. No alcohol dehydrogenase inhibition is indicated because the metabolite acetone is relatively nontoxic and excreted through the lungs. Hemodialysis is effective in removing isopropanol, but is reserved for prolonged coma, hypotension, and isopropanol levels higher than 400 or 500 mg/dL. Typically, patients progress well with supportive care alone.

Disposition

Isopropanol-intoxicated patients who are lethargic should be admitted, and asymptomatic children may be observed in the ED. Ingestion of over three swallows (15 mL) of 70% isopropanol by a 10-kg child (1.5 mL/kg) is an indication for several hours of observation.

SUGGESTED READINGS

Barceloux DG, Bond RG, Krenzelok EP, et al: American Academy of Clinical Toxicology Ad Hoc Committee: AACT practice guidelines on the treatment of methanol poisoning. *J Toxicol Clin Toxicol* 40:415–446, 2002.

Barceloux DG, Krenzelor E, Olson K, et al: American Academy of Clinical Toxicology Ad Hoc Committee: Guidelines on the treatment of ethylene glycol poisoning. *J Toxicol Clin Toxicol* 37:537–560, 1999.

Brent J, Lucas M, Kulig, et al: Methanol poisoning in a 6 week old infant. *J Pediatr* 118:644–646, 1991.

Brent J, McMartin K, Phillips S, et al: Fomepizole for the treatment of ethylene glycol poisoning. *N Engl J Med* 340:832–838, 1999.

Brent J, McMartin K, Phillips S, et al: Fomepizole for the treatment of methanol poisoning. *N Engl J Med* 344:424–429, 2001.

Brown MJ, Shannon MW, Woolf A, et al: Childhood methanol ingestion treated with fomepizole and hemodialysis. *Pediatrics* 108:E77, 2001.

Burkhart KK, Kulig KW: The other alcohols: Methanol, ethylene glycol and isopropanol. *Emerg Clin North Am* 8:913–928, 1990.

Erickson T: Toxic alcohol poisoning: When to suspect and keys to diagnosis. *Consultant* 40:1845–1856, 2000.

Haymond MW: Hypoglycemia in infants and children. *Endocrinol Metab Clin North Am* 18:211–252, 1989.

Jacobsen D, McMartin KE: Antidotes for methanol and ethylene glycol poisoning. *J Toxicol Clin Toxicol* 35:127, 1997.

Litovitz TL, Schwartz-Klein W, Rodgers GCS, et al: 2001 Annual Report of the AAPCC Toxic Exposure Surveillance System. *Am J Emerg Med* 20:391–452, 2002.

Liu JJ, Daya MR, Carrasquill O, et al: Prognostic factors in patients with methanol poisoning. *J Toxicol Clin Toxicol* 36:175, 1998.

Saladino R, Shannon M: Accidental and intentional poisoning with ethylene glycol in infancy: Diagnostic clues and management. *Pediatr Emerg Care* 7:93–96, 1991.

Woolf AD, Wynshaw-Boris A, Rinaldo P, et al: Intentional infantile ethylene glycol poisoning presenting as an inherited metabolic disorder. *J Pediatr* 120:421–424, 1992.

Wu AB, Kelly T, McKay C, et al: Definitive identification of an exceptionally high methanol concentration in an intoxication of a surviving infant: Methanol metabolism by first order elimination kinetics. *J Forensic Sci* 40:315–320, 1995.

48

Acids and Alkali

Diane P. Calello
Fred M. Henretig

HIGH-YIELD FACTS

- Pediatric caustic ingestions are more common but less severe than adult caustic ingestions because they tend to be accidental as opposed to deliberate.

- Acid and alkali ingestions do not differ significantly in severity or frequency of injury.

- Patients with no clinical signs or symptoms are unlikely to have significant esophageal or other organ injury.

- Decontamination techniques such as activated charcoal, gastric lavage, syrup of ipecac, and neutralization are contraindicated in caustic ingestions, but immediate dilution may have some benefit.

- The use of steroids to prevent strictures remains controversial, but appears most helpful in patients with second-degree esophageal burns.

- Severe pain and deep penetration despite minimal skin findings is the hallmark of a hydrofluoric acid burn. The mechanism of injury involves liquefaction necrosis and the formation of insoluble calcium and magnesium salts.

- The treatment of hydrofluoric acid injuries includes topical application or intradermal injection of calcium gluconate.

CASE PRESENTATION

A 19-month-old girl drank some drain cleaner, an 85% sulfuric acid solution, from a soda can in her home. The solution, a very concentrated industrial cleaner, was not intended for household use. She soon developed swollen lips and oral pain, and was brought to the emergency department (ED). In the ED she was found to be extremely uncomfortable and drooling; examination revealed erythematous perioral skin, edematous blistered lips, and a swollen tongue with some epithelial sloughing. Within 2 hours she developed stridor and dysphonia, which prompted direct laryngoscopic evaluation that revealed laryngeal and cricopharyngeal burns. Emergent tracheostomy was performed (Figure 48–1).

INTRODUCTION AND EPIDEMIOLOGY

Pediatric caustic ingestions have much in common with other pediatric poisonings. They often involve toddlers who ingest small volumes in the course of their exploratory behavior. Most occur in children under 6 years of age, with the average child being between 1 and 2 years old. Caustic exposures occur much more frequently in children than in adults, but usually have milder clinical consequences.

Regulatory legislation in the United States that governs packaging of hazardous materials has greatly influenced the epidemiology of pediatric caustic injury. In the 1960s, concentrated liquid lye became widely available in household preparations, and with it came a significant increase in both incidence and severity of pediatric caustic inges-

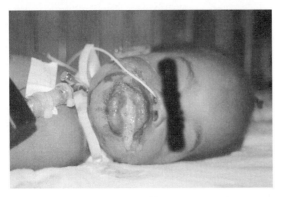

Fig. 48–1. A 19-month-old girl with emergency tracheostomy and severe oral and facial burns after a sulfuric acid ingestion.

Table 48–1. Dangers in the Home: Common Caustic Household Products[a]

Product Type	Caustic Ingredients
Drain cleaners	Sodium hydroxide
Oven cleaners	Sodium hydroxide, sulfuric acid
Porcelain cleansers, toilet bowl cleaners	Hydrochloric acid, sulfuric acid
Automatic dishwasher detergent	Phosphates
Hair relaxer: traditional	Sodium, potassium hydroxide
Hair relaxer: no lye	Calcium hydroxide
Clinitest, Efferdent tablets	Sodium hydroxide
Automobile battery acid	Sulfuric acid
Swimming pool cleaner	Cationic detergents, copper sulfate
Rust remover and etching compounds	Hydrofluoric acid

[a]Includes only products available in household concentrations. Does not include industrial-strength compounds for similar use. Products listed with their most common caustic ingredients. Individual products may vary.

tions heralded as the so-called lye epidemic. In response, the Federal Hazardous Substances Act and Poison Prevention Packaging Act of 1970 were enacted, requiring any caustic agent with a concentration greater than 10% to be sold in child-resistant containers. Further regulations were passed in 1973 requiring child-resistant packaging for all alkaline caustics of greater than 2% concentration. In addition, bleach and ammonia preparations, once packaged in high concentrations, are now available in much more dilute solutions for household use. The positive impact of these regulations is evident when considering the increased prevalence and severity of caustic injuries in children from countries without such regulations, as well as among U.S. children who have access to industrial-strength materials in unregulated settings, such as farms.

Although these regulations have decreased the availability of dangerous household caustics, the curious toddler may still encounter considerable hazards in the home. Table 48–1 provides a list of some common household products and the caustic materials they contain. Of special note in recent years is the mouthing by children of no-lye calcium hydroxide-based cream hair relaxer products. This typically cause mild burns of the lips and mouth, but rarely any serious pharyngeal, esophageal, or other visceral injury. A more complete discussion of hazardous and nonhazardous household products can be found in Chapter 46.

DEVELOPMENTAL CONSIDERATIONS

Exploratory ingestions in toddlers result from a complex interplay of developmental milestones. Between 7 and 9 months children develop the fine motor coordination required to pick up small objects. Most infants can crawl

at the age of 9 months and walk well by 15 months, and the once out-of-reach household caustic becomes accessible. The teething and curious toddler puts most objects encountered directly into his or her mouth. Social maturation creates the desire to mimic adult activity, such as drinking out of a soda can; many pediatric caustic ingestions occur when the substance is in a nonsafety container used originally for consumption.

Caustic injury in the adolescent patient is similar to the adult exposure. Ingestions are often intentional, involve large volumes, and as a result are much more severe. Access is not limited to household caustics; industrial-strength substances are also implicated. Thus, adolescents with caustic injury should be considered severely injured until proven otherwise.

CHEMISTRY: ACID–BASE CONCEPTS

Caustic is often used interchangeably with *chemical*, *corrosive*, *acid*, and *alkali*. In fact, acidic and alkaline materials may cause caustic injuries, but so may oxidizing and reducing agents, corrosives, desiccants, or vesicants. *Corrosion* is a nonspecific term that describes damage to the architecture of a tissue. It is therefore most accurate to refer to tissue damage from one of these agents as a *caustic* injury.

The inherent chemical characteristics of a substance determines the type and extent of tissue damage that it inflicts. The pH of a solution is the negative logarithm of the concentration of hydrogen ions: the lower the pH, the higher the concentration. For example, the pH of water is 7.0, so the hydrogen ion concentration is 10^{-7} mol; at a pH of 8.0, the concentration would be 10^{-8} mol. Exposure to agents with extreme acidity (pH < 2) or alkalinity (pH > 11.5) is associated with severe tissue damage. The concentration and strength of a solution influence its pH.

The strength of a substance reflects its tendency to dissociate. Acids dissociate to release hydronium (H_3O^+) ions, and bases release hydroxide (OH^-) ions. The more dissociated an acid or base in aqueous solution, the more readily it donates these ions, and the stronger it is. The pK_a of a solution is the pH at which it is 50% ionized. At a pH above its pK_a, an acid exists in increasingly more dissociated form. A base becomes more dissociated at a pH below its pK_a. The pK_a of a strong acid is very low, and the pK_a of a strong base is greater than 14.

Another property that influences the caustic potential of a given substance is its buffering capacity. For a basic solution, the amount of acid that must be added to restore the solution to a neutral pH is its buffering capacity, referred to as the *titratable alkaline reserve* (TAR), or *free alkalinity*. Similarly, the *titratable acid reserve* may be measured for acids. Just as the heat capacity of a material increases its ability to inflict a thermal burn, a higher titratable reserve implies greater caustic potential. This may be more significant in alkaline injuries.

Factors besides pH, pK_a, and TAR that influence the caustic potential of a substance include the volume ingested, whether the substance is a liquid or solid, and the viscosity, which influences transit time and thus tissue contact. The contents of the gastrointestinal (GI) tract may also mitigate caustic injury. In addition, some caustics inflict damage independent of their acid–base characteristics. For example, phenol, an antiseptic, has a neutral pH but causes cell death through desiccation. Zinc and mercuric chloride ($ZnCl_2$, $HgCl_2$), in addition to their caustic potential, may cause severe heavy metal toxicity. Of special note are Clinitest tablets, which inflict not only caustic but thermal injury.

PATHOPHYSIOLOGY

After an alkali ingestion, dissociated OH^- ions penetrate the esophageal squamous epithelium, causing protein dissolution, collagen destruction, fat saponification, cell membrane emulsification, and transmural thrombosis. This is referred to as *liquefaction necrosis*, and is somewhat unique to alkaline injuries. The alkali penetrates tissue until the OH^- concentration is lowered sufficiently and the solution is neutralized. Exothermic neutralization and dissolution of alkali causes thermal tissue injury. Severity of esophageal involvement varies from mild erythema to severe ulceration and necrosis. The oropharynx, larynx, and stomach are also potential sites of tissue damage. In contrast, after an acid ingestion, hydronium (H_3O^+) ions desiccate the epithelial cells and cause eschar formation and *coagulation necrosis*, which somewhat limits deeper penetration but causes edema, erythema, ulceration, and necrosis. In addition to esophageal injury, acid-induced pylorospasm leads to gastric outlet obstruction, antral pooling, and potentially, perforation. Dissociated anions of the acid (Cl^-, SO_4^{2-}, PO_4^{3-}) also act as reducing agents, further injuring tissue. Unlike alkali, ingested acids are systemically absorbed, creating a metabolic acidosis with either a normal or elevated anion gap. The resulting acidemia, in addition to that caused by tissue destruction, may have significant consequences including hemolysis, renal failure, extraintestinal organ damage, and death.

It was previously believed that, following acid ingestion, gastric burns were more prevalent than esophageal burns. However, studies have demonstrated that esophageal and gastric injury occur with equal frequency. In addition, although acids do not cause liquefaction necrosis, the incidence of perforation appears equal with acids and alkalis. In fact, patients with acid ingestions have a higher mortality rate, because ingestions are more often deliberate, involve large volumes of a substance, and are associated with severe metabolic derangements.

After any caustic ingestion, the resultant injury may range from mild and nonulcerative to severe, ulcerative, and necrotic. With significant esophageal injury, there is a predictable histologic progression. In the first 3 to 4 days, the exposed epithelium develops edema, erythema, ulceration, and necrosis, with associated bacterial invasion and tissue sloughing. Subsequently, neovascularization and fibroblast proliferation facilitate granulation and collagen cross-linking, which begins approximately 4 days after injury and corresponds to the time at which the tensile strength is lowest and the tissue is most vulnerable to perforation. As the healing process continues in the 3 to 6 weeks following the injury, fibrosis, contractures, and cicatrisation develop, and strictures may occur.

Classification of the extent of esophageal injury may help to determine the risks of stricture formation. Classification schema differ slightly, but in general group esophageal injury into first-, second-, and third-degree burns. First-degree burns (Type I) are characterized by hyperemia and edema. Second-degree (Type II) burns are ulcerated, and may be either discrete (IIa) or circumferential (IIb). Third-degree (Type III) burns are necrotic, with either scattered (IIIa) or extensive (IIIb) necrosis. Type I injuries are never associated with stricture, Type II develop strictures in up to 75% of cases, and Type III burns progress to stricture formation without exception.

CLINICAL PRESENTATION

Ingestion of a caustic substance is by far the most common route of exposure and the most significant cause of morbidity and mortality. The clinical progression of esophageal injury takes place in three phases, which correspond to the histopathologic stages described. Patients usually experience pain on contact with ingestion. Depending on the formulation ingested the patient may have burns of the mouth, lips, and oropharynx (Figure 48–2). Children may drool and refuse to drink. Evidence of upper airway injury may also present. Retrosternal chest pain, hematemesis, or abdominal pain may signify esophageal or gastric injury. Esophageal or visceral perforation is a dreaded and grave complication of caustic ingestion, par-

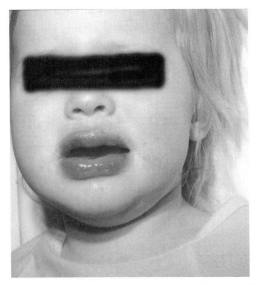

Fig. 48–2. A 3-year-old girl with oropharyngeal burns after ingesting a strong alkaline caustic (pipeline cleaner).

ticularly when part of the initial presentation. Fever, dyspnea, chest pain, and subcutaneous emphysema of the neck and chest herald mediastinitis. Caustic peritonitis may also be associated with viscous perforation. Other catastrophic complications include hemorrhage secondary to vessel erosion, aortoesophageal or tracheoesophageal fistulae, and pulmonary thrombosis. Ulceration and tissue sloughing may occur at approximately 72 hours or thereafter, rendering the tissue vulnerable to perforation.

During the latent phase, from 1 to 3 weeks postingestion, edema subsides and mucosal lesions heal; the patient is often asymptomatic. However, the granulation and collagen formation taking place provide the groundwork for stricture formation. Stricture formation and esophageal dysmotility characterize the chronic phase, usually developing within the first 4 to 8 weeks, but sometimes occurring months to years later.

Much has been written about historical and clinical predictors of esophageal injury. In the pediatric population, most ingestions involve small volumes; therefore, many patients have no esophageal or other organ injury, and recover without sequelae. Older standards of practice called for early endoscopy of all patients regardless of age, circumstances of ingestion, and presence of symptoms and signs. A number of earlier pediatric studies concluded that symptoms and signs were not predictive of endoscopy-demonstrated esophageal injury. However, these studies do not classify the severity or significance of endoscopic injury, making interpretation of these data difficult.

Recent literature has taken a more systematic approach. Gaudreault and colleagues retrospectively evaluated 378 children and concluded that, although children with symptoms were more likely to have significant esophageal burns (Type II or worse), 12% of asymptomatic children had Type IIa to IIIb injury. The study's retrospective design raises the question of symptom underreporting, and the symptoms evaluated did not include respiratory distress or stridor. Subsequent studies have demonstrated consistently that the complete absence of symptoms such as vomiting, prolonged drooling, abdominal pain, dysphagia, and refusal to drink, or signs such as oropharyngeal burns, respiratory distress, and stridor is highly predictive of the absence of significant esophageal injury. Predictors of significant injury include a history of ingestion of a strong acid or alkali, a deliberate or large-volume ingestion, and the presence of two or more of the symptoms described. Severity of injury on endoscopy appears not to differ significantly between acid and alkali ingestions.

Ocular or dermal exposure may cause burns and scarring of varying severity to affected tissues. Caustic eye injury can have devastating consequences, with blindness frequently resulting from extensive exposure. Inhalation exposure, whether isolated or as a result of concomitant ingestion, may involve the upper airway, with epiglottic and laryngeal edema and ulceration, or lower airways, with pneumonitis and impaired gas exchange. These patients, although not always symptomatic at the time of initial evaluation, often present with drooling, stridor, and respiratory distress. Laryngeal injury may progress quickly to life-threatening airway obstruction.

LABORATORY, RADIOGRAPHIC, AND ENDOSCOPIC EVALUATION

Any patient in whom a significant caustic ingestion is suspected should have a complete blood count, electrolytes, blood typing and cross-match, and blood urea nitrogen/creatinine. In addition, coagulation studies are indicated in severe caustic injury. A serum pH is useful both as an indicator of tissue necrosis, and to confirm systemic absorption of ingested acids. Progressive acidemia indicates severe tissue injury. Acids (e.g., sulfuric) produce an elevated anion gap acidosis; however, hydrochloric acid dissociates to form hydrogen and chloride ions, producing a hyperchloremic, normal anion gap acidosis.

Plain x-rays of the chest are obtained to assess possible esophageal perforation or mediastinitis. A lateral neck film may demonstrate laryngeal edema. Contrast esophagrams are not useful immediately after ingestion, and dye extravasation in the context of perforation may further complicate the clinical course. Contrast studies are more useful in the later stages of injury, to evaluate esophageal caliber and stricture formation (Figure 48–3).

The cornerstone of evaluation after caustic ingestion is endoscopic visualization of the upper GI tract. Endoscopy should be performed within the first 48 hours after ingestion, before the tissue becomes weakened and therefore at greater risk for iatrogenic perforation. Flexible endoscopy is preferred to minimize perforation risk and to permit visualization of areas distal to a first lesion; passage of a rigid scope through significantly injured areas is not advisable.

In general, endoscopy is indicated for any large-volume, intentional, or strong acid or alkali ingestion, as well as in any patient with respiratory distress, stridor, or hematemesis. In addition, two of any symptoms such as vomiting, prolonged drooling, abdominal pain, dysphagia, and refusal to drink are indications for endoscopic evaluation. Endoscopic classification of injury should guide further management and anticipation of sequelae.

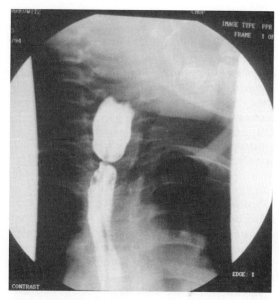

Fig. 48–3. Barium swallow demonstrating esophageal stricture from alkaline caustic ingestion.

MANAGEMENT

Initial Resuscitation

Caustic airway injury may rapidly progress to severe airway edema and compromise, so careful and constant attention to symptoms and signs of respiratory distress is imperative. Although no one clinical finding is consistently predictive of impending airway crisis, any patient with stridor or excessive drooling should have a radiographic evaluation and direct visualization of the laryngeal structures. Given the potentially rapid progression of airway edema, prophylactic intubation is often warranted, and should be done under direct or fiberoptic visualization. Blind and nasal intubation are contraindicated owing to the risk of perforation of injured laryngeal structures.

Decontamination

Any residual caustic is removed from the patient's clothing, skin, and eyes. Ocular and dermal lavage with copious sterile saline or water should be performed as soon as possible. The standard battery of GI decontamination methods often employed in poisoned patients has little use in the caustic ingestion. Emesis is contraindicated, because it reintroduces the offending substance to the esophagus, larynx, and oropharynx. Charcoal is also inappropriate because it does not bind most caustics, can induce emesis, and can obscure endoscopic visualization. Gastric lavage to lessen systemic absorption and toxicity is potentially useful, but only when a large-volume acid ingestion has occurred very recently; however, the risk of perforations associated with passage of a nasogastric or orogastric tube must be taken into consideration. Whole bowel irrigation is not an appropriate GI decontamination method for caustic ingestions.

Two other initial techniques that are sometimes advocated, especially with caustic household products, include neutralization and dilution. *Neutralization* is a process by which a weakly basic solution is given to the patient with acid ingestion—or the converse for alkali ingestion—in an attempt to neutralize the pH of the substance and minimize tissue damage. In fact, neutralization produces an exothermic reaction, and may exacerbate tissue injury. Furthermore, most caustic tissue damage occurs almost instantaneously after ingestion, rendering neutralization useless and potentially dangerous.

Dilution, through the administration of a neutral solution such as milk or water, may have some benefit in the home setting immediately after a caustic ingestion. In fact, this is often recommended as part of initial poison center protocol. This technique does not generate heat and cause thermal tissue damage, and may decrease transit time and diminish tissue contact with caustic substances. In vitro studies suggest a role for dilution, but clinical utility seems limited at most to the minutes immediately postingestion, before irreversible tissue damage has already occurred. The introduction of any substance into already injured esophageal tissue carries inherent risk of perforation, and vomiting may ensue, causing reinjury from the swallowed caustic. Dilution, therefore, should be attempted only immediately after ingestion in very cooperative children.

Surgical Exploration

Early surgical exploration has some role in the patient with known serious visceral caustic injury associated with perforation, mediastinitis, and severe acidosis. Fortunately, this is rare in pediatric caustic ingestions, and is largely confined to large-volume intentional ingestions in the adolescent and adult population.

Corticosteroids

The most controversial treatment modality after caustic ingestion is the use of corticosteroids to prevent the pathologic collagen cross-linking, shortening, and cicatrisation that give rise to esophageal stricture formation. Literature

suggests that although children with first-degree injuries do not develop strictures, and those with third-degree injuries almost always progress to strictures, those with second-degree injuries have variable outcomes and potentially benefit most from this therapy. A number of studies have attempted to analyze the benefit of corticosteroids after caustic ingestion. In 1990, Anderson and co-workers studied 60 children and demonstrated no decrease in stricture formation in the steroid versus the control group; however, there were insufficient numbers in this 18-year study to perform subgroup analyses of patients with second-degree injuries, the very patient population of most interest. Howell and associates conducted a meta-analysis of 361 children in 1992, which demonstrated a reduction in strictures in children with second-degree injuries or greater when treated with steroids (24% versus 52%); however, the nature of a meta-analysis' reliance on varied data leaves this conclusion still open for debate and further research. Although there are inconclusive data at this time, corticosteroids should be considered in patients with second-degree injuries, in whom the reduction in morbidity from esophageal stricture outweigh the risks of therapy. Methylprednisolone 2 mg/kg/d or dexamethasone 1 mg/kg/d is instituted ideally within 24 hours after ingestion. The increased risk of infection associated with steroid use must also be considered. Antibiotics should be given concurrently.

Hydrofluoric Acid

Hydrofluoric acid (HF) is commonly found in cleaning, etching, and rust-removing products and deserves special consideration. HF is a weak acid that behaves more like a strong alkali. External contact can result in severe dermal or ocular injury. Death has been reported with exposures affecting as little as 2.5% of the body surface area. Severe pain and deep penetration despite minimal skin findings is the hallmark of an HF burn. The mechanism of injury involves liquefaction necrosis and the formation of insoluble calcium and magnesium salts. Oral ingestions are frequently fatal. In cases of significant burns, systemic acidosis, hypocalcemia, hypomagnesemia, and hyperkalemia are common. Renal failure and hemolysis have been reported to occur.

In the prehospital setting, copious irrigation to decrease diffusion is indicated immediately after the exposure. In the ED, a topical calcium gluconate gel can be made by mixing 2.5 to 3.5 g of calcium gluconate powder in 5 ounces of water-soluble lubricant (K–Y jelly). Alternatively, 25 mL of a 10% calcium gluconate solution can be mixed in to create the gel. For hand burns, the

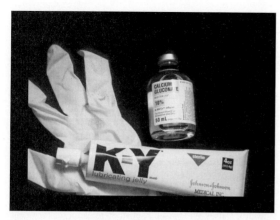

Fig. 48–4. A calcium gluconate gel can be easily mixed to treat hydrofluoric acid skin burns.

calcium gel can be filled into a latex glove, and worn by the patient (Figure 48–4). For minor burns not responsive to topical therapy, pain can also be alleviated by intradermal injection of 5% calcium gluconate 0.5 to 1.0 cm away from the burn site using a 27- or 30-gauge needle. Calcium chloride salt should be avoided because it can be corrosive to the skin. For severe extremity burns, intra-arterial administration of 5% to 10% calcium gluconate in 40 mL D_5W via the radial or ulnar artery has been shown to be beneficial in older children and adults. In cases of oral ingestion, intravenous calcium and magnesium are given on a milliequivalent per milliequivalent basis as needed.

Inhalation exposures to HF may be responsive to calcium gluconate nebulizer treatments (1.5 mL of 10% calcium gluconate in 4.5 mL of sterile water). For ocular exposures, 1% calcium gluconate prepared by adding 50 mL of 10% solution in 500 mL of normal saline can be used as an irrigation solution. However, prompt irrigation after exposure with sterile water or normal saline may be more important than the specific irrigant used with these potentially devastating injuries.

DISPOSITION

Asymptomatic children in whom a significant caustic exposure is suspected should have a 4- to 6-hour period of observation. Any child who is symptomatic after caustic ingestion is admitted to the hospital for further observation and evaluation by an appropriate specialist. Patients

with any respiratory or airway symptoms, significant acidosis, or suspected mediastinitis or perforation should be admitted to an intensive care unit, with surgical consultation. Those with symptomatic hydrofluoric acid injuries not responsive to topical therapy are admitted for observation and continued calcium therapy and burn care. Patients with severe hydrofluoric acid injuries should be admitted to an intensive care setting or designated burn unit.

SEQUELAE

Esophageal stricture is the most common long-term adverse outcome after caustic ingestion. A number of treatment methods have been suggested for the prevention of stricture formation, including corticosteroids and esophageal stenting. Unfortunately, strictures are inevitable in children with severe esophageal burns, and some may even develop multiple strictures of different caliber throughout the esophageal lumen. Feeding through a gastrostomy tube may be necessary, both in the immediate postingestion period, as well as long term. Treatment of strictures involves repeated esophageal dilations over months to years.

Other sequelae of caustic injury include scarring of any organ system originally affected, including the airway, face, eyes, and other viscera. Gastric outlet obstruction and dysmotility may occur. Longitudinal studies of patients with caustic ingestion have shown as high as a 1000-fold increase in the risk of esophageal and gastric carcinoma at an average of 40 years postingestion. Children in whom endoscopy reveals significant lesions require lifelong surveillance for development of malignancy.

CASE OUTCOME

Subsequent evaluation included endoscopy, which revealed multiple second-degree esophageal injuries. Corticosteroid and antibiotic therapy were instituted. The patient underwent gastrostomy tube placement on day 7. She was extubated without incident 1 week after the injury and discharged to a chronic rehabilitation facility the following week. Follow-up barium esophagram revealed no evidence of esophageal stricture.

CONCLUSION

Although pediatric caustic injuries are generally less severe than those in adults, there is still considerable potential for severe injury and life-long morbidity from these agents. Much has been done to determine the best methods to evaluate and treat these children; however, the importance of prevention, particularly the effective preventive legislation over the last 50 years, cannot be overemphasized.

SUGGESTED READINGS

Anderson KD, Rouse TM, Randolph JG: A controlled trial of corticosteroids in children with corrosive injury of the esophagus. *N Engl J Med* 323:637–640, 1990.

Appelqvist P, Salmo S: Lye corrosion carcinoma of the esophagus: a review of 63 cases. *Cancer* 45:2655–2658, 1980.

Bautista A, Varela R, Villanueva A, et al: Effects of prednisolone and dexamethasone in children with alkali burns of the oesophagus. *Eur J Pediatr Surg* 6:198–203, 1996.

Boldt GB, Carroll RG: Titratable acid/alkaline reserve is not predictive of esophageal perforation risk after caustic exposure. *Am J Emerg Med* 14:106–108, 1996.

Christesen HBT: Prediction of complications following unintentional caustic ingestion in children. Is endoscopy always necessary? *Acta Paediatr* 84:1177–1182, 1995.

Crain E, Gershel J, Mezey A: Caustic ingestions: symptoms as predictors of esophageal injury. *Am J Dis Child* 138:863–865, 1984.

Eaton H, Tennekoon GE: Squamous carcinoma of the stomach following corrosive acid burns. *Br J Surg* 59:382–386, 1972.

Edmonson MB: Caustic alkali ingestions by farm children. *Pediatrics* 79:413–416, 1987.

Gaudreault P, Parent M, McGuigan M, et al: Predictability of esophageal injury from signs and symptoms: a study of caustic ingestion in 378 children. *Pediatrics* 71:767–770, 1983.

Gorman RL, Khin-Maung-Gyi M, Klein-Schwartz W, et al: Initial symptoms as predictors of esophageal injury in alkaline corrosive ingestions. *Am J Emerg Med* 10:189–194, 1992.

Homan CS, Maitra S, Lane B, et al: Histopathologic evaluation of the therapeutic efficacy of water and milk dilution for esophageal acid injury. *Acad Emerg Med* 2:587–591, 1995.

Homan CS, Singer AJ, Thomajan C, et al: Thermal characteristics of neutralization therapy and water dilution for strong acid ingestion: an in-vivo canine model. *Acad Emerg Med* 5:286–292, 1998.

Homan CS, Maitra S, Lane B, et al: Effective treatment for acute alkali injury to the esophagus using weak-acid neutralization therapy: An ex-vivo study. *Acad Emerg Med* 2:952–958, 1995.

Homan CS, Maitra S, Lane B, et al: Therapeutic effects of water and milk for acute alkali injury of the esophagus. *Acad Emerg Med* 24:14–20, 1994.

Hopkins RA, Posthlethwait RW: Caustic burns and carcinoma of the esophagus. *Ann Surg* 194:146–148, 1981.

Howell J, Dalsey W, Hartsell F, et al: Steroids for the treatment of corrosive esophageal injury: A statistical analysis of past studies. *Am J Emerg Med* 10:421–425, 1992.

Lamireau T, Rebouissoux L, Denis D, et al: Accidental caustic ingestion in children: Is endoscopy always mandatory? *J Pediatr Gastroenterol Nutr* 33:81–84, 2001.

Maull KI, Osmand AP, Maull CD: Liquid caustic ingestions: an in vitro study of the effects of buffer, neutralization, and dilution. *Ann Emerg Med* 14:1160–1162, 1985.

Mutaf O, Ulman I: A critique of systemic steroids in the management of caustic esophageal burns in children. *Eur J Pediatr Surg* 8:71–74, 1998.

Nuutinen M, Uhari M, Karvali T, et al: Consequences of caustic ingestions in children. *Acta Paediatr* 83:1200–1205, 1994.

Previtera C, Giusti F, Guglielmi M: Predictive value of visible lesions in suspected caustic ingestion: may endoscopy reasonably be omitted in completely negative pediatric patients? *Pediatr Emerg Care* 6:176–178, 1990.

Rumack BH, Burrington JD: Caustic ingestions: a rational look at diluents. *Clin Toxicol* 11:27–34, 1977.

Seamens C, Seger D, Meridith T: Hydrofluoric acid. In: Ford M, Delaney K, Ling L, et al, eds: *Clinical Toxicology.* Philadelphia: Saunders; 2001:1019–1026.

Vergauwen P, Moulin D, Buts JP, et al: Caustic burns of the upper digestive and respiratory tracts. *Eur J Pediatr* 150:700–703, 1991.

49

Hydrocarbons

Bonnie McManus
Gregory Gaar

HIGH-YIELD FACTS

- Young children most frequently ingest hydrocarbons accidentally, whereas adolescents are more likely to abuse volatile substances or deliberately ingest hydrocarbons in suicidal gestures or attempts.

- Viscosity, volatility, and surface tension are physical properties that affect the type and extent of toxicity. Heavier compounds, such as mineral or baby oil, paraffin, and asphalt have a minimal risk of toxicity.

- The principal concern after most hydrocarbon ingestions is pulmonary toxicity.

- In general, ingestion of most petroleum distillates in a volume of less than 1 to 2 mL/kg body weight does not cause systemic toxicity.

- In a patient with any with a history of hydrocarbon ingestion, it is essential to try to identify the compound.

- Most sources discourage the use of gastrointestinal (GI) decontamination procedures in the case of accidental ingestions.

- Activated charcoal is not indicated in the vast majority of hydrocarbon ingestions.

- Glucocorticoids do not affect outcome and their use is not indicated.

CASE PRESENTATION

A 3-year-old girl presents to the emergency department (ED) 90 minutes after she was found in the backyard shed coughing and choking with the smell of gasoline on her breath and her clothes. The child is normally healthy. Vitals upon presentation reveal a respiratory rate of 40 breaths per minute; pulse of 120 bpm; blood pressure of 80/50 mmHg; and a temperature of 100.0°F. The patient was somewhat agitated. Her lung examination was remarkable for coarse breath sounds bilaterally.

INTRODUCTION

Hydrocarbons are organic compounds ubiquitous in daily life. Typical hydrocarbon products include gasoline, stove or lamp fuel, paints and paint thinners, glues, spot removers, degreasers, and typewriter correction fluid. In 2001, the National Data Collection System of the American Association of Poison Control Centers received 30,608 calls concerning hydrocarbons in patients younger than 20 years of age. Children under 6 years of age accounted for 73% of these calls. There were four pediatric deaths reported. Three of the cases involved teenagers who died following inhalation abuse, and one case involved a 12 month old who aspirated lamp oil. The hydrocarbons most frequently ingested in accidental childhood poisonings include gasoline, lubricating motor oil, lamp oil, kerosene, lighter fluid, mineral seal oil, and turpentine. The mechanism of exposure varies with age. Young children most frequently ingest hydrocarbons accidentally, whereas adolescents are more likely to abuse volatile substances or deliberately ingest hydrocarbons in suicidal gestures or attempts.

CLASSIFICATION AND PROPERTIES

Hydrocarbons are derived from petroleum distillation, which generates compounds composed of chains of varying lengths. The length of the chain affects the behavior of the hydrocarbon. At room temperature, short chains of carbons are gases such as methane and butane. Intermediate-length chains are liquids and account for most exposures seen in the ED. Compounds that are solids at room temperature, such as tar and paraffin, are long-chain hydrocarbons. The terpenes, which are derived from wood distillation, are toxicologically considered as hydrocarbons because of the similarity of their clinical effects.

There are three major classes of hydrocarbons. The *aliphatic*, or straight-chain compounds, include kerosene, mineral seal oil, gasoline, solvents, and paint thinners. Aliphatic compounds include halogenated hydrocarbons such as carbon tetrachloride and trichloroethane which are typically found in industrial settings as solvents. The *halogenated hydrocarbons* are well absorbed by the lung and gut, making them particularly dangerous. Centrilobular hepatic necrosis and renal failure are associated with ingestion of halogenated hydrocarbons, especially carbon tetrachloride. Fatal liver injury has been reported after ingestion of as little as 3 mL of carbon tetrachloride.

The *cyclic* or *aromatic compounds* contain a benzene ring, and are used in industrial solvents. The aromatics are highly volatile, and unlike the straight-chain hydrocarbons, benzene and its major derivatives toluene and xylene are well absorbed from the GI tract. Of the aromatics, benzene is the most toxic, with death reported after ingestion of as little as 15 mL. The terpene compounds consist mainly of cyclic terpene rings, and include compounds such as turpentine and pine oil.

Viscosity, volatility, and surface tension are physical properties that affect the type and extent of toxicity. *Viscosity* is resistance to flow and is the most important property in determining the risk of aspiration. The lower the viscosity (often expressed in Saybolt seconds universal), the higher the risk of pulmonary aspiration, and thus more toxic the compound. *Volatility* is the propensity of a substance to become a gas. If a compound is volatile, it displaces oxygen in the alveoli and causes transient hypoxia. *Surface tension* describes the propensity of a compound to adhere to itself at the liquid's surface. Low surface tension allows easy spread over a wide surface area. A substance with low surface tension may easily spread from the oropharynx to the trachea, promoting aspiration. Compounds that have low viscosity and low surface tension have the highest risk of aspiration.

Mineral seal oil has very low volatility but surprisingly low viscosity. When ingested it is likely to cause aspiration and pneumonia. Heavier compounds, such as mineral or baby oil, paraffin, and asphalt have a minimal risk of pulmonary toxicity. Gaseous hydrocarbons such as methane and butane can act as asphyxiants by displacing air in the lungs. They are also capable of crossing the capillary membrane and directly causing central nervous system (CNS) depression. Gasoline and naphtha have relatively high volatilities and can cause primary CNS depression after inhalation of fumes while causing minimal pulmonary damage.

PATHOPHYSIOLOGY

The principal concern after most hydrocarbon ingestions is pulmonary toxicity following aspiration into the lungs. Many studies in animal models involving gastric instillation of hydrocarbons suggest pulmonary toxicity does not occur through GI absorption alone. Very small amounts of an ingested compound may be aspirated and result in chemical or lipoid pneumonitis. Chemical pneumonitis may be due to direct destruction of lung tissue itself, depending on the type of hydrocarbon, or may be due to an aggressive inflammatory reaction. Delayed injury may be due to the destruction of surfactant, which results in decreased lung compliance and potentially significant atelectasis. Noncardiogenic pulmonary edema and bacterial superinfection can occur. Hemorrhagic pulmonary edema and respiratory arrest can occur within 24 hours. Following resolution of the acute insult, pulmonary dysfunction can persist for years. Lipoid pneumonia is seen frequently with high-viscosity hydrocarbons such as mineral oil and liquid paraffin. This lesion is more localized and less inflammatory than the reaction produced by low-viscosity petroleum distillates like kerosene. Hemorrhagic pneumonitis does not occur. Despite the less-aggressive inflammatory response, lipoid pneumonitis can take several weeks to resolve.

CNS compromise is frequently seen, but the factors responsible for this are unclear. Neurologic injury may be due to the direct effect on the CNS by the ingested hydrocarbon, but most authorities agree that asphyxiation and hypoxia are major contributors to CNS lesions.

The aromatic hydrocarbons have a high potential for causing major CNS depression. The terpenes are easily absorbed and typically cause mild CNS depression. The halogenated and volatile hydrocarbons may produce a euphoric state similar to alcohol intoxication. These products rapidly attain high concentrations in the CNS and can suppress ventilatory drive. This is most commonly seen in the adolescent glue sniffer, who appears intoxicated.

GI symptoms include nausea, vomiting, abdominal pain, and diarrhea. These symptoms are frequent but usually mild. Vomiting increases the risk of aspiration pneumonitis; therefore, it is important to limit emesis. Ingestion or chronic inhalation abuse can cause hematemesis. In general, ingestion of most petroleum distillates in a volume less than 1 to 2 mL/kg does not cause systemic toxicity.

When skin is exposed to hydrocarbons for an extended time, an eczematoid dermatitis develops owing to the drying and defatting action of these compounds. This is typically seen in adolescents abusing volatile substances and is known as *glue sniffer's rash*. It is predominantly located in the perioral area or midface regions. There may be significant skin erythema, inflammation, and pruritis. Gasoline and other hydrocarbons can cause full-thickness burns. Renal failure has been reported after the use of diesel fuel as a shampoo, strongly suggesting cutaneous absorption.

Fever is seen on presentation in 30% of cases. It does not correlate with clinical symptoms of infection and is possibly of central origin. Three fourths of patients defervesce within 24 hours. If fever persists for more than 48 to 72 hours, bacterial superinfection should be considered.

Organ system effects may also be due to compounds dissolved in a hydrocarbon solvent. Many anticholinesterase pesticides are combined with kerosene vehicles. A cholinergic crisis might be the cause of excessive bronchorrhea, salivation, lacrimation, or urinary incontinence. The classic bradycardia and miosis may be obscured by the tachycardia and mydriasis from hydrocarbon-induced hypoxia.

CLINICAL PRESENTATION

On presentation, patients may be completely asymptomatic or may suffer severe respiratory distress and CNS depression. A history of coughing or gagging is consistent with aspiration. In addition to cough, early signs of pulmonary toxicity include gasping, choking, tachypnea, and wheezing. Bronchospasm may contribute to ventilation–perfusion mismatch and exacerbate hypoxia. Cyanosis

may be present. In early stages, cyanosis is usually due to replacement of alveolar air by volatilized hydrocarbon. In later stages, it is due to direct pulmonary toxicity. CNS symptoms range from irritability, which can be a sign of hypoxia, to lethargy and coma.

After a significant oral ingestion, GI disturbance is common. In any patient with a history of hydrocarbon ingestion it is essential to try to identify the compound, because this information can have profound implications for management and prognosis.

LABORATORY STUDIES

In about 90% of patients with respiratory symptoms on presentation, the initial chest radiograph will be normal. However, radiographic abnormalities can occur as early as 20 minutes or as late as 24 hours after ingestion. Typical findings include increased bronchovascular markings and bibasilar and perihilar infiltrates (see Figure 24–9 for a representative chest radiograph). Lobar consolidation is uncommon. Pneumothorax, pneumomediastinum, and pleural effusions are rare. Pneumatoceles can occur and resolve over weeks. Oxygen saturation and arterial blood gas analysis help in determining pulmonary status. Depending on the severity of the ingestion, the patient's acid–base status, electrolyte balance, complete blood count, and hepatic profile should be followed. If an aromatic hydrocarbon like benzene is ingested, a complete blood count should be followed to rule out hematotoxicity.

MANAGEMENT
General

The mainstay of treatment for hydrocarbon exposure is supportive care. It essential to realize that although the vast majority of patients present with minimal if any symptoms, patients with respiratory compromise on presentation to the ED can suffer rapid deterioration. Thus, oxygenation and ventilation are initial priorities. Any patient with respiratory symptoms, including grunting, tachypnea, or cyanosis, is treated with humidified oxygen and requires an arterial blood gas evaluation. An abnormal alveolar–arterial gradient is frequently present in serious exposures. Nebulized β-2 agonists are the drugs of choice for patients with bronchospasm. Patients with respiratory failure require artificial ventilation. Because hydrocarbons solubilize surfactant, continuous positive airway pressure or positive end-expiratory pressure may be needed as a ventilatory adjunct. Extracorporeal membrane oxygenation (ECMO) has been reported to be successful in pediatric patients suffering hydrocarbon-induced pneumonitis who fail to respond to conventional ventilatory support (see Chapter 19).

Patients with altered mental status should have a bedside glucose test or be treated empirically with intravenous (IV) dextrose. Cyanosis is usually due to hypoxia, but may also be due to methemoglobinemia in cases where aniline or nitrobenzene has been ingested. Exposure to methylene chloride is a concern because it is frequently found in paint strippers. After exposure it is metabolized to carbon monoxide. Carbon monoxide poisoning must be considered in patients with persistent symptoms. Treatment consists of 100% oxygen. Depending on the degree of toxicity and the carboxyhemoglobin level, hyperbaric oxygen may be considered.

Gastric Evacuation

Most sources discourage the use of gastric decontamination procedures in cases of accidental ingestions. The risk of aspiration is generally higher than the risk of systemic absorption. Children are not likely to accidentally ingest sufficient quantities of hydrocarbons to cause significant systemic absorption.

The Cooperative Kerosene Poisoning Study concluded that gastric lavage was neither harmful nor beneficial. Pulmonary complications correlated better with the quantity of petroleum distillate ingested (>1 oz) or the fact that the patient vomited than with the use or omission of gastric lavage. Another study showed that in children in whom the time course of illness was known, 88% were symptomatic within 10 minutes of ingestion. Currently, gastric evacuation is not recommended in patients with minimal or no symptoms after accidental ingestion of a pure petroleum distillate or turpentine.

Gastric evacuation of most types of hydrocarbons is reserved for massive ingestions, which usually occur in adults or adolescents with intentional exposures. Although still controversial, recent ingestions of >4 to 5 mL/kg of naphtha, gasoline, kerosene, or turpentine probably justify evacuation. Other ingestions in which gastric evacuation is indicated are for those that contain dangerous additives such as benzene, toluene, halogenated hydrocarbons, heavy metals, camphor, pesticides, aniline, or other toxic compounds.

Ipecac is contraindicated, particularly if there is previous unprovoked emesis or any degree of neurologic, res-

piratory, or cardiac compromise. In cases where gastric lavage is indicated, the airway should be protected via endotracheal intubation with a cuffed tube. If the child is younger than 8 years old, inflate the cuff only during the lavage procedure. A nasogastric tube should be adequate to remove liquids. However, if a solid is ingested concomitantly, a small tube would be insufficient for adequate evacuation. Orogastric tubes, without the added protection of the airway by an endotracheal tube, are extremely controversial because insertion can induce gagging and vomiting, resulting in aspiration.

Activated charcoal is contraindicated in the vast majority of hydrocarbon ingestions. It does adsorb kerosene, turpentine, and benzene in vitro or in animal models. However, because it may induce vomiting, it is generally discouraged unless there is a coingestant known to be well adsorbed by charcoal. Its efficacy for other hydrocarbons is not documented.

Dermal Decontamination

In the event of a cutaneous exposure, all clothing is removed and the skin is irrigated and washed twice with soap and water. No special cleansers or solvents are usually necessary. Appropriate precautions should be taken by staff members to avoid becoming contaminated. It is important to remember that many of the hydrocarbons are flammable and pose a risk from fire.

Ancillary Therapy

IV hydration may be indicated for patients with significant vomiting or diarrhea and for patients with respiratory compromise who are unable to take oral fluids. Fluid replacement is restricted to a maintenance rate to diminish the risk of overhydration and the exacerbation of pulmonary edema. Glucocorticoids do not affect outcome and their use is not indicated. Antibiotics are reserved for patients with definite evidence of infection. The use of commercially available surfactants in animal models has been evaluated. At present no clear recommendations can be made for its use in human exposures.

DISPOSITION

A patient who accidentally ingests a hydrocarbon and presents to the ED without symptoms should be observed for 6 hours. If during that time they remain asymptomatic, and oxygen saturation and a chest radiograph are normal, discharge is appropriate. If symptoms develop during the 6-hour period of observation, hospital admission is indicated.

All patients who are symptomatic on presentation are admitted to the hospital. If respiratory compromise or hypoxia is present, admission to a pediatric intensive care unit is advised. Hospital admission is also indicated when there is risk of significant delayed organ toxicity as in the case of ingestion of carbon tetrachloride or other toxic additives. When they are medically stable, psychiatric evaluation is needed for adolescents who acted with suicidal intent.

VOLATILE SUBSTANCE ABUSE

Among adolescents, inhalation abuse of volatile hydrocarbons is a significant health hazard. Typically, solvent-containing fluids such as typewriter correction fluid, adhesives, and other halogenated hydrocarbons such as those found in gasoline and cigarette lighter fluid are abused. These substances are inexpensive, easily obtained, and readily concealed.

Volatile substance abuse typically involves more than just sniffing. Multiple deep inhalations are taken after the substance is poured into a plastic bag, which is known as *bagging*. Alternatively, a cloth is saturated and held to the face, which is known as *huffing*. Aerosolized products may be bubbled through water first to remove the unwanted product, and then the gases captured and inhaled.

The predominant acute risk of inhalation abuse is *sudden sniffing death*. It is believed that the myocardium is hypersensitized and a sudden outpouring of sympathetic stimulation leads to fatal cardiac dysrhythmias. There have been numerous case reports of patients abusing solvents and then collapsing shortly after beginning marked physical exertion or being startled. Other indirect effects of volatile abuse include trauma owing to impaired judgment, aspiration, and asphyxia associated with plastic bags.

As with alcohol, acute poisoning with volatile substances involves an initial period of euphoria and disinhibition, with further intoxication leading to dysphoria, ataxia, confusion, and hallucinations. There is rapid onset and recovery, but repeated inhalations can prolong the altered state. Because of the short half-life of these substances, patients rarely present acutely intoxicated. However, if this should be the case, take care not to stress or excite the patient because this may stimulate cardiac dysrhythmias. Treatment of the intoxicated patient consists of supportive measures. If resuscitation is necessary, standard advanced cardiac life support measures are indicated (see Chapter 59).

CASE OUTCOME

The child demonstrates worsening respiratory distress in the ED. A pulse oximetry reading of 88% is recorded. Following administration of IV midazolam, she is orally intubated without complications. Initial chest radiograph demonstrates good tube placement without evidence of infiltrate or consolidation. The patient is transported to the nearest tertiary care center pediatric intensive care unit (PICU) by helicopter. In the intensive care unit, she develops a fever 24 hours postingestion and radiographic evidence of an aspiration pneumonitis. Her white blood cell count is not elevated and her pulmonary status is not deteriorating. She received continued pulmonary supportive care but no antibiotics. After 36 hours in the PICU, she is transferred to the general pediatric floor and recovers uneventfully.

SUGGESTED READINGS

Anas N, Namasonthi V, Ginsburg CM: Criteria for hospitalizing children who have ingested products containing hydrocarbons. *JAMA* 246:840–843, 1981.

Anene O, Castello FV: Myocardial dysfunction after hydrocarbon ingestion. *Crit Care Med* 22:528–530, 1994.

Bandla HP, Davis SH, Hopkins NE: Lipoid pneumonia: A silent complication of mineral oil aspiration. *Pediatrics* 103:19, 1999.

Bass M. Sniffing gasoline. *JAMA* 255:2604–2605, 1986.

Carder JR, Fuerst RS: Myocardial infarction after toluene inhalation. *Pediatr Emerg Care* 13:117–119, 1997.

Dice WH, Ward G, Kelly J, et al: Pulmonary toxicity following gastrointestinal ingestion of kerosene. *Ann Emerg Med* 11:138–142, 1982.

Esmail A, Meyer L, Pottier A, et al: Deaths from volatile substance abuse in those under 18 years: Results from a national epidemiological study. *Arch Dis Child* 69:356, 1993.

Espeland KE. Inhalants: The instant, but deadly high. *Pediatr Nurs* 23:82–86, 1997.

Goldfrank LR, Kulgberg AG, Bresnitz EA: Hydrocarbons. In: Goldfrank LR, Flomenbaum NE, Lewin NA, et al, eds: *Goldfrank's Toxicologic Emergencies.* Norwalk, CT: Appleton & Lange; 1998:1383–1398.

Hart LM, Cobaugh DJ, Dean BS, et al: Successful use of extracorporeal membrane oxygenation (ECMO) in the treatment of refractory respiratory failure secondary to hydrocarbon aspiration (abstract). *Vet Hum Toxicol* 33:361, 1991.

Leikin JB, Kaufman D, Lipscomb JW, et al: Methylene chloride: Report of five exposures and two deaths. *Am J Emerg Med* 8:534, 1990.

Litovitz TL, Schwartz-Klein W, Rogers, GC, et al: 2001 Annual Report of the AAPCC Toxic Exposure/Surveillance System. *Am J Emerg Med* 20:391–452, 2002.

Machado B, Cross K, Snodgrass WR: Accidental hydrocarbon ingestion cases telephoned to a regional poison center. *Ann Emerg Med* 17:804, 1988.

McHugh MJ: The abuse of volatile substances. *Pediatr Clin North Am* 34:333–340, 1987.

Meadows R, Verghese A. Medical complications of glue sniffing. *South Med J* 89:455–462, 1996.

Steffee CH, Davis GJ, Nicol KK: A whiff of death: Fatal volatile solvent inhalation abuse. *South Med J* 89:879–884, 1996.

Subcommittee on Accidental Poisoning (SAP): Cooperative kerosene poisoning study: Evaluation of gastric lavage and other factors in treatment of accidental ingestion of distillate products. *Pediatrics* 29:648–674, 1962.

Widmer LR, Goodwin SR, Berman LS, et al: Artificial surfactant for therapy in hydrocarbon-induced lung injury in sheep. *Crit Care Med* 24:1524–1529, 1996.

50

Mothballs, Camphor, and Deodorizers

Howard A. Greller
Lewis S. Nelson

HIGH-YIELD FACTS

- Camphor is found in a variety of over the counter and home remedies, in which federal law mandates a concentration of less than 11%.

- The primary manifestation of camphor toxicity is seizure activity, which is generally brief and self-limited.

- The toxicities of naphthalene are primarily hematologic, manifesting in delayed hemolytic anemia or methemoglobinemia.

- Paradichlorobenzene is essentially nontoxic when ingested.

CASE PRESENTATION

A 3-year-old girl is brought to the emergency department (ED) after a witnessed generalized tonic–clonic seizure. The seizure lasted several minutes and at the time of presentation had not recurred. The child, who is developmentally normal, has had a mild cough, rhinorrhea, and congestion for a few days. There is no history of fever, rash, sick contacts, or known unintentional ingestion of prescription medication or household products. Her past medical history is unremarkable; there is no history of seizure or seizure disorder in the family; she is taking no medications and has no known allergies.

On physical examination she appears well, without pallor or cyanosis. Her heart rate is 110 bpm, respiratory rate 20 breaths per minute, blood pressure 110/75 mmHg, temperature 97.6°F, and pulse oximetry 100% saturation on room air. The finger stick blood glucose is 110 mg/dL. The child is mildly somnolent but arousable. There is no identifiable focality on neurologic examination and the neck is supple with a full range of motion. She has normal tone, reflexes, and follows simple commands. The child is covered in a strong-smelling, viscous gel from her neck to her lower extremities. The grandmother stated that the gel was Vicks Vapo-Rub, and that she applied it to the child to help with her congestion. The remainder of the physical examination is unremarkable.

INTRODUCTION AND EPIDEMIOLOGY

Camphor, a pleasant-smelling cyclic ketone (Figure 50–1), is an essential oil first produced by distillation of the bark of the camphor tree, *Cinnamomum camphora*. Camphor has been used widely as a fragrance, a bacteriostatic and fungistatic, an aphrodisiac, an antiseptic, a general remedy for cough and cold, a rubifacient, and a liniment. Historically, camphor was used as an abortifacient and suicidal agent. It was widely used as an insect and moth repellant in the early part of the twentieth century in the United States, until it was recognized as dangerous. In 1983, the U.S. Food and Drug Administration banned the nonprescription sale of camphorated oil and limited the concentration of camphor to less than 11% in regulated products. Despite recognition of its potential harm, it is still widely available both in the United States and abroad, in products ranging from camphor blocks to a variety of traditional remedies.

Naphthalene is a bicyclic aromatic compound (see Figure 50–1) that is the most abundant distillate of coal tar. It is commonly used as a fumigant against clothes moths, as a deodorizer in urinal scent disks, and in the manufacturing of dyes, resins, gunpowder, and lubricants.

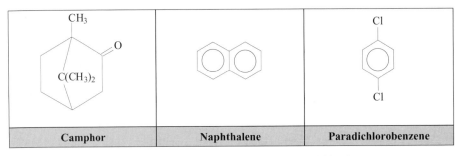

Fig. 50–1. Structures of camphor, naphthalene, and paradichlorobenzene.

Humans are therefore exposed to naphthalene through a wide variety of industrial, occupational, and environmental routes.

Paradichlorobenzene, a halogenated aromatic compound (see Figure 50–1), has replaced the prior two agents as the primary component of moth repellents, and is a very common component of deodorizers (e.g., urinal cakes) and disinfectants.

DEVELOPMENTAL CONSIDERATIONS

Newborns and patients with G-6-PD deficiency (an X-linked enzyme disorder) are at increased susceptibility to the toxicity of naphthalene. There are no specific developmental concerns unique to paradichlorobenzene. Older children have been reported to inhale and abuse mothballs and toilet deodorizers.

PHARMACOLOGY AND TOXICOKINETICS

There are few data concerning the pharmacology and toxicokinetics of camphor. It is rapidly and readily absorbed through dermal, GI, and inhalational exposure. It is very lipid soluble and metabolized in the liver via hydroxylation and glucuronidation, and then renally excreted. There is no consensus in the medical literature on the toxic dose of camphor.

Naphthalene exhibits a wide array of toxicity via ingestion, inhalation, and dermal routes. In humans, naphthalene undergoes metabolism through the cytochrome P450 system, through CYP2E1. The metabolites of naphthalene, and not the parent compound, are responsible for toxicity. The primary toxic metabolite of naphtha-

lene, α-naphthol, is thought to be responsible for the hematologic disorders. Further metabolism of α-naphthol to the reactive species 1,4-naphthoquinone and 1,2-naphthoquinone are thought to lead to the development of reactive oxygen species, with subsequent glutathione depletion, lipid peroxidation, and DNA damage. As with camphor, there is no consensus on the reported toxic dose, and as little as one naphthalene mothball in a child can be consequential.

There are no formal evaluations of the pharmacology or toxicokinetics of paradichlorobenzene. Exposures occur commonly through ingestion and inhalation.

PATHOPHYSIOLOGY

The exact mechanism by which camphor causes seizures is unknown. There is evidence that camphor noncompetitively inhibits nicotinic acetylcholine receptors but whether this leads to the neurotoxicity requires further investigation. Camphor, like many of the essential oils that cause seizure, shares an inhibitory effect on neuronal respiration, leading to cellular dysfunction and hyperexcitability.

Naphthalene causes both a hemolytic anemia and methemoglobinemia. The metabolites of naphthalene are responsible for the oxidative stress to the globin chains that lead to their denaturation and precipitation as Heinz bodies within red blood cells. These damaged cells are subsequently lysed by the reticuloendothelial system as they attempt to remove them from the blood. The primary mechanism by which the erythrocyte protects itself from oxidative stress involves the antioxidant glutathione. Patients deficient in glutathione, especially newborns and those with G-6-PD deficiency, are therefore more susceptible to the oxidative stress produced by naphthalene. Oxidative stress not only denatures hemoglobin leading to hemolysis, it also causes the oxidation of the iron in heme from the ferrous (Fe^{2+}) to the ferric (Fe^{3+}) state, forming methemoglobin. Methemoglobinemia and hemolysis can occur independently or simultaneously. Which of the two effects predominate when a patient is exposed to naphthalene cannot be reliably predicted. No particular route of exposure is associated with a particular toxicity.

Paradichlorobenzene is essentially nontoxic and there is scant evidence in the literature to relate paradichlorobenzene ingestion to anything more than minor gastrointestinal (GI) distress.

CLINICAL FINDINGS

Symptoms of camphor intoxication generally occur within 15 minutes of ingestion, and toxicity is usually seen within 2 hours of exposure. Mild toxicity includes GI symptoms of oral mucosal irritation, nausea and vomiting, and abdominal pain. There are case reports of hepatotoxicity following camphor exposure, although the mechanism is unknown. Central nervous system (CNS) depression is also common, but is not usually associated with respiratory depression. Seizures are the most serious manifestation of toxicity. Although they are usually brief and self-limited, status epilepticus may occur. Death is rare, and generally related to complications associated with status epilepticus.

Naphthalene toxicity causes headaches, restlessness, lethargy, nausea, vomiting, and anorexia. Hemolysis can occur, with associated fever, anemia, hyperkalemia, and acute renal failure. Jaundice and pallor may be present. Methoglobinemia can result; symptoms are generally vague, and include tachypnea, tachycardia, dyspnea, and malaise. CNS manifestations of toxicity include altered mental status, seizures, and coma. Cyanosis can also be present; oxygen saturation via pulse oximetry is typically around 85%. Neither cyanosis nor oxygen saturation is affected by the administration of supplemental oxygen (see Chapter 74). In animal models, naphthalene has produced cataracts and pulmonary epithelial damage. Toxicity is similar for both acute and chronic exposures. The metabolism to toxic metabolites delays the toxic effects, which usually develop within 1 to 2 days.

Paradichlorobenzene may cause GI upset, including nausea and vomiting, as well as irritation of the oropharyngeal mucosal.

LABORATORY AND DIAGNOSTIC TESTING

There are no rapidly and readily available tests that detect camphor, although the parent compound and its metabolites can be detected in both serum and urine. These tests are not useful in the acute management of a symptomatic patient, and levels are not known to correlate with toxicity.

Like camphor, naphthalene can be detected in both urine and serum, but there is no readily available diagnostic test. Anemia, unconjugated hyperbilirubinemia, elevated lactate dehydrogenase, or a urine dipstick positive for blood but a urinalysis negative for RBCs indicates hemolysis. Coombs testing in these patients, both direct and indirect, is negative. Peripheral blood smears show characteristic evidence of RBC destruction, including Heinz bodies, and early forms. Naphthalene-induced methemoglobinemia may be suggested by an abnormal pulse oximeter reading, and is quantified by cooximetry.

There are no readily available diagnostic tests for paradichlorobenzene, although it too can be detected in the serum and urine. Its nontoxic nature makes diagnostic testing unnecessary.

Mothball Identification

There have been a number of studies suggesting how to identify an unknown mothball (Figure 50–2). Paradichlorobenzene mothballs sink in both salt and fresh water, and camphor mothballs float in both salt and fresh water. Naphthalene mothballs sink in fresh water and float in water saturated with salt. Additionally, each of the products has different radioopacities. Paradichlorobenzene and naphthalene mothballs are radiopaque, with paradichlorobenzene being more strongly so. Camphor is radiolucent. When ignited with a match or Bunsen burner, paradichlorobenzene produces a green flame, and naphthalene burns with a blue coloration. None of these characteristics or tests are reliable enough to confirm the composition of the product, and in the absence of the package, the clinical findings guide management.

MANAGEMENT

GI decontamination has never been formally evaluated regarding exposure to camphor and naphthalene. For camphor, it is likely of limited utility, because the compound is rapidly absorbed. The propensity for seizures

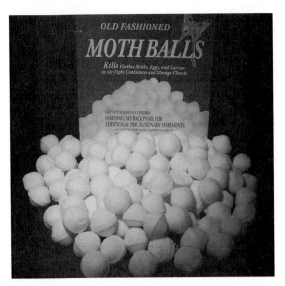

Fig. 50–2. It is important to identify whether unknown mothballs contain either camphor, naphthalene, or paradichlorobenzene.

contraindicates the administration of ipecac. With naphthalene ingestion, charcoal administration may be considered in some scenarios owing to the delayed nature of toxicity. If patients present with toxicity, consideration may be given to multiple-dose activated charcoal. Patients with paradichlorobenzene ingestion do not require decontamination.

Seizures from camphor are generally brief and self-limited; however, if the patient has a continuous or recurrent seizure, standard management including airway protection and supplemental oxygen is indicated. The first-line therapy for continued seizure activity is benzodiazepine administration. The metabolic consequences of seizure are addressed, and other causes of seizure are evaluated.

Depending on the exposure, most patients with an unintentional ingestion of a naphthalene-containing product do not require aggressive management. Patients with significant anemia should be treated with an appropriate therapy, packed red blood cells at an initial dose of 10 mL/kg. Symptomatic patients with significant methemoglobinemia (levels over 30%) may benefit from antidotal therapy with methylene blue 0.1 cc/kg of a 1% solution, slowly given intravenously.

DISPOSITION

The decision to admit a patient after exposure to one of these agents depends on the clinical situation and the agent ingested. A child who has a seizure after an exposure to a camphor-containing product is evaluated for sequelae of the seizure. If the patient has had no seizure, a normal mental status, and has been observed for a few hours, the patient may be safely discharged with close follow-up. Persistent alteration in mental status or other findings during evaluation should prompt admission and further work-up.

A child exposed to a naphthalene-containing product and in whom there is no evidence of methemoglobinemia or hemolytic anemia, should be reassessed in 48 hours. Patients and their caretakers should be cautioned for signs and symptoms of toxicity (dark urine, pallor, cyanosis, decreased exercise tolerance).

A child exposed to a paradichlorobenzene product can generally be discharged with routine follow-up with their pediatrician. All of these recommendations assume that the treating clinician believes that the home setting and caregivers offer an appropriate and safe environment for the child.

CASE OUTCOME

Wiping off the gel and gently washing the child with soap and warm water externally decontaminates the child. The Vicks Vapo-Rub is noted to have 4% camphor as an active ingredient. Over a short period of time, she becomes more arousable, and after an hour is at her baseline mental status. Laboratory examination is remarkable only for serum bicarbonate of 22 mEq/L, with an anion gap of 10. Noncontrast computed tomography of the head is unremarkable. She is observed for a few hours, and then discharged with close follow-up with her primary pediatrician in 24 hours. Careful instructions are given to the family regarding recurrence of seizure, as well as proper application and use of the product.

SUGGESTED READINGS

Abbott WS: Further work showing that paradichlorobenzene, naphthalene and cedar oils are ineffective as repellents against clothes moths. *J Econ Entomol* 28:493–495, 1935.

Burkhard PR, Burkhardt K, Haenggeli CA, et al: Plant-induced seizures: Reappearance of an old problem. *J Neurol* 246:667–670, 1999.

Committee on Drugs: Camphor revisited: Focus on toxicity. *Pediatrics* 94:127–128, 1994.

Ernst E. Adverse effects of herbal drugs in dermatology. *Br J Dermatol* 143:923–929, 2000.

Gidron E, Leurer J. Naphthalene poisoning. *Lancet* 1:228–230, 1956.

Höke H, Zellerhoff R. Metabolism and toxicity of diisopropyl-naphthalene as compared to naphthalene and monoalkyl naphthalenes: A minireview. *Toxicology* 126:1–7, 1998.

Kuffner EK: Camphor and moth repellents. In: Goldfrank LG, Flomenbaum N, Lewin N, et al, eds: *Goldfrank's Toxicologic Emergencies.* 7th ed. New York: McGraw-Hill; 2002:1295–1302.

Lahoud CA, March JA, Proctor DD: Campho-Phenique ingestion: An intentional overdose. *South Med J* 90:647–648, 1997.

Mackell JV, Rieders F, Brieger H, et al: Acute hemolytic anemia due to ingestion of naphthalene mothballs. *Pediatrics* 7:722–728, 1951.

Park TJ, Seo HK, Kang BJ, et al: Noncompetitive inhibition by camphor of nicotinic acetylcholine receptors. *Biochem Pharmacol* 61:787–793, 2001.

Santucci K, Shah B. Association of naphthalene with acute hemolytic anemia. *Acad Emerg Med* 7:42–47, 2000.

Schafer WB. Acute hemolytic anemia related to naphthalene. Report of a case in a newborn infant. *Pediatrics* 7:172–174, 1951.

Shannon K, Buchanan GR: Severe hemolytic anemia in black children with glucose-6-phosphate dehydrogenase deficiency. *Pediatrics* 70:364–369, 1982.

Stohs SJ, Ohia S, Bagchi D: Naphthalene toxicity and antioxidant nutrients. *Toxicology* 180:97–105, 2002.

Trevisan A, Rossi di Schio M, Pieno M: Haemolytic anaemia after oral self-giving of naphthalene-containing oil. *J Appl Toxicol* 21:393–396, 2001.

Uc A, Bishop WP, Sanders KD: Camphor hepatotoxicity. *South Med J* 93:596–598, 2000.

Valaes T, Doxiadis SA, Fessas P: Acute hemolysis due to naphthalene inhalation. *J Pediatr* 63:904–915, 1963.

Weintraub E, Gandhi D, Robinson C: Medical complications due to mothball abuse. *South Med J* 93:427–429, 2000.

Wilson AS, Davis CD, Williams DP, et al: Characterization of the toxic metabolite(s) of naphthalene. *Toxicology* 114:233–242, 1996.

Woolf AD, Saperstein A, Zawin J, et al: Radiopacity of household deodorizers, air fresheners, and moth repellents. *J Toxicol Clin Toxicol* 31:415–428, 1993.

Zinkham WH, Childs B: A defect of glutathione metabolism in erythrocytes from patients with a naphthalene-induced hemolytic anemia. *Pediatrics* 22:461–471, 1958.

51

Organophosphates, Carbamates, Pesticides, and Herbicides

Alexander Baer
Mark Kirk
Christopher Holstege

HIGH-YIELD FACTS

- Children are vulnerable to pesticide poisoning. They may be at greater risk of exposure owing to a higher ratio of body surface area to body mass and increased hand-to-mouth activity.

- Organophosphate and carbamate pesticides produce a distinct clinical syndrome (toxidrome) identified by the constellation of signs and symptoms, including bronchoconstriction, bronchorrhea, diarrhea, emesis, lacrimation, miosis, salivation, sweating, and urination.

- The diagnosis of pesticide poisoning may be difficult in children because they are more likely to present with mental status changes and seizures rather than the classic cholinergic toxidrome.

- Pesticide-related deaths in children are most often due to respiratory failure.

- Much higher doses of atropine than recommended for cardiac emergencies are often required to overcome severe muscarinic cholinergic effects. Pralidoxime is used to treat the nicotinic cholinergic effects.

- Pesticides mixed with a hydrocarbon vehicle may be labeled as *inert* on the container but may lead to chemical pneumonitis if aspirated.

CASE PRESENTATION

The 6-year-old son of a Hispanic farmer presents to the emergency department (ED) for the second time within the last 24 hours. On the first visit, the mother described the child as uncoordinated and sleepy after she found him in the garage with a spilled, unlabeled Mason jar. He was diagnosed with acute gastroenteritis. The child became difficult to arouse and the mother noted wheezing and white frothy secretions since being discharged from the ED earlier that day.

On physical examination the patient is lethargic with a pulse of 135 bpm; systolic blood pressure of 85 mmHg; respiratory rate of 16 breaths per minute; and an oral temperature of 37.4°C. Pupils are equal and pinpoint. Oral examination reveals copious secretions. Cardiac examination is significant for sinus tachycardia. Pulmonary auscultation reveals diffuse bilateral rales and wheezes. Hyperactive bowel sounds are appreciated on the abdominal examination.

INTRODUCTION AND EPIDEMIOLOGY

Pesticides are an important cause of pediatric poisoning because of the multitude of potential sources of exposure. Pediatric poisoning from organophosphates may be a challenge to the clinician because the child may present with subtle signs and symptoms. *Pesticide* is a broad term that incorporates many different chemicals. The focus of this chapter is on organophosphates, carbamates, and a brief review of other agents termed pesticides. According to 2001 data from the American Association

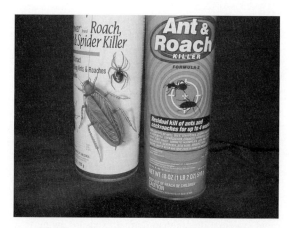

Fig. 51–1. Common household pesticide products.

of Poison Control Centers, there were 46,929 pediatric pesticide exposures and two fatalities. A survey by the U.S. Environmental Protection Agency found that 47% of all households with children had at least one pesticide stored in an unlocked cabinet within 4 feet of the ground. More than 120 pesticides that inhibit the acetylcholinesterase enzyme are commonly used in the home, garden, and on the farm (Figure 51–1). Child-resistant packaging and the development of safer products, like pyrethroids, have helped to decrease the number and severity of poisonings from pesticides. The most commonly used pesticides today include carbamates, organophosphates, pyrethroids and, with increasing rarity, organochlorines.

DEVELOPMENTAL AND AGE CONSIDERATIONS

Insecticides have teratogenic potential in laboratory animals, causing multiple structural abnormalities, but human data are extremely limited. There is a significant risk of toxicity in the fetus exposed to organophosphates, but the relationship between chronic exposure and risk of effects is still uncertain. Organophosphates cross the placenta. Fetal organophosphate levels have been detected on autopsy of fatalities from organophosphate poisoning. The neonate may also be more susceptible to the effects of cholinesterase inhibition because studies have found a 50% to 70% reduction of fetal red blood cell cholinesterase.

Toddlers are more prone to accidental poisonings, particularly if the pesticide containers are placed near the floor, or if they come in contact with floors that have been recently sprayed. Adolescent patients are more

prone to larger exposures owing to suicide attempts or from occupational exposures. Children may be the first affected in a family, acting as the "miner's canary," because of their particular physical and behavioral susceptibilities, namely a large surface area that causes increased exposure through dermal contact, hand-to-mouth activity, and playing in areas that are sprayed.

PHARMACOLOGY AND TOXICOKINETICS

Chlorpyrifos, diazinon, fenthion, malathion, and methyl parathion are some of the more common pesticides. Organophosphates are rapidly absorbed from the skin, gut, or lungs. The lipophilic structure of organophosphates lend to prolonged half-lives. Many agents, like malathion, have active metabolites that further prolong the half-life. For example, a methylparathion ingestion resulted in detectable levels of plasma methylparathion and parathion 27 days postexposure. The effect of organophosphates last longer than the half-life of the actual chemical because acetylcholinesterase needs to regenerate for the patient to improve clinically. The body is capable of synthesizing approximately 1% of acetylcholinesterase a day. Therefore it could take several weeks of respiratory support before enough neuronal acetylcholinesterase is generated to breathe independently.

PATHOPHYSIOLOGY

Organophosphate and carbamate insecticide poisoning result in excess release of acetylcholine. The clinical presentation is a reflection of acetylcholine accumulation at specific synapses when organophosphates and carbamates block the acetylcholinesterase enzyme. Acetylcholinesterase regulates acetylcholine action on nicotinic and muscarinic receptors by cleaving it into the inactive metabolites acetic acid and choline. The distinct clinical effects are explained by the activation of nicotinic and muscarinic synapses. The muscarinic or parasympathetic system, responsible for "rest and digest," may be stimulated when acetylcholine accumulates in the nicotinic ganglia. Conversely, increased acetylcholine in the sympathetic ganglionic synapses can stimulate sympathetic activity. Excessive acetylcholine in the nicotinic receptors along the motor end plate can lead to fasciculations, weakness, and paralysis. Excessive acetylcholine within the brain can cause seizures and coma.

A process called *aging* occurs when the bond between the organophosphate and acetylcholinesterase permanently renders the enzyme nonfunctional. This window before aging is an opportunity in which antidote therapy with pralidoxime can salvage the remaining acetylcholinesterase. Carbamates never form this permanent bond and eventually dissociate from acetylcholinesterase, usually within 24 hours.

CLINICAL PRESENTATION

The classic *cholinergic toxidrome* involves a combination of signs and symptoms caused by acetylcholine stimulation of central, autonomic, and peripheral nervous systems. Common mnemonics describing the cholinergic syndrome

DUMBELS (for Muscarinic Effects)

- *Diarrhea*
- *Urination*
- *Miosis*
- Bronchorrhea and Bronchospasm
- *Emesis*
- *Lacrimation*
- *Secretions*

CCC (for Central Nicotinic Effects)

- *Confusion*
- *Coma*
- *Convulsions*

The diagnosis of organophosphate poisoning can be challenging. Children often manifest only the central symptoms, which is one of the reasons that many of these cases are misdiagnosed at the outset. The majority of children actually present with tachycardia because the nicotinic effect on the sympathetic ganglion predominates over the classically described parasympathetic slowing of the heart rate. Miosis is an important clue because of the strong association with exposure, and its limited differential diagnosis.

Neurologic effects include agitation, seizures, or coma. Comatose patients may actually be suffering nonconvulsive seizures. Miosis is present in the majority of serious poisonings and is probably the most sensitive physical examination finding for diagnosing poisoning during the acute phase. It occurs early from vapor exposure, but maybe delayed in dermal exposures. Ciliary spasm may limit accommodation and cause ocular pain.

Respiratory effects are the most common cause of death. Organophosphate-poisoned patients are difficult to oxygenate and ventilate because of bronchoconstriction, increased tracheobronchial secretions, and respiratory muscle paralysis. Cardiac effects include bradycardia or tachycardia, depending on whether muscarinic or nicotinic effects predominate. Gastrointestinal (GI) effects include emesis and diarrhea. Dermatologic findings commonly include excessive diaphoresis. An isolated area of diaphoresis may be seen at the site of dermal exposure to the specific organophosphate. Muscular findings include fasciculations, which can progress to paralysis.

The route of exposure affects the temporal onset of symptoms. The respiratory route often produces a more rapid systemic illness than dermal exposure owing to a faster rate of absorption. Dermal exposures may present early with muscle fasciculations or sweating, whereas the inhalant route often produces central symptoms and miosis. Inhalation may lead to rapid onset of bronchospasm, bronchorrhea, and central nervous system (CNS) depression, which is the most common cause of death. Ingestion of organophosphates may cause nausea, vomiting, and diarrhea prior to other features. Often, several routes of exposure may cause mixed clinical effects. Eventually, systemic absorption by any route of exposure leads to severe toxicity that manifests in a cholinergic crisis.

Parents' occupation and hobbies are important historical aspects because children can receive a significant exposure from residual material on clothing. Suspicion may be raised if multiple people show up from the same gathering or meal with a cholinergic toxidrome. Storage of pesticides in unlabeled containers in the garage is often a source of exposure. Inappropriate use of agricultural insecticides for domestic fumigation has caused mass exposures and illness. Important historic questions to ask include whether there are other family members or pets that are sick, or if there was a prior sentinel case.

There are a few delayed effects that deserve brief mentioning. There is a well described *organophosphate-induced delayed neuropathy* that occurs 2 to 3 weeks postexposure and causes profound weakness of the lower extremities. This syndrome has been recognized for over a century, and was seen during prohibition during a major epidemic in which people consumed an alcohol extract of Jamaican ginger. This was known as *Jake's paralysis* and was the result of contamination with the pesticide tri-*o*-cresol phosphate. A delayed syndrome may also be found in rare case reports of children recovering from the cholinergic phase who become acutely stridorous from bilateral vocal cord paralysis approximately 1 to 4 days postexposure, and require several additional days of ventilatory support.

LABORATORY AND DIAGNOSTIC TESTING

A physician suspecting carbamate or organophosphate poisoning should begin treatment without waiting for supporting laboratory or diagnostic tests because of the risk of clinical deterioration. No diagnostic test is readily available to rapidly confirm the diagnosis of organophosphate poisoning. Plasma (serum) cholinesterase and erythrocyte acetylcholinesterase are surrogate markers that indicate acetylcholinesterase inhibition at the nerve synapse. Cholinesterase levels may be more a confirmation of exposure rather than a measure of clinical severity. A recent study showed no discernable difference between the serum cholinesterase obtained at outset in severely versus mildly poisoned patients. The cholinesterase activity should therefore be used to confirm a clinical suspicion of exposure rather than as a guide to initial treatment. Arterial blood gas analysis or pulse oximetry should be followed to assess the patient's oxygenation and acid–base status. Other laboratory work should be directed to end-organ dysfunction as indicated in any critically ill patient. An electrocardiogram may demonstrate a tachydysrhythmia or a bradydysrhythmia, depending on which group of nicotinic receptors predominate, sympathetic or parasympathetic. QT prolongation complicated by a tachydysrhythmia has been reported with organophosphate toxicity in children. Chest radiographs may look similar to noncardiogenic pulmonary edema, but more likely represent alveolar pooling of bronchorrhea. Metabolic acidosis is not typically seen, except in cases of concurrent seizure activity or hypoperfusion. These patients often undergo an extensive workup before the diagnosis is made. A strong clinical suspicion and a constellation of physical examination findings suggesting cholinergic poisoning are more useful than any diagnostic tests.

MANAGEMENT

Preventing further patient exposure and preventing secondary exposure to health care workers is paramount in the treatment of an organophosphate or carbamate poisoning. The person performing decontamination needs personal protective equipment appropriate for the agent involved. Surgical masks do not provide adequate pro-

tection from vapor exposure. Similarly, latex gloves provide inadequate protection from organophosphates and carbamates. Butyl rubber gloves and aprons provide a better barrier. Decontamination for a vapor inhalation requires removing the patient from the environment. Dermal exposures require the removal of clothing and cleansing of skin with soap and water. In cases of life-threatening ingestions, there may be a role of limited GI decontamination with gastric lavage. One must weigh the benefits of suctioning the residual pesticide aspirate with the risk of a chemical pneumonitis from aspiration of the hydrocarbon vehicle. There are no studies showing improved outcome with charcoal administration. Potential disadvantages of charcoal administration are an increased risk of vomiting and possible aspiration pneumonitis.

Basic life support is initiated concurrent to decontamination, with particular attention to the patient's airway. If the physical examination corroborates cholinergic poisoning, antidote therapy should be initiated.

Atropine sulfate (Figure 51–2) antagonizes the muscarinic receptors in the cardiac muscle, CNS, secretory gland cells, and smooth muscle. Indications for atropine are the presence of bronchorrhea and bronchoconstriction. Atropine is administered at 0.02 mg/kg intravenously (IV) every 5 to 10 minutes. The therapeutic endpoint is resolution of bronchospasm and drying of pulmonary secretions; therefore, doses should be repeated until clinical improvement is demonstrated in

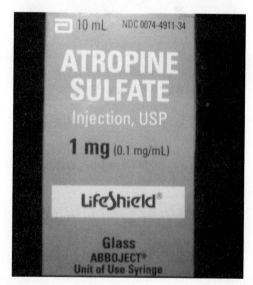

Fig. 51–2. Atropine sulfate antagonizes muscarinic receptors.

ventilation and oxygenation. Although it is ideally given IV, atropine may be administered by an intramuscular or endotracheal route. Large doses of atropine may be required to control muscarinic symptoms. Tachycardia and mydriasis are not contraindications to the administration of atropine. Atropine may be obtained through ophthalmology, veterinary, and emergency medical service sources if a hospital's supply is depleted during a mass casualty incident. The poison center may also be integral in networking between hospitals to arrange for redistribution of antidote inventories to help an overwhelmed hospital.

In moderate to severe cholinergic poisoning by organophosphates or an unknown agent, pralidoxime, 25 to 50 mg/kg over 30 minutes, should be infused (Figure 51–3). Pralidoxime chloride reactivates acetylcholinesterase by attacking the phosphorus moiety bound to acetylcholine-s-terase, causing an oxime phosphate bond. The earlier that the agent can be given, the smaller the proportion of acetylcholinesterase aging that occurs. This may need to be dosed again in 4 to 6 hours, if there are persistent nicotinic symptoms such as convulsions. An infusion may be initiated at 8 mg/kg/h. Some authors recommend withholding pralidoxime in cases of known carbaryl poisonings. However, it is best to empirically treat symptomatic patients when the exact agent cannot be identified, because the benefit from pralidoxime in organophos-

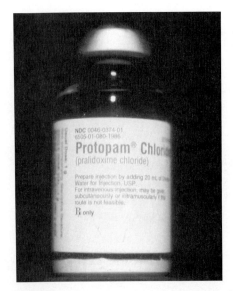

Fig. 51–3. Pralidoxime is indicated in organophosphate poisoning with cholinergic crisis.

phate poisoning is likely to be much greater than a theoretical adverse effect in carbaryl poisoning in humans.

Diazepam should be given to cases of seizure activity or in comatose patients in whom nonconvulsive seizures are suspected. Long-acting paralytics should be avoided so that seizure activity is not masked. An important consideration is that plasma cholinesterase is responsible for hydrolysis of some depolarizing agents like succinylcholine and mivacurium, so there may be prolonged paralysis if these agents are used during organophosphate or carbamate toxicity.

Nerve Agents

Potential pesticides synthesized in Germany under Nazi rule were recognized for their potential military use. Tabun, sarin, and soman were developed by the end of World War II. The British developed VX in 1952. Nerve agents are some of the more toxic substances known, with a LD_{50} as low as 10 mg for VX. Iraq used sarin against Kurdish refugees within their country in 1988, marking the first use of these agents as a weapon. In 1995, terrorists released sarin in Matsumoto and Tokyo, Japan. The United States has identified nerve agents as one of four likely agents to be used in a terrorist attack (see Chapter 15). Nerve agents are more potent than organophosphates used as pesticides. Tremendous financial resources are being devoted to various agencies to prepare for an act of chemical terrorism. Education regarding clinical recognition, decontamination, self-protection, and management are paramount. It is important to train in the use of personal protective equipment to help prevent injury. There were 11 reported fatalities from the inappropriate use of gas masks in Israel during the Iraqi missile offensive, 7 people suffocated from not removing the cover to the filter and 4 from myocardial infarctions.

Pyrethrins and Synthetic Pyrethroids

Pyrethrins, an extraction of *Chrysanthemum cinerariaefolium*, are much less toxic to humans than insects because they quickly undergo hydrolysis and inactivation by the liver. Their lethal effect to insects lies in the ability to delay sodium channel closure, thus allowing more sodium to enter the cells of the nervous system. This leads to hyperexcitability of the nervous system and eventually leads to the blocking of impulse propagation and paralysis. Pyrethroids are the synthetic form of pyrethrins. These agents may cause allergic reactions, especially in those allergic to ragweed pollen. Treatment is aimed at ending exposure by removing clothing and washing exposed skin with soap and water. These agents may be in a hydrocarbon vehicle, adding considerable risk of aspiration if gastric lavage is attempted. Allergic reactions should be treated with steroids, diphenhydramine, albuterol for respiratory symptoms, and epinephrine for severe systemic reactions.

Pyrethroids have caused seizures in animal models and humans with severe poisoning. Peripheral neuropathies have been reported with very large overdoses, but axonal repair occurs after ending the exposure.

Organochlorine

Organochlorines, such as DDT, chlordane, and lindane are effective pesticides because they cause neuroexcitation through either enhanced sodium channel conductance or inhibition of GABA$_A$ channels. Human toxicity, mainly in the form of seizures, increases in young children because of increased drug absorption from the skin or from frequent hand-to-mouth activity. Special attention to removing clothing and washing the skin with soap in water helps to decrease drug absorption in dermal exposures. Seizures should be treated with benzodiazepines, followed by barbiturates, in refractory cases, to enhance GABAergic activity.

DDT was credited in 1953 with having saved 50 million lives through control of the mosquito population worldwide, thus curbing malarial deaths. It was later banned by the Environmental Protection Agency in 1973 because of concerns that it persisted in the environment, and may effect certain predatory bird populations.

Low levels of chlordane exposure in an apartment complex sprayed for termites was associated with chronic neurotoxic effects, such as imbalance, delay in reaction time, and deficits in verbal recall when compared to controls. There is mixed evidence regarding the oncogenicity of organochlorines. There have been reports of neuroblastomas, blood dyscrasias, and biliary, liver, and breast cancer in various groups exposed to organochlorines, but the evidence is not definitive for causation.

Paraquat

Paraquat is an effective herbicide that causes severe lung injury in humans. GI absorption is the main route of toxic exposure with an initial caustic effect to the upper airway and the GI tract. The absorbed paraquat that circulates through the pulmonary vasculature undergoes cyclic reduction–oxidation reactions, producing superoxide radicals. This reaction sets off a cascade of events leading to the production of hydroxyl radicals. These paraquat radicals, superoxide radicals, and hydroxyl radicals interact with proteins, lipids, and DNA, ultimately halting cellular activity and leading to cell death. Life-threatening pulmonary edema and hemorrhage often result. Those who survive the lung injury will most likely develop pulmonary fibrosis.

Decontamination of the skin through removal of clothing and washing with soap and water is necessary for dermal exposures. GI decontamination should be instituted as quickly as possible in ingestions. Activated charcoal at a dose of 1 g/kg may be given. Volume replacement with IV fluids may be necessary. Oxygen is usually reserved for those with arterial oxygen tensions below 50 mmHg because of the concern that it will exacerbate free radical production. Mortality is extremely high from ingestion of paraquat, even in those who undergo lung transplantation.

Diquat belongs to the same class of herbicide as paraquat, but there are fewer cases of poisoning in the literature. Diquat has less pulmonary toxicity than paraquat because it is not actively taken up in the pulmonary alveolar epithelial cells. Most of the patients died from complications involving the GI tract, brain, and kidneys.

Aluminum and Zinc Phosphide

Aluminum and zinc phosphide usually comes in pellets that react with water or acid to produce phosphine gas, an effective pesticide used for stored grains. Phosphine inhibits cytochrome-c oxidase and catalase and stimulates superoxide dismutase, inducing oxidative toxicity and inhibition of cellular respiration. The clinical effect is widespread and involves cellular death in multiple organ systems, but the heart and kidney seem to be the major target organs. Patients may develop pulmonary edema if they inhale phosphine gas. Symptoms may be delayed several days after exposure.

No antidote exists for aluminum and zinc phosphide toxicity and treatment is largely supportive. Potential antidotes studied in animal models include anti-oxidants, like *N*-acetylcysteine, vitamin C, and vitamin E.

DISPOSITION

The safest approach to pesticide poisoning is to refer all cases to the nearest ED because of the serious risks associated with these agents. Symptomatic patients benefit from hospitalization. It is important to monitor patients even if they are asymptomatic, because there have been delayed cases of toxicity, particularly after dermal exposures.

CASE OUTCOME

The child was given atropine at 0.02 mg/kg every 5 minutes for a total of 20 mg to control the bronchorrhea and bronchoconstriction. The agent was never identified and 30 mg/kg of pralidoxime was administered before the results of any confirmatory tests. The pseudocholinesterase activity dropped from 30% to 15%, supporting the likely exposure to an acetylcholinesterase inhibitor. Profound weakness prompted mechanical ventilation and a repeat dose of pralidoxime was administered. The patient was weaned from the ventilator 3 days following exposure. He made a full recovery.

SUGGESTED READINGS

Aiuto LA, Pavlakis SG, Boxer RA: Life-threatening organophosphate-induced delayed polyneuropathy in a child after accidental chlorpyrifos ingestion. *J Pediatr* 122:658–660, 1993.

Aygun D, Doganay Z, Altintop L, et al: Serum acetylcholinesterase and prognosis of acute organophosphate poisoning. *J Toxicol Clin Toxicol* 40:903–910, 2002.

Bleich A, Dycian A, Koslowsky M, et al: Psychiatric implications of missile attacks on a civilian population. Israeli lessons from the Persian Gulf War. *JAMA* 268:613–615, 1992.

Dawson RM: Review of oximes available for treatment of nerve agent poisoning. *J Appl Toxicol* 14:317–331, 1994.

Ecobichon DJ, Ozere RL, Reid E, et al: Acute fenitrothion poisoning. *Can Med Assoc J* 116:377–379, 1977.

Gupta S, and Ahlawat, SK: Aluminum phosphine poisoning—A review. *Clin Toxicol* 33:19–24, 1995.

Holstege CP, Kirk M, Sidell FR: Chemical warfare. Nerve agent poisoning. *Crit Care Clin* 13:923–942, 1997.

Hsu C-H, Chi B-C: Phosphine-induced oxidative damage in rats: Role of glutathione. *Toxicology* 179:1–8, 2002.

John M, Oommen A, Zachariah A: Muscle injury in organophosphorous poisoning and its role in the development of intermediate syndrome. *Neurotoxicology* 24:43–53, 2003.

Karsenty E, Shemer J, Alshech I, et al: Medical aspects of the Iraqi missile attacks on Israel. *Isr J Med Sci* 27:603–607, 1991.

Kilburn K, Thornton J: Protracted neurotoxicity from chlordane sprayed to kill termites. *Environ Health Perspect* 103:691–694, 1995.

Kirk MA, Cisek J, Rose CR: Emergency department response to hazardous materials incidents. *Emerg Med Clin North Am* 12:461–481, 1994.

Litovitz TL, Klein-Schwartz W, Rodgers GC, et al: 2001 annual report of the American Association of Poison Control Centers Toxic Exposure Surveillance System. *Am J Emerg Med* 20:391–452, 2002.

Nel L, Hatherill M, Davies J, et al: Organophosphate poisoning complicated by a tachyarrhythmia and acute respiratory distress syndrome in a child. *J Paediatr Child Health* 38:530–532, 2002.

Okudera H: Clinical features on nerve gas terrorism in Matsumoto. *J Clin Neurosci* 9:17–21, 2002.

Okumura T, Takasu N, Ishimatsu S, et al: Report on 640 victims of the Tokyo subway sarin attack. *Ann Emerg Med* 28:129–135, 1996.

O'Malley M: Occupational medicine: Clinical evaluation of pesticide exposure and poisoning. *Lancet* 349:1161–1166, 1997.

Reigart JR, Roberts JR: Pesticides in children. *Pediatr Clin North Am* 48:1185–1198, 2001.

Selden BS, Curry SC: Prolonged succinylcholine-induced paralysis in organophosphate insecticide poisoning. *Ann Emerg Med* 16:215–217, 1987.

Sener EB, Ustun E, Kocamanoglu S, et al: Prolonged apnea following succinylcholine administration in undiagnosed acute organophosphate poisoning. *Acta Anaesthesiol Scand* 46:1046–1048, 2002.

Zwiener RJ, Ginsburg CM: Organophosphate and carbamate poisoning in infants and children. *Pediatrics* 81:121–126, 1988.

52

Rodenticides

Anthony M. Burda
Michael S. Wahl

HIGH-YIELD FACTS

- The labels of all indoor rodenticides currently approved by the Food and Drug Administration contain an EPA registration number, active ingredients, concentration, instructions for use, warnings, and first-aid information.

- An accidental ingestion or taste by pediatric patients of currently marketed-indoor rodenticides, such as the long-acting anticoagulants, bromethalin, cholecalciferol, or zinc phosphide, are not likely to result in serious toxicity.

- Treatment measures such as gastrointestinal (GI) decontamination, prophylaxis with vitamin K_1 or laboratory monitoring are unwarranted following accidental tastes of long-acting anticoagulant rodenticides.

- A single large ingestion or repeated small ingestions of long-acting anticoagulant (super warfarin) compounds may cause serious bleeding. Phytonadione (vitamin K_1) is the specific antidote. Active bleeding may require treatment with fresh frozen plasma (FFP).

- Very large ingestions of bromethalin may cause neurologic toxicity attributed to increased intracranial pressure. Cholecalciferol (vitamin D_3) may cause hypercalcemia. Zinc phosphide is converted to phosphine gas in the GI tract, resulting in pulmonary edema and multi-organ injury.

- Ingestions of any amount of very old, illegal, or products unapproved for indoor use should be considered extremely serious because these products may contain arsenic, strychnine, sodium monofluoroacetate, thallium, white phosphorus, aldicarb or other highly toxic chemicals.

CASE PRESENTATION

A 2-year-old child weighing 15 kg presents to the emergency department (ED) after ingesting an unknown amount of rat poison pellets. He is currently awake, alert, and in no visible distress. His vital signs are normal and physical examination unremarkable. He is currently taking amoxicillin for otitis media, but is otherwise healthy with no known allergies.

The parent states that approximately 1 hour ago, the child reached behind the kitchen stove and pulled out a cardboard tray of greenish rat poison pellets and ingested, at most, one mouthful. The child was caught immediately, his mouth was swept with a finger, and several granules were removed.

Unfortunately, the tray had no labeled brand name or ingredients. A building custodian had given the product to the parent in an unlabeled brown paper bag.

INTRODUCTION AND EPIDEMIOLOGY

Ingestion of rodenticide products by children account for a significant number of poisonings reported to the Toxic

Table 52–1. Ten-Year TESS Rodenticide Data, 1992–2001

Rodenticide Class	Age 0–6	Age 6–9
Anticoagulant, warfarin type	12,128	511
Anticoagulant, super warfarin	126,038	4373
Other non-anticoagulant	16,715	1590
Total	154,881	6474

Exposure Surveillance System (TESS) compiled by the American Association of Poison Control Centers. Between 1992 and 2001, TESS reported a total of 161,355 rodenticide poisonings in patients under 19 years of age (Table 52–1).

Deaths in this population were extremely rare, with only two (0.001%) reported. In one case, a 4-year-old girl died of pulmonary edema as a result of a family's misuse of aluminum phosphide pellets in the home. The second case involved the death of a 15 year old who committed suicide by ingesting zinc phosphide.

Several case reports of serious pediatric long-acting anticoagulant poisonings have been published. These cases were atypical in that the patients presented late in the course of illness, and a history of accidental poisoning was not the chief complaint. Circumstances in these cases included aspects of child abuse and neglect, as well as Munchausen syndrome by proxy.

Rodenticides pose significant risk for unintentional poisoning for at least two important reasons: (1) The toxicity is similar for humans and target rodents, because these products are specifically designed to kill mammals, and (2) the risk of accidental exposure to rodent baits is increased because rodents share environments with humans and other mammals.

The relative risk of toxicity following unintentional taste amounts of rodenticides is determined primarily by its composition and concentration of active ingredients. The U.S. Environmental Protection Agency (EPA) currently approves four rodenticides for indoor use: anticoagulants, cholecalciferol, bromethalin, and zinc phosphide (Table 52–2). A few granules of these chemicals ingested by a small child are unlikely to cause toxicity. Other outdated, illegal, or unapproved products for indoor use pose more danger to children and pets even from ingestions of small quantities. Examples of these highly toxic products include strychnine, arsenic, white phosphorus, and sodium monofluoroacetate (Table 52–3).

Oral and dermal contact between children and various glue traps has prompted parents to consult poison centers. These are generally composed of an adhesive material with an attractant. These products are considered to be nontoxic; however, multiple soap and water washings may be necessary to remove these sticky substances from skin and objects.

This chapter focuses on the anticoagulant products, because they are the most common rodenticides reported to regional poison control centers. Physicians must, however, not assume that all exposures involve these products. An improperly packaged and labeled poison or products obtained by other than legitimate means should raise suspicion for a potentially highly toxic chemical.

It is important to know that the Federal Insecticide Fungicide and Rodenticide Act regulations require all pesticide labels to contain the following information: an EPA registration number, active ingredients and concentration, first-aid statement, restrictions on use, environmental hazards, physical and chemical hazards, directions for use, net contents, and name and address of registrant. Products not meeting these labeling requirements may be among the more highly toxic formulations described in Table 52–3.

DEVELOPMENTAL CONSIDERATIONS

The TESS data shows that children under 6 years of age comprise the largest population at risk of rodenticide poisoning. Toddlers are attracted to the colorful appearance (usually green) of the pellets or cakes. Bait stations or trays are generally not child resistant and these products are often transferred from their original container to food bowls or dishes placed in reachable areas.

Children with a history of pica are at greater risk of chronic ingestions. The addition of denatonium benzoate (Bitrex), a bittering agent, to some products may limit the quantity ingested owing to unpalatability.

Adolescents and young adults may consume rodenticides intentionally in a suicide attempt. Mentally ill patients have been known to chronically eat these products as well. As a result, these two groups of patients are more prone to serious toxicity owing to ingesting larger amounts of the specific rodenticide.

PATHOPHYSIOLOGY

Most rodenticide exposures reported to poison control centers involve anticoagulants. Prior to 1980, most of

Table 52-2. Other Non-Anticoagulant Indoor Rodenticides

Rodenticide	Toxicology/Clinical Findings	Management/Antidotes
Bromethalin Bait 0.01% Assault, Clout All Weather Bait, Fastrac, Real Kill Rat and Mouse Killer, Top Gun, Vengeance	Uncouples oxidative phosphorylation resulting in decreased ATP production and increased fluid accumulation which interrupts nerve impulse conduction with resultant increased pressure on nerve axons; no established human lethal dose. *Symptoms*: large ingestions may cause headaches, confusion, tremors, myoclonic jerking, seizure, cerebral edema or coma. Toxicity may be delayed ≥8–12 owing to conversion to a more active metabolite.	Activated charcoal following ingestion of a large amount; no specific antidote; supportive care including measures to correct cerebral edema, i.e., hyperventilation, mannitol or furosemide, dexamethasone; benzodiazepines/phenobarbital for seizures; monitor cerebral spinal fluid pressure.
Cholecalciferol Bait 0.075% Quintox, Rampage	Mobilizes calcium from bones producing hypercalcemia, osteomalacia, and metastatic calcification of the cardiovascular system, kidneys, stomach, and lungs; toxicity may occur from a single large ingestion or chronic consumption; death occurs in animals in 2–5 days; however, serious human poisonings or fatalities from these rodent baits have yet to be reported. *Symptoms*: anorexia, nausea, vomiting, diarrhea or constipation, headache, fatigue, weakness, hypercalcemia, hyperphosphatemia, cardiac dysrhythmias, myocardial infarction, renal tubular injury.	See Chapter 33. Guidelines for the treatment of vitamin D toxicity: Activated charcoal following large ingestions; monitor serum calcium and phosphate carefully; some reference labs can measure vitamin D blood levels; institute a low calcium and vitamin D diet; manage significant hypercalcemia with prednisone 1 mg/kg/d to a max of 20 mg/d for 1–2 w, forced diuresis with IV normal saline and furosemide while maintaining normal potassium and magnesium levels, calcitonin (salmon calcitonin, Calcimar) 4 IU/kg q12h IM or SC for 2–5 d, dosage may be doubled if necessary (consult package insert), bisphosphonates may also be used; oral cholestyramine or multiple dose activated charcoal may possibly enhance vitamin D elimination.
Zinc phosphide Granules 2% Eraze, Mole Nots, and Mr. Rat Guard *Note*: aluminum phosphide is a fumigant not sold for household use.	Converted to phosphine gas on contact with acid or moisture; direct cellular toxin causing multiorgan injury by inhibiting cytochrome C oxidase, blocking the electron transport chain. In a series of 21 patients, those ingesting <1 g had a favorable outcome; lethal dose: 4 g in an adult. *Symptoms*: nausea, profuse vomiting and diarrhea (may be bloody); a decaying fish odor may be noted; headache, cough, tachypnea, dyspnea, dizziness, tremulousness, hypotension, shock, hypocalcemia, tetany, pulmonary edema, convulsions, cardiac dysrhythmias, renal damage, hepatotoxicity, acute pancreatitis, coma; death may occur in 12–24 h.	GI decontamination is controversial; lavage may release phosphine gas; activated charcoal may be given but is of questionable value; antacids, H₂ blockers, and proton pump inhibitors may be considered; ED staff should work in a well-ventilated area; no specific antidote; provide intensive supportive care including intubation at earliest sign of pulmonary edema, which may be delayed 24–72 h; give benzodiazepines/phenobarbital for seizures; monitor electrolytes, glucose, calcium, renal and hepatic function tests, magnesium, ABGs or pulse oximetry, chest x-rays

Abbreviations: ABGs, arterial blood gases; ATP, adenosine triphosphate; ED, emergency department; GI, gastrointestinal; IV, intravenous.

Table 52–3. Outdated, Illegal, and Unapproved Rodenticides for Indoor Use

Rodenticide[a]	Toxicology/Clinical Findings	Management/Antidotes
α-Naph-thylthiourea (2) ANTU Bait 1–3% Bontu	Damages pulmonary epithelium causing pulmonary edema; human lethal dose is estimated to be over 4 g/kg with no known reported human fatalities. *Symptoms:* dyspnea, cyanosis, noncardiogenic pulmonary edema and effusions, hypothermia; pulmonary edema may be delayed 24–72 h.	Activated charcoal; no known antidote; symptomatic care with oxygen and ventilatory support; monitor ABGs.
Arsenic (1) Arsenic trioxide	Combines with sulfhydryl (-SH) groups in many essential cellular proteins and enzymes; estimated fatal dose 1–4 mg/kg. *Symptoms:* garlic-like breath odor, profuse vomiting and diarrhea, hypotension and shock, cardiac dysrhythmias, renal tubular damage, pulmonary edema, delirium, seizures, coma. *Delayed symptoms:* peripheral neuropathy, alopecia, Mees lines, blood dyscrasias.	See Chapter 66. Orogastric lavage, activated charcoal; whole bowel irrigation if abdominal radiograph is positive; obtain blood, spot urine, and 24-h urine for arsenic; monitor electrolytes, ECG, renal function tests, CBC. *Antidotes:* IM dimercaprol (BAL) or PO succimer; supportive care with IV fluids, pressors, antidysrhythmics, hemodialysis.
Barium carbonate (1)	Soluble barium salts lower serum potassium and raise intracellular potassium; estimated lethal dose 20–30 mg/kg; barium sulfate is nontoxic. *Symptoms:* nausea, vomiting, diarrhea, paresthesias, weakness, paralysis, hypoglycemia, rhabdomyolysis, dysrhythmias, cardiac/respiratory failure.	Orogastric lavage with magnesium sulfate; frequent serum potassium levels, with IV potassium replacement as necessary; supportive care with antidysrhythmics; no specific antidote; barium level may confirm diagnosis.
Chloralose (2) (α-chloralose)	Has sedative effects similar to chloral hydrate and stimulant effect similar to strychnine. *Human toxic dose:* 1–4 g; *infants:* 20 mg/kg. *Symptoms:* increased salivation, sedation, coma, respiratory depression, myoclonis, seizures, hypotension, hypo- or hyperthermia, acidosis.	Activated charcoal; no specific antidote; supportive care for respiratory failure, hypotension, rhabdomyolysis; benzodiazepines/phenobarbital for seizures.
Norbormide (3) Bait 0.5–1	In rats it acts as an irreversible smooth muscle constrictor resulting in tissue anoxia; no known human toxicity; estimated lethal dose 5–15 g/kg; ingestion of smaller amounts may cause hypotension.	Activated charcoal for large ingestions; monitor BP and provide supportive care; no specific antidote.
Phosphorus (1) White or Yellow Stearns Chemical Paste 2.5%	Protoplasmic poison causing direct cell injury leading to multiorgan failure. *Lethal dose:* 1 mg/kg; mixed with peanut butter as bait. *Note:* red phosphorous found in matches is nontoxic. *Symptoms:* bloody vomiting, burns to entire GI tract, vomitus and stools may appear smoking or	Lavage and activated charcoal are controversial since phosphorous is corrosive; lavage with 1:5000 potassium permanganate has been suggested but no good clinical data to support its use; no specific antidote; supportive care with IV fluids and blood products; standard burn care; administer

luminescent and have a garlic like odor, delirium, coma, shock, hypocalcemia, hypoglycemia, pulmonary edema, hemorrhage, cardiovascular collapse. *Delayed symptoms:* myocardial, hepatic, and renal damage; dermally may cause partial and full thickness burns; mortality approaches 50%. | narcotics (e.g., morphine) for pain control; *N*-acetylcysteine may be hepatoprotective; ED staff must wear personal protective equipment to avoid contact with phosphorous.

Agent	Symptoms	Treatment
PNU (1) N-3-pyridylmethyl-N'-p-nitro-phenyl urea, Vacor Bait 0.5%, 2%	Similar to alloxan and streptozocin; destroys pancreatic β cells via interference with niacinamide (nicotinamide) metabolism. *Lethal dose:* 5 mg/kg; product introduced in 1975 and withdrawn in 1979. *Symptoms:* nausea, vomiting (peanut odor), hyperglycemia, diabetic ketoacidosis, sensory motor and autonomic neuropathies, GI perforation, cardiac dysrhythmias. *Permanent symptoms:* insulin-dependent diabetes mellitus and postural hypotension.	Orogastric lavage and activated charcoal. *Antidote:* early IM or IV niacinamide (nicotinamide) may prevent toxicity; however, parenteral products are not available in the U.S.; based on animal studies niacin (nicotinic acid) may not be effective; treat hyperglycemic ketoacidosis with insulin; monitor for GI perforation; mineralocorticoids (e.g., fludrocortisone) for persistent postural hypotension.
Red Squill (3) *Urginea maritima* Bait 100% or as 4.5% extract in bait	Contains scillaren A and B, which are cardiac glycosides; two bulbs has been fatal to an adult; intensely nauseating causing rapid vomiting, which limits toxicity. *Symptoms:* large amounts may cause nausea, vomiting, hyperkalemia, AV block dysrhythmias; however, cardiac toxicity is rare.	See Chapter 37; activated charcoal following large ingestions; monitor vital signs, serum potassium, and ECG; antidotes: atropine and digoxin immune Fab.
SMFA (1) Compound 1080 and Sodium fluoroacetamide Compound 1081	SMFA is converted to fluorocitric acid which blocks the tricarboxylic cycle of the Krebs cycle; estimated lethal dose 2–10 mg/kg; however, 1 mg may cause serious toxicity; SMFA is a white crystalline powder combined with nigrosin black dye as a colorant. *Symptoms:* nausea, vomiting diarrhea, seizures, acidosis, cardiac dysrhythmias, hypotension, hypocalcemia, hypokalemia, respiratory depression, coma.	Orogastric lavage and activated charcoal (adsorption may be insignificant); supportive care for hypotension, acidosis, dysrhythmias and seizures; IV calcium gluconate for hypocalcemia; no known effective antidote; experimental therapies with glycerol monoacetate or ethanol are ineffective.
Strychnine (1) Bait 0.3–0.5%	Acts by antagonizing glycine, an inhibitory neurotransmitter in the post synaptic motor neurons of the spinal cord; lethal dose 1–2 mg/kg, but may be as low as 5–10 mg in a child. *Symptoms:* rapid onset of nausea, vomiting, apprehension, painful tonic–tetanic spasms, trismus, opisthotonos, risus sardonicus (facial grimacing), seizures, respiratory paralysis, lactic acidosis, rhabdomyolysis, hyperthermia, cardiac arrest; patient is conscious until hypoxia leads to CNS depression.	Activated charcoal; avoid any stimulus that may trigger seizures; treat seizures with benzodiazepines, phenobarbital, general anesthesia with nondepolarizing agents; supportive care for acidosis, respiratory failure, rhabdomyolysis, and renal failure; no specific antidote, multiple dose activated charcoal possibly beneficial; urine acidification is contraindicated (may worsen renal toxicity).

(Continues)

Table 52–3. Outdated, Illegal, and Unapproved Rodenticides for Indoor Use

Rodenticide[a]	Toxicology/Clinical Findings	Management/Antidotes
Rodenticide: TETS (3) Tetramine (tetramethyl-enedisulfotetramine) Dushuqiang	TETS binds noncompetitively and irreversibly to GABA receptors on neuronal cell membranes and blocks chloride channels. Illegally imported from China. Two samples were analyzed to have 6.4% and 13.8%. LD_{50} in mammals: 0.10 – 0.3 mg/kg; 7–10 mg is lethal in humans. *Symptoms:* Refractory seizures, coma and possible ischemic changes on ECG.	Information is limited. No specific antidote is available. Supportive care. Seizures were refractory to benzodiazepines and phenobarbital in one pediatric case. Animal studies in China suggest benefit from IV pyridoxine and DMSA. Patients in China have been treated with charcoal hemoperfusion and hemodialysis.
Thallium sulfate (1)	Interferes with oxidative phosphorylation by binding with mitochondria sulfhydryl groups; banned in 1965; lethal dose 1 g. *Symptoms:* nausea, bloody vomiting and diarrhea followed by ileus, painful sensory neuropathy, respiratory failure, delirium, seizures, renal failure, optic neuritis, muscle weakness, lethargy, coma. *Delayed symptoms:* alopecia, Mees lines, neuropathies.	Orogastric lavage and activated charcoal; thallium may appear radiopaque on an abdominal radiograph; obtain blood and 24-h urine collection for thallium; no specific antidote; no chelators are safe and effective; potassium ferric ferrocyanide (Prussian blue) orally may enhance fecal elimination; a pharmaceutical-grade product of Prussian blue is available on a compassionate basis from REAC/TS in Oak Ridge, TN; multiple-dose activated charcoal may enhance fecal elimination of thallium; supportive care including IV fluids, blood products, hemodialysis.
Tres Pasitos (1) Aldicarb	Acts as a reversible inhibitor of cholinesterase enzymes; product is an approved carbamate insecticide sold illegally as a rodenticide; smuggled into U.S. from the Dominican Republic; LD_{50} in rats: 1 mg/kg. *Muscarinic Symptoms:* SLUDGEBAM. *Nicotinic Symptoms:* tachycardia, mydriasis, weakness, fasciculations, respiratory failure. *CNS Symptoms:* coma, seizures.	See Chapter 51; activated charcoal. *Antidotes:* IV atropine sulfate to reverse muscarinic symptoms, benzodiazepines for seizures, pralidoxime chloride is controversial; monitor RBC and plasma cholinesterase activities.

[a]The numbers (1), (2), or (3) refer to the acute LD_{50} in rats:

(1) *Highly Toxic:* LD_{50} less than 50 mg/kg, signal word *Danger.*

(2) *Moderately Toxic:* 50–500 mg/kg, signal word *Warning.*

(3) *Low Toxicity:* 500–5000 mg/kg, signal word *Caution.*

Expert clinical management information and product identification are available through the regional poison control center 1-800-222-1222 or the National Pesticide Information Center (NPIC) at 1-800-858-7378, web site: http://npic.orst.edu/. The NPIC is operated by Oregon State University and the U.S. Environmental Protection Agency (EPA) from 6:30 AM to 4:30 PM Pacific time, 7 days a week, excluding holidays. This service provides information including pesticide products, recognition, and management of pesticide poisoning, toxicology, and environmental chemistry

Abbreviations: ABG, arterial blood gases; AV, atrioventricular; CBC, complete blood count; CNS, central nervous system; DMSA, succimer; ECG, electrocardiogram; ED, emergency department; GABA, γ-aminobutyric acid; GI, gastrointestinal; IM, intramuscular; IV, intravenous; PO, orally; RBC, red blood cells; SMFA, sodium monofluoroacetate.

these poisonings contained warfarin as the causative agent. Typically, warfarin is found in rodenticide bait in a concentration of 0.025% to 0.050% or 25 to 50 mg/ 100 g of product. Two problems arose associated with warfarin use as a pesticide: (1) Several feedings of bait over a number of days by the target animal were required to reach a lethal dose; and (2) a genetic selection process led to the emergence of warfarin-resistant rats. These problems were overcome by the development and introduction of the *super warfarin*, or long-acting anticoagulant products, which are approximately 100 times more potent than warfarin and could kill the target animal with a single feeding.

The long-acting anticoagulants are classified in two groups: the 4-hydroxy coumarins and the indandiones (Table 52–4). Both short- and long-acting anticoagulants inhibit the activity of vitamin K_{2-3} epoxide reductase, a crucial enzyme in the synthesis of the active form of vitamin K. This leads to reduction of essential vitamin K–dependent blood clotting factors II, VII, IX, and X. Onset of anticoagulant toxicity is delayed until existing stores of active vitamin K are depleted and circulating factors are reduced. Factor VII has the shortest half-life, approximately 5 hours. Factor levels must fall 20% to 30% for prolongation of the prothrombin (PT) time to occur. Thus, three to four factor VII half-lives (15 to 20 hours) are necessary for effects to become evident.

Anticoagulants also damage capillaries and increase their permeability, thereby increasing the risk of hemorrhage. Indandione derivatives have caused cardiopulmonary and neurologic toxicity in animals.

In rats, the minimal amount of brodifacoum to depress PT activity was 0.1 mg/kg. Extrapolating to humans, this amounts to 1.5 mg for a 10-kg child or 30 g of a 0.005% bait.

PHARMACOLOGY AND TOXICOKINETICS

The pharmacokinetics of warfarin are well established. The toxicokinetics of the super warfarin rodenticides are not as well defined in humans. These agents are well absorbed orally. Toxicity following dermal exposure to low-concentration solid baits is unlikely; however, percutaneous absorption of concentrated industrial-strength products may result in toxicity. Warfarin is 99% bound to plasma proteins. Warfarin undergoes extensive hepatic metabolism with a therapeutic half-life of 35 hours. High lipid solubility and high concentrations in the liver account for the prolonged duration of action of the super warfarins. The half-life of brodifacoum is approximately 124 days in dogs and 6.5 days in rats. In one adult patient, the terminal half-life was 24 days. The half-life of chlorophacinone in four adult poisonings ranged from 6 to 11 days. Warfarin metabolites are eliminated in the urine and bile.

CLINICAL FINDINGS

Bleeding diathesis following unintentional ingestion of anticoagulant rodenticides by pediatric patients is unlikely, although mild PT prolongation has been noted. Clinical evidence of bleeding may occur, however, following acute intentional ingestions of large amounts or repeated ingestions as in the case of pica, child abuse, or Munchausen syndrome by proxy.

Table 52–4. Classification and Examples of Anticoagulant Rodenticides

Anticoagulant Class	Generic Name	Proprietary Name
Coumarin	Warfarin	D-Con Mouse Prufe, Fumarin, Hot Shot Rat and Mouse Killer, Kypfarin, Warfarin Plus
4-Hydroxycoumarin	Brodifacoum	D-Con Mouse Prufe II, Enforcer Rat Kill II,
	Bromodiolone	Final, Havoc, Talon-G Bromone, Contrac,
	Coumatetralyl	Maki, Ratimus, Super-Caid, Endox,
	Difenacoum	Endrocid, Endrocide, Racumin, Ratack
Indandiones	Chlorophacinone	Caid, Drat, Enforcer Rat Bait V, Liphadione,
	Diphacinone	Microzul, Ramucide, Ratomet, Raviac,
	Pindone	Rozol Contrax-D, Diaphacin, Ditrac,
		Liqua-Tox, Promar, Ramik, Tomcat
		Contract-P, Pival, Pivacin, Pivalyn, Tri-Ban

Signs and symptoms in toxic patients range from minor to life-threatening bleeding. These include epistaxis, easy bruising, gingival bleeding, petechiae, hematuria, hematemesis, melena, hemoptysis, extremity pain associated with compartment syndrome, vaginal bleeding, and intracerebral hemorrhage.

Clinical recovery following acute warfarin ingestion occurs in less than 1 week. Owing to greater affinity for hepatic binding sites and longer duration of action, second-generation super warfarins pose a more significant risk of coagulopathy, which may persist for weeks to months.

LABORATORY AND DIAGNOSTIC TESTING

No coagulation studies or other laboratory testing are necessary in the asymptomatic pediatric patient following a single unintentional ingestion of a small amount of an anticoagulant rodenticide. In the asymptomatic patient presenting soon after a single large intentional ingestion of an anticoagulant product, obtain a stat prothrombin time (PT) and partial thromboplastin time (PTT), and international normalized ratio (INR); reevaluate the patient at 24 and 48 hours. If an abnormal PT/PTT or INR is obtained from a clinically asymptomatic child, consider repeating the test to rule out a falsely elevated value from incomplete filling of the citrated blue-top tube.

In symptomatic patients or those demonstrating abnormal coagulation profiles consider obtaining the following:

- PT/PTT or INR every 6 to 12 hours until stabilized. Complete blood count; follow hemoglobin and hematocrit.
  Urinalysis to assess for hematuria.
  Stool hemoccult test.
  Type and screen; order type and cross if significant bleeding is present.
  Liver function tests to rule out hepatotoxicity as a cause of coagulopathy.

- Assays for long-acting anticoagulants may be performed by some reference laboratories. They may aid in confirmation of the diagnosis, but they are not routinely followed or used to guide therapy. Consider factor analysis if the cause of the coagulopathy is unknown; anticoagulants depress factors II, VII, IX, and X.

- Head CT if mental status changes are present.

- Endoscopy may be considered for the assessment of significant GI bleeding

MANAGEMENT

Identification of Product

It is imperative that every effort be made to identify the product involved in a rodenticide poisoning (Figure 52–1). Clearly document the brand name, active ingredients, and concentration. It also is important to keep in mind that the formulations of proprietary products periodically change. For example, an old formulation of Eraze contained warfarin 0.025%, but now contains zinc phosphide 2%. Mole Nots previously contained strychnine sulfate and now contains zinc phosphide 2%.

Patients who ingest any amount of the highly toxic rodenticides listed in Table 52–3 must be immediately referred to emergency care and promptly treated. Correspondingly, a child presenting soon after a rodenticide exposure with rapid onset of GI, neurologic, or cardiovascular symptoms should raise the suspicion of a very old, illicitly sold, or highly toxic pesticide.

Clinicians who become aware of covert sales or improper application of rodenticides should immediately report these incidents to local public health officials and to federal or state environmental protection agency pesticide divisions.

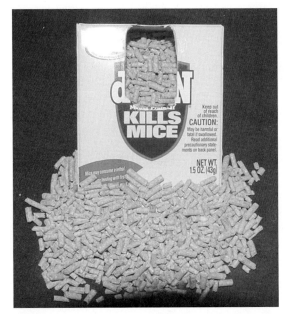

Fig. 52–1. It is important to identify the specific product involved in rodenticide exposures in order to identify the active ingredients.

Gastrointestinal Decontamination

Controversy exists regarding the benefits of home GI decontamination with syrup of ipecac or activated charcoal in the setting of unintentional pediatric long-acting anticoagulant rodenticide ingestions. Generally, no GI decontamination procedures are necessary following accidental trivial ingestions of these products.

For patients presenting soon after intentional ingestions of large amounts, give one dose of activated charcoal without a cathartic. Do not perform gastric lavage or induce vomiting in any patient actively bleeding or demonstrating an elevated PT or INR.

Fresh Frozen Plasma and Blood Products

For clinically significant active bleeding, FFP is essential to replenish all clotting factors (except platelets). The pediatric FFP dose is 10 to 25 mL/kg. The adult FFP dose is 2 to 4 U. This dose may be repeated as needed. Packed red cells, which do not supply clotting factors, may be given to correct severe anemia secondary to hemorrhage.

Specific Antidote: Vitamin K_1

Vitamin K_1 (Figure 52–2) is a specific antidote because it is a necessary cofactor that competes with warfarin and the long-acting anticoagulants to initiate formation of depleted clotting factors II, VII, IX, and X. Vitamin K_1

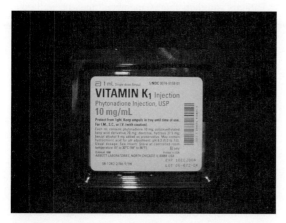

Fig. 52–2. Vitamin K is the antidote of choice with significant super warfarin or brodifacoum poisoning.

therapy is indicated for any patient experiencing active bleeding or demonstrating elevated PT or INR.

Prophylactic therapy is not indicated in asymptomatic patients with normal coagulation studies. Vitamin K_1 administration would merely provide a false sense of security for the prescribing physician, and only serve to delay the onset of anticoagulant effect of the rodenticide owing to its much longer duration of action. It is crucial to note that the only effective form of vitamin K is K_1 phytonadione (AquaMEPHYTON, Mephyton), which is the active form of the vitamin. Other forms of vitamin K, such as vitamin K_3, menadione (Synkayvite), are ineffective and should not be used.

Oral vitamin K_1 is the safest method of administration. It may be given with or without food. It has an onset of effect ranging from 6 to 12 hours. Vitamin K_1 is usually administered three to four times daily because it has a short therapeutic half-life. A human adult study showed an elimination half-life of 1.7 to 2.0 hours following intravenous (IV) administration. Following any adjustment in dose, the patient's PT or INR should be checked.

The only commercially available oral form of phytonadione is a 5-mg tablet. A 1 mg/mL suspension may be made by crushing six 5-mg tablets and adding 5 mL purified water and 5 mL 1% methylcellulose; mix well, add 70% sorbitol to a total volume of 30 mL, shake well, and refrigerate.

Phytonadione may be given parenterally via the intramuscular (IM), subcutaneous (SC), or IV routes. IM administration poses the risk of hematoma; therefore, the SC route may be a safer alternative. IV phytonadione offers the fastest onset of action (as little as 1 to 2 hours). Owing to the potential for significant adverse effects such as anaphylactoid reactions, IV administration is reserved for bleeding in which rapid correction of clotting is mandatory. Untoward reactions, which may occur even at correct dosages and rates, include flushing, hypotension, cyanosis, dizziness, diaphoresis, dyspnea, cardiac and/or respiratory arrest. Be prepared to resuscitate with epinephrine, antihistamines, and corticosteroid. Table 52–5 presents pediatric and adult dosing of phytonadione. Caution is advised in neonates because high doses of phytonadione (10 to 20 mg) may cause hyperbilirubinemia and severe hemolytic anemia. Because vitamin K_1 is a fat-soluble vitamin, concurrent administration of mineral oil as an emollient laxative may decrease oral absorption of this vitamin.

Following large ingestions of super warfarin products, antidotal therapy with large doses of vitamin K_1 (phytonadione), i.e., 50 to 100 mg/d, may be required for weeks to

Table 52–5. Pediatric and Adult Dosing of Phytonadione

Route	Pediatric Dose (mg)	Adult Dose (mg)	Comments
PO	5–10	15–25	Preferred route owing to safety. GI absorption is inconsistent. Daily maintenance doses of 50–200 g/d in 3–4 divided doses for weeks to months may be necessary.
SC	1–5	10–25	Safest and preferred parenteral route. Limited to 5 mL (50 mg) per administration site.
IM	1–5	5–10	Risk of hematoma and should avoided.
IV	0.5–5.0	Starting dose 10–25 mg. Repeated doses up to 400 mg have been used in maximally anticoagulated patients.	Most rapid onset of action. Reserved only for life-threatening bleeding when other routes are not feasible due to rare anaphylactoid reactions. Dilute in D_5W or 0.9% NS and give slowly, not to exceed 1 mg/min.

Abbreviations: IM, intramuscular; IV, intravenous; GI, gastrointestinal; NS, normal saline; PO, orally; SC, subcutaneously.

months. If a patient's medical condition, such as a prosthetic heart valve, requires the maintenance of therapeutic anticoagulation, place the patient on heparin until bleeding is controlled and PT is stabilized.

Enhanced Elimination

No definitive, clinically proven method of enhanced elimination exists for these agents.

DISPOSITION

For the pediatric patient with a reliable history of a taste amount of anticoagulant rodenticide bait, referral to a health care facility, home GI decontamination, and outpatient coagulation studies are not necessary. Caregivers should be advised to observe for signs of bleeding or easy bruising for several days and report any unusual symptoms to the physician or poison control center immediately.

For the pediatric patient suspected of eating large amounts of anticoagulant bait, home GI decontamination with activated charcoal may be considered, followed by a 48-h outpatient PT/PTT or INR. For the asymptomatic adolescent patient who presents soon after the intentional ingestion of a large amount of anticoagulant bait, give ac-

tivated charcoal, admit to a noncritical care unit, and monitor PT/PTT or INR at 24 and 48 hours.

For the asymptomatic patient presenting several days after a large acute ingestion, or in a patient with a history of chronic consumption with a an abnormal coagulation profile, admission to a noncritical care unit with frequent coagulation studies is reasonable. Initiate vitamin K_1 therapy as indicated. For any symptomatic patient who is actively bleeding, admit to a critical care unit for definitive care with FFP and vitamin K_1.

Patients and their family members must be well educated about the importance of full compliance with outpatient oral vitamin K_1 regimens and outpatient coagulation monitoring. The serious risk of bleeding must be thoroughly communicated. A social services investigation should be pursued following any suspicion of child neglect, abuse, or Munchausen syndrome by proxy.

CASE OUTCOME

The ED staff consults the regional poison control center. The product involved is presumed to be one of the more commonly used rodenticides, such as a long-acting anticoagulant, cholecalciferol, or bromethalin. No GI decontamination procedures or laboratory tests are advised pending information from building management

The custodian is reached by telephone. He identifies the rodenticide product as Talon G, which contains brodifacoum 0.005%. The assessment is that one mouthful of this long-acting anticoagulant in a small child is unlikely to be harmful. The patient is discharged and the family instructed to observe him for several days for evidence of bleeding or easy bruising.

SUGGESTED READINGS

Amr MM, Abbas EZ, El-Samra GM, et al: Neuropsychiatric syndromes and occupational exposure to zinc phosphide in Egypt. *Environ Res* 73:200–206, 1997.

Babcock J, Hartman K, Pedersen A, et al: Rodenticide induced coagulopathy in a young child. A case of Munchausen Syndrome by proxy. *Am J Pediatr Hematol Oncol* 15: 126–130, 1993.

Barrueto F, Nelson LS, Hoffman RS, et al: Poisoning by an illegally imported Chinese rodenticide containing tetramethylenedisulfotetramine—New York City. *MMWR Morb Mortal Wkly Rep* 52:199–201, 2003.

Blondell J: Epidemiology of pesticide poisonings in the United States with special reference to occupational cases. *Occup Med* 12:209–220, 1997.

Chugh SN, Aggarwal HK, Mahajan SK: Zinc phosphide intoxication symptoms: Analysis of 20 cases. *Int J Clin Pharmacol Ther* 36:406–407, 1998.

Favus MJ: Treatment of vitamin D intoxication. *N Engl J Med* 283:1468–1469, 1970.

Ingels M, Lai C, Manning BH, et al: A prospective study of acute, unintentional pediatric superwarfarin ingestions managed without decontamination. *Ann Emerg Med* 40: 73–78, 2002.

Jibani M, Hodges NH: Prolonged hypercalcaemia after industrial exposure to vitamin D_3. *BMJ* 290:748–749, 1985.

Johnson D, Kubic P, Levitt C: Accidental ingestion of Vacor rodenticide. *Am J Dis Child* 134:161–164, 1980.

Kanabar D, Volans G: Accidental superwarfarin poisoning in children—less is better. *Lancet* 360:963, 2002.

Mullins ME, Brands BL, Daya MR: Unintentional pediatric superwarfarin exposures: Do we really need a prothrombin time? *Pediatrics* 105:402–404, 2000.

Nelson LS, Perrone J, DeRoos F, et al: Aldicarb poisoning by an illicit rodenticide imported into the united states: Tres Pasitos. *J Clin Toxicol* 39:447–452, 2001.

Ramon A, Dong P, Perrone J et al: Poisonings associated with illegal use of aldicarb as a rodenticide—New York City, 1994–1997. *MMWR* 46:961–964, 1997.

Robinson RF, Griffith JR, Wolowich WR et al: Intoxication with sodium monofluoroacetate (compound 1080). *Vet Hum Toxicol* 44:93–95, 2002.

Rodengerg HD, Chang CC, Watson WA: Zinc phosphide ingestion: A case report and review. *Vet Hum Toxicol* 31:559–562, 1989.

Sheperd G, Klein-Schwartz W, Anderson B: Acute, unintentional pediatric brodifacoum ingestions. *Pediatr Emerg Care* 18:174–178, 2002.

Taketomo CK, Hodding JH, Kraus DM, eds: *Pediatric Dosage Handbook: Including Neonatal Dosing, Drug Administration & Extemporaneous Preparations.* 9th ed. Hudson, OH: Lexi-Comp; 2002.

Talcott PA, Mather GG, Kowitz EH: Accidental ingestion of a cholecalciferol-containing rodent bait in a dog. *Vet Hum Toxicol* 33:252–255, 1991.

Travis SF, Warfield W, Greenbaum BH, et al: Clinical and laboratory observations: Spontaneous hemorrhage associated with accidental brodifacoum poisoning in a child. *J Pediatr* 122:982–984, 1993.

van Lier RB, Cherry LD: The toxicity and mechanism of action of bromethalin: A new single-feeding rodenticide. *Fundam Appl Toxicol* 11:664–672, 1988.

Watts RG, Castleberry RP, Sadowski JA: Accidental Poisoning with a superwarfarin compound (brodifacoum) in a child. *Pediatrics* 86:883–887, 1990.

53

Drugs of Abuse

Sean M. Bryant

HIGH-YIELD FACTS

- It is important for medical personnel to understand the trends and epidemiologic data regarding the use of illicit substances in the pediatric population.

- It is commonly thought that drug abuse in pediatric patients is restricted to adolescents. However, even younger patients are vulnerable to drug abuse.

- The most common drugs abused by younger patients include amphetamines, cocaine, opioids, phencyclidine (PCP), cannabinoids, hallucinogens, tobacco, ethanol, inhalants, and anabolic steroids.

- Most drug abuse trends have remained steady over the last several years; however, use of the designer amphetamine MDMA (ecstasy) and inhalants has escalated.

The disturbing trends in drug abuse in the United States are not limited to the adult population. Pediatricians and emergency physicians are no doubt aware that children and adolescents abuse drugs for a variety of reasons. It is important for medical personnel to understand the trends and epidemiologic data regarding the use of these substances in the pediatric population.

It is commonly thought that drug abuse in pediatric patients is restricted to older children and adolescents. However, even younger patients are vulnerable to drug abuse. For example, this author was consulted on a 5-year-old patient who presented to the emergency department (ED) a second time with inebriation secondary to gasoline sniffing to get high. A variety of factors play a part in defining the risk factors in the epidemic of drug abuse in young patients. American society is greatly affected by the prevalence of risky behavior by this patient population. Emergency medical services (EMS) use reported by an urban academic ED recorded that approximately 15% of EMS transports were related to suicide, assault, alcohol, and drug intoxication. Data for the first 6 months of 2002 reported 29,846 drug-related ED visits for patients age 12 to 17. The Drug Abuse Warning Network (DAWN) study also reported a 17.1% increase in ED visits related to illegal drug use or nonmedical use of legal drugs between 1999 and 2001.

The most common drugs abused by younger patients include amphetamines, cocaine, opioids, PCP, cannabinoids, hallucinogens, tobacco, ethanol, inhalants, and anabolic steroids. Data recording trends of drug abuse are obtained from annual reports of the toxic exposure surveillance system (TESS) data published by the American Association of Poison Control Centers, DAWN, the National Household Survey on Drug Abuse (NHSDA), and national law enforcement agencies such as the National Institute for Drug Abuse. Each of these data sets provides valuable insight pertaining to drug abuse. However, each has important limitations. For example, TESS data records only those calls reported to a regional poison center. One can imagine a number of teenagers seen in the ED for illicit drug or ethanol-related reasons never get reported to the poison center. DAWN data may underreport drug-related episodes, because only cases in which a drug is part of the presenting problem are reported. The NHSDA data have the inherent limitations found in survey-acquired data. Collectively, however, these data shed significant light on the problem of drug abuse among America's youth.

EPIDEMIOLOGY

General

Drug use among minors continues to be significant, albeit lower than the highest recorded rate of abuse in 1979 (Figure 53–1). The peak annual use of any illicit drug by high school students was 54.2% in 1979, which subsequently dropped by approximately 50% in 1992. The National Institute on Drug Abuse Monitoring the Future (MTF) study has revealed a stable rate in drug abuse since 1992. According to the Department of Health and Human Service's Substance Abuse and Mental Health Services Administration's 1999 NHSDA, 9% of children between 12 and 17 years of age reported current use of an illegal drug in 1999, a 2% decline from 11.4% in 1997. The same survey found that the highest overall rate of drug abuse was in the 18- to 20-year-old range. Noteworthy substances of abuse include inhalants, which were distinguished as the most commonly abused poison among 12 year olds in 1999, whereas the favored drug of 14 year olds was reported to be marijuana.

Illicit Drugs

Initially used for nasal congestion and as a stimulant in World War II, amphetamines, and more specifically designer amphetamines like methamphetamine and methylenedioxymethamphetamine (MDMA or ecstasy), are now popular drugs of abuse. The NHSDS reported a significant rise in the rate of first time use among youths 12 to 17 years old from 1990 to 1998. According to the 2000 MTF survey, junior high school eighth graders showed a staggering past-year use increase of 82% and a past-month use rise of 75%. Both tenth and twelfth graders

had similar but less dramatic trends. In all age groups, the number of amphetamine-related deaths in the United States tripled from 1991 to 1994. ED visits related to methamphetamine use increased approximately 3.5 times from 1991 to 1994.

Cocaine is a commonly abused drug by patients of all ages and results in frequent drug-related ED visits in the United States. The annual number of new users of all forms of cocaine increased 45% from 1994 to 1999, with an overall threefold increase in the 12- to 17-year-old age group. One survey showed that almost 9.5% of students had used some form of cocaine during their lifetime. Another concerning trend is the rate of first-time use among those 12 to 17 years old, which was 5.1% in 1992, but increased to 13.1% in 1996. Poison center data indicate a relatively stable number of cocaine-related cases reported over the last 5 years among patients 6 to 19 years of age.

Opioids can be abused in a variety of forms. Nonmedical use of analgesic formulations like Oxycontin and Vicodin defines one subset of users; heroin is the most common illicit opioid abused. Heroin initiation in 12- to 17-year-old patients doubled from the mid 1980s to the late 1990s. In fact, 25% of all new users of heroin between 1996 and 1998 were reported to be younger than 18 years of age. For eighth and tenth graders, past-year use peaked in 1996 and 1997, respectively. However, among high school seniors, one survey reported a 275% increase for both past-year and past-month use. While insufflation (snorting) is the most popular route of administration in inner-city patients, intravenous use is prevalent among suburban dwellers.

PCP was used as an anesthetic in the 1950s and 1960s in both human and veterinary patients. Abuse of PCP be-

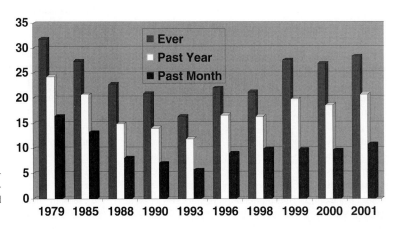

Fig. 53–1. Percentage of 12- to 17-year-olds reporting any illicit drug use as reported by the National Household Survey on Drug Abuse (NHSDA).

gan in the 1960s, becoming epidemic in the late 1970s. According to TESS data, poison center cases related to PCP have remained relatively stable over the last 5 years, with 30% consistently being associated with patients between 6 and 19 years of age.

Marijuana is the most popular of all illegal drugs in the United States. It is often touted as a gateway drug that leads to the use of more serious drugs like cocaine and heroin. ED visits related to marijuana increased over 40% from 1996 to 1998. Over 1 million adolescents 16 to 18 years of age reported driving at least once within 2 hours of illicit use. Poison center data reveal a steady rise in cases in the 6- to 19-year-old age group over the last 5 years. Male Caucasians appear to be the most prevalent group abusing marijuana. A report in 1998 indicated 85% of students had used marijuana at least once in their lifetime. Recent MTF data do, however, indicate that past-year use among eighth and tenth graders had decreased by 15% and 10%, respectively.

Hallucinogens include a variety of agents including lysergic acid diethylamide (LSD), GHB and its precursors, specific mushrooms, MDMA, marijuana, and plants such as jimsonweed. Use among all age groups decreased during the late 1970s and early 1980s. However, during the 1990s, there has been a resurgence in abuse. High school student use peaked in 1996. In 1999, over 14% of twelfth graders reported to have at least tried LSD, which was 5% higher than that reported 10 years earlier. The 2000 MTF study showed a declining trend in hallucinogen use among tenth and twelfth graders, and past-year and past-month use of LSD in twelfth graders decreased 10% and 44%, respectively. LSD use appears to be more prevalent in suburban communities. TESS data indicate that, over the last 5 years, 55% to 66% of LSD-related cases reported to poison centers involve patients between 6 and 19 years of age.

Other

Much like marijuana, ethanol, and inhalants, tobacco has been considered a particularly important gateway drug. In fact, patients 12 to 17 years of age who smoke are 7.3 times more likely to use illegal drugs than those who do not use tobacco, and 15% more likely to drink heavily than youths who do not smoke. The average age of smoking initiation is 10.7 years for boys and 11.4 years for girls. Each day more than 6000 patients 13 years of age or younger try their first cigarette. Although smoking trends in adults have declined, the rate of use in teens has remained steady over the last several years. One out of 10 middle school students and more than 25% of high

school students are currently regular smokers. Children in rural regions abuse tobacco products more often than their urban counterparts. Among eighth graders, rural students are twice as likely to have smoked cigarettes in the past month and 5 times more likely to have used smokeless tobacco when compared to urban children. Smokeless tobacco products have proven to be popular among the youth. In 1985, 10 million Americans were reported to have used these products, one-third being under 21 years of age.

Ethanol addiction appears to be, at least in part, related to the age of onset of drinking. Youth who drink ethanol prior to age 15 are roughly four times as likely to develop an addiction as are those who began drinking at the legal age. In 1999, close to 30% of U.S. citizens (10.4 million) 12 to 20 years of age were considered to be current ethanol users, 20% of whom binge drink, with 6% considered heavy drinkers. It is evident that young people use ethanol much more than illegal drugs. By eighth grade, almost half of all youth have tried ethanol, and over one-fifth have already been drunk once.

Solvent sniffing abuse has been noted since the 1950s, when it was found to be prevalent among adolescent males in California. Since then, an epidemic of inhalant abuse has spread nationwide in the form of sniffing, huffing, and bagging. Popular products include hydrocarbons, glues, cleaning fluids, typewriter correction fluid, fuels, refrigerants, deodorizers, and paints. Over the past 8 years, the rate of first-time inhalant use has more than doubled. Prevalence of use in the 12- to 17-year-old patient was reported to be 1.6%, 2%, and 0.9% in 1994, 1997, and 1999, respectively. By 2001 more than 14% of U.S. students had sniffed glue, abused aerosol spray cans, or inhaled paint fumes to get high.

When considering ergogenic abuse, like anabolic steroids, one generally associates it with participants in sports-related activity. The MTF study reported that use of steroids by tenth graders in 1999 to 2000 had increased by 29%. One survey of high school seniors documented 6.6% of boys who abused anabolic steroids; over one third of these students were not involved in organized athletics. The reported use of steroids by college football players is 20% to 30%, many of whom are under 20 years of age.

CONCLUSION

Many pediatric patients are regularly involved in using illicit drugs. Most drug abuse trends have remained steady over the last several years; however, use of MDMA and inhalants has escalated. It is important for the clinician to be aware of current epidemiologic trends in drug use to consider possible etiologies of presenting pathology, as well as to provide timely education and intervention.

SUGGESTED READINGS

Buckley WE, Yesalis CE 3rd, et al: Estimated prevalence of anabolic steroid use among male high school seniors. *JAMA* 260:3441–3445, 1988.

Dias PJ: Adolescent substance abuse assessment in the office. *Pediatr Clin North Am* 49:269–300, 2002.

Fine JS: Pediatric principles. In: Goldfrank LR, Flomenbaum NE, Lewin NA, et al, eds: *Goldfrank's Toxicologic Emergencies.* 7th ed. New York: McGraw-Hill; 2002:1667.

Johnston LD, O'Malley PM, Bachman JG: *National Survey Results on Drug Use From the Monitoring the Future Study, Volume I: Secondary School Students.* (NIH Publication No. 99-4660.) Rockville, MD: National Institute on Drug Abuse; 2000.

Litovitz TL, Klein-Schwartz W, Dyer KS, et al: 1997 annual report of the American Association of Poison Control Centers Toxic Exposure Surveillance System. *Am J Emerg Med* 16: 443–497, 1998.

Litovitz TL, Klein-Schwartz W, Caravati EM, et al: 1998 annual report of the American Association of Poison Control Centers Toxic Exposure Surveillance System. *Am J Emerg Med* 17:435–487, 1999.

Litovitz TL, Klein-Schwartz W, White S, et al: 1999 annual report of the American Association of Poison Control Centers Toxic Exposure Surveillance System. *Am J Emerg Med* 18: 517–574, 2000.

Litovitz TL, Klein-Schwartz W, White S, et al: 2000 annual report of the American Association of Poison Control Centers Toxic Exposure Surveillance System. *Am J Emerg Med* 19: 337–395, 2001.

Litovitz TL, Klein-Schwartz W, Rodgers GC, et al: 2001 annual report of the American Association of Poison Control Centers Toxic Exposure Surveillance System. *Am J Emerg Med* 20: 391–452, 2002.

National Center on Addiction and Substance Abuse at Columbia University (CASA): *No Place to Hide: Substance Abuse in Mid-Size Cities and Rural America.* Commissioned by the United States Conference of Mayors and Funded by the DEA with Support from the National Institute on Drug Abuse; January 1999.

National Institute on Alcohol Abuse and Alcoholism: *Advancing Knowledge through Research.* Fact Sheet; Fall 1999.

National Institute on Drug Abuse, University of Michigan: *Monitoring the Future 2002 Data From In-School Surveys of 8th, 10th, and 12th Grade Students.* December 2002.

Office of Juvenile Justice and Delinquency Prevention: *Drug Identification and Testing in the Juvenile Justice System.* May 1998.

Office of National Drug Control Policy: *National Drug Control Strategy.* February 2003.

Sapien RE, Fullerton L, Olson LM, et al: Disturbing trends: The epidemiology of pediatric emergency medical services use. *Acad Emerg Med* 6:232–238, 1999.

Substance Abuse and Mental Health Services Administration: *Emergency Department Trends From the Drug Abuse Warning Network, Preliminary Estimates January–June 2002.* December 2002.

Substance Abuse and Mental Health Services Administration/ Office of Applied Studies: *1999 National Household Survey on Drug Abuse.* Rockville, MD: Department of Health and Human Services; August 2000.

Substance Abuse and Mental Health Service Administration: *Results From the 2001 National Household Survey on Drug Abuse: Volume II, Technical Appendices and Selected Data Tables.* August 2002.

54

Amphetamines

Ernest Stremski
David D. Gummin

HIGH-YIELD FACTS

- Within the past 5 years, MDMA (ecstasy) use in the United States has increased at an alarming rate. This drug is very popular among adolescents at clubs hosting rave parties.

- The clinical syndrome associated with amphetamine toxicity consists of vasoconstriction, tachycardia, and hypertension, associated with agitation and central nervous system (CNS) excitation.

- Clinically, some amphetamines may have both stimulant (sympathomimetic) and hallucinogenic effects.

- Urine drug screening may be helpful to confirm amphetamine exposure. These screens are not specific to amphetamine, and false-positive results may occur with over-the-counter products such as pseudoephedrine, phenylpropanolamine, or ephedra.

- Tachycardia and hypertension may be seen in agitated patients. Benzodiazepine sedation may be required for treating cardiac stimulation.

- Patients with severe hyperthermia should be treated with aggressive, active cooling. Rhabdomyolysis is treated with volume diuresis and urinary alkalinization.

CASE PRESENTATION

A 16-year-old boy snorted a mixture of methamphetamine crystals in the company of friends at a party. The methamphetamine was obtained from an unknown source. The patient became agitated and tremulous within minutes of insufflation. He appeared sweaty and complained of feeling hot. He began speaking nonsensically. Friends were unable to control him as his agitation worsened. He then fell to the ground and began convulsing. Emergency medical services (EMS) was contacted.

On EMS arrival, he was noted to be diaphoretic and unresponsive. Active seizures were suspected, as he demonstrated facial twitching, extremity rigidity, and drooling. EMS assisted ventilations and administered 2 mg of lorazepam intravenously (IV).

On arrival to the Emergency Department (ED), the patient is unresponsive to deep pain. His blood pressure is 165/95 mmHg, heart rate 145 bpm, respirations are shallow at 22 per minute, core temperature is 100.8°F, and room air pulse oximetry is 93%. He continues to experience generalized tonic–clonic extremity movement. Rapid sequence intubation is performed with midazolam and rocuronium. Additional lorazepam is given IV over the next hour, to a total of 10 mg, which appears to stop the seizures. Other physical findings include dilated pupils and diaphoretic skin.

A computerized tomography (CT) scan of the brain is normal. Urine drug screen is positive for benzodiazepines, amphetamines, and cannabinoids. Initial electrolytes, glucose, and complete blood count are all within normal limits. Serum creatinine kinase level peaks at 6500 IU/L. Urinalysis is positive for myoglobin and trace red blood cells.

INTRODUCTION AND EPIDEMIOLOGY

Amphetamine and amphetamine-like stimulants have a long history of use in Western medicine. During the past century, amphetamines were prescribed for weight loss, depression, narcolepsy, and attention deficit disorder (ADD). They have also been used as analeptics and as general stimulants. Although medical use of amphetamines has waned, there has been a recent upsurge in both the number of children treated with stimulants for ADD, and in the number of pharmacologic preparations available to treat the disorder. Likewise, although amphetamine abusers constitute a minority of drug users, the available chemical derivatives of amphetamine continue to proliferate. The accessibility of chemical precursors for synthesis of designer amphetamines affords the drug counterculture opportunity to modify and experiment with a variety of new stimulant and hallucinogenic amphetamines.

According to the 2002 National Survey on Drug Use and Health, there are 1.2 million Americans abusing stimulants. Another 676,000 are current ecstasy users (defined as use within the past month). Among youths aged 12 to 17 years, lifetime prevalence of illicit amphetamine use increased from 0.7% to 4.3% between 1990 and 2002. Users of ecstasy (also known as 3,4-methylenedioxymethamphetamine or MDMA) and other stimulants totalled over 1.8 million, approaching the prevalence of cocaine use.

The most commonly abused illicit amphetamine is methamphetamine (commonly called *crystal, crank, ice,* and *meth*). Methamphetamine production and consumption is regional, concentrated primarily in the central Midwest and in the Western and Southwestern United States. Clandestine laboratories in the Southwest produce the lion's share of this drug. Since 1994, Mexican drug traffickers, operating super labs in Mexico and California, have controlled the production and distribution of most domestic methamphetamine.

The supply is augmented by synthesis of methamphetamine in small-scale laboratories operated by independent "cooks" who obtain ingredients from retail and convenience stores. Methamphetamine produced in these laboratories is generally for personal use or limited distribution. These clandestine laboratories typically substitute common items—pickle jars, coffee filters, hot plates, pillowcases, plastic tubing, and gas cans—for sophisticated laboratory equipment (Figure 54–1). The growing use of the Internet provides access to methamphetamine recipes. Coupled with increasing demand for high-purity

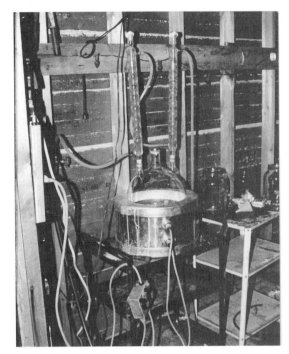

Fig. 54–1. Clandestine methamphetamine laboratory.

product, this sparked a substantial rise in the number of low-output clandestine laboratories throughout the United States; there were 7700 such labs in 2001.

An additional source of methamphetamine tablets is from Southeast Asia. Produced mainly by the *United Wa State Army* in Burma, the tablets are distributed throughout Southeast Asia, and smuggled and distributed as *yaba* among Southeast Asian ethnics.

A relatively newer form of methamphetamine has recently broached the illicit market. The clear, crystalline appearance is responsible for its street names—*crystal* or *ice.* Ice is precipitated in a purified crystalline form that is less likely to be adulterated. It can be smoked, injected, or nasally insufflated, and produces an immediate high similar to the rush of IV methamphetamine. Effects persist up to 24 hours. Auditory hallucinations, paranoid reactions, delirium, and violent behavior are reported to be more frequent with ice than with other forms of amphetamine.

Rave dance parties so commonly involve stimulant drug use, that the Drug Abuse Warning Network (DAWN) elected to issue reports on "Club Drug" abuse in 2000, and again in 2002. In both reports, methamphetamine was the most commonly abused drug. By the time of the latter report, the increasing use of MDMA made it the second most commonly encountered drug associated with these events. Within the past years, MDMA use in the United States has "increased at an alarming rate," according to the U.S. Drug Enforcement Agency. This drug is very popular among middle-class adolescents and young adults, and its use is on the rise, largely because many users view it as benign and nonaddictive. MDMA is sold at both legitimate nightclubs and at underground clubs that host all-night rave parties.

A typical Ecstasy tablet contains 70 to 120 mg of MDMA and sells for between $20 and $30 (Figure 54–2). The majority of MDMA consumed in the United States is clandestinely manufactured in Western Europe, particularly in the Netherlands or in Belgium. However, law enforcement agents seized 17 clandestine MDMA laboratories in the United States in 2001. DAWN estimates that MDMA use rose over 2000% between 1994 and 2001.

DEVELOPMENTAL CONSIDERATIONS

Amphetamine and amphetamine-like agents may be abused by women of childbearing age. Amphetamine agents share similar structures, and their physical properties allow them to cross the placenta and accumulate in fetal tissue. When injected IV into the pregnant ewe, methamphetamine crosses the placenta and is measurable in fetal tissue. Maternal doses of IV methamphetamine produce both maternal and fetal hypertension, as well as decreased uterine blood flow.

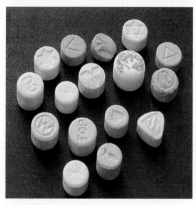

Fig. 54–2. MDMA (ecstasy) tablets.

A pregnant female may experience significant adverse cardiovascular effects from amphetamine use, particularly hypertension. Similar to other vasoconstrictive agents (like cocaine), this may induce eclampsia or spontaneous abortion. Fetal death has been associated with maternal methamphetamine use. Methamphetamine abuse may also elevate the risk of preterm labor, although other factors may also be contributory. Infants who had gestational exposure to methamphetamine have been shown to have lower birth weight, head circumference, and body length. Similar to the syndrome described in cocaine addiction, maternal abuse of amphetamine agents may lead to a neonatal withdrawal syndrome that includes agitation, tremor, poor feeding, and seizures.

A number of case reports and retrospective series describe teratogenic anomalies in infants born to maternal abusers of amphetamine, methamphetamine, and MDMA. Such effects included limb reduction, congenital heart disease, cleft palate, and biliary atresia. Although teratogenicity seems plausible, recent prospective series have not shown a significant increase in major congenital anomalies in these infants. In two prospective case series, infants of mothers who used MDMA had congenital heart disease in 2 of 78 cases and 1 of 49 cases, indistinguishable from rates seen in the general population.

Pregnant abusers of illicit amphetamines may also use other illicit compounds, ethanol, or nicotine. They may have relatively poor nutrition and inadequate prenatal care. Adverse fetal outcomes owing to amphetamine use during pregnancy, therefore, may be multifactorial, and are difficult to attribute solely to an illicit amphetamine compound.

Amphetamines are secreted into breast milk. The American Academy of Pediatrics considers amphetamine agents to be contraindicated for women who are breastfeeding (see Chapter 4).

PHARMACOLOGY AND PATHOPHYSIOLOGY

Chemically, amphetamines are phenylethylamines. The basic amphetamine structure mimics that of epinephrine, or more closely, that of norepinephrine (Figure 54–3). Pharmacologic properties parallel those of the endogenous catecholamines. Clinically, some amphetamines may be both stimulant (sympathomimetic) and hallucinogenic. Pharmacologic activity is classically described as being indirect because amphetamines prevent packaging of catecholamine neurotransmitters in presynaptic vesicles, causing more endogenous bioamine to be available for synaptic transmission. But many amphetamine derivatives and congeners have direct neurotransmitter activity as well, and directly agonize adrenergic receptors.

Amphetamines are α-adrenergic agonists, and cause stimulation of vascular smooth muscle, resulting in vasoconstriction. Centrally, amphetamines stimulate both cortical and medullary centers to increase sympathomimetic outflow. Peripherally, amphetamines cause release of norepinephrine and also directly stimulate both α- and β-adrenergic receptors. β-Adrenergic activity increases cardiac contractility and heart rate. Amphetamines may also inhibit endogenous catecholamine breakdown by inhibition of monoamine oxidase. In toxic patients, these sympathomimetic effects are exaggerated.

Designer amphetamines, in general, possess serotonergic properties. This may explain the hallucinations seen in both recreational use and in toxicity. Ecstasy, in particular, possesses both norepinephrine-like and serotonin-like moieties (see Figure 54–3). Toxic effects combine both sympathomimetic and serotonergic features.

Amphetamine and methamphetamine are rapidly and completely absorbed from the oral mucosa and gastrointestinal (GI) tract. Ecstasy is also well absorbed by ingestion, with onset of effects at 30 to 60 minutes, and effects peak at approximately 90 minutes. Bioavailability of methamphetamine is on the order of 90% when smoked.

A sizeable fraction of most amphetamines is excreted in the urine. However, most also undergo hepatic deamination, hydroxylation, and dealkylation to various metabolites. Noteworthy among these metabolites is α-methyl tyramine, which is a potent hallucinogen, and may be responsible for amphetamine-induced psychosis. Elimination half-life of amphetamines varies with the specific drug, but is generally between 10 and 30 hours. Onset of activity relates to the dose, route, and degree of absorption. Duration of toxicity is more variable. Elimination depends not only on the dose and the agent consumed, but also on urinary pH, a key determinant of the rate of elimination. Elimination kinetics appear to be nonlinear. Duration of clinical toxicity need not correlate with the drug's kinetics, particularly where active metabolites are involved. In the setting of severe toxicity, a more prolonged duration of effects should be anticipated.

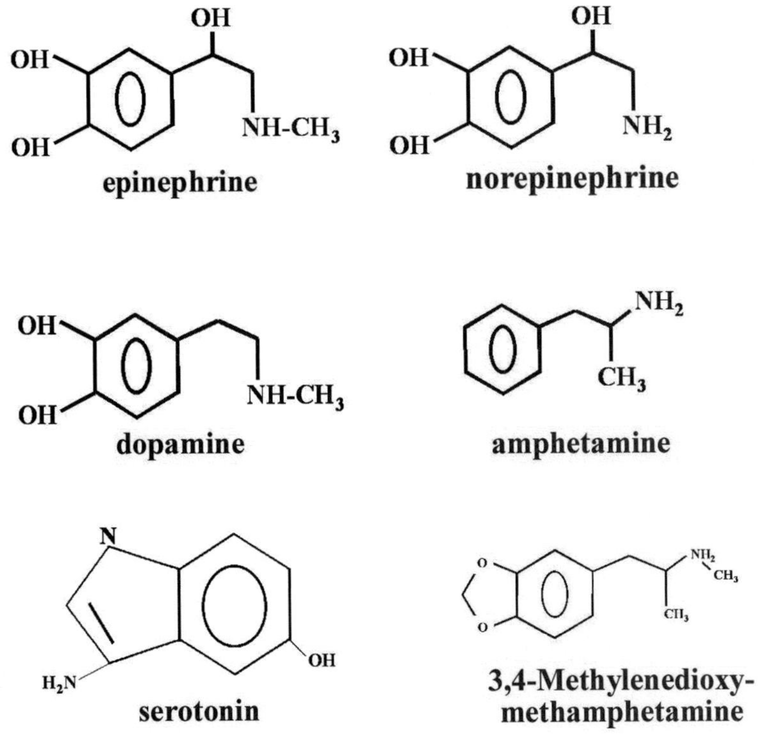

Fig. 54–3. The basic amphetamine structure is similar to that of epinephrine and norepinephrine.

DIAGNOSIS

The clinical syndrome associated with amphetamine toxicity consists of vasoconstriction, tachycardia, and hypertension, associated with agitation and CNS excitation. In acute toxicity, cardiovascular and CNS complications require immediate attention. Dysrhythmias, cerebrovascular accidents, seizures, hyperthermia, and acute psychotic delirium are not uncommon. Neurologic signs involve a spectrum from mild agitation to violent or catatonic behavior, seizures, and stroke. Mild hypertonicity is common. Acute, and often fatal, nontraumatic cerebral edema is reported as a complication associated with hyperthermia after MDMA use.

Hemodynamic signs range from mild to severe hypertension, and may lead to stroke, renal insufficiency, or cardiac compromise. Myocardial ischemia or infarction, aortic dissection, and ventricular dysfunction have been reported in overdose. This may occur in young, previously healthy patients. In massive overdose or severe toxicity, cardiovascular collapse heralds a very poor prognosis.

A plethora of respiratory tract pathology has been reported after either nasal insufflation or smoking of amphetamines. These include nasal septal perforation, and pulmonary complications including pulmonary edema, hemorrhage, infarct, and eosinophilic pulmonary infiltrates. The degree to which any single physiologic mechanism accounts for this pathology remains elusive. Contributing factors include forced Valsalva, smoke irritation, or direct toxicity from drug or adulterants.

Orally ingested amphetamines cause local vasoconstriction in the gut, and may result in varying degrees of tissue damage. Ischemic complications include acute abdominal pain, bloody diarrhea, and shock from mesenteric ischemia.

Mild amphetamine-induced hyperthermia is common in overdose, and likely relates to agitation and increased metabolic demands. Severe hyperthermia ($>40°C$) is probably of multifactorial origin, and is predictive of fulminant hepatic necrosis, rhabdomyolysis, and possible cardiovascular collapse. Although the specific mechanism of stimulant-induced hyperthermia is unknown, the prognosis is poor once it occurs. Hyperthermia in this setting should be treated aggressively with external cooling measures. Antipyretics are of no benefit.

Dermatologic signs of amphetamine toxicity include early piloerection and cutaneous vasoconstriction. Overt toxicity is associated with diaphoresis. Parenteral administration may leave track marks or scarring from healing of recurrent local injections or infections.

Amphetamine toxicity should be suspected in a patient who exhibits signs and symptoms consistent with sympathomimetic stimulation. The sympathomimetic toxidrome may be difficult to clinically distinguish from anticholinergic toxicity. Both toxidromes are associated with CNS excitation, mydriasis, tachycardia, hypertension, and hyperthermia. Unlike sympathomimetic toxicity, however, anticholinergic agents cause acute urinary retention. Further, sympathomimetic toxicity is associated with normal bowel sounds and with diaphoresis, whereas anticholinergic overdose causes hypoactive bowel sounds, and dry skin and mucous membranes.

LABORATORY TESTING

Routine laboratory and other diagnostic studies are generally not helpful in amphetamine toxicity. In moderate to severe toxicity, a complete blood count, serum electrolytes, glucose, blood urea nitrogen, and creatinine are indicated. An anion gap metabolic acidosis may be seen in significantly intoxicated individuals. Hyponatremia-induced seizures have been described in individuals using MDMA. This may result from dehydration, excessive water consumption, or elevated antidiuretic hormone levels. A clinical assessment of volume status is critical in determining the etiology of hyponatremia.

In patients who are severely toxic, hyperthermic, or suffering seizures, the clinician should consider obtaining initial liver enzymes and bilirubin, as well as coagulation parameters. Marked hyperpyrexia may lead to acute hepatic failure and disseminated intravascular coagulopathy (DIC), similar to that seen in environmental heat stroke. Sympathomimetic agents associated with hyperpyrexia and DIC include cocaine, methamphetamine, MDMA, other MDMA-like designer amphetamines, and ephedra.

The urine drug screen may be helpful in confirming amphetamine exposure. These screens are not specific to amphetamine, and often detect over-the-counter products such as pseudoephedrine, phenylpropanolamine, or ephedra, as amphetamines. Designer amphetamines that contain the phenylethylamine structure typically cause the urine drug screen to be positive for amphetamines. However, these qualitative screens do not identify the specific amphetamine, nor are they useful in quantifying exposure. Individuals who are intoxicated with sympathomimetic agents used in the treatment of ADD develop the amphetamine toxidrome, yet fail to test positive on the amphetamine assay. These agents, including methylphenidate, pemoline, and atomoxetine, do not possess the phenylethylamine structure, and will not show up on the amphetamine screen. Adderall (D,1-amphetamine) is detected as a true positive on this screen (see Chapter 20).

Quantitative serum or urine levels for the more common amphetamine agents can be obtained through reference laboratories. Levels frequently do not correlate with presence or severity of toxicity. Further, prolonged turnaround time from reference laboratories typically limits the clinical utility of these levels.

In the setting of severe agitation, obtundation, or hyperthermia, rhabdomyolysis is possible, and serum creatinine and urine myoglobin are indicated. The urine dipstick provides a readily available screen for urine myoglobin. An acellular urine that tests positive for blood on the dipstick is strongly suggestive of the presence of urine myoglobin.

Continuous electrocardiographic and core temperature monitoring are indicated for patients who demonstrate or develop vital sign abnormalities. This monitoring should be continued through resolution of abnormal vital signs.

A CT scan of the brain is performed on all patients suspected of stimulant abuse who present with an abnormal mental status to exclude cerebral edema, stroke, and intracranial hemorrhage.

MANAGEMENT

Paramount to the treatment of any intoxicated individual is attention to protecting the airway and maintaining adequate ventilation. Supplemental oxygen and/or endotracheal intubation may be required for obtunded or seizing patients. Benzodiazepines, short-acting barbiturates, propofol, and nondepolarizing paralytics may be used for rapid sequence intubation.

There is no specific antidote for stimulant toxicity. Mild amphetamine-induced toxicity generally requires no intervention. Patients should be observed until signs of toxicity normalize. Benzodiazepines are considered safe and may be useful to control dysphoria or agitation.

More severe toxicity such as agitation, hypertension, or tachycardia can be managed with benzodiazepines as well. Agitation may be safely controlled with titrated, multiple, IV boluses of diazepam or lorazepam. Often, larger amounts of benzodiazepines are required than with standard sedative-hypnotic dosing. Diazepam is dosed at 0.2 to 0.5 mg/kg, and repeated every 5 minutes if needed.

Lorazepam is similarly administered, but dosed at 1/10th to 1/5th the diazepam dose, 0.05 to 0.1 mg/kg, every 5 to 10 minutes. These same agents are considered first line for involuntary motor activity, dystonia, or seizures induced by stimulants. Refractory convulsions may require an IV phenobarbital load. In addition, continuous IV drips of midazolam or propofol may be beneficial for patients requiring mechanical ventilation.

Activated charcoal is effective at binding amphetamines and amphetamine-like stimulants and, if provided within the first 1 to 2 hours after a large oral ingestion, may be useful for GI decontamination. There is no role for activated charcoal if the stimulant was administered parenterally, smoked, or nasally insufflated. No data support the use of multiple-dose activated charcoal to enhance elimination of these agents. Whole bowel irrigation decreases intestinal transit time and may be indicated in body stuffers or body packers (see below).

Mild tachycardia and hypertension may be seen in agitated patients. Benzodiazepine sedation may be all that is required for treating mild cardiac stimulation. In hemodynamically unstable patients, labetolol, which blocks both α- and β-adrenergic receptors, may control hypertension. Monotherapy with β-specific antagonists is relatively contraindicated, because unopposed α stimulation can exacerbate hypertension. Sodium nitroprusside may be required for refractory hypertension. A calcium channel antagonist, such as diltiazem, may be required for tachydysrhythmias. Benzodiazepines and coronary vasodilators (e.g., nitroglycerin) are the treatments of choice in managing acute coronary syndrome induced by stimulants.

Patients with severe hyperthermia should be treated with aggressive, active cooling. Rhabdomyolysis is treated with volume diuresis. Alkalinization of the urine may be required. Variable protein binding and generally large volumes of distribution hinder hemodialysis or other means of extracorporeal elimination. In the past, clinicians sought to exploit the weak alkalinity of most amphetamines, and recommended acid diuresis to enhance elimination. Metabolic disturbances caused by serum acidification, as well as worsening of renal failure with rhabdomyolysis, led to current recommendations to avoid acidification of the serum or urine.

BODY STUFFERS AND PACKERS

Body stuffers may swallow amphetamines when confronted by authorities. *Body packers* intentionally swallow or pack body orifices with drug to conceal and illegally transport the product. To avoid inadvertent packet rupture, body packing typically entails more elaborate methods of packaging the substance. Conversely, body stuffing implies poorly wrapped drug, which threatens to become bioavailable. The clinician should attempt to gather enough information regarding the dose ingested and the type of packaging to assess the potential for toxicity.

In body stuffers, gastric decontamination with syrup of ipecac or gastric lavage is relatively contraindicated, because either may rupture packets. Whole bowel irrigation with polyethylene glycol-electrolyte lavage solution can enhance drug transit through the GI tract. This mode of decontamination is intended to decrease transit time and minimize systemic absorption of the toxicant. It is important to ensure that all ingested packets pass before the patient is discharged. To ensure this may require a gastrograffin swallow or abdominal CT. In symptomatic body stuffers, surgical consultation is indicated, because laparotomy may be required.

DISPOSITION

Patients with asymptomatic or mild cases of amphetamine toxicity can adequately be observed for 4 to 6 hours in the ED. Patients with moderate to severe symptoms are admitted to a monitored bed. Body stuffers should be observed in a monitored setting until all packets have passed. All patients manifesting stimulant toxicity should be observed until sympathomimetic signs and vital signs normalize.

CASE OUTCOME

Over the next 16 hours, the patient is admitted to a critical care unit, where he requires further doses of IV midazolam for control of agitation. He remains tachycardic, with a heart rate in the 140s, is mildly hypertensive, and reaches a T_{max} of 101.2°F. No antihypertensive agents are required. Fanning and a cooling blanket are intermittently used to control elevated body temperature.

The patient is discharged from the hospital on day 3, alert and with no apparent sequelae. He admitted to past use of ice and ecstasy, along with ethanol, tobacco, and marijuana. He states that he never in the past experienced seizures or syncope following use of these agents. He denies suicidal intent and eventually enrolls in outpatient drug rehabilitation.

REFERENCES

Albertson TE, Derlet RW, Van Hoozen BE: Methamphetamine and the expanding complications of amphetamines. *West J Med* 170:214–219, 1999.

Albertson TE, Walby WF, Derlet RW: Stimulant-induced pulmonary toxicity. *Chest.* 108:1140–1149, 1995.

Burchfield DJ, Lucas VW, Abrams RM, et al: Disposition and pharmacodynamics of methamphetamine in pregnant sheep. *JAMA* 265:1968–1973, 1991.

Cook CE, Jeffcoat AR, Hill JM, et al: Pharmacokinetics of methamphetamine self-administered to human subjects by smoking S-(+)-methamphetamine hydrochloride. *Drug Metab Dispos* 21:717–723, 1993.

The DAWN Report (DHHS Publication). Rockville, MD: SAMHSA Office of Applied Studies; December 2000.

The DAWN Report (DHHS Publication). Rockville, MD: SAMHSA Office of Applied Studies; October 2002.

de la Torre R, Farre M, Ortuno J: Non-linear pharmacokinetics of MDMA ('Ecstasy') in humans. *Br J Clin Pharmacol* 49:104–109, 2000.

Derlet RW, Heischober B: Methamphetamine: Stimulant of the 1990s? *West J Med* 153:625–628, 1990.

Emergency Department Trends from the Drug Abuse Warning Network, Final Estimates 1994–2001 (DHHS Publication No. SMA 02-3635). Rockville, MD: SAMHSA Office of Applied Studies; 2002.

Felix RJ, Chambers CD, Dick LM, et al: Prospective pregnancy outcome in women exposed to amphetamines. *Teratology* 61: 441, 2000.

Little BB, Snell LM, Gilstrap LC: Methamphetamine abuse during pregnancy: Outcome and fetal effects. *Obstet Gynecol* 72:541–544, 1988.

McElhatton PR, Bateman DN, Evans C, et al: Congenital anomalies after prenatal ecstasy exposure. *Lancet* 154:1441–1442, 1999.

Oro AS, Dixon SD: Perinatal cocaine and methamphetamine exposure: Maternal and neonatal correlates. *J Pediatr* 111: 571–578, 1987.

Overview of Findings from the 2002 National Survey on Drug Use and Health (DHHS Publication No. SMA 03-3774). Rockville, MD: SAMHSA Office of Applied Studies; 2003.

Schwartz RH, Miller NS: MDMA (Ecstasy) and the rave: A review. *Pediatrics* 100:705–708, 1997.

Sherman MP, Wheeler-Sherman J: Cranky babies: Outcomes associated with maternal methamphetamine abuse. *J Perinatol* 20:478, 2000.

Stek AM, Baker RS, Fisher BK, et al: Fetal responses to maternal and fetal methamphetamine administration in sheep. *Am J Obstet Gynecol* 173:1592–1598, 1995.

Stek AM, Fisher BK, Baker RS, et al: Maternal and fetal cardiovascular responses to methamphetamine in pregnant sheep. *Am J Obstet Gynecol* 169:888–897, 1993.

Steiner E: Amphetamine secretion in breast milk. *Eur J Clin Pharmacol* 27:123–124, 1984.

Traub S, Hoffman R, Nelson L: The "ecstasy" hangover: Hyponatremia due to 3,4 methylenedioxymethamphetamine. *J Urban Health* 79:594–554, 2002.

United States Drug Enforcement Agency. *Drug Trafficking in the United States.* DEA Brief, 2003. Available from: http://www.dea.gov/concern/drug_trafficking.html

Van Tonningen MR, Garbis H, Reuvers M: Ecstasy exposure during pregnancy. *Teratology* 58:33A, 1998.

55

Androgenic Anabolic Steroids and Athletic Performance-Enhancing Substances

Peter A. Chyka

HIGH-YIELD FACTS

- The use of athletic performance-enhancing drugs is increasing among adolescent athletes and nonathletes of both genders.

- Androgenic anabolic steroids can produce undesirable effects such as acne, hirsutism, combativeness, and tendon rupture. Permanent changes include gynecomastia, clitoral hypertrophy, stunted growth, and baldness in adolescents.

- Other agents to consider if exposure to athletic performance-enhancing substances is suspected include dietary supplements that may be adulterated with agents such as thyroid hormone, caffeine, heavy metals, unlabeled plant products, and prohormones of androgenic anabolic steroids.

- Most athletic performance-enhancing substances are not detected on routine urine drug screens. Targeted analysis by a reference or specialized laboratory is required if confirmation or identification is necessary.

- Unless the athletic performance-enhancing substance has been recently ingested, there is no value to routine gastric decontamination.

- Risks of parenteral anabolic steroid use and needle sharing include infections such as human immunodeficiency virus (HIV), hepatitis, and endocarditis, as well as complications from particulate emboli.

CASE PRESENTATION

A 15-year-old boy presents to the emergency department complaining of sharp pain in his right shoulder for the past 2 hours. He describes the initial pain as a searing sensation with abrupt onset during a high school wrestling tournament. The pain is now a continuous throbbing sensation with sharp pain upon movement. Ice was applied to the area after the injury. He is a well-developed, well-nourished boy who has a muscular upper torso. His vital signs and oxygen saturation are within normal limits. He claims that he takes no medication, has no known allergies, and is otherwise healthy. The remainder of the physical examination is essentially normal and unremarkable except for pronounced acne on his back and chest, a 5-cm nodule of diffuse tenderness and ecchymosis on his left upper arm; his right shoulder is swollen with minimal range of motion.

INTRODUCTION AND EPIDEMIOLOGY

Androgenic anabolic steroids have been used since the 1950s by elite athletes in hopes of improving athletic performance. In recent years, androgenic anabolic steroids have also been increasingly used by adolescents in hopes of enhancing athletic performance and physical appearance. The availability of an increasingly greater number of athletic performance-enhancing substances was facilitated by the passage of the Dietary Supplement Health and Education Act of 1994, which allows dietary supplements to be sold with less stringent safety, purity, and marketing regulations compared to drugs. The widespread use of the Internet has also greatly increased the availability of these substances. In the past, athletic performance-enhancing substances were available mainly by importation from foreign countries, theft from pharmacies, prescription by unscrupulous providers, diversion from veterinarians, or manufacture by clandestine laboratories. They are now available via shopping malls, and marketed through mainstream print and electronic media.

Characterizing the toxicity of athletic performance-enhancing substances in adolescents is difficult because there are many such substances available, a variety of regimens are employed, and the product may be adulterated. In addition, factors such as extreme physical exercise, unusual diets, and extreme temperatures could explain many of the ill effects. An estimated 4% to 5% of high school students have used androgenic anabolic steroids. Of these, 16% to 36% do not even participate in sports. Both genders use these drugs, with boys' use being three times more frequent than girls. The extent of use of other athletic performance-enhancing substances is unknown, but many are likely to be equally or more prevalent than that for androgenic anabolic steroids (Table 55–1). Risk factors associated with adolescent use of androgenic anabolic steroids include the use of other illicit drugs, alcohol, and tobacco. High-risk groups include athletes engaged in football, wrestling, weight lifting, and body building, and individuals who participate in risk-taking behavior such as driving under the influence of alcohol or carrying a gun. These characteristics

Table 55–1. Some Substances Used for Purported Athletic Performance Enhancement

Amphetamines and related stimulants
Androgenic anabolic steroids
Androstenedione
β-Adrenergic agonists
β-Adrenergic blockers
Caffeine (guarana)
Cocaine
Creatine
DHEA
Ephedra (ma huang) and bitter orange
Erythroid stimulants (epoetin α, darbepoetin α)
Ethanol
γ-Hydroxybutyrate
Human chorionic gonadotropin
Human growth hormone
Marijuana
Opioids

Abbreviation: DHEA, dehydroepiandrosterone.

may prompt a clinician to initiate a discussion about the use of athletic performance-enhancing substances.

This chapter focuses on androgenic anabolic steroids as athletic performance-enhancing substances, but there are many other substances promoted and used for this indication (see Table 55–1). There are approximately 40 different androgenic anabolic steroids available worldwide. Some common oral products include methandrostenolone (Dianabol), methyltestosterone oxandrolone (Oxandrin), oxymetholone (Anadrol), and stanozolol (Winstrol). Some products for parenteral administration include boldensone undecylenate (Equipose, a veterinary drug), nandrolone decanoate (Deca-durabolin), nandrolone phenproprionate (Durabolin), and testosterone cypionate (Depo-testosterone). Two commonly used dietary supplements (androstenedione and dehydroepiandrosterone) are metabolic precursors to testosterone (Figure 55–1) and can act as prohormones when taken in excess. An analysis of off-the-shelf nutritional supplements commissioned by the International Olympic Committee in 2002 found that 15% of 634 products worldwide and 19% of 240 U.S. products were adulterated with prohormones that could produce a positive urine test and could be consumed unknowingly by an athlete. In the United States, dietary supplements may be adulterated or contaminated with drugs such as thyroid supplements, alprazolam, caffeine, heavy metals, and unlabeled plant products. Purity and potency cannot be assured.

Individuals who chronically use androgenic anabolic steroids may use other substances to mask or minimize the adverse effects of the drugs. Substances that purportedly minimize the estrogen effects of excessive exposure of androgenic anabolic steroids include tamoxifen, saw palmetto, and chrysin. Drugs that purportedly minimize the effects on decreased spermatogenesis and sexual drive include clomiphene, mesterolone, and human chorionic gonadotropin.

DEVELOPMENTAL CONSIDERATIONS

The developmental effects on children from chronic exposure to androgenic anabolic steroids can be profound. In addition to the general adverse effects on body development (Table 55–2), young boys may develop precocious puberty and young girls may exhibit contrasexual precocity. Based on anecdotal reports from female Soviet athletes who were given androgenic anabolic steroids throughout childhood, infertility may result. In young children and adolescents, androgenic anabolic steroids

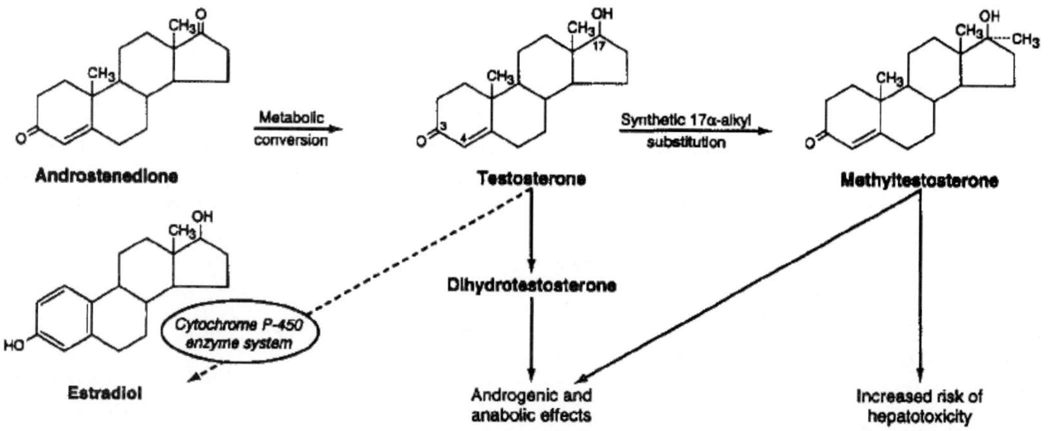

Fig. 55–1. Relationship of testosterone, precursors, synthetic analogs, and metabolites to effects. *Source:* Reprinted from Chyka PA: Androgenic-anabolic steroids. In: Ford M, Delaney K, Ling L, et al, eds: *Clinical Toxicology.* Philadelphia: Saunders; 2001:597.

can stunt growth by the premature closure of the epiphyseal growth plates of bones.

Exposure to androgenic anabolic steroids during pregnancy has been reported to produce abnormal differentiation of external genitalia in animals and humans. Androgenic anabolic steroids are contraindicated during pregnancy and are in the U.S. Food and Drug Administration's Pregnancy Category X. Experiences of androgenic anabolic steroid use during lactation have not been reported. Many athletic performance-enhancing substances would be expected to cross into maternal milk and supplementation of normal dietary intake of these substances should be avoided during lactation.

PATHOPHYSIOLOGY AND PHARMACOLOGY

Androgenic anabolic steroids are synthetic forms of testosterone that react with androgen receptors to produce androgenic and anabolic effects. Many of the adverse effects from androgenic anabolic steroids are exaggerations of the pharmacologic and physiologic effects of testosterone (see Table 55–2) owing to the superphysiologic 10- to 100-fold doses used for prolonged periods. Excess stimulation of androgen receptors by exogenous androgenic anabolic steroids can produce negative feedback on the release of gonadotropin-releasing hormone from the hypothalamus and luteinizing and follicle-stimulating hormones from the anterior pituitary, thereby de-

creasing spermatogenesis and sexual libido. A small proportion of testosterone is metabolized to estradiol (see Figure 55–1), which can lead to feminizing effects in men when taken in excess. Several androgenic anabolic steroids were developed to be orally bioavailable by 17-α alkyl substitution on the steroid ring. This chemical manipulation has been associated with a greater frequency of cholestatic jaundice compared to other agents.

CLINICAL FINDINGS

Individuals who chronically use androgenic anabolic steroids rarely seek medical attention until the drug-induced changes become disturbing or embarrassing. Patients also present with trauma as a secondary injury or problem. Most abusers exhibit varying degrees of the hormonal effects including disproportionate muscular development of the upper torso, minimal body fat, and acne on the chest and back (see Table 55–2). Some individuals exhibit aggressive and combative behavior from androgenic anabolic steroid use that may also be attributable to abuse of other substances such as cocaine and hallucinogens or to antisocial adolescent behavior. With increased muscle strength and size, many individuals may suffer rupture, inflammation, or tears of tendons, and present with acute localized pain. Complications from the parenteral administration of androgenic anabolic steroids including cellulitis, septicemia, hepatitis, and HIV infection may prompt the need for medical attention.

Table 55–2. Possible Adverse Effects of Anabolic-Androgenic Steroid Abuse

Hormonal system

Men:	Infertility
	Breast development
	Testicular atrophy
	High-pitched voice
Women:	Enlargement of the clitoris
	Excessive growth of body hair
	Low-pitched voice
	Reduced breast size
Both genders:	Male-pattern baldness

Musculoskeletal system

    Short stature with childhood use
    Tendon rupture

Cardiovascular system

    Myocardial infarction
    Left ventricular hypertrophy

Liver

    Elevated liver function tests
    Peliosis hepatis
    Tumors

Skin

    Acne and cysts
    Oily scalp

Infection

    HIV/AIDS
    Hepatitis

Psychiatric effects

    Rage and mania
    Delusions

Adapted from National Institute on Drug Abuse Research Report. Anabolic steroid abuse. NIH publication number 00-3721, April 2000. Available at: www.steroidabuse.org. Accessed on March 28, 2003.

Sudden death in young athletes may be due to the interaction of a variety of factors that can be exacerbated by androgenic anabolic steroid use. These include exercise-induced exacerbation of genetic cardiac disease such as hypertrophic cardiomyopathy, coronary artery anomalies, and the consequences of commotio cordis. The influence of external factors during exercise or competition such as extreme conditioning, heat exposure, dehydra-tion, specialized diets, drugs, and dietary supplements are other contributing factors.

A single, acute exposure to androgenic anabolic steroids is unlikely to produce noticeable or significant effects. The acute or chronic effects of exposure to other performance-enhancing substances are evaluated on an individual basis. The adverse effects of selected dietary supplements used as athletic performance-enhancing substances are listed in Table 55–3.

LABORATORY TESTING

Androgenic anabolic steroids are not detected on routine urine drug screens performed in a hospital-based clinical laboratory. Some athletic performance-enhancing substances, such as ephedra and amphetamines, can be detected by routine preliminary urine drugs screens, but most substances are not included in the assay panel. Targeted analysis of the urine for a specific compound or group of compounds will need to be performed by a reference or specialized laboratory. The results are often reported weeks to months after collection and are not useful in the emergency management of these patients. If adverse effects of androgenic anabolic steroids, growth hormone, or erythroid-stimulating agents are suspected, consultation with a pediatric endocrinologist or hematologist on specific laboratory tests is recommended.

MANAGEMENT

Depending on the condition and symptoms of the patient, emergent care for those suffering adverse effects from athletic performance-enhancing substances is typically focused on supportive care, stabilization of injuries, assessment for the presence of other substances, and subsequent referral to a specialist. A true emergency exists for the patient who is hyperthermic and dehydrated. Immediate measures to rehydrate with intravenous fluids, restore electrolyte balance, and achieve an acceptable body temperature of 38.5°C rectally (101.3°F) through evaporation, mist, cooling blankets, and iced lavage are critical to avoid life-threatening cardiovascular and neurologic complications. If the adolescent patient has ingested the substance within 1 to 2 hours of presentation, oral administration of activated charcoal should be considered. If a preschool-aged child unintentionally ingests an athletic performance-enhancing substance, general approaches for the management of an acute poisoning are observed. If an older teenaged

Table 55–3. Adverse Health Effects Associated With Selected Dietary Supplements Used for Enhancement of Athletic Performance

Substance	Adverse Effect
Androstenedione	Elevated HDL, increased estradiol, virilization in women, feminization in men
Caffeine (guarana)	Dependency and withdrawal, CNS stimulation, tachycardia, jitteriness, mild diuresis upon initiation
Creatine	Weight gain owing to water retention, increased compartmental pressure, muscular cramps, rare reports of renal dysfunction
DHEA	Elevated HDL, increased estradiol
Ephedra and bitter orange	Hypertension, tachycardia, stroke, seizures, CNS stimulation

Abbreviations: CNS, central nervous system; DHEA, dehydroepiandrosterone; HDL, high-density lipoprotein.
Sources: Data are complied from Congeni J, Miller S: Supplements and drugs used to enhance athletic performance. *Pediatr Clin North Am* 49:435–461, 2002; Juhn MS: Popular sports supplements and ergogenic aids. *Sports Med* 33: 921–939, 2003; and Koch JJ: Performance-enhancing substances and their use among adolescent athletes. *Pediatr Rev* 23:310–317, 2002.

patient is overly combative and aggressive, benzodiazepines are indicated for sedation.

DISPOSITION

After the initial assessment and management of urgent conditions by the emergency physician, patients should be advised to consult with their pediatrician to evaluate the potential adverse effects of athletic performance-enhancing substances. Referrals should be considered for specialists in orthopedics, pediatric endocrinology, infectious diseases, and adolescent psychiatry, depending on the patient's complaints and the pediatrician's evaluation.

CASE OUTCOME

A radiograph of the right shoulder reveals normal-appearing bones and joints with no apparent fractures. During discussions with a nurse, the boy admits to using nutritional supplements, creatine, and occasional intramuscular steroids. The tentative diagnosis of a tendon rupture is made. The nodule in his left bicep is thought to be a local reaction from a recent intramuscular injection of a veterinary steroid obtained via the Internet. His right shoulder is immobilized with a sling and he is advised to use acetaminophen or ibuprofen for pain control. He is referred to an orthopedic sports medicine specialist for evaluation of his shoulder. He is asked to make an appointment with his pediatrician to evaluate other potential consequences of his use of athletic performance-enhancing substances.

SUGGESTED READINGS

American Academy of Pediatrics. Committee on Sports Medicine and Fitness: Adolescents and anabolic steroids: A subject review. *Pediatrics* 99:904–908, 1997.

American College of Sports Medicine Position Stand: The use of anabolic-androgenic steroids in sports. *Med Sci Sports Exerc* 19:534–539, 1987.

Chyka PA: Androgenic-anabolic steroids. In: Ford M, Delaney K, Ling L, et al, eds: *Clinical Toxicology.* Philadelphia: Saunders; 2001:595–601.

Chyka PA, Banner W Jr: Hematopoietic agents. In: Dart RC, ed:. *Medical Toxicology.* 3rd ed. Philadelphia: Lippincott Williams & Wilkins; 2004:605–614.

Congeni J, Miller S: Supplements and drugs used to enhance athletic performance. *Pediatr Clin North Am* 49:435–461, 2002.

Grunbaum JA, Kann L, Kinchen SA, et al: Youth risk behavior surveillance—United States, 2001. In: *Surveillance Summaries,* June 28, 2002. *MMWR* 51(No. SS-4):1–66, 2002.

Juhn MS: Popular sports supplements and ergogenic aids. *Sports Med* 33:921–939, 2003.

Koch JJ: Performance-enhancing substances and their use among adolescent athletes. *Pediatr Rev* 23:310–317, 2002.

Maron BJ: Sudden death in young athletes. *N Engl J Med* 349:1064–1075, 2003.

National Institute on Drug Abuse Research Report: *Anabolic Steroid Abuse.* (NIH publication number 00-3721), April 2000. Available at: www.steroidabuse.org. Accessed March 28, 2003.

Schänzer W: Analysis of non-hormonal nutritional supplements for anabolic-androgenic steroids—An international study. Available at: http://multimedia.olympic.org/pdf/en_report_324.pdf. Accessed September 29, 2003.

56

Cannabinoids

Carson R. Harris

CASE PRESENTATION

A 14-year-old boy is brought to the emergency department after he was noted to be acting strangely at school. The patient was found sitting in the school bathroom rocking back and forth repeating, "I didn't do it." He refused to answer the principal's questions, and an ambulance was called.

On physical examination, he is alert and in no acute distress. He repeats, "I didn't do it," and occasionally speak of unrelated topics when questioned. His pulse is 110 bpm, respiratory rate 24 breaths per minute, blood pressure 108/66 mmHg. His pupils are equal and reactive and the remainder of his neurologic examination is normal. The conjunctivae are injected. The lung and heart examination are unremarkable except for tachycardia.

INTRODUCTION AND EPIDEMIOLOGY

The cannabis or hemp plant (*Cannabis sativa*) has been grown for several hundred years not only for recreational use of the leaf and flower as marijuana, but also for use of the stem in making hemp for clothing and rope. The dried, compressed resin of the plant is known as hashish, which is smoked. Each day more than 3000 people try marijuana for the first time. During the 1990s, there was a steady increase in the use of cannabis among adolescents. The rise in the use of cannabis has been accompanied by a dramatic increase in its concentration of tetrahydrocannabinol (THC), the predominant psychoactive ingredient in the plant.

DEVELOPMENTAL CONSIDERATIONS

Infant and toddlers may be passively exposed to marijuana smoked in the home, or ingest cakes, cookies, or brownies prepared with marijuana or hashish. Young children may be neglected by caretakers using marijuana or hashish and therefore be at risk for accidental injuries in the household.

Many teenagers view marijuana as having little to no significant health risk, and as having fewer negative effects than other drugs, and thus are more willing to experiment with its use. The risk factors for initiation of use of cannabis include peer pressure, drug availability, low self-esteem, a parent with a mental disorder or early parental death, and previous experience with legal drugs.

Nearly 24% of adolescents report that they have tried marijuana by the time they were in eighth grade. Approximately one third of cannabis-related admissions to substance abuse treatment programs are patients between the ages of 12 and 17. Based on data from the National Survey on Drug Abuse, it is the age at first use of marijuana that is the most predictive of future need for treatment of illicit drug abuse. Complications from the use of cannabinoids include graduating to the use of and addiction to other illicit drugs such as cocaine, heroin, and prescription narcotics, and the development of physical and cognitive disorders. Chronic use of cannabis during adolescence increases the likelihood of developing schizophrenia in adulthood.

PHARMACOLOGY AND TOXICOKINETICS

The lethal dose of cannabis is unknown, but has been estimated to be 30 mg/kg. To achieve this dose an adolescent would have to smoke 600 joints in a single sitting. Between 18% and 50% of the available THC is absorbed with inhalation smoking. Heavy users tend to absorb more than light users. The onset of action is 6 to 12 minutes, and the duration of effect is 2.5 to 4.0 hours. If a child ingests the substance, only 5% to 10% of the available THC is absorbed. An effect can be seen in 20 to 30 minutes, and may last up to 6 hours postingestion.

PATHOPHYSIOLOGY

The cannabis plant contains over 60 cannabinoids and 300 other substances. The primary psychoactive substance of cannabis is delta-9-tetrahydrocannabinol (delta-9-THC). The behavioral effects of cannabinoids are probably mediated by cannabinoid, (CB_1 and CB_2), catecholamine (dopamine, norepinephrine, serotonin, and choline), and GABA receptor sites. The CB_1 receptors are found primarily in the brain, and mediate the majority of the psychoactive effects.

THC is highly protein bound (97% to 99%) and lipophilic. The volume of distribution of approximately 10 L/kg. Because of its high lipid solubility, the apparent volume of distribution is 500 L/kg. It is primarily metabolized in the liver, and metabolites are detected in the urine for several days; they can be detected for up to 6 weeks in frequent users. The elimination half-life is 25 to 36 hours.

Smoking marijuana cigarettes causes much more carbon monoxide and tar insult to the respiratory system than tobacco. Marijuana cigarettes contain roughly 30% to 50% more tar than tobacco cigarettes, and the tar in marijuana cigarettes contains more carcinogens.

CLINICAL PRESENTATION

Pediatric ingestions of hashish or marijuana are typically accidental, and can cause rapid onset of drowsiness, hypotonia, mydriasis, and, rarely, coma. Respiratory arrest has been reported in children who have ingested 1.0 to 1.5 grams of hashish, or several marijuana cigarette butts.

The purpose of recreational use of cannabinoids is to attain a certain level of intoxication. The speed of arriving at a specific level of intoxication depends on the THC concentration of the substance used. Intoxication may be mild, moderate, or severe.

With mild intoxication, the patient typically displays mild euphoria, a relaxed feeling of well-being, heightened sensory awareness, altered time perception, and drowsiness. Moderate intoxication is associated with short-term memory impairment, inability to follow conversation, depersonalization, decreased inhibitions, and a sense of increased interpersonal closeness. The patient may also experience laughing episodes or giddiness, and withdrawn behavior. With severe intoxication, the patient may experience incoordination, ataxia, slurred speech, poor concentration, lethargy, and increased reaction time. Other physical findings of cannabinoids are noted in Table 56–1. Adulterants may also contribute to the overall symptoms.

Several cases of uvulitis have been seen in heavy cannabis smokers, occasionally resulting in airway obstruction. This appears to be rare, but nevertheless, potentially life threatening.

Withdrawal Syndrome

Marijuana use has a subtle but definite withdrawal syndrome that is not as profound as alcohol or heroin. The symptoms include restlessness, abdominal cramps and nausea, irritability, and mild agitation. The patient may experience insomnia and disturbance of sleep electroencephalogram. The symptoms typically last for 3 to 4 days.

LABORATORY AND DIAGNOSTIC TESTING

The presence of cannabinoids can be determined qualitatively with urine immunoassay for THC and its metabo-

Table 56–1. Clinical Findings Associated With Cannabinoid Use

System	Findings
Vitals signs	Hypothermia or hyperthermia
HEENT	Mydriasis, conjunctivitis, chemosis, nystagmus, decrease intraocular pressure, uvular edema, dry mouth
Cardiovascular	Tachycardia, postural hypotension, increased cerebral blood flow
Pulmonary	Bronchial irritation, cough, respiratory depression
GI	Increased appetite, decreased bowel sounds, abdominal pain (ingested or IV), nausea, vomiting
Genitourinary	Urinary retention, decreased sperm count and motility, abnormal sperm morphology (chronic use)
CNS	Confusion, amnesia, dizziness, proconvulsive, euphoria, emotional lability (inappropriate laughter), incoordination/ataxia, coma
Psychiatric	Psychosis, depersonalization, apathy, adjustment disorder, depression, anxiety

Abbreviations: CNS, central nervous system; GI, gastrointestinal; HEENT, head, eyes, ears, nose, and throat; IV, intravenous.

lites. However, immunoassays can be adulterated with various substances to produce false-negative results. Commonly, patients may add soap, vinegar, Visine, bleach, or goldenseal to their urine to hide the presence of THC and its metabolites. Confirmation of qualitatively positive results should be done with gas chromatography mass spectrometry or mass spectrometry with liquid chromatography.

Enzyme immunoassays are capable of detecting urine levels of 20 to 100 ng/mL, depending on the test used. A single use of marijuana may be detected up to 4 days in the urine; moderate use will yield a positive test up to 10 days. Because marijuana is deposited in body fat, the drug can be detected for up to 4 to 6 weeks in heavy users. Passive exposure to marijuana smoke typically yields a negative result unless the nonsmoker is in a small, enclosed, and heavily smoke-filled environment.

Urine toxicology screen may not routinely screen for THC. There are no known drugs that cause false positive results on immunoassay screen or on GC/MS.

MANAGEMENT

Generally management of the patient involves supportive care. For acute psychosis or severe agitation requiring chemical restraint, benzodiazepines are preferred. Uvulitis has been successfully treated with corticosteroids and antihistamines. Chemical dependency intervention is advised, as well as social service evaluation of environmental and family dynamics.

DISPOSITION

Most adolescents can be discharged to their home with their parents or a responsible caretaker after a period of observation. Children with severe intoxication may require observation over night. Any child suspected of being neglected is admitted for social service and child protection agency intervention.

CASE OUTCOME

The patient is admitted and has an uneventful course during the night. The next morning he admits that he had smoked marijuana prior to coming to school; however, he cannot recall events leading to his arrival to the ED. He is referred for substance abuse counseling before discharge.

SUGGESTED READINGS

Boyce SH, Quigley MA: Uvulitis and partial airway obstruction following cannabis inhalation. *Emerg Med (Fremantle)* 14:106–108, 2002.

Gfroerer JC, Epstein JF: Marijuana initiates and their impact on future drug abuse treatment need. *Drug Alcohol Depend* 54:229–237, 1999.

Fried PA: Postnatal consequences of maternal marijuana use in humans. *Ann NY Acad Sci* 562:123–132, 1989.

Jones SD, Howland MA, Kulig K, et al: Plants—Marijuana. In: *Thomson POISINDEX.* Micromedex Healthcare Series, Vol. 115; expires 3/2003.

Joy JE, Watson SJ Jr, Benson JA: *Marijuana and Medicine: Assessing the Science Base.* Institute of Medicine, Division of Neuroscience and Behavioral Health. Washington, DC: National Academy Press; 1999.

Lynskey MT, Heath AC, Bucholz KK, et al: Escalation of drug use in early-onset cannabis users vs co-twin controls. *JAMA* 289:427–433, 2003.

Nahas GG: Lethal cannabis intoxication. *N Engl J Med* 284:792, 1971.

von Sydow K, Lieb R, Pfister H, et al: What predicts incident use of cannabis and progression to abuse and dependence? A 4-year prospective examination of risk factors in a community sample of adolescents and young adults. *Drug Alcohol Depend* 68:49–64, 2002.

Witter FR, Niebyl JR: Marijuana use in pregnancy and pregnancy outcome. *Am J Perinatol* 7:36–38, 1990.

Wu TC, Tashkin DP, Djahed B, et al: Pulmonary hazards of smoking marijuana as compared with tobacco. *N Engl J Med* 318:347–351, 1988.

57

Cocaine

David D. Gummin
Steven E. Aks

HIGH-YIELD FACTS

- Approximately 2.7% of Americans aged 12 to 17 have used cocaine, and 15.4% of Americans aged 18 to 25 have used cocaine.

- Behavioral and cognitive developmental abnormalities, craniofacial anomalies, cardiac anomalies, necrotizing enterocolitis, hypospadias, and other genitourinary abnormalities have all been linked to maternal cocaine use.

- In overdose, cocaine causes a sympathomimetic toxidrome manifested by agitation, diaphoresis, hypertension, tachycardia, and hyperthermia.

- Myocardial infarction has been seen in normal adolescents after cocaine use with clean coronary arteries. A mechanism including vasospasm has been implicated.

- Benzodiazepines are the first line agent for reversing mild to moderate cocaine-induced sympathetic symptoms.

CASE PRESENTATION

A 15-year-old boy presents to your office delirious and agitated. He complains of diffuse abdominal pain. His father states that the patient was out all night. Dad states that the boy was brought home by police officers, and that he believes that the boy has been using drugs. The patient has no significant past medical history, is on no medications, and has no known allergies.

Clinical examination reveals a diaphoretic and warm young man, who is somewhat uncooperative. His vital signs are blood pressure, 156/94 mmHg; heart rate, 126 bpm; respiratory rate, 24 breaths per minute; and oral temperature: 39°C. Room air pulse oximetry is 96%. His pupils measure 5 mm and are sluggishly reactive. The mucous membranes are moist. Lung sounds are clear. Heart is tachycardic without murmur or extra heart sounds. The bowel sounds are slightly hyperactive, but the abdomen is soft and nontender. Extremities are moist. The pulses are bounding and symmetric, but with poor capillary refill. Neurologic examination reveals that he is uncooperative, oriented only to self. His strength is normal in all extremities, but he appears fidgety and unable to sit still. There are repetitive, involuntary writhing and twisting movements of the hands, and occasionally the legs. He is diffusely hyperreflexic.

Your nurse, because of the patient's abdominal pain, has obtained a urine dipstick. She informs you that the dipstick was positive for "large blood." You call 911.

INTRODUCTION AND EPIDEMIOLOGY

In the late nineteenth century, cocaine was commonly used as an oral medicinal for rapid pain relief, and as an additive to cola drinks (Figure 57–1). Presently, cocaine is an insidious cause of toxic morbidity and mortality in North America. Unlike the many available synthetic agents today, the sole source of cocaine remains refinement from the coca plant (*Erythroxylum coca*). Cocaine is widely abused by adolescents and adults as a recreational drug. Small children may be exposed intentionally or inadvertently, typically to cocaine being abused by others. Toddlers may become toxic through second-hand smoke, from crack cocaine, or may inadvertently

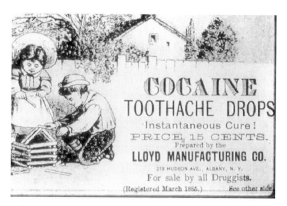

Fig. 57–1. A late 19th-century advertisement for cocaine-containing toothache drops.

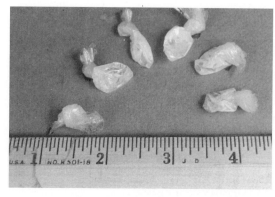

Fig. 57–2. Dime bags of cocaine.

ingest the drug. Seizures may occur in breastfed infants whose mothers abuse cocaine. In one study, 2.4% of children in a group of inner-city preschoolers tested positive for the cocaine metabolite (benzoylecgonine) in their urine.

Approximately two thirds of illicit cocaine enters the United States across its Southwest border. Cocaine is readily available in nearly all major American cities. Organized crime groups operating in Colombia control the worldwide supply, but traffickers in Mexico now control wholesale cocaine distribution throughout the Western and Midwestern United States. The average purity of street cocaine provided to secondary wholesalers is 73%, but varies with each shipment. Typically, cocaine hydrochloride is converted into crack cocaine, or *rock*, by the secondary wholesaler or retailer. Crack cocaine is often packaged in vials, glassine bags, zip-lock bags, or film canisters (Figure 57–2). The size of a crack rock can vary, but generally ranges from 0.1 to 0.5 g. Rocks can sell for as low as $3 to as high as $50, but prices generally range from $10 to $20.

As of 2002, 19.5 million Americans (8.3% of the population over age 11) are illicit drug users. Of these, 2 million admit to using cocaine in the past month. Over half a million use crack cocaine. Approximately 2.7% of Americans aged 12 to 17 have used cocaine. This is overshadowed by the 15.4% of young adults aged 18 to 25 who have used the drug. After 1965, the incidence of cocaine use rose steadily, to peak at 1.7 million new users in 1983. The incidence declined through the 1980s to 0.7 million new users in 1992, but rebound during the 1990s to reach over 2 million users in 2002. The average age of cocaine initiates rose from 17.2 years in 1967 to 23.8 years in 1991, but declined again to 20.0 years by 2000. These epidemiologic data from the National Survey on Drug Use and Health are reinforced by the findings of the Monitoring the Future study of school-aged children.

The Drug Abuse Warning Network (DAWN) of the Substance Abuse and Mental Health Services Administration monitors 458 hospital emergency departments (EDs) in 21 metropolitan areas of the United States. The most current available data derives from 196,268 annual drug of abuse encounters in metropolitan EDs. Cocaine is the most frequently reported drug in ED visits (in 76 visits per 100,000 population). Additionally, DAWN monitors mortality data from medical examiners and coroners from 128 jurisdictions in 42 metropolitan areas of the United States. In over 80% of municipalities, cocaine is the most commonly implicated illicit agent in drug-related deaths. DAWN trends from 1994 to 2001 reveal a progressive increase in both mortality and in ED visits related to cocaine use. There has been a 35% rise in cocaine-related ED visits from 1994 to 2001. Almost a quarter of these involved crack cocaine.

DEVELOPMENTAL CONSIDERATIONS

Cocaine is considered to be in the U.S. Food and Drug Administration's Pregnancy Category C for medicinal use, and in Category X for recreational use. Because of its propensity to induce vasospasm, cocaine abuse has been associated with a number of complications of pregnancy, including placental abruption, low birth weight, preterm delivery, and pregnancy loss.

Additionally, a myriad of birth defects have now been associated with prenatal cocaine abuse. These include craniofacial anomalies, congenital cardiac anomalies, necrotizing enterocolitis, hydronephrosis, hypospadias and other genital abnormalities, and behavioral and cognitive developmental abnormalities. Although the risk of fetal malformations cannot be precisely quantified, some authors suggest that the incidence may be as high as 15% to 20% in chronic maternal abusers.

PHARMACOLOGY AND PATHOPHYSIOLOGY

Chemically, cocaine is benzoylmethylecgonine, a naturally occurring anesthetic and sympathomimetic (Figure 57–3). Processing involves precipitating the drug as crystalline cocaine hydrochloride. This substance is rapidly absorbed from mucus membranes, lung tissue, and somewhat less rapidly from the gastrointestinal (GI) tract. The crystalline structure of cocaine hydrochloride is heat labile, and undergoes pyrolitic degradation when heated or smoked. Conversely, cocaine that has been suspended and precipitated from an alkaline medium crystallizes as the alkaloid "free base." This crystalline alkaloid is heat stable when smoked.

Numerous mishaps involving volatile solvents in the illicit preparation of freebase led to a simple and cheap street method of adding water and baking soda to the cocaine hydrochloride salt. When water evaporates from this solution, a crude form of freebase precipitates as a rock. This lower purity form of alkalinized cocaine is hard, crumbly, fragmented, and is both smokeable and potent. In fact, the euphoric potency of the aptly named crack cocaine is reportedly about 10-fold that of hydrochloride salt. In addition, delivery to the central nervous system (CNS) after smoking crack cocaine is as rapid and reported to be more pleasurable than intravenous (IV) administration of cocaine hydrochloride.

Pharmacologically, cocaine is a local anesthetic which blocks fast sodium channels in both the CNS and in the peripheral nervous system. It is also a potent vasoconstrictor, causing α-adrenergic stimulation of vascular smooth muscle. Toxicologically, cocaine is primarily a sympathomimetic, blocking the presynaptic reuptake of catecholamines such as epinephrine, serotonin, and particularly dopamine and norepinephrine. In large doses, cocaine is directly cardiotoxic, likely through its effects on myocardial fast sodium channels. Its primary target organs are the CNS, the cardiovascular system, the lungs, gastrointestinal tract, skin, and the thermoregulatory center.

Clinically, cocaine causes CNS stimulation that can result in agitation, hallucinations, abnormal movements, and convulsions. Paradoxically, children may present with lethargy. Both ischemic and hemorrhagic strokes have been reported.

In toxicity, cardiovascular manifestations predominate, including sinus tachycardia and both supraventricular and ventricular dysrhythmias. Elevations in blood pressure can range from mild to fulminant hypertension associated with stroke. Myocardial ischemia, including myocardial infarction, is described in otherwise healthy individuals with normal coronary arteries. Age is not a reliable risk factor; acute coronary syndromes are seen in patients as young as 19 years of age. Interestingly, cardiovascular manifestations are not predictably dose related, and, although uncommon, fatalities have occurred after as little as 25 mg of topically applied cocaine.

Multiple pulmonary effects from inhalation of cocaine have been described. These include exacerbation of asthma, pulmonary infarction, pneumomediastinum (see Figure 24–7), pneumothorax, and respiratory failure.

Orally ingested cocaine can cause ischemic complications in the GI tract, which include acute abdominal pain, hemorrhagic diarrhea, and shock from mesenteric ischemia. In association with agitation and hypertension, cocaine-induced hyperthermia may occur. Potential complications of hyperthermia include rhabdomyolysis, disseminated intravascular coagulation, and fulminant hepatic necrosis. Cocaine-induced rhabdomyolysis can also occur in the absence of hyperthermia. The mechanism for this is unknown. Severe hyperthermia ($>40°C$) correlates with high mortality, and should be treated aggressively.

The dermatologic manifestations of cocaine abuse are primarily related to IV injection and skin popping,

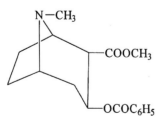

Fig. 57–3. Chemically, cocaine is benzoylmethylecgonine, a naturally occurring anesthetic and sympathomimetic.

including localized areas of necrosis, infection, and eventual scarring. Acute cocaine intoxication may be associated with diaphoresis and pallor from peripheral vasoconstriction.

CLINICAL FINDINGS

Cocaine toxicity is likely in a patient who exhibits signs and symptoms consistent with sympathomimetic stimulation. Occasionally, the sympathomimetic toxidrome is difficult to distinguish from that caused by anticholinergic toxicity. Both toxidromes are associated with CNS excitation, mydriasis, tachycardia, hypertension, and hyperthermia. Unlike sympathomimetic toxicity, however, anticholinergics cause acute urinary retention and decreased bowel sounds. Also, sympathomimetic toxicity is often associated with diaphoresis, whereas anticholinergic overdose is associated with dry skin.

LABORATORY STUDIES

In patients in whom cocaine toxicity is suspected, the urine drug screen may help to confirm the ingestion and rule out coingestants. Serum cocaine levels are not readily available, and are rarely clinically useful. Because there are multiple mechanisms of toxicity, and because cardiotoxicity is unpredictable, quantitative cocaine levels do not correlate with severity of toxicity. Cocaine itself is rarely detectable in the urine more than 24 hours after typical recreational use. Most commercial urine assays take advantage of the fact that cocaine metabolites undergo more prolonged elimination. The most widely available urine assays test for the presence of the major metabolite of cocaine, benzoylecgonine. Benzoylecgonine (Figure 57–4) can usually be detected in urine for up to 72 hours after cocaine use, and in some cases for up to a week.

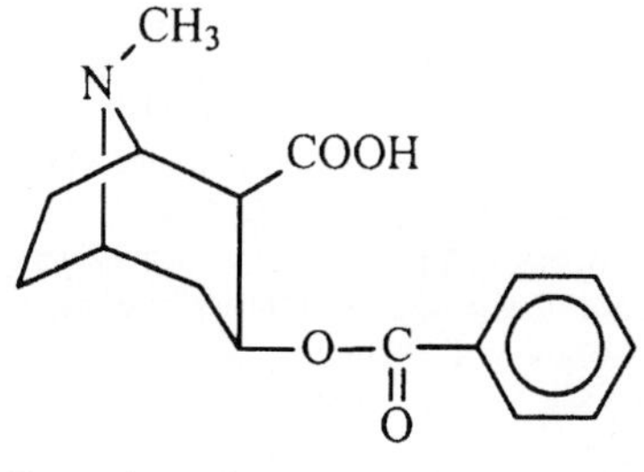

Fig. 57–4. Benzoylecgonine can be detected in urine for up to 72 hours after cocaine use.

Electrocardiographic monitoring is essential to evaluate the patient for dysrhythmias. Patients who complain of chest pain require a 12-lead electrocardiogram. In patients with chest pain a radiograph is useful to exclude a pneumothorax, pneumomediastinum, or infiltrate.

Laboratory studies help to establish a baseline and are useful in patients with significant toxicity. These include a complete blood count, serum electrolytes, glucose, and blood urea nitrogen and creatinine levels. If a urine dipstick is positive for blood but microscopy is negative for red blood cells, the patient should be evaluated for rhabdomyolysis with a serum creatinine phosphokinase (CPK) and urine myoglobin.

A computed tomographic (CT) scan of the brain is indicated in patients with a severe headache or neurologic deficit to investigate the possibility of a cocaine-induced cerebrovascular accident.

MANAGEMENT

Mildly toxic patients generally require no specific therapy. Moderate to severe agitation typically responds to benzodiazepines, which are also the drugs of choice for seizures. Persistent seizure activity may require loading with phenobarbital. Phenytoin is probably only indicated if a structural lesion is present. Rarely, status epilepticus requires paralysis. Patients with persistent seizures may suffer from a structural CNS lesion or from toxicity by a coingestant.

Benzodiazepines are also effective treatment for most patients with mild to moderate hypertension. In more severe cases, labetolol, which has both α- and β-blocking characteristics, may be effective. Because the α and β effects are not in a 1:1 ratio, response may be variable. Sodium nitroprusside is an effective vasodilator that can effectively lower the blood pressure. β-Blockers are relatively contraindicated, because unopposed α stimulation can theoretically exacerbate hypertension. Benzodiazepines and coronary vasodilators such as nitroglycerin are useful in managing cocaine-induced chest pain. Some authors advocate the use of phentolamine to promote coronary vasodilation and reduce blood pressure in cocaine-induced acute coronary syndromes.

Patients with severe hyperthermia are treated with aggressive, active cooling measures. The urine should be alkalinized in patients with moderate to severe rhabdomyolysis. Activated charcoal absorbs unpackaged or poorly packaged, orally ingested cocaine, and is useful for gastric decontamination.

BODY STUFFERS AND PACKERS

Body stuffers may swallow cocaine in an attempt to avoid prosecution when confronted by the police. *Body packers* intentionally swallow or pack body orifices with drug, in an attempt to conceal and illegally transport the product. Body packing often entails very elaborate methods of packaging the substance to avoid inadvertent rupture of the packets. Conversely, body stuffing implies poorly wrapped cocaine, which is likely to become bioavailable (see Figure 57–2). Even carefully packaged packets can rupture, and this setting typically involves potentially lethal doses of cocaine. Types of packages most likely to rupture are paper, aluminum foil, or poorly secured plastic bags. The physician may be able to gather enough information regarding the amount of cocaine ingested and the type of packaging to assess the potential for toxicity.

Abdominal radiographs are generally not useful for body stuffers, but may be positive is approximately 80% of body packers. A gastrograffin swallow or CT scan of the abdomen with contrast may reveal ingested packets in cases where plain radiographs are negative, but suspicion of ingestion is high.

In body stuffers and packers, gastric decontamination with syrup of ipecac or gastric lavage is contraindicated, because both may cause rupture of the packets. Whole bowel irrigation with polyethylene glycol electrolyte lavage solution can be used to enhance transit through the GI tract. It is important to be sure that all ingested packets pass before the patient is discharged. To do so may require a gastrograffin swallow or abdominal CT. In symptomatic body stuffers who are refractory to initial attempts at pharmacologic management, surgical consultation is indicated. Laparotomy may be a necessary life-saving intervention to remove the leaking cocaine packets.

DISPOSITION

In asymptomatic or mild cases of cocaine toxicity 4 to 6 hours of observation in the ED is adequate. Patients with moderate to severe symptoms should be admitted to a monitored bed. Body stuffers and packers are observed in a monitored setting until all packets have passed.

CASE OUTCOME

In the ED the patient has a heart rate of 134 bpm with a blood pressure of 150/92 mmHg and a temperature of 40°C. His is given an IV of 0.9 normal saline bolus of 1 L over 30 minutes, and is placed on oxygen 2 L by nasal cannula. On the cardiac monitor the patient is in sinus tachycardia. The ED team administers lorazepam in 2-mg increments to a total dose of 10 mg. Additionally, he is sprayed with water mist and placed under high-power fans. The only laboratory of significance is his CPK of 2324 mg/dL. In 1 hour his temperature is 37.2°C, his heart rate is 104 bpm, and his blood pressure is 125/74 mmHg. He is admitted to a monitored setting for IV hydration and monitoring. His CPK decreases to 204 mg/dL by 36 hours of hospitalization and he otherwise recovers uneventfully.

SUGGESTED READINGS

Albertson TE, Walby WF, Derlet RW: Stimulant-induced pulmonary toxicity. *Chest* 108:1140–1149, 1995.

Amin M, Gabelman G, Karpel J, et al: Acute myocardial infarction and chest pain syndromes after cocaine use. *Am J Cardiol* 66:1434–1437, 1990.

Overview of Findings from the 2002 National Survey on Drug Use and Health (DHHS Publication No. SMA 03-3774). Rockville, MD: SAMHSA Office of Applied Studies, 2003.

Bateman DA, Heagarty MC: Passive freebase cocaine ('crack') inhalation by infants and toddlers. *Am J Dis Child* 143:25–27, 1989.

Chaney NE, Franke J, Wadlington WB: Cocaine convulsions in a breast-feeding baby. *J Pediatr* 112:134–135, 1988.

Conway EE, Mezey AP, Powers K: Status epilepticus following the oral ingestion of cocaine in an infant. *Pediatr Emerg Care* 6:189–190,1990.

The DAWN Report (DHHS Publication). Rockville, MD: SAMHSA Office of Applied Studies, October, 2002.

Emergency Department Trends from the Drug Abuse Warning Network, Final Estimates 1994–2001 (DHHS Publication No. SMA 02-3635). Rockville, MD: SAMHSA Office of Applied Studies, 2002.

Eng JG, Aks SE, Waldron R, et al: False-negative abdominal CT scan in a cocaine body stuffer. *Am J Emerg Med* 17:702–704, 1999.

Garland JS, Smith DS, Rice TB, et al: Accidental cocaine intoxication in a nine-month-old infant: Presentation and treatment. *Pediatr Emerg Care* 5:245–247, 1989.

Gay GR: Clinical management of acute and chronic cocaine poisoning. *Ann Emerg Med* 11:562–572, 1982.

Geggel RL, McInerny J, Estes NA: Transient neonatal ventricular tachycardia associated with maternal cocaine use. *Am J Cardiol* 63:383–384, 1989.

June R, Aks SE, Keys N, et al: Medical outcome of cocaine bodystuffers. *J Emerg Med* 18:221–224, 2000.

Johnston LD, O'Malley PM, Bachman JG: *Monitoring the Future national survey results on adolescent drug use: Overview of key findings, 2001* (NIH Publication No. 02-5105). Bethesda, MD: National Institute on Drug Abuse; 2002.

Johnston LD, O'Malley PM, Bachman JG: *Monitoring the Future national survey results on adolescent drug use: Overview of key findings, 2002* (NIH Publication No. 03-5374). Bethesda, MD: National Institute on Drug Abuse; 2003.

Kharasch SJ, Glotzer D, Vinci R, et al: Unsuspected cocaine exposure in young children. *Am J Dis Child* 145:204–206, 1991.

Minor RL, Scott BD, Brown DD, et al: Cocaine-induced myocardial infarction in patients with normal coronary arteries. *Ann Intern Med* 115:797–806, 1991.

Mortality Data from DAWN: 2000 (DHHS Publication No. SMA 02-3633). Rockville, MD: SAMHSA Office of Applied Studies, 2002.

Mortality Data from DAWN: 2001 (DHHS Publication No. SMA 03-3781). Rockville, MD: SAMHSA Office of Applied Studies, 2003.

Perez-Reyes M, Di Guiseppi S, Ondrusek G, et al: Free-base cocaine smoking. *Clin Pharmacol Ther* 32:459–465, 1982.

Riggs D, Weibley RE: Acute hemorrhagic diarrhea and cardiovascular collapse in a young child owing to environmentally acquired cocaine. *Pediatr Emerg Care* 7:154–155, 1991.

Riggs D, Weibley RE: Acute toxicity from oral ingestion of crack cocaine: A report of four cases. *Pediatr Emerg Care* 6:24–26, 1990.

Rivkin M, Gilmore HE: Generalized seizures in an infant due to environmentally acquired cocaine. *Pediatrics* 84:1100–1102, 1989.

Sand IC, Brody SL, Wrenn KD, et al: Experience with esmolol for the treatment of cocaine-associated cardiovascular complications. *Am J Emerg Med* 9:161–163, 1991.

Schardein JL: *Chemically Induced Birth Defects.* 3rd ed. New York: Marcel Dekker; 2000.

Seaman ME: Acute cocaine abuse associated with cerebral infarction. *Ann Emerg Med* 19:34–37, 1990.

Shaw GM, Malcoe LH, Lammer EJ: Maternal use of cocaine during pregnancy and congenital cardiac anomalies (Letter). *J Pediatr* 118:167–168, 1991.

Sofuoglu M, Brown S, Babb DA, et al: Effects of labetalol treatment on the physiological and subjective response to smoked cocaine. *Pharmacol Biochem Behav* 65:255–259, 2000.

Tomaszewski C, Vorhees S, Wathen J, et al: Cocaine adsorption to activated charcoal in vitro. *J Emerg Med* 10:59–62, 1992.

Traub SJ, Hoffman RS, Nelson LS: Body packing—The internal concealment of illicit drugs. *N Engl J Med* 349:2519–2526, 2003.

United States Drug Enforcement Agency (DEA): *Drug Trafficking in the United States.* DEA Brief, 2003. Available from http://www.dea.gov/concern/drug_trafficking.html.

Van der Woude FJ: Cocaine use and kidney damage. *Nephrol Dial Transplant* 15:299–301, 2000.

Weiss RJ: Recurrent myocardial infarction caused by cocaine abuse. *Am Heart J* 111:793, 1986.

Welch RD, Todd K, Krause GS: Incidence of cocaine-associated rhabdomyolysis. *Ann Emerg Med* 20:154–157, 1991.

Wetli CV, Mash D, Karch SB: Cocaine-associated agitated delirium and the neuroleptic malignant syndrome. *Am J Emerg Med* 14:425–428, 1996.

58

LSD and Other Hallucinogens

Leon Gussow

HIGH-YIELD FACTS

- The major effects of LSD are perceptual and sympathomimetic.
- The drugs of choice for a patient agitated after taken a hallucinogen who cannot be talked down are benzodiazepines and, if necessary, haloperidol.
- MDMA is the hallucinogen associated with the most fatalities in recent years.
- High-risk manifestations of MDMA toxicity include hyperthermia, seizure, and rhabdomyolysis.

CASE PRESENTATION

A 17-year-old boy is brought to the emergency department (ED) by paramedics for a panic reaction. He had been at an all-night rave and dance party, where a local rock group call the Toxic Mushrooms were playing. He suddenly became dizzy, and noted that lights, shapes, and colors at the club were pulsating and merging with one another. He felt that the floor was turning into a shimmering pool of water and that he would drown. He says that he knows these thought disturbances were caused by a drug that he had purchased at the club and ingested 45 minutes before the symptoms started, that was sold as a *microdot*. He took two doses. Still, he was terrified that these illusions would never disappear.

On examination, the patient is alert and oriented but very anxious. Pulse rate is 115 bpm, respiratory rate 22 breaths per minute, blood pressure 150/105 mmHg, temperature 99.1°F. Skin is mildly diaphoretic. Pupils are dilated but sluggishly reactive. There is no nystagmus. The remainder of the physical examination is unremarkable.

EPIDEMIOLOGY

Hallucinogens have been defined as substances that primarily alter perception and cognition without producing delirium or other changes in mental status. Naturally occurring hallucinogenic substances, mostly of plant origin, have been used for millennia by many cultures, often as adjuncts to religious rituals. The first synthetic hallucinogen, LSD-25, was derived from the rye fungus (*Claviceps purpurea*) by Albert Hofmann in 1938. The psychogenic properties of this derivative became apparent 5 years later, when Hofmann inadvertently absorbed the preparation topically and developed striking distortions of perception. Lysergic acid diethylamide (LSD) was later marketed for a number of indications, including facilitation of psychiatric treatment, but because of its widespread abuse during the "hippie" era of the 1960s, it was classified as a Schedule I controlled substance in 1966.

LSD is a tasteless, colorless, and odorless powder that can be dissolved in water and distributed on various carrier vehicles such as gelatin squares (*window panes*), sugar cubes, or colored paper (*blotter acid*). Although its popularity has waxed and waned since the 1960s, it is still produced illegally and used predominantly by high school and college students. A study of patients treated during Chicago-area rock concerts in the summer of 1994 found that LSD use was prevalent during concerts by the Grateful Dead, but not those by Pink Floyd or the Rolling Stones.

The 1990 National Institute of Drug Abuse household survey found that 7.6% of the United States population over 12 years of age admitted to using hallucinogens at some time in their lives, 1.1% during the previous year. A survey of over 18,000 households in 1993 found that 8.7% of respondents admitted using hallucinogens; of these, 5.5% had used LSD and 3% had used mescaline. It is most likely that statistics from surveys such as these underestimate the true prevalence of drug use. Data from the Toxic Exposure Surveillance System reveal that in 2002, 208 LSD exposures were reported to Poison Control Centers in the United States. Of these only one was in a child younger than 6. There were 18 exposures to peyote/mescaline in children younger than 6. Neither of these drugs was associated with a death in any age group during that year. Exposure to hallucinogenic amphetamines, however, was reported in 2185 cases, 23 of which were in children younger than 6 years. There were 15 deaths overall, although it is not clear from the data how many of these were in children.

AGE AND DEVELOPMENTAL CONSIDERATIONS

Exposure to hallucinogens in children younger than 6 is usually accidental and rarely involves major morbidity. Previous concern that LSD might cause chromosomal damage appears to be unfounded. There is no evidence that LSD is teratogenic or produces fetal abnormalities.

PHARMACOLOGY AND TOXOKINETICS

There are two major classes of hallucinogens. The *indoleamines* include LSD, lysergic acid hydroxyethylamide (*morning glory*), psilocybin, bufotenine, and AMT. This class also includes the various tryptamines, such as DMT and *foxy-methoxy*. The *phenethylamine*s include peyote/mescaline and the hallucinogenic amphetamine derivatives such as MDMA (*ecstasy*).

LSD is rapidly absorbed by the gastrointestinal (GI) tract and metabolized in the liver. Onset of action is 30 to 90 minutes, with sympathomimetic signs and symptoms often appearing before the occurrence of perceptual and cognitive distortion. Peak effects occur at 2 to 5 hours with duration up to 16 hours. Tolerance to the psychogenic effects of LSD can develop with frequent use, but disappears shortly after regular use is stopped. There is no withdrawal syndrome.

LSD acts primarily on serotonin (5-HT) receptors in the central nervous system (CNS), which regulate mood, perception, personality, and affect. The most important target is the 5-HT$_{2A}$ receptor, which is found throughout the cerebral cortex. There is a strong correlation between the affinity of various hallucinogens for 5-HT$_{2A}$ receptors and the magnitude of their effects on perception and cognition. 5-HT$_{2A}$ receptors are also abundant in the locus ceruleus, a structure located in the upper pons that receives and coordinates sensory and visceral input for projection to the cortex.

CLINICAL PRESENTATION

LSD has mild sympathomimetic effects that can precede the onset of perceptual distortions. These include tachycardia, tachypnea, hypertension, mydriasis, and hyperthermia. Dizziness is common. Because LSD usually causes alteration in the perception of real sensation rather than the experience of sounds or vision with no basis in reality, some argue that it should be called an *illusogen* rather than a *hallucinogen*. The acute perceptual effects of LSD include a heightened sense of sound, shape, and color. Lights and other objects may seem to be surrounded by halos. Moving objects may leave a trail of discrete afterimages in the visual field. Time sense is distorted. An unusual perceptual change is *synesthesia*, the illusion that stimulation of one of the five senses is experienced through another sensory modality. For example, sound may be experienced as shifting patterns of light and color. This was the inspiration for the light shows that were often shown during rock concerts in the 1960s.

Acute psychiatric reactions caused by LSD include severe anxiety and panic attacks. Ordinary thoughts and perceptions can seem grandiose or profound, sometimes leaving the user with the impression that he or she has discovered the meaning of life or the secret of the universe. Sensations of paranoia, depersonalization, and ego fragmentation can be terrifying, leading to the so-called "bad trip." Usually, however, the user is alert, oriented, and aware that the perceptual distortions and illusions are the result of drug ingestion.

The effects of LSD are usually not life threatening. When morbidity and, rarely, mortality occur, they typically result from self-induced trauma. However, more serious reactions possibly caused by LSD have been reported. Klock and associates described eight patients aged 19 to 39 years who presented shortly after intranasal snorting of a white powder containing LSD. Six patients were comatose, and three progressed to respiratory arrest. Four patients were hyperthermic up to 107°F. Testing revealed platelet dysfunction in all eight patients, four of whom had evidence of abnormal bleeding. All patients recovered. Similar cases related to LSD have not been reported in the literature, and it does not appear from the report that extensive testing was done to rule out other coingestants.

Flashbacks

Flashbacks are perceptual distortions and hallucinations that occur in a user of LSD after the acute drug effects have worn off. Often, they repeat the user's previous hallucinogenic experience with LSD, and have been reported to occur up to 5 years after acute drug use. They can be persistent or short lived, and may be precipitated by stress, illness, fatigue, and the use of alcohol or marijuana. The etiology of flashbacks is not clear. A more recent term for this phenomenon is *hallucinogen-persisting perception disorder.*

OTHER HALLUCINOGENS

Mescaline

Mescaline is a phenethylamine alkaloid found naturally in the buttons on top of the peyote cactus, which grows in the southwestern United States and northern Mexico. The buttons are collected, dried, and ingested. Mescaline can also be synthesized in the laboratory. Like other phenethylamines such as MDMA, it has sympathomimetic properties similar to those of amphetamines, as well as the ability to cause hallucinations and perceptual distortion. Nausea and vomiting begin approximately 1 hour after ingestion, along with mydriasis, sweating, tachycardia, and hypertension. The perceptual and cognitive effects follow.

Morning Glory Seeds

The psychoactive alkaloids in morning glory seeds were first isolated in 1960 by Albert Hofmann, the chemist who had synthesized LSD in 1938. The effects are similar to those of LSD and are dose related. At higher doses significant GI discomfort, nausea, and vomiting occur, which often discourage repeated experimentation with this product.

MDMA/MDEA

MDMA, a popular drug at some dance clubs and rave parties, is also called *ecstasy, XTC,* or *Adam.* It was first synthesized in 1914 for use as an appetite suppressant, but not actually marketed until 1972 when it was used as an adjunct to psychotherapy. Because its abuse quickly became widespread, it was reclassified as a Schedule I controlled substance in 1985. In 2002, five deaths involving MDMA in patients under 19 years of age were reported to U.S. poison centers.

Effects are dose related, and include nausea, sweating, tachycardia, hypertension, tremor, and perceptual distortions. Patients can present looking like methamphetamine overdose with severe agitation, delusions, and paranoia. A finding described as characteristic of MDMA intoxication is *bruxism,* or jaw clenching and grinding of teeth. Fatalities are usually associated with severe hyperthermia, seizure, and rhabdomyolysis.

After MDMA ingestion, the urine drug screen may read positive for amphetamine. Serum sodium level may be significantly reduced as a result of volume loss, rehydration with free water, and inappropriate release of antidiuretic hormone.

There has been a large body of medical literature claiming that use of MDMA, even for brief periods, could cause significant neurologic damage and persistent deficits. Recently many of those studies have been criticized for severe flaws in methodology, and five related papers were withdrawn from publication.

Foxy-Methoxy

5-MeO-DIPT is a synthetic tryptamine with structure and effects similar to those of psilocybin. It was classified as a Schedule I controlled substance in April 2003. It has the street names *foxy-methoxy* or *foxy,* most likely because of its reputed aphrodisiac properties. It has GI and neurologic effects, including nausea, vomiting, diarrhea, restlessness, and mydriasis. Larger doses cause perceptual effects similar to those of LSD. It has been supplied as a purple tablet, a capsule, or on a sugar cube or blotting paper. It is rapidly absorbed, with onset at 20 minutes, peak effect at 1.5 hours, and duration of 3 to 6 hours.

LABORATORY AND DIAGNOSTIC TESTING

Any patient with a significantly altered mental status, especially if associated with increased muscle tone or activity, requires determination of core (rectal) temperature. Most routine urine drug screens do not test for LSD. Other hallucinogens may appear on toxicology screens, including phencyclidine and MDMA (which shows up as amphetamine). Any patient with altered mental status should have a glucose level determined with a rapid bedside test. Measuring serum blood urea nitrogen and creatinine, creatine kinase, and a urinalysis may reveal onset of rhabdomyolysis and renal failure, a risk for patients with hyperthermia or increased muscle activity. Other laboratory tests that may be helpful include complete blood count, electrolytes, liver function tests, and serum alcohol level.

MANAGEMENT

The goal in treating a patient having a bad trip from LSD or other hallucinogens is to reduce anxiety, reinforce the patient's awareness that the unpleasant effects being experienced will wear off before long, and provide a quiet, nonthreatening environment. The term for this is *talking the patient down.* Unfortunately, in the ED, there is often neither the space nor available staff to successfully accomplish this. Benzodiazepines are very effective at relieving anxiety, decreasing agitation, and reducing sympathetic outflow from the CNS. When agitation does not respond adequately to benzodiazepines, haloperidol can be used. Phenothiazines are not recommended, because they can lower the seizure threshold and induce dystonic reactions. Severe hypertension that does not respond to benzodiazepines can be treated with phentolamine or nitroprusside. Physical restraints should be avoided if at all possible; if they are necessary, they should be replaced at the earliest possible time with adequate sedation. Because hallucinogens such as LSD are rapidly absorbed after ingestion, GI decontamination is not indicated and may serve only to increase the patient's agitation. Severe hyperthermia can be treated with hydration, supportive care, and standard cooling methods. Patients experiencing flashback phenomena can be managed with reassurance and benzodiazepines. They should also be advised to avoid precipitating factors, such as stress, use of marijuana or alcohol, and fatigue.

DISPOSITION

Admission is often not necessary for patients who present to the ED after exposure to a hallucinogen. After perceptual distortions and anxiety have resolved, the patient can be discharged if accompanied by a competent friend or relative. A 24-hour course of oral benzodiazepines can be considered. If necessary, the patient can be admitted to an observation unit. If severe acute symptoms do not resolve, the diagnosis is unclear, other etiologies have not been ruled out, or there are significant concurrent medical problems (such as severe hypertension, hyperthermia, or rhabdomyolysis) hospital admission may be required. Children who have had inadvertent exposure to a hallucinogen should be referred to social service. Older children can be referred to a drug treatment program, if available.

CASE OUTCOME

An acute panic reaction following ingestion of LSD is diagnosed. Reasonable efforts to talk the patient down by providing calming reassurance in a quiet environment fail. He is given diazepam 10 mg by mouth and over the next half hour improves dramatically. After being observed for 6 hours, he is discharged to the care of his parents.

SUGGESTED READINGS

Abraham HD, Aldridge AM: Adverse consequences of lysergic acid diethylamide. *Addiction* 88:1327, 1993.

Abraham HD, Aldridge AM, Gogia P: The psychopharmacology of hallucinogens. *Neuropsychopharmacology* 14:285–298, 1996.

Aghajanian GK, Marek GJ: Serotonin and hallucinogens. *Neuropsychopharmacology* 21:16S–23S, 1999.

Brady ET: A note on morning glory seed intoxication. *Am J Hosp Pharm* 25:88, 1968.

Brown RT, Braden NJ: Hallucinogens. *Pediatr Clin North Am* 34:341–347, 1987.

Buchanan JF, Brown CR: 'Designer drugs': A problem in clinical toxicology. *Med Toxicol* 3:1–17, 1988.

Callaway CW, Clark RF: Hyperthermia in psychostimulant overdose. *Ann Emerg Med* 24:68, 1994.

Cohen S, Ditman KS: Complications associated with lysergic acid diethylamide (LSD-25). *JAMA* 181:161–162, 1962.

DuPont RL, Verebey K: The role of the laboratory in the diagnosis of LSD and ecstasy psychosis. *Psychiatr Ann* 24:142, 1994.

Erickson TB, Aks SE, Koenigsberg M: Drug use patterns at major rock concert events. *Ann Emerg Med* 28:22–26, 1996.

Hanrahan JP, Gordon MA: Mushroom poisoning: Case reports and a review of therapy. *JAMA* 251:1057, 1984.

Hofmann A: How LSD originated. *J Psychedelic Drugs* 11:53–60, 1979.

Ingram AL: Morning glory seed reaction. *JAMA* 171:1342–1344, 1959.

Klock JC, Boerner U, Becker CE: Coma, hyperthermia and bleeding associated with massive LSD overdose: A report of eight cases. *West J Med* 120:183, 1973.

Kulig K: LSD. *Emerg Med Clin North Am* 8:551–558, 1990.

Leikin JB, Krantz AJ, Zell-Kanter M, et al: Clinical features and management of intoxication due to hallucinogenic drugs. *Med Toxicol Adverse Drug Exp* 4:423–450, 1989.

Lyttle T, Goldstein D, Gartz J: Bufo toads and bufotenine: Fact and fiction surrounding an alleged psychedelic. *J Psychoactive Drugs* 28:267–290, 1996.

McNeil DG: Research on ecstasy is clouded by errors. *NY Times* December 2, 2003.

Markel H, Lee A, Homes RD, et al: LSD flashback syndrome exacerbated by selective serotonin reuptake inhibitor antidepressants in adolescents. *J Pediatr* 125:817–819, 1994.

Miller PL, Gay GR, Ferris KC, et al: Treatment of acute, adverse psychedelic reactions: "I've tripped and I can't get down." *J Psychoactive Drugs* 24:277–279, 1993.

Passie T, Seifert J, Schneider U, et al. The pharmacology of psilocybin. *Addition Biol* 7:357–364, 2002.

Schultes RE: Hallucinogens of plant origin. *Science* 163:245–254, 1969.

Schwartz RH: LSD: Its rise, fall, and renewed popularity among high school students. *Pediatr Clin North Am* 42:403–413, 1995.

Schwartz RH, Smith DE: Hallucinogenic mushrooms. *Clin Pediatr* 27:70–73, 1988.

Shannon M: Methylenedioxymethamphetamine (MDMA, "Ecstasy"). *Pediatr Emerg Care* 16:377, 2000.

Smith DE, Seymour RB: LSD: History and toxicity. *Psychiatric Ann* 24:145, 1994.

Ulrich RF, Patten BM: The rise, decline, and fall of LSD. *Perspectives Biol Med* 34:561–578, 1991.

Watson WA, Litovitz TL, Rodgers GC, et al: 2002 annual report of the American Association of Poison Control Centers Toxic Exposure Surveillance System. *Am J Emerg Med* 21:390, 2003.

59

Inhalants

Heather Long
Lewis S. Nelson

HIGH-YIELD FACTS

- The median age of first use of inhalants is 13 years; lifetime prevalence among girls now equals that of boys.

- Commonly abused substances include volatile hydrocarbons, nitrous oxide or whippets, and amyl nitrite.

- The cardiovascular and central nervous systems are most vulnerable to the effects of inhalants.

- Signs and symptoms of inhalant use may be subtle, tend to vary widely among individuals, and generally resolve within 2 hours of exposure. Unique clinical manifestations occur with abuse of some agents, including toluene, *n*-hexane, nitrous oxide, and amyl nitrite.

- A thorough history and physical examination and careful questioning of the patient's friends and family are probably more helpful in diagnosing cases of suspected inhalant abuse than laboratory testing.

- Initial management of the patient begins with the ABCs; the patient's presenting signs and symptoms direct further management and diagnostic testing.

CASE PRESENTATION

A previously healthy 17-year-old boy presents to the emergency department (ED) with weakness and pain in his arms and legs for 1 day. He describes the pain as *crampy* and states he is unable to walk because of the weakness. He has no fever or chills, no nausea, vomiting, or diarrhea, and no history of recent illness. There is no difficulty urinating, no change in bowel habits, and no change in sensation. He has no previous medical or surgical history, and has no history of trauma, recent travel, or use of prescription medications. The patient denies use of illicit drugs, herbal medications, or dietary supplements.

On physical examination, he appears well and vital signs are normal. His examination is remarkable for musculoskeletal strength of 1/5 in the lower extremities bilaterally and 3/5 in the upper extremities bilaterally. He is symmetrically hyporeflexic. There are no sensory deficits. Cranial nerves II to XII are intact.

Laboratory and diagnostic studies reveal: sodium 140 mEq/L, potassium 1.7 mEq/L, magnesium 1.9 mEq/L, and creatine phosphokinase 4800 IU/L. An electrocardiogram (ECG) reveals a normal sinus rhythm; and U waves are present.

INTRODUCTION AND EPIDEMIOLOGY

Inhalant abuse is the deliberate inhalation of vapors for the purpose of changing one's consciousness, or becoming high. It is also referred to as *volatile substance abuse* and was first described in 1951. Inhalants are appealing to adolescents because they are cheap, readily available, and sold legally. Initially, inhalant abuse was viewed as physically harmless, but reports on sudden sniffing death began to appear in the 1960s. Shortly thereafter, evidence of other significant morbidities, including organic brain syndromes and peripheral neuropathy, began to appear.

The 2002 Monitoring the Future Study found that more than 2 million youths aged 12 to 17 had used inhalants at least once in their lifetime. The 2000 National Household Survey on Drug Abuse showed that the number of new inhalant users in the United States increased more than 50% between 1994 and 2000, from 618,000 to 979,000. Youths aged 12 to 17 had higher rates of past-year use than adults aged 18 and over. The lifetime prevalence of inhalant use peaked among eighth graders at 15%.

The median age of first use is 13 years. Although long considered to be a problem among boys, there has been a steady increase of inhalant abuse among girls, and their lifetime prevalence now equals that of boys. The problem is greatest among lower socioeconomic groups. Non-Hispanic white adolescents are the most likely to abuse inhalants and black adolescents the least. Although inhalant use is a problem in both urban and rural communities, its prevalence is higher in rural settings. This is probably related to the easier access to other drugs in urban areas.

Inhalant abuse includes the practices of sniffing, huffing, and bagging. *Sniffing* entails the inhalation of a volatile substance directly from a container, as occurs with airplane glue or rubber cement. *Huffing* involves pouring a volatile liquid onto fabric (e.g., a rag or sock) and placing it over the mouth and/or nose while inhaling. Huffing is the method used by over 60% of volatile substance abusers. *Bagging* refers to spraying a solvent into a plastic or paper bag and rebreathing from the bag several times; spray paint is among the agents commonly used by this method.

Agents Used

There are a multitude of inhalational substances abused (Table 59–1), most of which are volatile hydrocarbons. Commonly inhaled hydrocarbons include gasoline, spray paints, lighter fluid, and glue. Of inhalant cases reported to two regional poison centers, spray paint and gasoline accounted for more than 61%. In many cases, the class of the substance is identified rather than the specific chemical. Because exact components may vary between products, this method is inaccurate and imprecise.

The volatile hydrocarbons can be further divided into the aliphatic hydrocarbons, the aromatic hydrocarbons, halogenated hydrocarbons, and the alkyl nitrites. The *alkyl nitrites* include amyl, butyl and isobutyl nitrite, and are sold in sex and drug paraphernalia shops. Amyl nitrite is contained in small glass capsules known as *poppers*. When covered in gauze and crushed, the capsules release the nitrite and make a characteristic sound. Amyl, butyl, and isobutyl nitrites are sold as room deodorizers or liquid incense in small vials typically containing 10 to 30 mL.

Table 59–1. Common Inhalational Substances and Their Chemical Constituents

Inhalant	Chemical
Glues/adhesives	Toluene, *n*-hexane, benzene, xylene, trichloroethane, trichloroethylene, tetrachloroethylene, ethyl acetate, methylethyl ketone, methyl chloride
Spray paint	Toluene, butane, propane
Hair spray, deodorants, room fresheners	Butane, propane, fluorocarbons
Lighter fluid	Butane
Paint thinner	Toluene, methylene chloride, methanol
Gasoline	Aliphatic and aromatic hydrocarbons
Dry cleaning agents, spot removers, degreasing agents	Tetrachloroethylene, trichloroethane, trichloroethylene
Typewriter correction fluid	Trichloroethane, trichloroethylene
Nail polish remover	Acetone
Paints, lacquers, varnishes	Trichloroethylene, toluene
Poppers	Amyl nitrite
Room deodorizers	Butyl nitrite, isobutyl nitrite
Whipped cream dispensers (whippets)	Nitrous oxide

The most commonly used nonhydrocarbon inhalant is nitrous oxide. Nitrous oxide or laughing gas is used therapeutically as an inhalational anesthetic. Cartridges of the compressed gas, known as *whippets*, are sold for commercial use in whipped cream dispensers. These battery-sized metal containers of compressed gas are punctured using a cracker and the escaping gas is either inhaled directly or collected in a balloon and then inhaled.

PHARMACOLOGY AND PATHOPHYSIOLOGY

Inhalants, which are generally highly lipophilic agents, gain rapid entrance into the central nervous system (CNS).

The exact mechanism by which various inhalants exert their neurologic effects are poorly understood. Some agents like toluene and trichloroethane produce effects similar to subanesthetic concentrations of the general anesthetics and CNS depressants like ethanol and barbiturates. These effects are likely mediated through stimulation of the GABA receptor complex, the primary system responsible for inhibitory neurotransmission within the CNS. In addition, there is evidence suggesting toluene, like ethanol, may inhibit excitatory transmission by interfering with glutamate at the NMDA receptors. In animals, toluene, as with other drugs of abuse, has been found to activate dopaminergic neurons within the mesolimbic region of the brain, suggesting a mechanism for its rewarding/reinforcing effects.

Acute Toxicity

The CNS is the intended target of the inhalants and most susceptible to adverse effects. Early CNS effects include euphoria, visual and auditory hallucinations, as well as headache and dizziness. As intoxication progresses, CNS depression develops and patients may manifest slurred speech, confusion, tremor, and weakness. Further CNS depression is marked by ataxia, lethargy, seizures, coma, respiratory depression, and death.

Acute cardiotoxicity is manifested most dramatically in sudden sniffer's death. In witnessed cases, sudden death occurred when sniffing was followed by some physical activity like running or wrestling, or in a stressful situation like being caught sniffing by parents or police. It is thought that the inhalant sensitizes the myocardium, producing a substrate within the heart for dysrhythmia propagation; activity or stress then causes a catecholamine surge that initiates the dysrhythmia. Cardiac dysrhythmias following use of inhalational anesthetics have been documented since the early 1900s, particularly with the chlorinated hydrocarbons, and this association was confirmed in animal and human studies. Hypoxia, hypokalemia, and ethanol consumption all have been shown to increase the likelihood of dysrhythmias.

Serious pulmonary toxicity associated with volatile hydrocarbons is most often due to aspiration following attempted ingestion of a liquid hydrocarbon. Reports of asphyxiation initially ascribed to inhalant abuse were later found to be due to plastic bag suffocation, not specifically to the inhaled vapor. Inhalational use can, however, induce coughing, dyspnea, bronchospasm, and chemical pneumonitis, probably via its irritant effects. Hydrocarbon pneumonitis is characterized by rales/rhonchi on lung auscultation, tachypnea, fever, leukocytosis, and radio-

graphic abnormalities. Rebreathing of exhaled air, as occurs with bagging, may lead to hypercapnia and hypoxia.

Hepatotoxicity has been associated with carbon tetrachloride and other halogenated hydrocarbons including chloroform, trichloroethane, and trichloroethylene, as well as toluene. Although carbon tetrachloride can cause a potentially fatal centrilobular necrosis, most of the other agents are associated with elevated liver enzymes that generally return to baseline with 2 weeks of abstinence.

Renal toxicity has been most frequently described following inhalation of toluene, which is found in spray paints and glues. Classically, prolonged toluene inhalation causes a distal renal tubule acidosis (RTA) and a resultant hypokalemia. Although distal RTAs are associated with a hyperchloremic metabolic acidosis and a normal anion gap, some patients have been found to have an increased anion gap following toluene inhalation. This is explained by toluene's metabolism to hippuric acid and benzoic acid by an inducible cytochrome P450 enzyme. It is hypothesized that patients with renal insufficiency may have decreased ability to excrete these organic acids, resulting in an increased anion gap. Additionally, these patients may have microscopic pyuria, hematuria, and proteinuria.

Methylene chloride, most commonly found in paint removers and degreasers, differs from other halogenated hydrocarbons in that it is metabolized by cytochrome P450 to carbon monoxide. Carboxyhemoglobin levels may be significantly elevated and may not rise for several hours after exposure, because of the time required for metabolism.

Inhalation of amyl, butyl, and isobutyl nitrites may cause methemoglobinemia. These agents also cause peripheral vasodilatation and can result in orthostatic hypotension and syncope.

Chronic Toxicity

Given the high lipophilicity of most inhalants, the neurotoxic effects following chronic use may be striking. Cerebral and cerebellar functions appear especially vulnerable, and chronic inhalant abusers may have marked deficits in memory, attention, auditory discrimination, and visual-motor function.

Toluene is lipophilic and a well-recognized white matter toxin. Prolonged inhalation is known to cause a leukoencephalopathy characterized by dementia, ataxia, eye movement disorders, and anosmia. *n*-Hexane, a solvent found in lacquers and glues, causes a sensorimotor peripheral neuropathy. Distal sensory abnormalities predominate initially, but with progression, motor symptoms develop distally and move proximally. Toxicity is produced via a metabolite, 2,5 hexanedione, which inhibits neuronal microtubular function resulting in axonal death.

Chronic abuse of nitrous oxide can result in a peripheral neuropathy, characterized initially by symmetric sensory deficits, and ataxia owing to abnormal proprioception. With prolonged abuse there is lower extremity spasticity. Toxicity is mediated via interference with metabolism of vitamin B_{12}.

Tolerance has been observed with weekly usage in as few as 3 months. Withdrawal symptoms including sleep disturbances, nausea, tremor, and irritability lasting 2 to 5 days after last use have been described. Whether this represents a true withdrawal syndrome or residual effects of the inhalant is unclear.

CLINICAL MANIFESTATIONS

Signs and symptoms of inhalant use may be subtle, tend to vary widely among individuals, and generally resolve within 2 hours of exposure (Table 59–2). Following acute exposure, there may be a distinct odor of the abused substance on the patient's breath or clothing. Depending on the agent used and the method, there may be discoloration of skin around the nose and mouth. Mucus membrane irritation may cause sneezing, coughing, and tearing. Patients may complain of dyspnea and palpitations. Gastrointestinal complaints include nausea, vomiting, and abdominal pain. After an initial period of euphoria, patients may have headache and dizziness.

Table 59–2. Clinical Manifestations of Inhalant Use

Distinctive odor on breath, clothing
Discoloration around nose/mouth
Mucus membrane irritation: sneezing, coughing, tearing.
Dyspnea, wheezing
Palpitations
GI complaints: nausea, vomiting, abdominal pain
Huffer's eczema (chronic)
Euphoria, intoxication
Headache, dizziness
Progressive CNS depression

Abbreviations: CNS, central nervous system; GI, gastrointestinal.

Syncope is one of the more serious clinical events that may occur with inhalant abuse. Patients can arrive at the ED with a persistent altered level of consciousness following syncope and can rarely suffer cardiorespiratory arrest. The most common causes of such events include hypoxia from simple asphyxiation, profound respiratory depression, and malignant dysrhythmia. Determining the exact cause of syncope or death is difficult, because most events are unwitnessed. Clinical testing and autopsy generally reveal little information.

Consequential but less frequent acute effects noted in inhalant abusers include marked weakness and loss of deep tendon reflexes (toluene-induced hypokalemia), cyanosis (methemoglobinemia from alkyl nitrites), headache, or findings related to carbon monoxide poisoning (methylene chloride) and clinical hepatitis (chlorinated hydrocarbons).

With chronic inhalant abuse, patients may develop severe drying and cracking around the mouth and nose known as *huffer's eczema*. Patients with a history of prolonged use of nitrous oxide or *n*-hexane may present with sensory deficits suggestive of a peripheral neuropathy. Leukoencephalopathy from chronic hydrocarbon inhalation, most notably toluene, is characterized by dementia, ataxia, eye movement disorders, and anosmia.

LABORATORY AND DIAGNOSTIC TESTING

Routine urine toxicology screens are not able to detect inhalants or their metabolites. Most volatile agents can be detected using gas chromatography for up to 10 hours after exposure, but this is not readily available at many institutions, and is of little utility in most clinical situations. A thorough history and physical examination and careful questioning of the patient's friends and family are probably more helpful in cases of suspected inhalant abuse than laboratory testing.

Depending on the patient's signs and symptoms additional diagnostic testing may be indicated, including an ECG, chest x-ray, and blood tests. The patient's presenting complaint should guide decisions regarding further diagnostic testing.

Some inhalants present with unique diagnostic considerations (Table 59–3). The potassium level should be measured in patients manifesting weakness and decreased deep tendon reflexes. Hypokalemia may represent a toluene-induced distal RTA. Diagnosis of a distal RTA is suggested by a hyperchloremic metabolic acidosis with a normal anion gap, as well as hypophosphatemia,

Table 59–3. Inhalants: Common Sources and Special Considerations

Agent	Found in	Special Considerations
Toluene	Spray paints, glues/adhesives, paint thinners	Hypokalemia Hyporeflexia Distal RTA Elevated LFTs *Chronic:* leukoencephalopathy
Tricholoroethane, trichloroethylene	Typewriter correction fluids, degreasers, spot removers	Elevated LFTs
Methylene chloride	Paint thinner	CO poisoning
Alkyl nitrites (amyl, butyl, isobutyl)	Poppers, room deodorizers	Methemoglobinemia
n-Hexane	Glues/adhesives	*Chronic:* peripheral neuropathy
Nitrous oxide	Whippets, inhalational anesthetic	*Chronic:* peripheral neuropathy

Abbreviations: CO, carbon monoxide; LFTs, liver function tests; RTA, renal tubular acidosis.

hypokalemia, and aciduria. A carboxyhemoglobin level should be drawn initially and repeated several hours after methylene chloride exposure. A methemoglobin level may be indicated following exposure to amyl, butyl, or isobutyl nitrites. Liver function tests may be indicated following exposure to toluene, trichloroethylene, and trichloroethane.

Electromyography may be useful in cases of suspected peripheral neuropathy. Routine laboratory testing, including cerebrospinal fluid analysis, is unremarkable in patients with inhalant-induced leukoencephalopathy. Computed tomographic scanning of the head is generally normal until late in the disease, when diffuse hypodensity of white matter becomes evident. T_2-weighted magnetic resonance imaging with its superior resolution of white matter is the diagnostic study of choice.

MANAGEMENT

As always, management begins with assessment and stabilization of the patient's airway, breathing, and circulation. Place the patient on a pulse oximeter and cardiac monitor. Administer oxygen and treat with nebulized albuterol if the patient is wheezing. Early consultation with a regional poison control center may assist with identification of the toxin and patient management. Cardiac dysrhythmias associated with inhalant abuse carry a poor prognosis.

Sudden death following inhalant use is not limited to the new users. There appears to be no premonitory signal to the user, and the effect of the inhalant on the my-

ocardium lingers after inhalation has stopped. It is also important to consider an electrolyte abnormality in the treatment of dysrhythmia. Although there are no evidence-based treatment guidelines for the management of inhalant-induced cardiac dysrhythmias, avoidance of sympathomimetic agents like epinephrine is generally recommended. Agents with β-blocking activity are thought to offer some cardioprotective effects to the sensitized myocardium. Amiodarone and esmolol have both been used successfully in resuscitations of ventricular fibrillation arrests following inhalant abuse.

Fluid and electrolyte abnormalities are corrected. Complications including methemoglobinemia and elevated carboxyhemoglobin are managed with standard therapy. Patients with respiratory symptoms that persist beyond the initial complaints of gagging and choking are evaluated for hydrocarbon pneumonitis and treated supportively. Neither prophylactic antibiotics nor steroids have ever been proved beneficial.

Agitation, either from acute effects of the inhalant or from withdrawal, is safely managed with diazepam or lorazepam. In the vast majority of patients, symptoms resolve quickly and hospitalization is not required. The potential toxicity of inhalants should be reinforced, and the patient referred for counseling. Subsets of users meet criteria for inhalant dependence and inhalant-induced psychosis. These patients require inpatient psychiatric care. Pharmacotherapy with carbamazepine or an antipsychotic like haloperidol or risperidone appears beneficial in some cases. Drug use treatment programs for inhalant abuse are scarce and few providers have special training in this area.

CASE OUTCOME

Immediate intravenous hydration and potassium supplementation is begun. The patient receives a total of 100 mEq of potassium chloride over the next 24 hours and his symptoms resolve completely. After further questioning, the patient admits he had been huffing paint thinner several times a day for 4 days and that he had been using inhalants on and off for 5 years.

SUGGESTED READINGS

Adgey AAJ, Johnston PW, McMechan S: Sudden cardiac death and substance abuse. *Resuscitation* 29:219, 1995.

Balster RL: Neural basis of inhalant abuse. *Drug Alcohol Depend* 51:207, 1998.

Bass, M: Sudden sniffing death. *JAMA* 212:2075, 1970.

Beauvais F, Wayman JC, Jumper-Thurman P, et al: Inhalant abuse among American Indian, Mexican American, and non-Latino white adolescents. *Am J Drug Alcohol Abuse* 28:171, 2002.

Brouette T, Anton R: Clinical review of inhalants. *Am J Addict* 10:79, 2001.

Flowers NC, Horan LG: Nonanoxic aerosol arrhythmias. *JAMA* 219:33, 1972.

Garriott J, Petty CS: Death from inhalant abuse: toxicological and pathological evaluation of 34 cases. *Clin Toxicol* 16:305, 1980.

Hernandez-Avila CA, Ortega-Soto HA, Jasso A, et al: Treatment of inhalant-induced psychotic disorder with carbamazepine versus haloperidol. *Psychiatr Serv* 49:812, 1998.

Kono J, Miyata H, Ushijima S, et al: Nicotine, alcohol, methamphetamine, and inhalant dependence: A comparison of clinical features with the use of a new clinical evaluation form. *Alcohol* 24:99, 2001.

Kurtzman TL, Otsuka KN, Wahl RA: Inhalant abuse by adolescents. *J Adolesc Health* 28:170, 2001.

McGarvey EL, Clavet GJ, Mason W, et al: Adolescent inhalant abuse: Environments of use. *Am J Drug Alcohol Abuse* 25:731, 1999.

Misra LK, Kofoed L, Fuller W: Treatment of inhalant abuse with risperidone. *J Clin Psychiatry* 60:620, 1999.

National Institute on Drug Abuse: *NIDA InfoFacts: Inhalants.* Available from www.drugabuse.gov/infofax/inhalants.html. Updated March 5, 2004; accessed March 2003.

Nelson LS: Toxicological myocardial sensitization. *J Toxicol Clin Toxicol* 40:867, 2002.

Neumark YD, Delva J, Anthony JC: The epidemiology of adolescent inhalant drug involvement. *Arch Pediatr Adolesc Med* 152:781, 1998.

Press E, Done AK: Solvent sniffing: The physiological effects and community control measures for intoxication from the intentional inhalation of organic solvents I. *Pediatrics* 39:451, 1967.

Press E, Done AK: Solvent sniffing: The physiological effects and community control measures for intoxication from the intentional inhalation of organic solvents II. *Pediatrics* 39:611, 1967.

Riegel AC, French ED: Abused inhalants and central reward pathways. *Ann NY Acad Sci* 965:281, 2002.

Shepherd RT: Mechanism of sudden death associated with volatile substance abuse. *Human Toxicol* 8:287, 1989.

Spiller HA, Krenzelok EP: Epidemiology of inhalant abuse reported to two regional poison centers. *J Toxicol Clin Toxicol* 35:167, 1997.

U.S. Department of Health and Human Services, Substance Abuse and mental health Services Administration: *Drugs.* Available from: www.samhsa.gov/oas/drugs.htm#Inhalants. Updated March 5, 2004; accessed March 2003.

60

Opioids

Timothy B. Erickson

HIGH-YIELD FACTS

- The classical triad of central nervous system (CNS) depression, respiratory depression, and pinpoint pupils characterizes opioid toxicity.

- Some opioids such as methadone and diphenoxylate-atropine (Lomotil), can have delayed or prolonged effects.

- Certain opioids can cause acute lung injury in severe overdoses.

- Toxicity from proxyphene, meperidine, and tramadol, as well as neonatal opioid withdrawal, can result in seizure activity.

- Airway management and the use of the pure opioid antagonist naloxone are the mainstays of opioid toxicity treatment.

- Longer-acting opioid antagonists, such as nalmefene, may be effective in non–opioid-dependent children.

CASE PRESENTATION

A 3-year-old boy is found unresponsive at his uncle's house. The paramedics are notified, and the child is transported to the nearest emergency department. Upon arrival, the child is noted to be unresponsive, with a pulse of 70 bpm, a respiratory rate of 8 breaths per minute; a blood pressure of 80/40 mmHg; a temperature of 95°F, and a pulse oximetry reading of 82%. There are no signs of obvious trauma. The child is noted to have pinpoint pupils, with no gag reflex appreciated.

INTRODUCTION AND EPIDEMIOLOGY

Opioids are naturally occurring or synthetic drugs that have activity similar to that of opium or morphine. *Opiate* refers only to those drugs derived from natural opium, including morphine, codeine, and thebaine. *Narcotic* is derived from the Greek word for *stupor*, and was originally used to describe any drug that could induce sleep, but became erroneously associated with opioids alone. Some have defined narcotics as those substances that bind opiate receptors, whereas others refer to any illicit substances as narcotics. The poppy plant *Papaver somniferum* is the source of all opium alkaloids. This plant was originally grown in the Mediterranean region as early as 5000 BC, but is now cultivated in several temperate countries throughout the world.

Heroin was first synthesized from morphine in 1874. Commercial production of heroin as a pain remedy first began in 1898. Although it received widespread acceptance from the medical profession, physicians remained unaware of its abuse potential and addictive properties for years. The first comprehensive control of heroin occurred with the Harrison Narcotic Act of 1914. Today heroin is considered to be an illicit substance having no medicinal utility, and is categorized in the United States as a Schedule I drug. The United States ranks first in the world in thebaine utilization. Thebaine is not used therapeutically, but is converted into a variety of substances, including naloxone.

Opioids are used clinically for analgesia, anesthesia, as cough suppressants, and to alleviate diarrhea. These drugs are widely available for medical and illicit use in oral, inhalational, parenteral, transdermal, and suppository forms. According to the latest U.S. Drug Enforcement Agency sources, more than 500 tons of opium are legally imported into the United States annually for legitimate medical use. Codeine is the most widely used, naturally occurring narcotic in the world.

Since 1990, there has been a threefold increase in morphine products in the United States. In 1990, 3 tons of oxycodone was produced. In the 2000, 47 tons were manufactured. In 2001, oxycontin, a sustained-release synthetic morphine product, was one of the leading prescribed drugs in the United States. As a result, usage, addictions, and fatalities have risen to epidemic proportions.

According to the 2001 annual report of the American Association of Poison Control Centers, in children younger than 20 years of age there were 789 exposures to codeine, 164 to meperidine, 293 to methadone, 428 to morphine, 841 to oxycodone, 32 to pentazocine, and 125 to propoxyphene. According to this database, there were 11 pediatric opioid-related deaths. One of the fatalities involved a 9-month-old girl who was admitted to the hospital for a surgical procedure. Following surgery, an order was written for her to receive 0.5 mg of parenteral morphine every 2 hours for pain control. A decimal point was misplaced, and the child died after receiving two doses of 5.0 mg morphine. A recent survey by the National Institute on Drug Abuse documents an 80% increase in opioid use among high school students over the past decade, heralding a resurgent heroin epidemic in the adolescent population.

AGE AND DEVELOPMENTAL CONSIDERATIONS

Neonates can experience lethargy at birth if there was recent maternal opioid use, or if large doses of an opioid agent were iatrogenically administered to the mother during labor. Additionally, the neonate is prone withdrawal symptoms during the newborn period if the mother exhibited chronic dependency during her later prenatal stages. Toddlers are prone to opioid poisoning if their environment permits exposure, most often from unintentional ingestions. For example, powdered heroin, methadone and codeine tablets, long-acting morphine derivatives, and fentanyl patches may be readily available to the younger child. Unlike the chronically exposed newborn, withdrawal symptoms are rarely encountered in younger children unless the child is utilizing opioids for chronic pain management. Adolescents tend to experiment with different routes of exposure, such as inhalational (smoking), intranasal (snorting), ingestion, or intravenous (IV) administration. In a suicide attempt, they are potentially exposed to life-threatening doses. In addi-

tion, the opioids may have synergistic effects with other drug combinations such as ethanol, benzodiazepines, and γ-hydroxybutyrate, or opposing effects when mixed with sympathomimetic agents like cocaine and amphetamines. Chronically addicted teenagers are also prone to acute withdrawal states, particularly when treated with naloxone.

PHARMACOLOGY AND TOXICOKINETICS

Opium is broken down into alkaloid constituents. These alkaloids are divided into two distinct chemical classes, phenanthrenes and isoquinalines. The principle phenanthrenes are morphine, codeine, and thebaine. The isoquinolines have no significant CNS effects and are not federally regulated. Opioids produce clinical effects by interacting with specific receptors located throughout the central and peripheral nervous system and the gastrointestinal (GI) tract. Opioid activity resembles the body's three endogenous opioid peptides: enkephalins, endophins, and dynophins. The three main receptors are mu (μ), kappa (κ), and delta (δ). Most analgesia results from supraspinal μ_1 receptors. It is the only opioid receptor in the brain and is primarily responsible for the opioid-induced euphoria and sedation. μ_2 is responsible for spinal analgesia, respiratory depression, miosis, physical dependence, and decreased gut motility. κ_1 produces spinal analgesia, and miosis (although less pronounced than μ_2). κ_2 results in dysphoria and disorientation. The δ receptor produces spinal analgesia and is the least defined of the three receptors. Sigma is no longer considered to be an opioid receptor, because it is not antagonized by the pure opioid antagonist naloxone.

The pharmacokinetics for morphine and morphine derivatives in children aged 1 to 15 years are comparable to adults. Most opioids are completely absorbed from the GI tract and peak within 60 to 90 minutes, with a duration of effect lasting 3 to 6 hours. Exceptions range from fentanyl, with a duration of effect approximating 1 hour, to methadone, which lasts up to 24 to 48 hours. Many of the other oral agents, such as codeine, sustained-release morphine (e.g., MS Cotin, Oxycontin), oxycodone, and Lomotil (an antidiarrheal agent containing diphenoxylate and atropine), also demonstrate a delayed effect of up to 4 to 12 hours.

Pharmacokinetics are also dependent of the route of exposure. For example, IV users experience a peak effect within 1 to 5 minutes, but have a duration of effect of about 30 minutes. Fentanyl, a synthetic opioid approximately 80 times more potent than morphine, causes toxi-

Table 60–1. Common Opioids With Generic and Trade Names

Generic Name	Trade Names
Morphine	MS-Contin, Oramorph SR, MSIR, Roxanol, Kadian, RMS
Hydromorphine	Dilaudid
Codeine	Tylenol #3, #4, Tylenol with codeine
Oxycodone	OxyContin, Oxyl, Percodan (ASA) Percocet (APAP)
Hydrocodone	Anexsia, Hycodan, Hycomine, Lorcet, Lortab, Tussinex, Tylox, Vicodin, Vicoprofen
Meperidine	Demerol, Mepergan, MPPP, MPTP
Methadone	Dolophinel, ORLMM
Buprenophine	Buprenex
Propoxyphene	Darvon
Pentazocine	Talwin, Talwin Nx (with naloxone)
Butorphanol	Stadol, Torbugesic, Torbutol
Fentanyl	Sublimaze (80× more potent than morphine)
Fentanyl patch	Durgesic patch
Fentanyl citrate	Actiq (solid on a stick for oral use)
Sufentanil	Sufenta (1000× more potent than morphine)
Carfentanil	Wildnil (10,000× more potent than morphine)

city with extremely small doses. Fentanyl is available in IV form, as a transdermal patch, and as fentanyl citrate on a popsicle stick. Table 60–1 provides a list of commonly prescribed opioid compounds and their generic and trade names.

Most ingested opioids result in significant first pass metabolism, resulting in low bioavailability. Protein binding varies from 20% to 40% in morphine and up to 90% in methadone. Hepatic biotransformation is the primary route of metabolism. Therefore, patients with severe liver disease who ingest opioids have an increased risk of toxicity. The active metabolites of morphine, meperidine, and propoxyphene are renally excreted. Renal dysfunction can therefore contribute to toxicity owing to accumulation of these metabolites.

The development of *tolerance* is characterized by a shortened duration and a decreased intensity of analgesia, euphoria, and sedation, which creates the need to consume progressively larger doses to attain the desired effect. Tolerance does not develop uniformly for all actions of these drugs, giving rise to a number of toxic effects. *Physical dependence* refers to physiologic and psychological changes that necessitate the continued presence of a drug to prevent a withdrawal syndrome. The intensity and character of the physical symptoms experienced during withdrawal are directly related to the particular drug of abuse, the total daily dose, the interval between doses, the duration of use, and the underlying health of the user. In general, shorter-acting narcotics tend to produce shorter, more intense withdrawal symptoms, whereas longer-acting narcotics produce a withdrawal syndrome that is protracted but tends to be less severe. Although unpleasant, withdrawal from narcotics is rarely life threatening.

PATHOPHYSIOLOGY

By binding to the μ, κ, and δ receptors, opioid agonists cause specific G proteins to be activated. G proteins reduce the capacity of adenylate cyclase to produce cyclic adenosine monophosphate. These proteins also close calcium ion channels that reduce the signal to release neurotransmitters inhibiting norepinephrine release, and open potassium channels which hyperpolarize the cell, indirectly reducing cell activity. Each mechanism depends on the receptor subtype (μ, κ, δ), the location of the receptor (pre/postsynaptic), as well as the specific neuron within the central or peripheral system.

Opioid-induced respiratory depression is primarily mediated through the μ_2 receptors. When opioid agonists bind to these receptors, ventilatory drive is reduced by diminishing the sensitivity of the medullary chemoreceptors to hypercapnea. Acute lung injury, classically described with severe opioid overdose, results from hypoxia secondary to ventilatory compromise, which causes precapillary pulmonary hypertension. This results in increased pulmonary capillary permeability, which causes an extensive fluid leak. This variation of acute lung injury (described in other sources as *noncardiogenic pulmonary edema*) may also be due to direct hypersensitivity or alveolar membrane toxicity.

The mechanism by which opioids induce miosis is controversial. Morphine specifically causes stimulation of parasympathetic pupilloconstrictor neurons in the oculomotor nerve. Other opioids mediate inhibitory neurotransmission, causing hyperpolarization of inhibitory neurons to the parasympathetic neurons, resulting in the classic pinpoint pupils associated with opioid use. Constipation is a common side effect of both therapeutic and recreational opioid use. This is mediated by the μ_2 receptors within the smooth muscle of the intestinal wall.

Opioid-induced seizure activity is most often secondary to profound hypoxia. However, a proconvulsant effect has also been demonstrated in animal models treated with morphine, which is not inhibited by naloxone, suggesting that the mechanism may be unrelated to opioid receptor binding. Morphine-induced seizures in neonates may also be related to incomplete formation of the newborn blood–brain barrier, resulting in greater CNS toxicity. Certain opioids cause cardiotoxicity via conduction system dysfunction. Propoxyphene blocks myocardial sodium channels, with a quinidine-like effect similar to cyclic antidepressants. As a result, propoxyphene is consistently listed among the leading causes of drug overdose-related fatalities by forensic medical examiners.

CLINICAL PRESENTATION

Opioid poisoning classically presents with an altered level of consciousness. The triad of acute toxicity consists of CNS depression, respiratory depression, and pupillary constriction. CNS depression ranges from mild sedation to stupor and coma. Patients are typically hypotensive, hypothermic, bradycardic, and hyporeflexic. Many patients experience central-mediated vomiting. This, coupled with respiratory depression and a diminished gag reflex, places the patient at risk for aspiration pneumonitis. Other respiratory effects may also include bronchospasm from histamine release induced by insufflating or inhaling fumes of opioid compounds cut with impurities or adulterants. In massive overdoses, respiratory toxicity can also cause severe hypoxia, hypercarbia, and acute lung injury.

Although miotic or pinpoint pupils are a classic opioid-induced clinical finding, mydriasis or pupillary dilation has been described with meperidine, propoxyphene, and diphenoxylate-atropine (Lomotil) overdoses. With Lomotil overdose, a two-phase toxicity has been described. Phase one manifests with anticholinergic symptoms such as dry mouth, flushing, and mydriasis; phase two consists of opioid effects of respiratory and CNS depression with associated miosis.

Less common effects of opioid toxicity include generalized seizure activity following overdose of propoxyphene, meperidine, tramadol, fentanyl, or pentazocine. Neonates receiving continuous IV morphine can also suffer seizures from mere toxicity or during acute opioid withdrawal.

Dermatologic effects include flushing and pruritis sec-

ondary to histamine release. GI effects include decreased gut motility and constipation. Finally, medical complications common among chronic users arise from adulterants found in street drugs and the nonsterile practices of injecting drugs. Patients who chronically use opioids IV or by skin popping can contract bacterial endocarditis, septic pulmonary emboli, skin infections, tetanus, wound botulism, hepatitis, and human immunodeficiency virus infection.

LABORATORY AND DIAGNOSTIC TESTING

Patients presenting with suspected opioid toxicity should have their oxygenation status continually monitored. If severe respiratory compromise and hypoxia continue despite antidote therapy and oxygen administration, an arterial blood gas analysis is obtained to rule out hypercarbia and acidosis. If a child presents with a depressed level of consciousness, a rapid bedside serum glucose is measured to rule out hypoglycemia. If head trauma is suspected, a computed axial tomographic scan of the brain is indicated. With severe respiratory distress, acute lung injury or aspiration pneumonitis should be suspected, and confirmed with a chest radiograph. With a propoxyphene overdose, an electrocardiogram and QRS complex is assessed.

Toxicology screens are not helpful in the initial management of the child with an opioid overdose. Serum assays may only detect opioid compounds for up to 6 hours. Urinary qualitative screens may be useful in ruling out an opioid exposure in a child presenting with altered mental status. These are typically positive for up to 48 to 72 hours postexposure. Most urinary screens lack sensitivity, and may not detect many of the synthetic opioids including methadone, hydrocodone, and propoxyphene. In addition, routine screens may not detect potent opioids such as fentanyl, because standard detection or cut-off limits are usually set at around 2000 ng/mL. Toxicology screens may also result in false-positive screens following dietary ingestion of poppy seeds. Along with other routine baseline laboratory tests, serum acetaminophen and salicylate levels should be measured, because many opioid compounds like hydrocodone and codeine also contain these common analgesics.

MANAGEMENT

The primary management of opioid poisoning includes

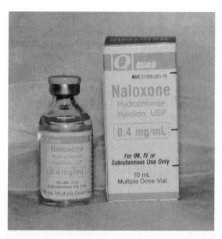

Fig. 60–1. Naloxone is the most commonly administered opioid antagonist.

stabilization of the airway and administration of the pure opioid antagonist naloxone (Figure 60–1). If adequate doses of this antidote are given in a timely fashion, intubation can be avoided, because the onset of action for naloxone is usually within 1 minute of administration. However, if there is no response to naloxone, and oxygenation cannot be maintained with bag–valve–mask ventilations, the patient's airway is secured by endotracheal intubation.

According to the most recent American Association of Poison Control Centers database, naloxone was the third most commonly administered antidote. Naloxone is derived from thebaine, a minor constituent of opium. In addition to IV administration, naloxone can be given via the endotracheal tube, subcutaneously, intramuscularly or by nebulizer, with a comparably rapid onset of action. Clinical trials have demonstrated that slower absorption via the subcutaneous route was offset by the delay in establishing IV access, particularly in young children. Intramuscular administration has also been demonstrated to be safe and efficacious in an urban prehospital adult patient population. In the overdose setting, the dose of naloxone is 0.1 mg/kg in children from birth to 5 years of age or in children weighing less than 20 kg. In older children, or in the setting of life-threatening toxicity, a rapid 2-mg dose is recommended. Naloxone can be administered in any IV fluid in varying concentrations. If there is no response, repeat doses of 2 mg every 2 to 3 minutes can given to older children and adolescents, up to a maximum of 10 mg. If no response occurs, other causes for CNS and respiratory depression should be considered.

Naloxone doses up to 4 mg/kg have been given to human adult volunteers with minimal to no adverse side effects. An exception to this rule is in the chronic opioid abusing adolescent, in whom an acute withdrawal syndrome can be precipitated. In this setting, doses of 0.1 to 0.4 mg can be given to relieve the respiratory depression without precipitating florid withdrawal symptoms. If the patient experiences acute withdrawal symptoms, general supportive care measures are indicated, because opioid withdrawal is not a life-threatening situation. In the newborn setting, however, withdrawal seizures have been well documented among neonates born to opioid-dependent mothers.

Naloxone's duration of action is 20 to 30 minutes, which is shorter than most opioid agents, except fentanyl. Thus, repeat doses may be indicated, particularly when dealing with opioids with longer duration of action, such as oxycodone, methadone, and Lomotil (diphenoxylate). Titrated doses administered every 3 to 5 minutes may be initially required. If repeat doses of naloxone are necessary, a continuous IV infusion of naloxone can be instituted. The drip rate can be calculated by using two thirds of the initial dose required to reverse the patient's respiratory depression and administering this amount hourly. The infusion rate may vary, however, depending on the specific opioid and the patient's level of physical dependence.

The new longer-acting antagonist nalmefene may be useful in younger, non–opioid-dependent children who are exposed to longer-acting agents. Although studies of this agent in the pediatric population are limited, it has been safely administered in the clinical setting by reversing iatrogenically induced opioid sedation in children, with no reported adverse side effects. Doses of 0.5 to 2.0 mg have been reported to be safe and effective, with a duration of effect up to 8 hours. Nalmefene would be most clinically efficacious in younger children not experiencing withdrawal symptoms. In the setting of chronically addicted adolescents, a shorter-acting antagonist like naloxone would be a more humane approach, because withdrawal symptoms would be shorter in duration.

In patients who have ingested oral narcotics, gastric lavage may be performed if the patient presents within 1 hour after the ingestion. Attention must paid to the patient's mental status owing to the risk of respiratory depression. An initial dose of activated charcoal is advised following any oral ingestion, particularly in opioids that have delayed absorption, such as diphenoxylate-atropine (Lomotil) and sustained-release morphine products.

As with cyclic antidepressant overdose, cardiotoxicity from propoxyphene demonstrating a widened QRS complex may be responsive to IV administration of sodium bicarbonate.

Children who present as body packers or stuffers of heroin- or opioid-containing drugs may require GI decontamination with whole bowel irrigation using polyethylene glycol (PEG) solution to enhance elimination of drug packets. The PEG dose is 25 mL/kg/h, which often requires orogastric tube insertion. Contraindications to whole bowel irrigation include unstable vital signs, respiratory compromise, and lack of bowel sounds or gut motility. Activated charcoal should be given prior to whole bowel irrigation to adsorb any leaking drug from the packets. Charcoal noted later in the rectal effluent indicates successful whole bowel irrigation.

DISPOSITION

Any young pediatric patient presenting with CNS and respiratory depression from opioid poisoning who is responsive to naloxone should be admitted for observation, because most of the opioids demonstrate longer duration of action than naloxone and repetitive dosing or continuous naloxone infusion may be required. Long-acting agents such as methadone and the antidiarrheal agent Lomotil are much more likely to demonstrate recurrence of CNS and respiratory depression. Because of the potential delays in toxicity, young children should be observed in a monitored setting for at least 24 hours. However, most recurrences are evident within 2 hours of presentation.

Adolescents presenting with CNS depression from heroin overdose who quickly respond to naloxone administration can be discharged home with reliable caretakers after 4 to 6 hours of observation. In patients who continue to demonstrate respiratory compromise or require repeated doses of naloxone, it would be prudent to observe these patients for a longer period of time. In patients demonstrating chronic addiction patterns, detoxification programs and appropriate counseling referrals should be arranged.

CASE OUTCOME

The child is administered 100% oxygen by face mask. IV access is delayed owing to difficulties locating an adequate site. Therefore, 1 mg of subcutaneous naloxone is administered. The child begins to awaken and cry with spontaneous eye opening within 1 minute. Pulse oximetry improves to 92%. A rapid bedside serum glucose of 120 mg/dL is measured. When IV access is obtained, the child is given a repeat dose of 1 mg of naloxone. The

patient becomes completely alert and pulse oximetry increases to 98%. The child's uncle then presents to the emergency department and admits that he is on methadone, and had inadvertently left his medication out the night before. The child is admitted to the intensive care unit. One hour later, the child requires a subsequent dose of IV naloxone; the longer-acting antidote, nalmefene, is given. The child remains alert over the next 10 hours and requires one more subsequent dose of nalmefene. He is discharged uneventfully the next day, 36 hours after presentation to the hospital.

SUGGESTED READINGS

Binchy JM, Molyneux EM, Manning J: Accidental ingestion of methadone by children in Merseyside. *BMJ* 308:1335–1336, 1994.

Chamberlain JM, Klein BL: A comprehensive review of naloxone for the emergency physician. *Am J Emerg Med* 12:650–660, 1994.

Chumpa A: Nalmefene hydrochloride. *Pediatr Emerg Care* 15:141–143, 1999.

Chumpa A, Kaplan RL, Burns MM, Shannon MW. Nalmefene for elective reversal of procedural sedation in children. *Am J Emerg Med* 19:545–548, 2001.

Cohen MR, Cohen RM, Pickar D, et al: Behavioral effects after high-dose naloxone administration to normal volunteers. *Lancet* 2:1110, 1981.

Cone EJ, Fant RV, Rohay JM, et al: Oxycodone involvement in drug deaths: a DAWN-based classification scheme applied to an oxycodone postmortem database containing over 1000 cases. *J Anal Toxicol* 27:57–67, 2003.

Crain SM, Shen KF: Modulation of opioid analgesia, tolerance and dependence by Gs-coupled, GM1 ganglioside-regulated opioid receptor functions. *Trends Pharmacol Sci* 19:358–365, 1998.

Cutler EA, Barrett GA, Craven PW, et al: Delayed cardiopulmonary arrest after Lomotil ingestion. *Pediatrics* 65:157–158, 1980.

De la Fuente L, Barrio G, Royuela L: Heroin smoking by "chasing the dragon": Its evolution in Spain. *Addiction* 93:444–446, 1998.

Glare PA, Walsh TD: Clinical pharmacokinetics of morphine. *Ther Drug Monit* 13:1–23, 1991.

Hoffman JR, Schriger DL, Luo JS: The empiric use of naloxone in patients with altered mental status: A reappraisal. *Ann Emerg Med* 20:246–252, 1991.

Ginsburg CM, Lomotil (diphenoxylate and atropine) intoxication. *Am J Dis Child* 125:241–242, 1973.

Glick C, Evans OB, Parks BR: Muscle rigidity due to fentanyl infusion in the pediatric patient. *South Med J* 889:1119–1120, 1996.

Goldfrank L, Weisman RS, Errick JK, et al: A dosing nomogram for continuous infusion intravenous naloxone. *Ann*

Emerg Med 15:566–570, 1986.

Kaplan JL, Mark JA, Calabro JJ, et al: Double-blind, randomized study of nalmefene and naloxone in emergency department suspected narcotic overdose. *Ann Emerg Med* 34:42–50, 1999.

Kauffman RE, Banner W, Blumer JL, et al: Naloxone dosage and route of administration for infants and children. *Pediatrics* 86:484, 1990.

Kleinschmidt KC, Wainscott M, Ford M: Opioids. In: Ford M, Delaney KA, Ling L, et al, eds: *Clinical Toxicology.* Philadelphia: Saunders; 2001:627–639.

Koren G, Butt W, Pape K, et al: Morphine-induced seizures in newborn infants. *Vet Hum Toxicol* 27:519, 1985.

Lewis JM, Klein-Shwartz W, Benson BE, et al: Continuous naloxone infusion in pediatric narcotic overdose. *Am J Dis Child* 138:944–946, 1984.

Litovitz TL, Schwartz-Klein W, Rodgers GCS, et al: 2001 annual report of the American Association of Poison Control Centers Toxic Exposure Surveillance System. *Am J Emerg Med* 20:391–452, 2002.

McCarron MM, Challoner RR, Thompson GA: Diphenoxylateatropine (Lomotil) overdose in children: An update. *Pediatrics* 87:694–700, 1991.

Medical Letter: Oxycodone and oxycontin. *Med Lett Drugs Ther* 43:80–81, 2001.

Meyer FP, Rimasch H, Glaha B, et al: Tramadol withdrawal in a neonate. *Eur J Clin Pharmacol* 53:159–160, 1997.

Minami M, Satoh M: Molecular biology of the opioid receptors: Structures, functions and distributions. *Neurosci Res* 23:121–145, 1995.

Moore RA, Rumack BH, Conner CS, et al: Naloxone. *Am J Dis Child* 134:156–158, 1980.

Nelson L: Opioids. In: Goldfrank LR, Flomenbaum NE, Lewin NA, et al, eds: *Goldfrank's Toxicologic Emergencies.* 7th ed. New York: McGraw-Hill; 2002:901–923.

Pasterak GW: Pharmacologic mechanisms of opioid analgesics. *Clin Neuropharmacol* 16:1–18, 1993.

Rumack BH, Temple AR: Lomotil poisoning. *Pediatrics* 53:495–500, 1974.

Schneir AB, Vadeboncoeur TF, Offerman SR, et al: Massive oxycontin ingestion refractory to naloxone therapy. *Ann Emerg Med* 40:425–428, 2002.

Sporer KA: Acute heroin overdose. *Ann Intern Med* 130:584–590, 1999.

Sporer KA, Firestone J, Isaacs M: Out of hospital treatment of opioid overdoses in an urban setting. *Acad Emerg Med* 3:600–667, 1996.

Stork CM, Redd JT, Fine K, Hoffman RS: Proxyphene-induced wide QRS complex dysrhythmia responsive to sodium bicarbonate: A case report. *Clin Toxicol* 33:179–183, 1995.

U.S. Drug Enforcement Administration (DEA): *Narcotics.* Available from http://www.dea.gov/pubs/abuse/index.html. 2003.

Utecht MJ, Stone AF, McCarron MM: Heroin body packers. *J Emerg Med* 159:750–754, 1993.

Wagner K, Brough L, MacMillan I, et al: Intravenous vs subcutaneous naloxone for out-of-hospital management of presumed opioid overdose. *Acad Emerg Med* 5:293–299, 1998.

Watson WA, Steele MT, Muelleman RL, et al: Opioid recurrence after an initial response to naloxone. *Clin Toxciol* 36:11–17, 1998.

61

Drug-Facilitated Sexual Assault

Kirk L. Cumpston

HIGH-YIELD FACTS

- Ethanol is the most common date rape drug.

- γ-Hydroxybutyrate (GHB), flunitrazepam (Rohypnol), and ketamine are other drugs used to facilitate rape.

- All of these drugs can incapacitate a person in 15 to 20 minutes and lose effect hours later, leaving the victim with either incomplete or no recollection of the past events.

- γ-Butyrolactone (GBL) and 1,4-butanediol (1,4 BD) are precursors that are metabolized to GHB after ingestion, resulting in the same effects.

- Collecting blood within 24 hours and urine within 72 hours of the rape and refrigeration of the sample can detect a few select date rape drugs if analyzed in a specialized laboratory.

- Prevention tips: (1) Do not accept drinks from strangers, (2) Do not leave your drink uncovered, (3) When returning to your table get a fresh drink, and (4) Have your designated driver monitor your group.

CASE PRESENTATION

A 14-year-old girl presents to the emergency department at 7:00 AM stating she thinks she might have been raped last night. She was out with one female friend and two older male friends, and she admits to drinking more than 6 cans of beer that night. She denies any other drug use. She states that she passed out twice but has large gaps in her memory. Her last recollection of the night is getting a ride home with the two men. When she awoke this morning she noticed bruises on her arms and the sensation that she had had intercourse, but she cannot remember clearly. Her past medical history is unremarkable, she takes no medications, and has no allergies.

On physical examination, all vital signs are within normal limits. She was a well-developed, well-nourished female in no apparent distress. Pupils are midrange and reactive, mucous membranes moist, and breath notable for ethanol odor. The heart has a regular rate and rhythm with normal heart sounds and no murmur. The lungs are clear to auscultation. The abdomen appears scaphoid, with active bowel sounds, is nontender to palpation, and has no rebound, guarding, rigidity, or masses. The pelvic examination reveals no trauma, tenderness, blood, discharge, or masses. Her skin has superficial scratches and abrasions on both arms. The neurological examination is without focal deficits and she has normal reflexes.

INTRODUCTION AND EPIDEMIOLOGY

Date rape refers to nonconsensual sex facilitated by the use of a sedative or mind-altering drug. It is estimated that 1 in 4 women in the United States will be raped during their lifetimes, and 3 in 4 women will know their assailant. To facilitate the deception of their acquaintance, the rapist may use quick-acting pharmaceuticals to sedate the victim and erase any memory of the event. The drugs most commonly associated with date rape are ethanol, GHB, flunitrazepam, and ketamine.

Date rape was first described in the 1950s in 13% to 21% of college-aged women. Two different surveys in 1993 and 1995 found the prevalence of date rape in high school students was 20% and 26%, respectively. In another study with a more diverse sample, the prevalence of date rape ranged from 22% to 68%, with the highest percentage in female street youth. The racial group most often reported was Caucasian (16%).

Risk factors for women becoming a victim of date rape include an acceptance of violence toward women, the belief that rape is justified, the ages from 16 to 19 years, early menarche and initiation of sex, use of alcohol beginning in the eighth or ninth grade, any substance abuse, prior voluntary use of flunitrazepam, and past sexual victimization. The most common location for date rape is an apartment or private house; dormitories or parked cars are second. Because date rape has become such a common event, it is also of significant importance when young women are asked to compare it to other health issues. Of African American women 18 to 22 years old, 62% strongly agree that date rape is relevant to their lives. Of students participating in a mixed gender workshop on date rape prevention, 97% believed it is a worthy topic.

GHB, flunitrazepam, and ketamine are the drugs most commonly implicated in date rape. This is exemplified by the largely publicized deaths of Hillory Farias and Samantha Reid after they died from the effects of GHB during their dates. As a result of their deaths, the bill HR2130, named the Hillory Farias and Samantha Reid Date-Rape Drug Prohibition Act of 2000 was signed by President Clinton on February 18, 2000, making GHB a schedule I drug. Although GHB is a commonly used date rape drug, other substances are involved in the majority of date rapes. Several studies have tested urine samples of rape victims within 72 hours of assault. Alcohol was by far the most common substance detected in the urine (38% to 70%), and second was tetrahydrocannibinol (18% to 30%). Less than 5% of the urine samples reported GHB, and 0.0% to 0.5% of the samples were positive for flunitrazepam. None of the studies tested for ketamine. There is a long list of drugs that have the potential to be used for date rape (Table 61–1).

THE AGENTS

γ-Hydroxybutyrate

GHB was first isolated by the French chemist Henry Laborit in 1960. It is an endogenous four-carbon chain similar to γ-aminobutyric acid (GABA) in structure and clinical effects. It was discovered in an effort to find a substance like GABA that could be used by anesthesiologists to sedate patients. It is now known that GHB has

Table 61–1. Drugs Used to Facilitate Sexual Assault

Alcohol	Imidazolines
Alprazolam	Ketamine
Barbiturates	Lorazepam
1,4 Butanediol	Marijuana
Cocaine	MDMA
γ-Butyrolactone	Meprobamate
Cannabis	Methamphetamine
Carisoprodol	Midazolam
Chloral hydrate	Opiates
Chlordiazepoxide	Oxazepam
Clonazepam	Phencyclidine (PCP)
Cyclobenzaprine	Propoxyphene
Diazepam	Scopolamine
Diphenhydramine	Secobarbital
Flunitrazepam (Rohypnol)	Temazepam
Fluazepam	Triazolam
γ-Hydroxybutyrate	Zoplidem

its own receptors, can act at GABA B receptors, and may modulate other neurotransmitters such as dopamine, acetylcholine, GABA, and endogenous opioids. GHB is metabolized to harmless carbon dioxide by the tricarboxylic acid cycle, and eliminated by respiration.

The enthusiasm for GHB waned when anesthesia was found to be inconsistent and analgesic properties absent. Seizures were also reported as a side effect. In the United States, GHB was used as a dietary supplement by body builders because it was erroneously thought GHB could increase muscle mass. GHB was also touted by the herbal drug industry as a sedative after L-tryptophan was banned. In the late 1980s and early 1990s GHB increased in popularity as a club drug and date rape drug. Some common street names for GHB are listed in Table 61–2. Because of the alarming numbers of people using GHB and the potential harmful effects, in 1990 the Food and Drug Administration issued a ban on the production of GHB in the United States. However, like cannabis, GHB is now a schedule I and III drug, because it is approved for the treatment of narcolepsy, under the trade name Xyrem.

GHB is distributed as a liquid, powder, and gel. Most commonly it is ingested in the liquid form. It has a soapy or salty taste. It is a lucrative street product that is sometimes sold at $5 to $10 a capful, offering the buyer the same effect as alcohol for a small amount of money. The desired effect sought by most users is to enhance disinhi-

Table 61–2. Street Names for Classic Drugs Used in Sexual Assault

GHB	1,4 BD	GBL	Flunitrazepam	Ketamine
Biosky	Enliven	Blue Nitro	Circles	K
Blue nitro	GHRE	Blue Nitro-Vitality	Darkene	Green
Cherry fX bombs	NRG3	Gamma G	The "Drop Drug"	Jet
Cherry meth	Revitalize Plus	GH Revitalizer	Forget pill	Kay
Coke	Serenity	Remforce	La roche	Keets
Easy lay	Somatopro	RenewTrient	Mexican valium	Mauve
Everclear	Thunder Nectar	Revivarant	Mind erasers	Purple
Firewater	Weight belt-cleaner	Revivarant G	Pappas	Special K
Gamma G		Pine needle oil	Pastas	Special LA Coke
Gammo-OH			Peanuts	Super acid
GBH			Poples	Super C
Georgia Home Boy			R05-4200	
G.II. Revitalizer			R-2	
GHB			Reynol	
Gib			Rib	
Goops			Roaches	
Great Hormones at Bedtime			Roachies	
Grievous Bodily Harm			Robinol	
G-riffick			Roche	
Growth Hormone Booster			Roches	
Insom-X			Roches Dos	
Invigorate			Rohibinol	
Lemon fX drops			Rohypnol	
Liquid X			Roofenol	
Liquid E			Roofies	
Longevity			Roopies	
Natural sleep-500			Ropanol	
Nature's Quaalude			Rophies	
Orange fX rush			Ropes	
Organic Quaalude			Ropies	
Oxy-sleep			Roples	
Poor man's heroin			Row-shay	
Remforce			Rubies	
Salt water			Ruffies	
Scoop			Ruffiew	
Soap			Trip and fall	
Somatomax PM			Whiteys	
Somsanit			Wolfies	
Vita-G				
Water				
Wolfies				
Zonked				

bition, and allow the individual to relax and dance. The onset of action is 15 to 20 minutes, making it ideal for the person desiring to sedate a potential rape victim quickly. The amnestic properties prevent the victim from clearly recalling the rape. It therefore confers difficulty in prosecuting the rapist.

The classic clinical picture of GHB intoxication is CNS and respiratory depression, sometimes to the point of coma. In one study, 60% of patients presented with a GCS <9. The CNS depression often reverses abruptly and without warning, and the patient's mental status may oscillate between somnolence and agitation with combativeness. It is not uncommon for the patient to become aroused during intubation, or suddenly awaken afterward, and remove the endotracheal tube themselves. Other signs of GHB intoxication include seizures, myoclonus, ataxia, nystagmus, bradycardia, hypotension, emesis, and mild hypothermia. The duration of action is dose dependent, but anywhere from 1 to 4 hours has been reported. Doses of 10 mg/kg cause amnesia and hypotonia and 50 to 70 mg/kg lead to anesthesia, coma, seizures, and respiratory depression. Most clinical symptoms resolve within 7 hours. There are almost always coingestants with GHB.

Because GHB was made illegal in 2000, distributors of GHB have circumvented the law by selling precursors to GHB, such as GBL and 1,4 butanediol (BD). Both of these agents are metabolized in the human body to GHB (Figure 61–1). GBL is a solvent used commercially for the production of paint, beer, plastics, textiles, nail polish remover, and floor strippers. BD is sold as a nutritional supplement. Common street names of these products are listed in Table 61–2. The clinical effects of both of these precursors are the same as GHB. BD is metabolized by alcohol dehydrogenase to GHB; this may be inhibited by ingestion of alcohol. Clinically, mental status depression may occur in a bimodal presentation or last longer than expected, because the first mental status change results from the alcohol, and the second from the formation of GHB from the BD. GBL is metabolized to GHB by lactonase. In 2000, GBL and BD became classified as List I chemicals, which requires anyone who imports, exports, or distributes these products to register them with the Drug Enforcement Agency (DEA).

There are no consistently effective antidotes for GHB overdoses. Some sources recommend the use of physostigmine. However, its use in the setting of GHB toxicity remains controversial. Treatment is primarily supportive. Protecting the airway, maintaining hemodynamic stability, and seizure precautions are the primary goals of treatment.

The possibility of being exposed to GHB or its precursors in a date rape scenario is significant. Health-risk behaviors increase from 5% to 10% per year between sixth and twelfth grades. GHB should be discussed as

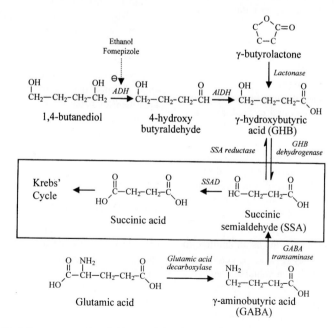

Fig. 61–1. Precursors such as 1,4 butanediol and γ-butyrolactone are metabolized to GHB.

part of the HEADSS (home life, education, activities, drugs, suicide, sex) assessment during the social history of all teenage patients.

Flunitrazepam

Flunitrazepam (Rohypnol) is a fast-acting benzodiazepine, 10 times more potent than diazepam, manufactured by Hoffman-LaRoche. Flunitrazepam is not produced in the United States, but is prescribed in Mexico, South America, Asia, and Australia for the treatment of insomnia. In the United States it is most commonly seen in the states on the Mexican border. Until 1996 it was legal to bring an unopened 90-day supply of flunitrazepam across the border. Now it is illegal to prescribe, sell, or import flunitrazepam in the United States. The Drug-Induced Rape Prevention and Punishment Act, passed in 1996, makes the use of flunitrazepam for the purposes of rape punishable by imprisonment for a maximum of 20 years.

Flunitrazepam is frequently sold as white tablets in blister packs, with the Roche insignia imprinted on the surface. The tablets are either swallowed, ingested with a carbonated beverage, dissolved under the tongue, sprinkled on marijuana, or crushed and snorted. One survey found that use averaged 1 to 2 times per week, along with alcohol. Flunitrazepam is also used with heroin to attenuate withdrawal symptoms, and with cocaine to modulate the stimulant effects. Popular street names of flunitrazepam are listed in Table 61–2.

The onset of action of a 2-mg dose is 15 to 20 minutes. Effects can last 8 to 12 hours. Like other benzodiazepines, flunitrazepam acts by facilitating the binding of GABA at its receptor. Flunitrazepam is used in the date rape scenario because it causes fast sedation and prolonged amnesia of the event. It has been found to have a greater amnestic effect than diazepam, and a more rapid onset of sedation than lorazepam.

Hoffman-LaRoche has taken steps to decrease the use of this drug in date rapes by making the pills dissolve more slowly in liquids, turning clear beverages bright blue, and making dark beverages appear murky. The company also has a hotline available if there is a need to analyze urine to detect flunitrazepam.

Flumazenil has been recommended as an antidote to flunitrazepam. This antidote may reverse the central nervous system depression, making it a valuable diagnostic and therapeutic agent. Caution must be taken when flumazenil is used in the setting of a possible tricyclic antidepressant overdose, in the benzodiazepine-depend-

Fig 61–2. Chemical structures of PCP and ketamine.

ent patient, and in patients with seizure disorders. Otherwise, like GHB, the treatment is support of airway and hemodynamic status.

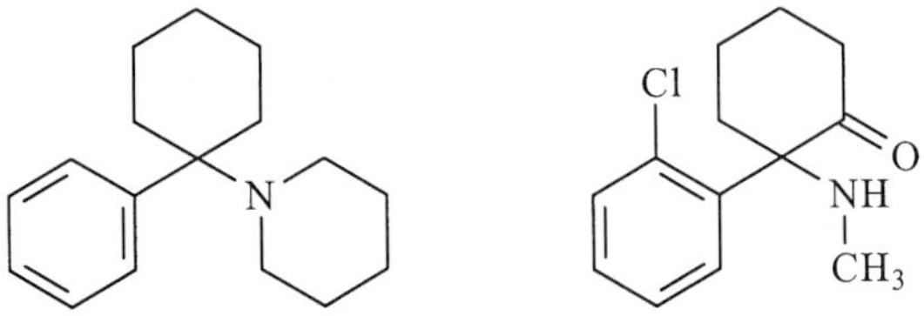

Ketamine

Ketamine is a dissociative anesthetic that is used in human and veterinary medicine. It is registered with DEA as a schedule III drug. It has a structure similar to PCP and LSD (Figure 61–2) and is used illicitly for a similar effect. It is distributed as an injectable drug, but it can also be snorted, swallowed, and smoked. Common street names are listed in Table 61–2. It is believed that the first case report of date rape with ketamine was in Florida in 1993. However, there are actually few case reports of ketamine used for date rape. Many studies that reported the drugs detected in the urine samples of date rape victims did not test for ketamine. The onset of anesthetic effects is 15 to 20 minutes, and effects last for 20 to 45 minutes. Side effects of ketamine include hypertension, vomiting, hypersalivation, dizziness, disorientation, hallucinations, vivid dreams, nystagmus, and emergence nightmares. Treatment of ketamine intoxication is supportive. If the victim is hallucinating decrease, external stimuli. Benzodiazepines may be needed for agitation.

LABORATORY EVALUATION

γ-Hydroxybutyrate

GHB is rapidly eliminated from the body, and is undetectable in the plasma and urine after 8 and 12 hours, respectively. Urine samples are analyzed for GHB by either gas chromatography–mass spectrometry or high-performance liquid chromatography. Because GHB is an endogenous substance, an investigation tested urine samples to determine if endogenous GHB levels could increase over 6 months to levels considered indicative of illicit drug use. It was discovered that none of the subjects obtained a level consistent with exogenous GHB use. On the contrary, citrate buffer in the collection tube can falsely elevate GHB to levels seen in exogenous use. As a resullt, it is recommended that blood specimens be collected in grey-top (sodium fluoride/potassium oxalate) tubes. Other methods of detection are sweat and hair samples. A sweat patch may be effective if applied less than 12 hours after the alleged rape. The patch is left on for 3 to 7 days and the contents are extracted and analyzed. This method has been successful in the laboratory, but has not been tested in a single-dose scenario like date rape. Hair analysis has actually been used to convict an assailant. In the case, a woman who suspected date rape waited 1 month for her hair to grow and had it analyzed by Gas chromatography/mass spectrometry/mass spectrometry. The level of GHB detected was significantly greater than the levels in controls without GHB exposure.

Flunitrazepam

Flunitrazepam has an elimination half-life of 19 to 22 hours, and its two metabolites norflunitrazepam and 7-aminoflunitrazepam allow detection up to 2 days in the blood and 4 days in the urine. Usually, a standard EMIT urine toxicology screen is negative for benzodiazepines if flunitrazepam has been taken. The sample must be screened for the specific flunitrazepam metabolites.

In general, collection of blood within 24 hours and the urine within 3 days is the upper limit of time to detect some of the drugs that are used in date rape. Any blood or urine sample needs to be collected as soon as possible and refrigerated. Most of these samples will need to be analyzed by a special laboratory. It is important to include these analyses in suspected cases of drug-facilitated sexual assault because it may assist forensically and for counseling.

In 10 volunteers who ingested 2 mg of flunitrazepam, half were found to have 7-aminoflunitrazepam detected in their hair 24 hours later. In two of the subjects, this metabolite was detected at 14 days and in two subjects at 21 days. The longest time from ingestion that 7-aminoflunitrazepam was detected in the hair was 28 days.

CONCLUSION

Drug-facilitated sexual assault is not a new phenomenon. However, it has been recognized since the 1990s, with

Table 61–3. Drug-Facilitated Sexual Assault Prevention Guidelines

- Do not accept unopened beverages offered by strangers
- Make sure your date is drinking from the same punch bowl
- Avoid drinking games
- Do not drink alcoholic beverages more than 2 drinks every hour
- In an unfamiliar bar directly observe your drink being poured
- If your drink tastes, looks, or smells different, do not drink it
- When returning to your table, obtain a new drink
- Use your designated driver to observe for any suspicious activity and watch for quick inebriation of members of your group

the explosion of GHB and flunitrazepam abuse. These drugs are used because of the rapid onset of sedation, disorientation, and amnesia. In addition to the injury caused by the sexual assault, the deep sedation can lead to hypoventilation and death. Advanced laboratory technology does allow detection of these drugs, if the specimens are collected early and in the proper container, and refrigerated. Other samples such as sweat and hair show promise for the future. Media attention may focus on illegal drugs such as GHB, flunitrazepam, and ketamine, but legal drugs like alcohol are used in the majority of date rapes. It is important for pediatricians to include questioning about drugs and date rape in the assessment of adolescents. Prevention through education is a necessity (Table 61–3).

CASE OUTCOME

Laboratory values are significant for a negative urine pregnancy test, and a negative urine toxicologic screen for opiates, cocaine, amphetamines, cannabis, methadone, benzodiazepines, and barbiturates. A serum ethanol level was 109 mg/dL. All other laboratory tests are within the normal range. After obtaining informed consent, urine and blood samples are collected for the purpose of analysis for date rape drugs by the state laboratory. The police are contacted, and all evidence collected during the examination is turned over to their custody. Because of the high-risk behavior of this patient, she is admitted to the hospital for further counseling.

SUGGESTED READINGS

Calhoun SR, Wesson DR, Galloway GP at al: Abuse of Flunitrazepam (Rohypnol) and other benzodiazepines in Austin and South Texas. *J Psychoactive Drugs* 28(2):183–189, 1996.

Couper FJ, Logan BK: Determination of gamma-hydroxybutyrate (GHB) in biological specimens by gas chromatography-mass spectrometry. *J Analyt Toxicol* 24:1–7, 2000.

Druid H, Holmgren P, Ahlner J: Flunitrazepam: An evaluation of use, abuse and toxicity. *Forens Sci Int* 122:136–141, 2001.

Dyer J: Gamma-Hydroxybutyrate: A health-food product producing coma and seizurelike activity. *Am J Emerg Med* 9: 321–324, 1991.

Elian AA: A novel method for GHB detection in urine and its application in drug-facilitated sexual assaults. *Forens Sci Int* 109:183–187, 2000.

ElSohly MA: Drug-facilitated sexual assault. *South Med J* 94: 655–666, 2001.

ElSohly MA, Salamone SJ: Prevalence of drugs used in cases of alleged sexual assault. *J Analyt Toxicol* 23:141–146, 1999.

Ford DS, Goode CR: African American college students' health behaviors and perceptions of related health issues. *J Am Coll Health* 42:206–210, 1994.

Kilpatrick DG, Acierno R, Resnick HS, et al: A 2-year longitudinal analysis of the relationships between violent assault and substance use in women. *J Consult Clin Psychol* 5: 834–847, 1997.

Kintz P, Cirimele V, Jamey C, et al: Testing for GHB in hair by GC/MS/MS after a single exposure. Application to document sexual assault. *J Forens Sci* 48:195–200, 2003.

LeBeau M, Andollo W, Hearn WL, et al: Recommendations for toxicological investigations of drug-facilitated sexual assaults. *J Forens Sci* 44:227–230, 1999.

LeBeau MA, Miller ML, Levine B: Effect of storage temperature on endogenous GHB levels in urine. *Forens Sci Int* 119: 161–167, 2001.

LeBeau M, Montgomery MA, Jufer RA: Elevated GHB in citrate-buffered blood. *J Analyt Toxicol* 24:383–384, 2000.

LeBeau M, Montgomery MA, Wagner JR, et al: Analysis of biofluids for flunitrazepam and metabolites by electrospray liquid chromatography/mass spectrometry. *J Forens Sci* 45: 1133–1141, 2000.

Lee DC: Sedative-hypnotic agents. In: Goldfrank LR, Flomenbaum NE, Lewin NA, et al, eds: *Goldfrank's Toxicologic Emergencies.* 7th ed. New York: McGraw-Hill; 2002:929.

Leikin JB, Paloucek FP: Flunitrazepam. In: Leikin JB, Paloucek FP, eds: *Leikin and Paloucek's Poisoning & Toxicology Handbook.* 3rd ed. Hudson, OH: Lexi-Comp; 2002:584.

Mason PE, Kerns WP: Gamma hydroxybutyric acid (GHB) intoxication. *Acad Emerg Med* 9:730–739, 2002.

Negrusz A, Moore CM, Hinkel KB, et al: Deposition of 7-aminoflunitrazepam and flunitrazepam in hair after a single dose of Rohypnol(r). *J Forens Sci* 46:1143–1151, 2001.

Nicholson KL, Blaster RL: GHB: A new and novel drug of abuse. *Drug Alcohol Depend* 63:1–22, 2001.

Nordenberg T: The death of the party, all the rave, GHB's hazards go unheeded. *FDA Consumer* March–April:15–19, 2000

O'Connell T, Kaye L, Plosay JJ: Gamma-hydroxybutyrate (GHB): A newer drug of abuse. *Am Fam Physician* 62:2478–2483, 2000.

Payne-James J, Rogers D: Drug-facilitated sexual assault, 'ladettes' and alcohol. *J R Soc Med* 95:326–327, 2002.

Placement of gamma-butyrolactone in List I of the Controlled Substances Act. *Federal Register* 65:21645–21647, 2000.

Reif CJ, Elster AB: Adolescent preventative services. *Adolesc Med* 25:1–21, 1998

Rhynard J, Krebs M, Glover J: Sexual assault in dating relationships. *J School Health* 67:89–93, 1997.

Rickert VI, Vaughan RD, Weimann CM: Adolescent dating violence and date rape. *Curr Opin Obstet Gynecol* 14:495–500, 2000

Rickert VI, Wiemann CM: Date rape among adolescents and young adults. *J Pediatr Adolesc Gynecol* 11:167–175, 1998.

Ropero-Miller JD, Goldberger BA: Recreational drugs: Current trends in the 90s. *Clin Lab Med* 18:727–746, 1998.

Schwartz RH, Milteer R, LeBeau MA: Drug-facilitated sexual assault ('date rape'). *South Med J* 93:558–561, 2000.

Simmons MM, Cupp MJ: Use and abuse of flunitrazepam. *Ann Pharmacother* 32:117–119, 1998.

Slaughter L: Involvement of drugs in sexual assault. *J Reprod Med* 45:425–430, 2000.

Smith KM: Drugs used in acquaintance rape. *J Am Pharm Assoc* 39:519–525, 1999.

Stillwell ME: Drug-facilitated sexual assault involving gamma-hydroxybutyric acid. *J Forens Sci* 47:1133–1134, 2002.

62

Phencyclidine and Ketamine

In-Hei Hahn

HIGH-YIELD FACTS

- Patients with phencyclidine (PCP) poisoning may present with the triad of acute behavioral changes, sympathomimetic signs, and nystagmus.

- Emergence reactions from ketamine occur more frequently in older pediatric patients and can be treated with benzodiazepines.

- Severely agitated or violent patients intoxicated with PCP often require sedation with benzodiazepines.

- Urinary acidification is not recommended for increased elimination of PCP.

- PCP may cause rhabdomyolysis with associated electrolyte disturbances, metabolic acidosis, and acute renal failure.

CASE PRESENTATION

A 13-year-old boy presents to the emergency department (ED) after smoking a marijuana joint. His friends state that the patient is hearing and seeing things that he never experienced before when smoking marijuana, and became violent while he was trying to run away from them. He sustained a large laceration to his arm but did not seem to notice. His past medical history is unremarkable and he is not taking any medications nor does he have any known allergies. The patient denied ever using any illicit drugs except for marijuana.

On physical examination, he appears catatonic and trance-like and is slow to communicate. His vital signs reveal a temperature 100.6°F, pulse 120 bpm, blood pressure of 110/70 mmHg, and a respiratory rate of 22 breaths per minute. His physical examination is significant for rotatory nystagmus, moist mucous membranes, tachycardia, and diaphoresis. The patient does not seem to realize that he is in the ED, and does not recognize his friends. The rest of his examination is normal. Laboratory studies are pending.

INTRODUCTION AND EPIDEMIOLOGY

Phencyclidine (PCP), (1-phenylcyclohexyl-piperidine), otherwise known as *angel dust*, *crystal joint*, *elephant* or *horse tranquilizer*, and *hog*, is a commonly abused drug (Table 62–1). It is often used to enhance the effects of other drugs, especially marijuana. The marijuana cigarette is often sprinkled with PCP powder, or dipped in a solution containing PCP, and is commonly referred to as a *happy* or *wicky stick*.

PCP was first marketed under the trade name *Sernyl* by Parke Davis Pharmaceutical Company as a sedative and surgical anesthetic in the late 1950s. Because of the postoperative side effects consisting of psychotomimesis and hallucinations, the drug was removed from the market. In 1967, PCP returned as *Sernylan* and was marketed as a veterinary tranquilizer, hence the nicknames referring to the drug as an animal tranquilizer. In 1967, the first report of its illicit street appearance occurred from San Francisco, where it was referred to as the *PeaCe Pill*. Although PCP is not as widely abused as cocaine and heroin, it still remains in today's society as a major drug of abuse. According to the reports of the DAWN Emergency Departments from 1994 to 2001, the numbers range from 3441 to 6102 exposures. The manufacture of PCP was prohibited in 1978, after the drug was added

Table 62–1. Street Names for PCP and Ketamine

PCP	Ketamine
Angel	Cat valium
Angel dust	Green
Boat	Honey oil
Crystal joint	Jet
Dummy dust	K
Elephant or horse tranquilizer	KitKat
Hog	Purple
Illy	Special K
Love boat	Special LA coke
PeaCe pill	Super acid
Supergrass	Super C
Zombie	Vitamin K

to the Federal Controlled Substance Act of 1970. The Controlled Substance Analogue Enforcement Act of 1986 made PCP and its derivatives illegal, and made the precursor, piperidine, a chemical requiring mandatory reporting.

The only legal analogs that are used clinically for sedation and anesthesia are ketamine and tiletamine. Only ketamine, [2-(ortho-chlorophenyl)-2-methylaminocyclohexanone], a chloroketone analog, is medically used for humans. It is also abused recreationally, and has nicknames such as *Special K*, *K*, *KitKat*, and *vitamin K* (see Table 62–1). Ketamine is used regularly at all-night raves and nightclubs because of its hallucinatory effects and out of body/near-death experiences. The drug is fairly inexpensive, and has a duration of action of approximately 15 to 45 minutes. Its toxicity is similar to PCP, it but is far less potent. Unlike PCP, ketamine is not typically manufactured illegally. It is obtained from diverted veterinary, dental, and medical sources. Ketamine was classified as a controlled substance in 1999.

DEVELOPMENTAL CONSIDERATIONS

Several authors report adverse neurobehavioral effects in neonates exposed to PCP in utero. These include extreme jitteriness, course flapping movements in response to slight auditory or tactile stimuli, nystagmus, poor visual tracking, and hypertonicity. A study by Howard and associates following the growth and development of 12 infants exposed prenatally to PCP showed that that the mean birth weight and mean frontal-occipital head cir-

cumference were in lower 10th percentile, and the mean crown-to-heel length was in the lower 25th percentile. All infants were normocephalic, without obvious congenital anomaly. The infants in this study developed the neurobehavioral symptoms mentioned within 24 hours of birth. Symptoms lasted between 2 and 14 days, and were relieved with either a trial of conservative measures such as swaddling, use of a pacifier, decreased stimulation, or chemical sedation with benzodiazepines, phenobarbital, or paregoric. Five PCP-exposed preterm infants experienced more frequent respiratory illnesses and slower weight gain, which subsequently contributed to prolonged hospitalizations, which averaged 24 days (control group, 10 days). Seven PCP-exposed full-term neonates had an average hospital stay of 8.0 days (control group, 2.5 days). This case series suggests that PCP-exposed infants are at risk for prolonged hospitalization regardless of their gestational age.

Developmental outcome for these infants was followed after their delivery and placement in foster homes. PCP-exposed infants were found to be delayed in abnormal fine motor skills, suffer from eye movements consisting of persistent nystagmus and darting, and to have less enjoyment with social interactions with adults. This study also suggests that PCP use during pregnancy may cause persistent developmental abnormalities.

Adolescents engaging in PCP use include those with unintentional exposure, those for whom it is the drug of choice, and those who engage in polysubstance abuse. All groups have reported hallucinations, paranoia, dysphoria, bizarre experiences, violence, threatening behaviors, and lack of control. PCP use does not seem to cause classical physiologic tolerance and physical withdrawal symptoms. However, it does produce drug cravings, and users develop a compulsion to repeat the PCP experience. A personality type has not been linked to PCP preference. One study suggests that disturbed adolescents who prefer PCP as their drug of choice have severe depression, feelings of hopelessness, powerlessness, and dysphoria prior to PCP use and that the drug offers them the feelings of power and invulnerability. However, there is still no satisfactory reason to explain why some adolescents with this profile abuse PCP and others do not.

PATHOPHYSIOLOGY AND TOXICOKINETICS

PCP is classified as a dissociative anesthetic, because in the anesthetized state the patient remains conscious but has a glazed stare, flat affect, and is immobile, colloquially known as the *lights on, nobody home effect.* The patient experiences a feeling of dissociation from themselves or an out-of-body sensation after being administered the drug.

The drug binds to many sites including, GABAnergic, cholinergic, μ opiate receptor systems, and at the neuronal membrane-associated Na/K channels; however, the interactions of these sites occur at serum PCP levels that would be considered lethal or unobtainable clinically. The only three sites that have been identified in serum or tissue concentrations as clinically relevant are the *N*-methyl-D-aspartic acid (NMDA)-type glutamate receptors, the neuronal dopamine/norepinephrine/serotonin (DA/NE/5HT) reuptake complex site, and the sigma opiate receptor complex. It is hypothesized that when PCP inhibits the NMDA glutamate transmitter system, the overall hypofunction is responsible for the schizophrenic-like symptomatology. PCP also binds to the neuronal DA/NE/5HT reuptake site and may modulate the dopaminergic and catecholaminergic effects seen in PCP poisoning. Finally PCP binds to the sigma opiate receptor, which may contribute to its analgesic and sedative properties.

The drug is a highly lipophilic, a weak base, soluble in water and ethanol, and rapidly absorbed after all routes of use throughout the tissues. Absorption occurs in the upper intestine rather than the stomach, and has an unusual enterogastric circulation such that it is actively secreted in the stomach and absorbed in the small intestine. The enterogastric recirculation can cause symptoms to recur in a cyclic fashion. Owing to ion trapping, the concentration of PCP in the stomach is 50 times greater than the serum and 9 times greater in the brain than the plasma. The volume of distribution is 6.2 L/kg, and the drug is 78% bound to plasma proteins (Table 62–2). This may account for the persistent effects and long duration of action.

The drug is metabolized by the liver and renally excreted. Approximately 10% remains unchanged when renally eliminated. There is also significant first-pass metabolism in the liver when PCP is ingested. In general, 0.1 μ/mL of PCP is considered a toxic level, and a fatal dose of PCP is 1 mg/kg.

Ketamine is often used for the induction of anesthesia, especially in the setting of status asthmaticus or for the adult experiencing severe chronic obstructive pulmonary disease exacerbation. Conscious sedation with ketamine is often utilized in the ED for elective procedures. The onset of action is rapid. Clinically, the patient's eyes glaze over in a dissociative state, which can be seen within seconds to a minute. Muscular tone may become increased, and purposeless movements of the extremities

Table 62–2. Pharmacokinetics of PCP and Ketamine

	PCP	Ketamine
pKa	8.6–9.4	7.5
V_d (L/kg)	6.2	1.8 ± 0.7
Routes of absorption	PO, IM, IV, SC, smoking, insufflation	PO, IM, IV, SC, smoking, insufflation
Elimination	Renal	Renal
Elimination half-life (h)	21 ± 3	2.3 ± 0.5
Onset of action (min)		
IV/inhalation		1
GI	2–5	30
IM	30–60	5

Abbreviations: GI, gastrointestinal; IM, intramuscular; IV, intravenous; PO, orally.

often occurs. Pharyngeal and laryngeal reflexes remain intact, depression of the cough reflex may occur, and increased salivary secretions may develop. The increase in secretions may be minimized by concurrent administration of an anticholinergic agent such as glycopyrrolate or ipratropium bromide.

CLINICAL FINDINGS

Patients may present to the ED with a history of using PCP or ketamine recreationally. Frequently, it is misrepresented as a more exotic hallucinogen such as mescaline, psilocybin, or tetrahydrocannabinol, or it can be used as an adulterant to other drugs without the knowledge of the user. The presentation depends on dose, route of use, concomitant drug use, and the individual's underlying medical condition. Patients typically present with the triad of abnormal vital signs, nystagmus, and acute psychomotor abnormalities.

The vital signs often show mildly elevated blood pressures with tachycardia and elevated temperatures caused by psychomotor agitation. Hypertension and vasospasm can lead to cerebral hemorrhage. Cardiac dysrhythmias have been reported in PCP-poisoned animals, but this has not been seen in humans. Ketamine has been found to cause dysrhythmias in animals, but has not been seen in cardiac patients undergoing surgery or catheterization. Respiratory drive is maintained and hypoventilation is uncommon unless extremely high doses of PCP or ketamine are involved. Ketamine has bronchodilatory effects, and may help prevent patients from being intubated in refractory asthma. Rarely, high doses of ketamine or fast infusions have been reported to cause respiratory depression and apnea. Slowing the infusion to occur over 1 to 2 minutes decreases the respiratory effects. Ketamine stimulates salivary and tracheobronchial secretions. Both laryngeal and pharyngeal reflexes are hyperactive, and a risk of laryngospasm exists for both PCP and ketamine. Children younger than 6 months to 1 year old are at greater risk for laryngospasm. Laryngospasm is generally reversed with oxygen administration and assisted ventilation.

All types of nystagmus, including vertical, horizontal, and rotatory, can be present in the PCP- or ketamine-exposed patient. Pupils may be small or large, but are reactive; patients may complain of diplopia. Neuropsychological effects vary widely and can include disorientation, confusion, depersonalization, dissociative thought, and catatonic trance. Some patients exhibit violent behavior, tremendous strength, feelings of omnipotence, and profound euphoria (Tables 62–3 and 63–4). Because PCP and is an anesthetic agent, patients are often unaware of injuries, such as fractures, lacerations, and even enucleation. Patients who have taken more than 10 mg are usually comatose, and may remain so for hours or even days. PCP-induced psychotic states may be long-lasting and flashbacks may recur.

Psychological dependence in the absence of physical symptoms has been described. Animal studies suggest physiologic dependence. There is some evidence that chronic PCP abuse may lead to withdrawal symptoms

Table 62–3. Behavioral Effects of PCP Toxicity

Violent behavior
Hallucinations
Apparent tremendous strength owing to lack of pain
  perception
Disorientation
Depersonalization
Dissociative thought
Catatonic trance-like state
Euphoria
Omnipotence
Sociability
Sexual prowess
Irrational thinking
Perseveration
Uncommunicative

Table 62–4. Clinical Effects of PCP Toxicity

Rotatory, horizontal, or vertical nystagmus
Hypertension
Ataxia
Slurred speech
Sweating
Muscle rigidity
Blank dissociative stare
Analgesia
Anesthesia

characterized by depression, anxiety, irritability, restlessness, anergia, sleep disturbance, and disturbed thoughts after 1 day of abstinence. Long-term neuropsychiatric effects of chronic PCP abuse seems to affect the ability to perform integrated higher-order function such as flexibility of thinking, formulation of simple and complex abstractions, and to cause incidental memory loss. Impaired fine motor function has also been reported.

LABORATORY AND DIAGNOSTIC TESTING

PCP exposure is often diagnosed clinically, and does not require diagnostic testing unless child abuse or foul play is suspected. Many hospitals have qualitative tests for PCP available as part of their urine toxicology screen. PCP is detected by an enzyme immunoassay. Positive PCP urine metabolites are present for at least 7 days postexposure in more than 90% of users. Chronic PCP users may test positive for urine metabolites 4 weeks postexposure. Quantitative testing is rarely used, because serum concentrations do not correlate with clinical presentations. Although urine is most often used in this assay, gastric and serum contents can be analyzed. Other nonspecific laboratory values have been used to support PCP exposure. They include leukocytosis, hypoglycemia, and elevation of creatinine phosphokinase (CPK), myoglobin, blood urea nitrogen, and creatinine.

There is no commercially available immunoassay for ketamine. If diagnostic testing needs to be done, gas chromatography mass spectroscopy may be performed. Hair analysis is another qualitative test that has been used to identify ketamine exposure. Ketamine has been reported to cross-react with the PCP urine immunoassay, although this has not been confirmed by PCP immunoassay manufacturers. Drugs that have been known to cause a false-positive reading for the PCP immunoassay include dextromethorphan, diphenhydramine, ibuprofen, imipramine, meperidine, mesoridazine, thioridazine, and venlafaxine.

MANAGEMENT

Agitation

Most patients presenting with PCP or ketamine intoxication require supportive care addressing their airway, circulation, and thermoregulation. Airway compromise from increased salivation and tracheobronchial secretions or laryngospasm may rarely require intubation. Other adverse reactions include emergence reactions, agitation, and persistent incoherence. Benzodiazepines may be used for the agitation and dysphoria associated with emergence. Prospective evaluation of adjunctive use of benzodiazepines for prophylaxis against emergence reactions during conscious sedation found no benefit to such use.

Extremely agitated or violent patients with PCP intoxication often require chemical restraints with benzodiazepines such as diazepam or lorazepam. In severe cases, neuroleptic agents such as haloperidol may be necessary for sedation. Physical restraints may also become necessary to avoid patient self-harm and to protect the medical staff. However, physical restraints should monitored vigilantly because they can contribute to hyperthermia, dehydration, rhabdomyolysis, with resulting myoglobinuria and renal damage in severely agitated patients. Ketamine toxicity induced iatrogenically should be managed conservatively.

Decontamination and Enhanced Elimination

Patients presenting to the hospital with a recent ingestion of PCP or ketamine may merit the administration of activated charcoal as long as there is no contraindication. Urinary acidification with ammonium chloride to enhance renal elimination of PCP is currently not recommended. Acidifying the urine will only marginally increase the excretion of PCP, and can decrease the excretion of myoglobin, which increases the risk of acute renal tubular necrosis in patients with rhabdomyolysis. Urinary acidification also decreases uric acid solubility, predisposing to uric acid nephropathy. A review of 27 confirmed PCP-poisoned cases found 3 patients developed rhabdomyolysis, with 2 of the 3 cases progressing to acute renal failure. Both of these patients received acidification measures before diagnosis. Overall, it is important to establish adequate hydration, monitor urinary output, and treat patients symptomatically without causing harm.

DISPOSITION

Patients suffering adverse reactions to ketamine, such as an iatrogenically poisoned patient, can be monitored in the ED until signs and symptoms have normalized. Management by supportive care is typically all that is required. PCP-intoxicated patients demonstrating hyperthermia, rhabdomyolysis, or severe agitation require admission to a monitored or intensive care setting. Adolescents brought in for recreational exposure to PCP or ketamine toxicity should medically managed as mentioned, and then discharged with adequate follow-up to involve drug counseling.

CASE OUTCOME

The patient became violent and paranoid while in the ED. The security guards noted that he seemed to have superhuman strength and did not seem to feel any pain when being restrained. The patient was sedated with 2 mg lorazepam IV and became less fearful and paranoid. He seemed catatonic and stopped speaking, eventually falling asleep. When he awoke, he did not understand why he felt so suspicious and could not understand his reaction to the marijuana. His urine toxicology test was positive for PCP. The patient admitted that he did not know the friend who gave him the joint and was not surprised to hear that it was laced with PCP. After the psychiatry consult was obtained and arrangements were made for drug counseling the patient was subsequently discharged to the care of his parents.

SUGGESTED READINGS

Akunne HC, Reid AA, Thurkauf A, et al: [3H]1-[2-(2-thienyl)-cyclohexyl)]piperidine labeled two high-affinity binding sites in human cortex: Further evidence for phencyclidine binding sites associated with the biogenic amine reuptake complex. *Synapse* 8:289–300, 1991.

Aronow R, Miceli JN, Done AK: Clinical observations during phencyclidine intoxication and treatment based on ion-trapping. *NIDA Res Monogr* 21:218–228, 1978.

Bailey DN: Phencyclidine detection during toxicology testing of a university medical center patient population. *J Toxicol Clin Toxicol* 25:517–526, 1987.

Chen G, Ensor CR, Russell D, et al: The pharmacology of (1-(1-phenylcyclohexyl)_piperidine hydrochloride. *J Pharmacol Exp Ther* 127:241–250, 1959.

Done AK, Aronow R, Miceli JN: The pharmacokinetics of phencyclidine in overdosage and its treatment. *NIDA Res Monogr* 21:210–217;1978.

Fram DH, Stone N: Clinical observations in the treatment of adolescent and young adult PCP users. *NIDA Res Monogr* 64:252–265, 1986.

Gaillard Y, Pepin G: Evidence of polydrug use using hair analysis: A fatal case involving heroin, cocaine, cannabis, chloroform, thiopental and ketamine. *J Forensic Sci* 43:435–438, 1998.

Hartness C, Buchan J, Bayer M: Phencyclidine. *Top Emerg Med* 7:33–38, 1985.

Howard J, Kropenske V, Tyler R: The longterm effects on neurodevelopment in infants exposed prenatally to PCP. Phencyclidine: An update. *NIDA Res Monogr* 64:237–251, 1986.

Kochhar MM: The identification of ketamine and its metabolites in biologic fluids by gas-chromatography-mass spectrometry. *Clin Toxicol* 11:265–275, 1977.

Kotz A, Merkel P: *J Prakt Chem* 113: 49, 1926.

Litovitz TL, Klein-Schwartz W, White S, et al. 1997 annual report of the American Association of Poison Control Centers. *Am J Emerg Med* 16:443–497, 1998.

Litovitz TL, Klein-Schwartz W, White S, et al. 1998 annual report of the American Association of Poison Control Centers. *Am J Emerg Med* 17:435–487, 1999.

Litovitz TL, Klein-Schwartz W, White S, et al: 1999 annual report of the American Association of Poison Control Centers. *Am J Emerg Med* 18:517–574, 2000.

Litovitz TL, Klein-Schwartz W, White S, et al: 2000 annual report of the American Association of Poison Control Centers. *Am J Emerg Med* 19:337–395, 2001.

Litovitz TL, Klein-Schwartz W, White S, et al: 2001 annual report of the American Association of Poison Control Centers. *Am J Emerg Med* 20:391–452, 2002.

Lundberg GD, Gupta RC, Montgomery SH: Phencyclidine: Patterns seen in street drug analysis. *Clin Toxicol* 9:503–510, 1976.

McCarron MM, Schulze BW, Thompson GA, et al: Acute phencyclidine intoxication: Incidence of clinical findings in 1000 cases. *Ann Emerg Med* 10:237–242, 1981.

Misra AL, Pontani RB, Bartolomeo J: Persistence of phencyclidine and metabolites in brain and adipose tissue and implications for long-lasting behavioral effects. *Res Commun Chem Pathol Pharmacol* 24:431–435, 1979.

Olmedo R: Phencyclidine and ketamine. In: Goldfrank LR, Flomenbaum NE, Lewin NA, et al, eds: *Goldfrank's Toxicological Emergencies.* 7th ed. New York: McGraw-Hill; 2002:1034–1041.

Olney JW, Newcomer JW, Farber NB: NMDA receptor hypofunction model of schizophrenia. *J Psych Res* 33:523–533, 1999.

Rainey JM, Crowder MK: Prevalence of phencyclidine in street drug preparations. *N Engl J Med* 290:466–467, 1974.

Simpson GM, Khajawall AM, Alatorre E, et al: Urinary phencyclidine excretion in chronic abusers. *J Toxicol Clin Toxicol* 19:1051–1059, 1982.

Wright RO, Woolf AD: Phencyclidine. In: *Clinical Management of Poisoning and Drug Overdose.* 3rd ed. Philadelphia: Saunders; 1998:552–559.

Wolfe SA, De Souza EB: Sigma and phencyclidine receptors in the brain-endocrine-immune axis. *NIDA Res Monogr* 133: 95–123, 1991.

63

Tobacco

Carl R. Baum

HIGH-YIELD FACTS

- Smokers create a hazard for children in their care. Environmental tobacco smoke is implicated in numerous childhood diseases, including sudden infant death syndrome (SIDS). It is a known human carcinogen.

- Cigarette smoking is highly addictive: a puff on a cigarette leads to peak nicotine levels within 10 seconds, and dependence is common after as few as 100 cigarettes.

- Despite efforts to curb smoking among children, 12- to 17-year-olds smoke more than 900 million packs per year. Approximately one third of the more than 700,000 children who became regular smokers in 2003 will die prematurely from their disease.

- Tobacco smoking is the leading preventable cause of morbidity and mortality in the United States.

- According to the World Health Organization, there are 1 billion smokers worldwide; each day, there are more than 10,000 tobacco-related deaths, representing 4% of all deaths.

CASE PRESENTATION

A 6-year-old boy presents to the pediatric emergency department of an urban teaching hospital with a chief complaint of difficulty breathing. His work of breathing at home has worsened overnight despite the use of nebulized albuterol treatments every 2 hours. He has a history of asthma, for which he has been admitted to the hospital 39 times. The attending physician orders a nebulized albuterol/ipratropium treatment as well as a loading dose of oral corticosteroids. He notices the distinct odor of cigarette smoke in the room and asks whether there are any smokers in the home. "Yes," replies the mother defensively, "but I only smoke outside."

INTRODUCTION AND EPIDEMIOLOGY

Tobacco is a drug of abuse. It shares many features with other drugs of abuse: addiction, disease and premature death, and enormous costs to society. In the early 1990s, the U.S. Food and Drug Administration (FDA) explored the possibility of regulating tobacco, the consumer product that was—and remains today—the leading preventable cause of death in this country (Figure 63–1). The FDA commissioner at the time, pediatrician David Kessler, proposed a paradigm shift—smoking should be considered a pediatric disease rather than a mere adult problem: "For while the epidemic of disease and death from smoking is played out in adulthood, it begins in childhood." Contrary to Big Tobacco's claims that the decision to smoke is freely made, Kessler maintained that "addiction is freedom denied." The FDA had no doubts about the dangers of cigarettes, but the question at the time was strategic: should the FDA attempt to regulate tobacco and nicotine as drugs, and cigarettes as drug delivery devices?

The FDA faced the reality that manufacturers of tobacco directed highly effective advertising at children. For example, one study of product logo recognition demonstrated that cigarette advertising made a significant impression on young children. Thirty percent of 3-year-old children recognized the Joe Camel cartoon

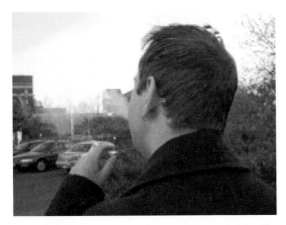

Fig. 63–1. Tobacco is the leading preventable cause of death in the United States.

character, used to promote Camel cigarettes, and matched the character with a picture of a cigarette. Recognition rates in this study rose with age: 91.3% of the 6-year-olds made the correct match. Another study compared recognition of Joe Camel in two groups: high school students (grades 9 through 12) versus adults (21 years of age and older). The ability of the students to correctly identify the Camel product was significantly better than that of the adults (93.6% versus 57.7%; P <.0001). These findings are consistent with tobacco industry documents that such advertising is meant to encourage addiction in children. Another study of 534 adolescents (ages 11 to 18 years) revealed that the most commonly smoked cigarette brands in this age group—Marlboro and Camel—also provided the most popular advertisements.

Ironically, tobacco warning labels modeled after the successful Joe Camel campaign and introduced years later demonstrated that children and adolescents found warnings bearing a cartoon animal character more believable than plain text warnings.

In 1996, the FDA asserted jurisdiction over tobacco in an attempt to eliminate sales to minors. The assertion was challenged, culminating in a Supreme Court ruling 4 years later that the FDA would require congressional approval for such jurisdiction. To date, the FDA has no authority to regulate nicotine, tobacco, or tobacco-delivery devices.

Children may find other ways to self-administer tobacco: in 2001, 22% of male high school students and 8.5% of female students used cigars. The hazards of tobacco, however, are not isolated to the cigarette or cigar smoker. In 1986, following the release of a government report that smokeless tobacco was not a safe substitute

for cigarettes and in fact caused cancer, Congress passed a law that required the surgeon general's warning to appear on all smokeless products. In 2001, however, almost 15% of male high school students still used smokeless tobacco. In 2003, after years of fighting FDA regulation, Philip Morris USA testified before Congress in support of increased agency oversight while announcing plans to market two new reduced-risk products: a less-harmful cigarette, and a cigarette-like device that electrically heats tobacco. Critics charged that the tobacco company was seeking a stamp of approval for newer products. The Cancer Prevention Study II provided an opportunity to investigate the effect of smoking *intensity* (cigarettes/day) versus *duration* on lung cancer. An analysis of a subset of adults, aged 40 to 79 years, who smoked no more than 40 cigarettes per day reveals that years of smoking is of much greater significance in predicting lung cancer risk than the number of cigarettes smoked per day. This study has critical implications for individuals who initiate smoking in childhood, and may therefore have many decades of exposure ahead.

Tobacco is a growing concern worldwide. The World Health Organization estimated in 2003 that cigarette smoking is annually responsible for 5 million deaths, a figure that may increase to 10 million by 2020. The World Health Assembly meeting in Geneva adopted the first-ever global health treaty, known as the Framework Convention on Tobacco Control, intended to decrease smoking and associated deaths.

Exposure to tobacco is not always intentional. Evidence has been mounting that environmental tobacco smoke (ETS) represents a hazard for individuals who live and work in the vicinity of smokers. In an evidence-based position statement, the American College of Occupational and Environmental Medicine summarized convincing epidemiologic evidence that implicated ETS as a cause of lung cancer and respiratory disease, adding to the burden from smokers themselves.

DEVELOPMENTAL CONSIDERATIONS

Numerous effects of smoking during pregnancy arise in the newborn period. The incidence of low-birth-weight (LBW) infants as reported on birth certificates, for example, is double the rate compared to infants whose mothers did not smoke. Even light smoking (fewer than 5 cigarettes daily) is associated with LBW. Smokeless tobacco is not a safe alternative to smoking, and women who use snuff during pregnancy, for example, are at increased risk for preeclampsia and preterm delivery.

Infants born to women who smoked during pregnancy have a fivefold risk of death from SIDS. Rodent studies conducted at Arizona State University have revealed a possible explanation: in utero exposure to nicotine leads to an increased number of the GABA receptors in the brainstem. Oversensitivity to GABA ensues, and neural activity in respiratory circuits diminishes. Smoking during pregnancy may have long-term impact: first-void urine samples obtained from neonates born to mothers who smoked during pregnancy reveal the presence of the nitrosamine tobacco metabolite NNAL, a potent rat lung carcinogen derived from 4-(methylnitrosamino)-1-(3-pyridyl)-1-butanone (NNK). A pilot study conducted in two pediatric EDs revealed detectable levels of NNAL in children 0 to 36 months of age who were exposed to smokers at home.

Older children may be exposed to ETS at home and in the workplace. The International Labor Office estimates there are 250 million child laborers worldwide. It is often in these workplace settings that children are exposed to smokers, and therefore vulnerable to early initiation of smoking.

PHARMACOLOGY AND TOXICOKINETICS

Nicotine is a highly toxic, rapidly acting, addictive drug. It occurs naturally in the leaves of *Nicotiana tabacum* and *N. rusticum* in concentrations of 2% to 8%; the tobacco industry processes nicotine from the dried leaves, and routinely manipulates the concentration of nicotine in tobacco products. Dermal absorption occurs and may cause significant toxicity. Absorption from mucous membranes or the lungs is particularly rapid, and a puff on a cigarette leads to peak nicotine concentrations within 10 seconds; a single smoked cigarette elevates blood nicotine concentration as high as 0.05 mg/L. Only 100 cigarettes may produce dependence in a smoker. Nicotine, however, is not a carcinogen.

PATHOPHYSIOLOGY

Nicotine addiction creates the link between smoking and lung cancer. The individual who smokes—or inhales ETS—is exposed to the carcinogens NNK and polycyclic aromatic hydrocarbons. Human metabolism activates these carcinogens, which—unless detoxified—create DNA adducts and induce mutations in critical genes. Although DNA repair capacity exists in humans to return altered DNA to its normal state, prolonged exposures

presumably have the ability to overcome these processes in some individuals.

As a result of synergy between cigarette smoke and radon gas, smokers who are exposed to radon have at least 15 times the risk of developing lung cancer compared to nonsmokers. The U.S. EPA publishes a radon risk comparison chart that describes exposure to various radon levels to lifetime risk of lung cancer. A number of measures may be undertaken to reduce the entry of radon gas from soil and rock into buildings, or to expedite its exhaust. Although exposure to radon should be minimized, the EPA's present action level of 4 picoCuries (pCi)/L represents a balance between the very real risk of exposure and the practical limits of mitigation technology to reduce gas concentration.

CLINICAL FINDINGS

Although smokers tolerant to the drug enjoy its calming effects, symptoms of acute overdose may include nausea, vomiting, fasciculations, tachycardia, and seizures.

LABORATORY AND DIAGNOSTIC TESTING

A nicotine metabolite, cotinine, is often measured in studies of ETS exposure. When quantitated in the serum or urine of smokers or ETS-exposed individuals, cotinine serves as a proxy for exposure to nicotine but has no toxicity itself. Bioassays of tobacco-derived carcinogens are more clinically relevant, although the extremely short half-life of the nitrosamine NNK is not conducive to accurate measurement. Measurements of NNK metabolites NNAL and NNAL-glucuronide require specialized equipment and are therefore limited to research studies.

MANAGEMENT

Although the toxicity of tobacco is primarily chronic, young children occasionally ingest discarded cigarette butts, or entire cigarettes that contain residual amounts of nicotine. Symptoms and signs of acute toxicity, including nausea, vomiting, fasciculations, and seizures, can occur within 60 to 90 minutes. Poison control centers usually follow the "three-butt" rule: a toddler who ingests at least three cigarette butts or one fresh cigarette is referred to a health care facility for gastrointestinal decontamination with activated charcoal, monitoring, and appropriate supportive care. Hypotension is treated with fluid administration. If vomiting is intractable, antiemetics such as prochloraperazine or ondansetron can be administered. Sinus tachycardia and hypertension are transient, and usually do not require treatment. Seizure activity is generally responsive to benzodiazepine therapy. Atropine can be used to control excessive bronchial secretions from parasympathetic stimulation.

The management of tobacco addiction is challenging. Many who use tobacco are unwilling to quit their habit, although educational efforts about the dangers of tobacco and ETS may convince them otherwise. Even individuals who want to quit smoking may have difficulty.

DISPOSITION

Children ingesting less than one cigarette usually do not require treatment, and can be observed at home. Children ingesting larger quantities should be evaluated at a health care facility. Symptoms generally develop within 1 to 2 hours, and resolve within 12 to 24 hours. Children with seizures or cardiovascular instability require admission.

Chronic smokers should be referred to their primary care provider for assistance with smoking cessation. Programs exist that use various combinations of behavioral and pharmacologic (nicotine transdermal patches, bupropion) interventions to help smokers quit. Most states have established tobacco prevention programs, and many receive financial support from the 1998 multistate settlement, known as the Master Settlement Agreement, of lawsuits that 46 state attorneys general had brought against major tobacco companies. Total payments were projected to be $246 billion over the first 25 years. Although statewide tobacco prevention programs have been proven to reduce tobacco use significantly, the fifth anniversary report of the agreement revealed that most states fail to adequately fund the programs, and many governors divert settlement funds for other uses.

CASE OUTCOME

The attending physician discusses with the patient's mother the dangers of secondhand smoke. He describes its role in asthma, respiratory infections (upper and lower), and SIDS, adding that the EPA classifies secondhand smoke as a known human carcinogen. The mother would like to quit smoking, but her attempts in the past were associated with significant weight gain and ultimately failed. The physician refers her to her primary care provider for information about smoking cessation strategies, and provides her with the state's toll-free telephone "Quit Line."

SUGGESTED READINGS

American College of Occupational and Environmental Medicine: *Evidence based statements: epidemiological basis for an occupational and environmental policy on environmental tobacco smoke.* Available at http://www.acoem.org/guidelines/article.asp?ID=8. Accessed April 29, 2003.

American Academy of Pediatrics, Committee on Environmental Health: Environmental tobacco smoke: A hazard to children. *Pediatrics* 99:639–642, 1997.

American Academy of Pediatrics, Committee on Substance Abuse: Tobacco's toll: implications for the pediatrician. *Pediatrics* 107:794–798, 2001.

Arnett JJ, Terhanian G: Adolescents' responses to cigarette advertisements: Links between exposure, liking, and the appeal of smoking. *Tob Control* 7:129–133, 1998.

Baum CR, Listman DA, Hsiao AL, et al: Detection of a tobacco-specific carcinogen in the urine of children exposed to environmental tobacco smoke. *J Toxicol Clin Toxicol* 41:733, 2003.

Budavari S, ed: *The Merck Index.* 11th ed. Rahway, NJ: Merck & Co; 1989.

Campaign for Tobacco-Free Kids. Available from: http://www.tobaccofreekids.org. Accessed November 19, 2003.

DiFranza JR, Richards JW, Paulman PM, et al: RJR Nabisco's cartoon camel promotes Camel cigarettes to children. *JAMA* 266:3149–3153, 1991.

Duffy SA, Burton D: Cartoon characters as tobacco warning labels. *Arch Pediatr Adolesc Med* 154:1230–1236, 2000.

England LJ, Levine RJ, Mills JL, et al: Adverse pregnancy outcomes in snuff users. *Am J Obstet Gynecol* 189:939–943, 2003.

Fischer PM, Schwartz MP, Richards JW Jr, et al: Brand logo recognition by children aged 3 to 6 years. Mickey Mouse and Old Joe the Camel. *JAMA* 266:3185–186, 1991.

Flanders WD, Lally CA, Zhu BP, et al: Lung cancer mortality in relation to age, duration of smoking, and daily cigarette consumption: Results from Cancer Prevention Study II. *Cancer Res* 63:6556–6562, 2003.

Hecht SS: Tobacco smoke carcinogens and lung cancer. *J Natl Cancer Inst* 91:1194–1210, 1999.

Kessler D: *A Question of Intent: A Great American Battle With a Deadly Industry.* New York: Public Affairs; 2001.

Langely A: World health meeting approves treaty to discourage smoking. *The New York Times* May 22, 2003:A11.

Leikin JB, Paloucek FP, eds: *Poisoning & Toxicology Handbook.* 3rd ed. Hudson, OH: Lexi-Comp; 2002.

Matyunas N, Rodgers GC: Nicotine poisoning. In: Ford M, Delaney K, Ling L, et al, eds: *Clinical Toxicology.* Philadelphia: Saunders; 2001:985–989.

Paulos JA: *Innumeracy: Mathematical Illiteracy and its Consequences.* New York: Hill and Wang; 2001.

Prenatal nicotine: a role in SIDS? *Sci News* 163:270, 2003.

Tomar SL: Trends and patterns of tobacco use in the United States. *Am J Med Sci* 326:248–254, 2003.

U.S. Environmental Protection Agency: Radon risk comparison charts. Available from http://www.epa.gov/iaq/radon/riskcht.html. Accessed October 29, 2003.

Ventura SJ, Hamilton BE, Mathews TJ, et al: Trends and variations in smoking during pregnancy and low birth weight: Evidence from the birth certificate, 1990–2000. *Pediatrics* 111:1176–1180, 2003.

Wei Q, Cheng L, Amos CI, et al: Repair of tobacco carcinogen-induced DNA adducts and lung cancer risk: A molecular epidemiologic study. *J Natl Cancer Inst* 92:1764–1772, 2000.

Woolf AD: Health hazards for children at work. AAPCC/WHO Symposium. *J Toxicol Clin Toxicol* 40:477–482, 2002.

64

Withdrawal Syndromes

Rotem Freide
Timothy B. Erickson

HIGH-YIELD FACTS

- Neonatal abstinence syndrome (NAS) usually results from maternal drug abuse. It is characterized by central nervous system (CNS) hyperirritability, gastrointestinal (GI) dysfunction, respiratory distress, and autonomic dysfunction.

- Ethanol withdrawal syndrome in adolescents can be life-threatening if not properly recognized and treated.

- Acute withdrawal from benzodiazepines can present with agitation, tremors, delirium, and seizures.

- Patients with cocaine withdrawal can present with fatigue, insomnia, anxiety, depression, and drug-craving behavior.

- Owing to its increased use over the past years many cases of γ-hydroxybutyrate (GHB) withdrawal have been reported. This syndrome has been described with higher doses as well as chronic use in association with abrupt cessation.

- Nicotine and caffeine withdrawal can be a common presenting complaint in adolescents.

CASE PRESENTATION

The patient is 2-day-old male infant born prematurely at 32 weeks. In the hospital nursery, he is found to be irritable, agitated, and demonstrates poor feeding. The baby's heart rate is 180 bpm, respiratory rate is 48 breaths per minute, and temperature is 100.1°F rectally. The nightshift nurse observes the newborn to have myoclonic jerking and a brief episode of generalized tonic–clonic seizure activity that is self-limited. The mother of the infant had previously admitted to daily heroin use during her second and third trimesters of pregnancy.

NEONATAL WITHDRAWAL OR ABSTINENCE SYNDROME

NAS results from prenatal maternal drug abuse, and is most commonly described with opioids. These include heroin and methadone, but other less potent opiates and even nonopiate CNS depressants have been implicated (Table 64–1). It is characterized by CNS hyperirritability, GI dysfunction, respiratory distress, and autonomic dysfunction. The condition develops as a result of the abrupt removal of the drug after the newborn is delivered.

Developmental Considerations

Intrauterine narcotic exposure causes passive addiction, and is associated with lower birth weight and smaller head circumference. Infants with this syndrome have significantly higher rates of neurobehavioral complications. However, there is little evidence that the prenatal exposure results in cognitive defects in the affected newborns later in life.

Pharmacology and Pathophysiology

The syndrome often begins within 24 to 48 hours of birth. However, symptoms can vary depending on the drug being used by the mother, the quantity, frequency,

Table 64–1. Drugs Associated With Neonatal Abstinence Syndrome

- Opiates and narcotics
  - Codeine
  - Fentanyl
  - Heroin and methadone
  - Meperidine (Demerol)
  - Morphine
  - Pentazocine
  - Propoxyphene
- Other drugs
  - Barbiturates
  - Caffeine
  - Chlordiazepoxide
  - Cocaine
  - Diazepam and lorazepam
  - Diphenhydramine
  - Ethanol
  - Marijuana
  - Nicotine
  - Phencyclidine

and duration of intrauterine exposure, as well as the timing of the withdrawal prior to the delivery. For example, the withdrawal from methadone tends to occur later compared with heroin because of the longer half-life of methadone. The exact cause of the syndrome is unclear, but evidence suggests that noradrenergic hyperactivity may play a role.

Clinical Presentation

Neonates can experience lethargy at birth if there was recent maternal opioid use, or if large doses of an opioid agent were iatrogenically administered to the mother during labor. Additionally, the neonate is prone to withdrawal symptoms during the newborn period if the mother exhibited chronic dependency during her later prenatal stages. Withdrawal symptoms in the dependent neonate may also be iatrogenically precipitated by the administration of the pure opioid antagonist naloxone.

CNS symptoms of the withdrawal syndrome include irritability, restlessness, tremor, high-pitched cry, increased muscle tone, myoclonic jerks, exaggerated Moro reflex, and decreased duration of sleep between feedings. Respiratory distress is characterized by tachypnea, nasal flaring, nasal stuffiness, and sneezing. GI dysfunction includes vigorous but uncoordinated sucking, postfeeding regurgitation, and loose and watery stools. Autonomic symptoms include fever, sweating, and skin mottling.

Laboratory Testing

The use of serum and urinary drug screens is unreliable for assessing neonatal withdrawal because the drug may have been metabolized and excreted prior to birth. The exception to this is methadone, which has a long half-life and generally higher maternal doses. Recent studies have documented that the use of meconium testing may be a superior sampling method to detect exposure to abusable drugs in utero.

Other conditions that must be recognized and excluded in the differential diagnosis include sepsis, hypoglycemia, electrolyte abnormalities, hyperthyroidism, hypocalcemia, and intracranial hemorrhage.

The most widely accepted scale to evaluate the newborn for NAS is the modified version of a scale developed by Finnegan (see Chapter 7). This scale uses 31 items, and allows a semiquantitative measure of the degree to which the newborn is experiencing symptoms of withdrawal. This scale can also be used to assess the resolution of signs and symptoms after initiating treatment. To obtain a daily average score, measurements are performed every 4 hours until the patient is stable. If three consecutive scores are equal to or greater than 8, treatment for withdrawal is started. These infants are best cared for in a unit with experienced personnel who can recognize problems, perform constant evaluations, and institute the necessary interventions.

Management

The published incidence of neonatal withdrawal requiring pharmacotherapy ranges from 60% to 80%. Rapid diagnosis and treatment of neonatal withdrawal are imperative because of the risk of seizures and cardiovascular collapse. Many agents have been used in the past as treatment. These include tincture of opium, paregoric, diazepam, chlorpromazine, and phenobarbital. There is no consensus as to the best treatment for withdrawal in the opiate-exposed infant. Currently the most commonly used pharmacologic agents include opiates (diluted tincture of opium, paregoric), or barbiturates (phenobarbital) (see Table 7–5). An opiate is preferred by most neonatologists because it is more physiologic, and substitutes for the drug causing the withdrawal. Phenobarbital is a reasonable alternative, but it does little to ameliorate some of the specific opiate-related symptoms, such as diarrhea and poor feeding.

Disposition

Neonates with clinical evidence of neonatal withdrawal syndrome or maternal history of chronic drug abuse should be observed and given symptomatic care in a neonatal intensive care setting until the baby stabilizes. Mothers with prenatal addiction should be referred for drug counseling. The state department of children and family services should be notified for ongoing social setting evaluation.

ETHANOL

Although most commonly associated with adult chronic alcoholics, alcohol withdrawal symptoms have been described in adolescent patients who started drinking regularly at a young age. In addition to alcohol-containing beverages such as beer, wine, and hard liquors, children have access to mouthwashes that can contain up to 75% ethanol, colognes and perfumes (40% to 60% ethanol) and, over 700 ethanol-containing medicinal preparations.

Pharmacology and Pathophysiology

Ethanol undergoes hepatic metabolism via two metabolic pathways: alcohol dehydrogenase and the microsomal ethanol-oxidizing system. Alcohol dehydrogenase pathway is the major metabolic pathway and the rate-limiting step in converting ethanol to acetaldehyde. In general, nontolerant individuals metabolize ethanol at 10 to 25 mg/dL/h and alcoholics metabolize up to 30 mg/dL/h. Children may ingest large amounts of ethanol in relation to their body weight, resulting in rapid development of high blood alcohol concentrations. In children under 5 years of age, the ability to metabolize ethanol is diminished owing to immature hepatic dehydrogenase activity.

Clinical Presentation

Clinical presentation of ethanol withdrawal has been described in four distinct stages: tremulousness, seizures, hallucinations, and delirium. The range of symptoms, however, usually presents in more of a continuum. Tremors, agitation, and irritability may manifest within 6 to 8 hours from the last drink, and are common initial symptoms of acute alcohol withdrawal. Alcohol withdrawal-related hallucinations occur at 24 to 36 hours. Hallucinations are mostly visual, and appear to occur in patients with insufficient thiamine stores. Another com-

mon trait is formication, or the sensation of ants crawling on the skin. This often promotes itching and excoriation.

Alcoholic seizures may occur between 7 and 48 hours of withdrawal, and peak within 24 hours. They are usually self-limited, tonic–clonic events with a short postictal period. Status epilepticus is uncommon. One third of patient who develop delirium tremens (DTs) have alcoholic seizures as a precipitating event. Adolescents with new-onset seizures should be evaluated for possible acute withdrawal from ethanol. DTs is seen within 3 to 5 days of abstinence, but may be observed as late as 14 days.

Management

Acute alcohol withdrawal manifesting as delirium tremens has a 5% mortality if aggressive therapy is not instituted. This includes proper cooling and fluid resuscitation. Adolescents manifesting alcohol withdrawal symptoms should be admitted for thiamine and nutritional replenishment, benzodiazepine administration, supportive care, and seizure precautions. Ethanol withdrawal seizures often require large doses of benzodiazepines with diazepam or lorazepam. Anticonvulsant agents such as phenobarbital may also be necessary. Once stabilized, the patient should be referred to an adolescent alcohol detoxification program.

SEDATIVE-HYPNOTICS

Sedative-hypnotics such as benzodiazepines are frequently prescribed for anxiety, sleep, and panic disorders. Additionally, they may be used for conscious sedation, seizures, and muscle relaxation. The common effects of these drugs are sedation and disinhibition. Often times these agents are coingested with other substances such as ethanol, which act synergistically. Alcohol and cocaine withdrawal symptoms may be diminished with the use of sedative-hypnotics.

Pharmacology and Pathophysiology

Sedative-hypnotics act by binding to the γ-aminobutyric acid (GABA)$_A$ receptor. Sedative hypnotics lead to frequent opening of the GABA$_A$ receptor. Binding increases the flow of calcium ions into the cells resulting in an inhibitory effect. Consequently, withdrawal leads to disinhibition.

Withdrawal symptoms are variable and may present early or late based on the half-life of the drug. Additionally, time of onset also depends on duration of use and the extent of the patient's dependence.

Clinical Presentation

Withdrawal can present with delirium, agitation, and seizures. Patients experience anxiety, depression, irritability, insomnia, headache, tremor, nausea, anorexia, and heightened sensory perception. Symptoms are more severe with short-acting agents and in people taking large doses over long periods of time. Acute benzodiazepine withdrawal can also be precipitated iatrogenically when administrating the antidote flumazenil in chronically benzodiazepine-dependent patients.

Treatment

Patients are kept calm and well hydrated, and vital signs stabilized. Pharmacologic management is achieved with a cross-reactive benzodiazepine such as diazepam or lorazepam, which can then be tapered every 1 to 2 days. Subsequent doses may be needed for breakthrough symptoms such as tremulousness, perceptual disturbances, tachycardia, or hypertension. Data also suggest that anticonvulsants such as carbamazepine, valproic acid, and gabapentin may be used to ameliorate the symptoms of withdrawal.

γ-HYDROXYBUTYRATE

GHB was introduced as an anesthetic in the 1960s. However, its use has significantly increased in the last few years. Currently, it is being used as an anabolic agent, sexual enhancer, euphoriant, and date rape drug. It has also recently been approved for the treatment of narcolepsy, and is being studied for its use in the treatment of alcohol and opiate withdrawal.

In the 1990s, the sale of GHB was banned by the U.S. Food and Drug Administration. GHB can be obtained over the Internet and its precursors can be bought as dietary supplements. Its precursors include γ-butrylactone and 1,4 butanediol. 1,4 Butanediol is oxidized by alcohol dehydrogenase to γ-hydroxybutyraldehyde, and then by aldehyde dehyrogenase to GHB. γ-Butyrolactone is hydrolyzed by a peripheral lactonase. GHB has many street names such as Grievous Bodily Harm, Liquid Ecstasy, Liquid X, Scoop, and Salty Water.

Pharmacology and Pathophysiology

GHB has a similar structure to GABA and glutamic acid. It exhibits properties of a neuromodulator by neuroinhibition. GHB can cross the blood–brain barrier and induce sedation and anesthesia.

There have been many reports of the pharmacologic similarities of between GHB and ethanol. Ethanol increases levels of GHB and acts synergistically with GHB to produce CNS depression and respiratory depression. Owing to its rapid absorption, symptoms develop within 15 minutes. Absorption, however, is limited, and therefore increasing the dose leads to increased time to peak levels. Elimination is also saturable. Therefore, for dependence to occur, frequent, prolonged dosing is required.

Laboratory Testing

Laboratory detection of GHB is difficult. Most GHB is transformed into carbon dioxide and expired, with only about 5% eliminated in the urine. However, if urine is collected within 12 hours of last ingestion, γ-butyrolactone can be detected by reference laboratories.

Clinical Presentation

Symptoms of GHB intoxication include bradycardia, myoclonic movements, seizures, coma, and respiratory depression. Other symptoms include drowsiness, euphoria, confusion, dizziness, temporary amnesia, increased libido, headache, nausea, vomiting, and mild acute respiratory acidosis.

Owing to its increased use over the past years, many more reports of GHB withdrawal have been reported in the literature. This syndrome has been reported with higher doses as well as chronic use in association with abrupt cessation. The syndrome is characterized by early symptoms of insomnia, anxiety, and tremors. More severe symptoms of disorientation, paranoia, and auditory and visual hallucinations develop. After 2 or 3 days of abstinence, autonomic instability is manifested by tachycardia, diaphoresis, extraocular movement impairment, and hypertension. As the syndrome progresses patients become combative, confused, and disoriented. Often the syndrome is not recognized in the early phases.

GHB withdrawal syndrome can mimic withdrawal from ethanol and sedative-hypnotics. It can also mimic intoxication with sympathomimetic agents, serotonin syndrome, and neuroleptic malignant syndrome (NMS). Thyroid storm and pheochromocytoma should also be considered.

Management

Withdrawal is usually treated with supportive care and long-acting benzodiazepines in high doses. Sedation is necessary to prevent injury, hyperthermia, and rhabdomyolysis. In addition to benzodiazepines, propofol, and barbiturates, often required in high doses, have been shown to be effective. GHB is thought to act in a manner similar to ethanol, and its withdrawal syndrome has many of the same features as alcohol withdrawal; consequently it is treated in a similar manner.

COCAINE

Cocaine is widely abused by adolescents and adults as a recreational drug. Small children can also be exposed to cocaine being abused by others. Seizures may occur in the breastfed infant whose mother abuses cocaine. Toddlers may become toxic through second-hand smoke, or may inadvertently ingest the drug.

Pharmacology and Pathophysiology

Cocaine stimulates the sympathetic nervous system by preventing clearance of stimulatory neurotransmitters, and by causing direct CNS stimulation. The desire for the euphoria of cocaine and the tolerance that develops from continued use contribute to cocaine dependence. Cocaine withdrawal develops within a few hours to a few days after stopping or reducing cocaine use that has been heavy and prolonged.

Clinical Presentation

Patients present in one of three phases. The syndrome is characterized by dysphoria and two or more physiologic changes including fatigue, vivid and unpleasant dreams, insomnia or hypersomnia, increased appetite, and psychomotor agitation or retardation. Anhedonia and craving for cocaine can be a part of the withdrawal syndrome. Depression and suicidal ideation are the most serious complications. Patients may present in the initial crash phase, where the patient experiences fatigue, insomnia, alteration of mood, and depression. Patients may also experience symptoms that persist for a longer period of time, including dysphoria, anxiety, impotence, and craving. These symptoms are followed by a longer extinction phase, but they may recur and be associated with intense feelings of craving for cocaine.

Management

Treatment for cocaine withdrawal is mainly supportive. However, these patients should be evaluated for the complications of long-term cocaine use, including intracranial hemorrhage; cerebrovascular ischemia; cardiovascular ischemia; and GI complications and rhabdomyolysis. Long-term treatment requires counseling and management by a drug treatment center. There is a high rate of relapse in adolescents who have cocaine addiction.

NICOTINE

Tobacco smokers create a hazard for children in their care. Environmental nicotine smoke is implicated in numerous childhood diseases, including sudden infant death syndrome, and is a known human carcinogen. Tobacco is a drug of abuse. It shares many features with other drugs of abuse: addiction, disease and premature death, and enormous costs to society. Cigarette smoking is highly addictive: a puff on a cigarette leads to peak nicotine levels within 10 seconds, and dependence is common after as few as 100 cigarettes. Tobacco smoking is the leading preventable cause of morbidity and mortality in the United States. Besides cigarettes, children can have nicotine exposure from cigars, smokeless tobacco, and second-hand smoke.

Pharmacology and Pathophysiology

The potential of nicotine withdrawal to cause discomfort is well recognized. This may be secondary to the ability of nicotine to stimulate specific nicotinic receptors leading to dopamine release. However, this is likely not the only mechanism accounting for the affects of nicotine withdrawal.

Clinical Presentation

Patients present with anxiety, craving, tremor, depressed mood, weight gain, and bradycardia. Because there are only mild physiologic symptoms, morbidity is quite low.

Withdrawal symptoms begin after approximately 6 to 12 hours of cessation and peak in 1 to 3 days. Symptoms may last as long as 4 weeks. Onset and symptoms do not appear to be associated with amount and duration of smoking.

Management

The management of tobacco addiction is challenging. Many who use tobacco are unwilling to quit their habit, although educational efforts about the dangers of tobacco convince them otherwise. Even adolescents who want to quit smoking often have difficulty.

Symptoms may be somewhat alleviated with nicotine patches, chewing gums, and nasal sprays; these agents do appear to help patients quit. Buproprion has also been shown to be effective in smoking cessation in a dose-dependent manner. However, it is not completely effective; there is a high rate of failure.

CAFFEINE

Caffeine is widely consumed throughout the world, and is probably the most frequently ingested pharmacologically active substance. It is commonly found in beverages, chocolates, diet aids, energy drinks, and prescription and over-the-counter medications. Children are often unaware they are even consuming caffeine when drinking certain brands of carbonated soda.

Pharmacology and Pathophysiology

Caffeine withdrawal occurs 12 to 24 hours after the last dose of caffeine and resolves within 2 to 4 days. It is not life threatening.

Clinical Presentation

Patients with caffeine withdrawal usually present with headaches, sleeplessness, drowsiness, impaired concentration, school or work difficulty, and flu-like symptoms. Withdrawal headaches with nausea and vomiting can occur in moderate or sporadic users of caffeine products. Other withdrawal symptoms include nausea, yawning, drowsiness or lethargy, rhinorrhea, irritability, nervousness, and poor attention in school. Patients generally present with a depressed mood and affect. This depressive presentation is seen in heavy users of caffeine products (>750 mg/d).

Management

Treatment consists of reassurance that the symptoms will subside within 2 to 4 days. Acetaminophen or non-steroidal anti-inflammatory agents can be used treat headache. Low-dose caffeine pills or beverages also ameliorate symptoms. The patient should be encouraged to either abstain or moderate their daily caffeine intake with a gradual reduction over a few day period.

CASE OUTCOME

The 2-day-old neonate responds well to paregoric and phenobarbital in the NICU. His baseline labs are normal,

sepsis is ruled out, and toxicology screen is positive for opioids and methadone. The mother admitted to snorting heroin during her active labor period to dull the pain of contractions.

The infant is observed for 7 days and given supplemental doses of paregoric and phenobarbital. He tolerates formula feedings and begins to gain weight. The mother is given psychosocial referral for opioid detoxification and follow-up for her chronic addiction. The child is placed in foster care until the mother can document abstinence from her opioid habit. The child recovers apart from being consistently measured at the lower 10% on the pediatric growth chart for the first year of life.

SUGGESTED READINGS

American Academy of Pediatrics, Committee on Substance Abuse: Tobacco's toll: Implications for the pediatrician. *Pediatrics* 107:794–798, 2001.

Bell GL, Lau K: Perinatal and prenatal issues in substance abuse. *Pediatr Clin North Am* 42:261, 1995.

Cheesebrow D: Caffeine. In: Harris CR, ed: *Emergency Management of Selected Drugs of Abuse*. Dallas: ACEP; 2000.

Chiang C, Wax P: Withdrawal syndromes. In: Ford M, Delaney K, Ling L, et al, eds: *Clinical Toxicology*. Philadelphia: Saunders; 2001:582–590.

Erwin WE, Williams DB, Speir WA: Delirium tremens. *South Med J* 91:425–432, 1998.

Farrell M: Opiate withdrawal. *Addiction* 89:1471–1475, 1994.

Field AS, Laurienti PJ, Yen YF, et al: Dietary caffeine consumption and withdrawal: Confounding variables in quantitive cerebral perfusion studies? *Radiology* 227:129–135, 2003.

Ford RPK, Schluter PJ, Mitchell EA, et al: Heavy caffeine intake in pregnancy and sudden infant death syndrome. *Arch Dis Child* 78:9–13, 1998.

Hughs JR, Higgins ST, Bickel WK: Nicotine withdrawal versus other drug withdrawal syndromes: Similarities and dissimilarities. *Addiction* 89:1461, 1994.

Hurt RD, Sachs DP, Glover ED, et al: Comparison of sustained release bupropion and placebo for smoking cessation. *N Engl J Med* 337:1195, 1997.

Greenberg OA: Ethanol and sedatives. *Neurol Clin* 11:523–534, 1993.

Little PJ, Price RR, Hinton RK, et al: Role of noradrenergic hyperactivity in neonate opiate abstinence. *Drug Alcohol Dependence* 4:47, 1996.

Mendelson JH, Mello NK: Management of cocaine abuse and dependence. *N Engl J Med* 334:965, 1996.

Miller NS, Gold MS: Management of withdrawal syndromes and relapse prevention in drug and alcohol dependence. *Am Fam Physician* 58:139–146, 1998.

Nawrot P, Jordan S, Eastwood J, et al: Effects of caffeine on human health. *Food Addit Contam* 20:1–30, 2003.

Roy-Byne PP, Sullivan MD, Cowley DS, et al: Adjunctive treatment of benzodiazepine discontinuation syndrome: A review. *J Psychiatric Res* 27(suppl 1):143–153, 1993.

Strain EC, Griffiths RR: Caffeine dependence: Fact or fiction? *J R Soc Med* 88:427, 1995.

Theis JG, Selby P, Ikizler Y, Koren G: Current management of the neonatal abstinence syndrome: A critical analysis of the evidence. *Biol Neonate* 74:345, 1997.

Tomar SL: Trends and patterns of tobacco use in the United States. *Am J Med Sci* 326:248–254, 2003.

65

Metals

Carl R. Baum

HIGH-YIELD FACTS

- Heavy metals are durable and reactive, and tend to persist both in the environment and in humans.

- Assessment of heavy metal toxicity must consider the developmental stage of the child at risk.

- The lay public often blames heavy metals for chronic medical disorders such as childhood autism.

- Inaccuracies can occur in the collection and interpretation of laboratory tests for heavy metals.

Prized for their utility, strength, electrical conductivity, magnetism, plasticity, and esthetics, metals are known especially for their durability. In the earth's crust, metals occur naturally in the form of relatively stable ores such as cinnabar (mercuric sulfide), galena (lead sulfide), pyrite (iron sulfide), and hematite and magnetite (iron oxides). The affinity of some metals for sulfide groups relates directly to their toxicity in the human context. For example, the divalent cation of mercury binds to, and disrupts the function of, sulfhydryl protein groups. Heavy metals, which humans are unable to metabolize, cause pathology because they combine with reactive groups on which normal physiology depends. Heavy metals induce hepatic production of the metallothioneins, a family of low-molecular-weight proteins that both regulate the transport of essential metals and mitigate the effects of toxic ones.

The familiar periodic table, which dates back to the nineteenth century, provides a framework in which to understand heavy metals (Figure 65–1). The table arranges more than 100 elements in rows and columns according to properties such as atomic weight and the number of bonds that may be formed by *neutral atoms*. Some scientists believe that the periodic table should be redesigned to include *charged ions*, which better reflects the actual occurrence and behavior of all matter, including heavy metals. According to this concept, an element may appear in multiple positions on the table if there are various forms that exhibit different properties. Mercury, for example, appears on the table as the elemental form Hg^0, as intermediate cations Hg^+ and Hg^{2+}, and as a soft cation that binds to carbon. Thus, mercury may exist as liquid metal, as inorganic mercurous and mercuric salts, and as organic compounds, such as ethyl- and methylmercury.

Mercury and lead are two examples of durable heavy metals that are widely dispersed in the environment from a variety of sources. Prevailing winds may carry mercury originating in a Midwestern United States power plant to a lake near the east coast over a thousand miles away. Lead-containing paint scraped from a house settles into the surrounding soil, later exposing a toddler playing in the yard. Heavy metals are also biologically persistent. As an example, although humans are capable of excreting lead from the central blood compartment, the elimination half-life from bony stores is on the order of a decade.

DEVELOPMENTAL CONSIDERATIONS

Assessment of the toxicity of a metal must take into account not only its physical and chemical properties but also the age-specific behavior of the child who may en-

1 **H** 1.008																	2 **He** 4.003
3 **Li** 6.941	4 **Be** 9.012											5 **B** 10.81	6 **C** 12.011	7 **N** 14.007	8 **O** 15.999	9 **F** 18.998	10 **Ne** 20.179
11 **Na** 22.99	12 **Mg** 24.305											13 **Al** 26.981	14 **Si** 28.086	15 **P** 30.974	16 **S** 32.06	17 **Cl** 35.453	18 **Ar** 39.948
19 **K** 39.098	20 **Ca** 40.08	21 **Sc** 44.956	22 **Ti** 47.88	23 **V** 50.942	24 **Cr** 51.996	25 **Mn** 54.938	26 **Fe** 55.847	27 **Co** 58.933	28 **Ni** 59.69	29 **Cu** 63.546	30 **Zn** 65.38	31 **Ga** 69.72	32 **Ge** 72.59	33 **As** 74.922	34 **Se** 78.96	35 **Br** 79.904	36 **Kr** 83.80
37 **Rb** 85.468	38 **Sr** 87.62	39 **Y** 173.04	40 **Zr** 91.22	41 **Nb** 92.91	42 **Mo** 95.94	43 **Tc** 98	44 **Ru** 101.07	45 **Rh** 102.91	46 **Pd** 106.42	47 **Ag** 107.87	48 **Cd** 112.41	49 **In** 114.82	50 **Sn** 118.69	51 **Sb** 121.75	52 **Te** 127.60	53 **I** 126.90	54 **Xe** 131.29
55 **Ca** 132.91	56 **Ba** 137.33	* 57–71	72 **Hf** 178.49	73 **Ta** 180.95	74 **W** 183.85	75 **Re** 186.21	76 **Os** 190.2	77 **Ir** 192.22	78 **Pt** 195.08	79 **Au** 196.97	80 **Hg** 200.59	81 **Tl** 204.38	82 **Pb** 207.2	83 **Bi** 208.98	84 **Po** 209	85 **At** 210	86 **Rn** 222
87 **Fr** 223	88 **Ra** 226.03	† 89–103	104 **Unq** 261	105 **Unp** 262	106 **Unh** 263												

	57 **La** 138.91	58 **Ce** 140.12	59 **Pr** 140.91	60 **Nd** 144.24	61 **Pm** 145	62 **Sm** 150.36	63 **Eu** 151.96	64 **Gd** 157.25	65 **Tb** 158.93	66 **Dy** 162.50	67 **Ho** 164.93	68 **Er** 167.26	69 **Tm** 168.93	70 **Yb** 173.04	71 **Lu** 174.97
*															
†	89 **Ac** 227.03	90 **Th** 232.04	91 **Pa** 231.04	92 **U** 238.03	93 **Np** 237.05	94 **Pu** 244	95 **Am** 243	96 **Cm** 247	97 **Bk** 247	98 **Cf** 251	99 **Es** 252	100 **Fm** 257	101 **Md** 258	102 **No** 259	103 **Lr** 260

Fig. 65–1. Periodic table of the elements.

counter it. For example, the crawling infant with hand-to-mouth activity may encounter lead dust on the floor of an older home, whereas the curious toddler with a well-developed pincer grasp may discover an improperly secured container of prenatal iron prescribed for her pregnant mother. A history of recent seafood consumption or daily well water exposure in any age child may explain the finding of organic arsenic on laboratory testing. As clarified in Chapter 66, organic arsenic compounds are potentially much less harmful than are the inorganic forms.

MOST COMMON TOXINS

Subsequent chapters review the toxicology of four heavy metals that most commonly present risk to children: arsenic, iron, lead, and mercury. Table 65–1 summarizes additional information regarding other heavy metals that children are less likely to encounter, including cadmium, copper, nickel, thallium, and zinc.

There is a tendency for the lay public to blame heavy metals for a variety of ills without understanding the specific nature of their toxic effects. Many parents turn to the Internet to conduct a search targeted at heavy metal poisoning. Thus, a parent who has claimed to have done the research often lacks the scientific sophistication to synthesize the information appropriately. Furthermore, there is a natural tendency to ascribe causality to situations or forces that are temporally associated with the effect. For example, parents of children diagnosed with autism may observe a temporal association between the emergence of this disorder and the administration of childhood preventive vaccines. Desperate to find a cure for this debilitating condition, parents may conclude that vaccine preservatives, such as the mercury-containing thimerosal, or other environmental contaminants are responsible, and seek advice from health care professionals who claim to have expertise in the diagnosis and treatment of heavy metal poisoning (Table 65–2). A number of errors or inaccuracies can be made in the collection or interpretation of biological samples such as blood, hair, or urine screens for heavy metals. These tests are performed to justify or monitor chronic chelation therapy that is intended to reduce an individual's body burden. Common pitfalls are summa-

Table 65–1. Toxicity of the Heavy Metals Cadmium, Copper, Nickel, Thallium, and Zinc

Metal	Occurrence	Toxic Mechanism	Clinical Effects
Cadmium (Cd)	Rechargeable batteries, cigarette smoke, button batteries, metalworks, jewelry	Irritant and systemic effects Renally concentrated	Gastroenteritis Pneumonitis (inhalation) Renal tubular dysfunction Osteomalacia Pulmonary carcinogen
Copper (Cu)	Batteries, coins, electrical wires, pipes, fungicides, wood preservatives, chemistry sets	Generates oxidative stress and inhibits key metabolic enzymes Participates in redox reactions leading to mitochondrial and membrane dysfunction	Acute gastroenteritis Acute renal failure Hepatotoxicity Hemolysis
Nickel (Ni)	Rechargeable batteries, jewelry, clothing fasteners	Direct irritant effects Cellular debris accumulates in alveolar sacs	Contact dermatitis Respiratory tract irritation Pneumonitis
Thallium (Tl)	Semiconductors, radiopharmaceuticals, pesticides (banned by EPA in 1972)	Handled intracellularly (like potassium) Inhibits oxidative phosphorylation Altered protein and heme synthesis	Severe gastroenteritis Sensorimotor neuritis Motor weakness Cardiotoxicity Alopecia Mees' lines
Zinc (Zn)	Coins, vitamins, construction nails, welding, soldering flux, rodenticides	Oxidant stress or inactivation of natural antioxidant systems Direct damage to epithelial, pulmonary endothelial cells and mucosa	Caustic GI injury, renal tubular necrosis, interstitial nephritis Pneumonitis, metal fume fever (zinc oxide)

rized in Table 65–3. The timing of the test with respect to chelation therapy may be a critical factor. Consider the example of a child without baseline studies who receives a dose of a chelating agent, and then is screened for heavy metals. Assuming the collection and analytical techniques are sound, the presence of detectable concentrations of heavy metals in the urine may be of questionable clinical significance. Other pitfalls include the choice of test, such as urine lead levels for organic lead exposure, versus blood levels for inorganic lead, or a 24-h urine collection for arsenic preferred over an isolated, spot urine assay. In addition, environmental contamination of a biologic sample may occur. Proper urine collection requires a plastic, hydrochloric acid-washed, low-metal container. Hospital- or community-based lab-oratories may not be capable of heavy metal assays and therefore send samples to outside reference laboratories, with variable reliability.

SUMMARY

Heavy metals are durable and persistent, and their toxicity in humans relates to a tendency to combine with reactive biological systems. Children may be at particular risk for toxicity because their development brings them into contact with heavy metals in a variety of situations. The assessment of exposure is emotionally charged and often fraught with inaccuracies. The subsequent chapters describe the toxicology and management of selected heavy metals that children are most likely to encounter.

Table 65–2. Heavy Metal Treatment

Cadmium	Supportive therapy, remove from source of exposure. Possible chelation therapy with DMSA (succimer) BAL may be detrimental by increasing renal tissue levels of cadmium
Copper	Supportive measures CaNa-EDTA, BAL plus penicillamine used as potential chelators
Nickel	Dermal decontamination Antidote: diethyldithiocarbamate (experimental)
Thallium	Gastric decontamination: gastric lavage and activated charcoal if recent ingestion. *Antidote:* oral Prussian blue (potassium ferric hexacyanoferrate) exchanges potassium ions for thallium in the gut lumen. *Hemodialysis:* possible role if within first 48 hours of exposure.
Zinc	Supportive care, hydration Possible role for CaNa-EDTA therapy Corticosteroids for metal fume fever

Table 65–3. Common Pitfalls in the Collection and Interpretation of Biological Samples for Heavy Metals

Pitfall	Examples
Timing of test versus therapy	Prechelation test offers more representative baseline Postchelation test reflects heavy metals mobilized from body burden
Choice of test	Sample type *Urine:* preferred for organic lead *Blood:* preferred for inorganic lead Sample collection period *Urine:* 24-h usually preferred over spot
Environmental contamination	*Urine:* should be collected in a plastic, hydrochloric acid-washed, low-metal container
Reference laboratory	Variable reliability of analytical techniques
Interpretation of results	Detectable concentrations may not imply clinically significant body burden

SUGGESTED READINGS

Bania T: Thallium and other metals. In: Ford MS, Delaney K, Ling L, et al, eds: *Clinical Toxicology*. Philadelphia: Saunders; 2001:744–748.

Baum CR: Treatment of mercury intoxication. *Curr Opin Pediatr* 11:265–268, 1999.

Goho A: The nature of things: Attempts to change the periodic table raise eyebrows. *Sci News* 164:264–265, 2003.

Hardman JG, Limbird LE, eds: *Goodman & Gilman's The Pharmacologic Basis of Therapeutics.* 10th ed. New York: McGraw-Hill; 2001.

Leikin JB, Paloucek FP, eds: *Poisoning & Toxicology Handbook.* 3rd ed. Hudson, OH: Lexi-Comp; 2002.

Offit PA, Jew RK: Addressing parents' concerns about vaccine additives. *Pediatrics* 112:1394–1401, 2003.

Wilford JN: Oldest planet is revealed, challenging old theories. *The New York Times.* July 11, 2003.

66

Arsenic

Rachel Haroz
Michael I. Greenberg

HIGH-YIELD FACTS

- Acute arsenic poisoning can result in garlicky breath, gastrointestinal (GI) symptoms such as vomiting, watery diarrhea or rice water stools, cardiovascular toxicity, renal failure, and acute neurologic manifestations.

- Arsine gas may cause immediate death when present in very high concentrations. In lower concentrations, exposure to arsine may lead to GI and neurologic symptoms as well as renal failure and hemolysis.

- Chronic arsenic toxicity results in a variety of dermatologic manifestations including hyperpigmentation, dermatitis, and hyperkeratosis. Patients can develop transverse white bands in the nail beds (Aldrich-Mees lines) in the chronic setting.

- A 24-h urine collection for arsenic is recommended for diagnosis when acute intoxication is suspected.

- Because urine arsenic testing can be confounded by the ingestion of seafood, speciation of test specimens is recommended.

- Serum arsenic levels are not useful in determining acute or chronic intoxication.

- British Anti-Lewisite (BAL) is the initial chelating agent of choice. The recommended dose for BAL is 3 mg/kg by intramuscular injection (IM) every 4 hours.

CASE PRESENTATION

A 4-year-old girl is brought to the emergency department (ED) by her grandmother with complaints of vomiting and diarrhea for 1 day. The grandmother is concerned because she found the child the day prior to admission in the garage with a old, half empty box of ant poison containing arsenic, but did not think at the time that the child had ingested any. The patient has no significant past medical history, no known allergies, and is currently taking no medications.

Physical examination reveals a pale girl who appears lethargic. She vomits in the ED twice producing yellow emesis with some streaks of blood. Her temperature is 37.4°C; heart rate, 140 bpm; blood pressure is 70/40 mmHg; and respiratory rate is 30 breaths per minute. The ear-nose-throat examination reveals dry mucous membranes and slightly pale conjunctiva. The cardiovascular examination reveals no murmurs, rubs, or gallops. Her lungs are clear bilaterally. The abdomen is tender diffusely with hyperactive bowel sounds. Extremities have full range of motion and capillary refill is 3 seconds. The skin is flushed, and there are no rashes. The neurologic exam is nonfocal; however, the patient is lethargic, unable to answer questions appropriately for her age, and appears confused.

Laboratory studies reveal a bicarbonate level of 13 mmol/L, WBC of 2.5 K/μL, hemoglobin of 9.4 g/dL, and platelets of 100 K/μL. A spot urine arsenic level is sent and a 24-h urine collection is started. The patient is aggressively hydrated, and based the history of probable arsenic ingestion, BAL at 3 mg/kg IM is started. The patient is admitted to the intensive care unit (ICU) and monitored.

INTRODUCTION AND EPIDEMIOLOGY

Arsenic may have been derived from the Greek word *arsenikon*, meaning *potent*, or from the Arabic word *azzernikh*, meaning *king's gold*. Historically, arsenic has found benevolent as well as malevolent uses. Fowler's solution, available on the U.S. market until the 1950s, contained 1% potassium arsenite, and was routinely used to treat asthma and psoriasis, as well as leukemia. Prior to the advent of penicillin, syphilis was routinely treated using arsenic-containing medications. Even today, the drug Melarsoprol, which contains trivalent arsenic, is the preferred treatment for African trypanosomiasis in the meningoencephalitic stage. Recently, arsenic trioxide (Trisenox) has been used to treat acute promyelocytic leukemia.

Arsenic is perhaps most widely recognized for its potentially harmful capabilities as a suicidal or homicidal agent. Tasteless, odorless, and sugar-like in appearance, arsenic may cause chronic as well as acute intoxication, and can be lethal. Pope Pius III, Charles Frances Hall, and Napoleon Bonaparte were all theorized to have died as a result of arsenic exposure. Arsenic has also played a role as a component of certain chemical warfare agents, including adamsite and lewisite. Arsenic has been responsible for several civilian mass poisonings, primarily due to contamination events.

Arsenic is recognized to be the most common acute heavy metal poisoning, and the second most common source of chronic heavy metal poisoning. A 200- to 300-mg intake of arsenic in humans may represent a lethal ingestion. In 2001, there were 1680 arsenic exposures reported by the American Association of Poison Control Centers. Of these cases, 161 involved children younger than 6 years of age.

Arsenic exists in both organic and inorganic forms. Organic sources for arsenic are primarily the earth's crust, seawater, and seafood, which contain arsenobetaine and arsenocholine. The inorganic arsenic compounds are more potentially harmful than are the organic forms. Potential exposure sources are listed in Table 66–1.

Chromated copper arsenate (CCA) has been used to treat certain commercially available woods as a preservative and pesticide. Recently concerns have been expressed regarding the potential for human exposure through sawdust from CCA-treated wood, as well as exposure from skin and oral contact. Currently, there is no reliable scientific data to support the development of disease resulting from these exposures. Nonetheless, public concern has led to a cessation of the manufacture of CCA-treated wood for most consumer use. A specific focus of concern with regard to CCA-treated wood involves potential exposure to arsenic in children who frequent playgrounds where the equipment may have been made using CCA-treated wood. This concern has recently led to the banning of CCA in wood used to construct playground equipment.

DEVELOPMENTAL CONSIDERATIONS

Arsenic crosses the placenta and can thus be found in the fetus under some circumstances. High levels of arsenic may be linked to premature delivery and fetal loss. Even with high maternal levels, arsenic is not excreted in breast milk in medically important amounts. Arsenic has been linked to several neoplastic processes including lung, bladder, and skin cancer, and may also be linked to some chromosomal aberrations. A single article by Calderon and associates refers to the possibility that chronic exposure under certain circumstances may be linked to some lower verbal IQ scores, poorer linguistic abstraction, and long-term memory loss. However, these possibilities remain unproven.

Table 66–1. Possible Sources of Inorganic Arsenic

Coal combustion	Contaminated well water	Cattle and sheep dips
Semiconductors	Insecticides (prior to 1970)	Microelectronics
Fossil fuel burning	Rodenticides (prior to 1970)	Defoliants
Metal alloys	CCA-treated wood	Glass clarifier
Fertilizers	Metal and glass smelting	Feed additives
Pesticides	Fungicides	
Paint and dye pigments	Desiccants	
Agricultural waste burning	Glass and ceramics	

PHARMACOLOGY AND TOXICOKINETICS

The toxicity of arsenic depends on the nature and degree of exposure, the degree of absorption, the dose absorbed, and the valence form. Arsenic exists in several forms including metalloid $As[^0]$, inorganic trivalent As $[^{3+}]$, and pentavalent $As[^{5+}]$, and in organic forms such as arsenobetaine, arsenocholine, and as arsine gas. Arsine gas is virtually odorless and colorless, and the most potentially harmful to humans of all the arsenic forms. The elemental metalloid is insoluble in water, and not generally harmful to humans. Organic arsenic has minimal potential to cause human disease. The inorganic forms are soluble and responsible for most of the potentially harmful medical effects known.

Absorption of arsenic can occur via the GI and respiratory tracts as well as through the skin and mucosa. GI absorption can be substantial. Soluble trivalent and pentavalent forms may exhibit up to 60% to 90% absorption. Respiratory absorption is largely dependent on particle size and solubility and is less important than GI absorption. Skin absorption is the least medically important, but may be increased with repeated exposures. Arsenic is rapidly cleared from the blood and distributed to various tissues.

Metabolism of arsenic is accomplished primarily by methylation in the liver. Pentavalent arsenic can be first reduced to trivalent arsenic and then methylated to monomethylarsonic acid and dimethylarsinic acid. Excretion of arsenic is primarily accomplished via renal mechanisms, but inorganic compounds and their metabolites may be found in feces and bile.

PATHOPHYSIOLOGY

The mechanism of arsenic toxicity appears to vary based on the chemical form. Trivalent arsenic (arsenite) exerts its potentially harmful effects by binding to sulfhydryl groups, leading to inhibition of key biochemical processes. These include the pyruvate dehydrogenase complex, the citric acid cycle, fatty acid oxidation, and other enzyme systems. The result may be decreased ATP production, and decreased levels of NADH, FADH2, and glutathione. Arsenite can also affect glucose metabolism leading to a possible association between some arsenic exposures and the development of diabetes mellitus.

Pentavalent arsenic (arsenate) acts by substituting arsenate for phosphate. These complexes rapidly hydrolyze, leading to disruption of oxidative phosphorylation. These two separate mechanisms can cause cellular toxicity and can result in tissue hypoxia and capillary damage leading to vasodilation and transudation.

Arsine gas, the most potentially harmful chemical form of arsenic, acts by binding to hemoglobin and causing rapid hemolysis. Arsine gas is largely an occupational exposure and hence almost never seen in pediatric patients.

CLINICAL PRESENTATION

The symptoms of arsenic poisoning are multifold. They vary depending on whether an exposure is acute or chronic, as well as the amount ingested, rate and degree of absorption, excretion, metabolism, and the arsenic form.

Acute Toxicity

The onset of symptoms after an acute ingestion is usually rapid, within 30 to 60 minutes, but may be delayed if ingested with food. Patients may initially complain of garlicky breath or stool, a metallic taste, fever, dry mouth, and dysphagia. GI symptoms are common, and patients usually have nausea, vomiting, abdominal pain, and profuse watery diarrhea or rice water stools. Hematemesis or hematochezia can occur. Cardiovascular collapse can occur owing to capillary leakage, plasma transudation, and extravascular fluid loss. Patients may develop ventricular arrhythmias, prolonged QT, ST depression, torsades de pointes, cardiomyopathy, and acute respiratory failure. Acute neurologic symptoms can include changes in mental status, seizures, delirium, and encephalopathy. Bone marrow failure can occur leading to pancytopenia, hemolytic anemia, dysfunctional erythropoietin, and karyorhexis. Renal failure can occur and can lead to acute tubular necrosis and interstitial fibrosis. Other symptoms can include skin flushing, toxic erythroderma, and exfoliative dermatitis. Arsine gas may cause immediate death when present in very high concentrations. In lower concentrations, exposure to arsine can lead to GI and neurologic symptoms, as well as renal failure and hemolysis.

Subacute and Chronic Toxicity

The onset of chronic arsenic poisoning is insidious. Patients can develop jaundice, liver dysfunction, and hepatomegaly with portal hypertension. Histology may reveal fatty infiltration, central necrosis, and cirrhosis. Diabetes and pancreatitis can occur. Axonal degeneration with peripheral neuropathies can develop, as well as an ascending paralysis similar to Guillian-Barré syndrome. Patients can under certain circumstances develop headaches and cranial nerve palsies. Proximal renal tubule degeneration and papillary and cortical necrosis sometimes occur. Other patients present with a dry cough, hemoptysis, and patchy lung infiltrates. Hematologic abnormalities similar to those seen in acute toxicity can develop, along with basophilic stippling of red blood cells.

Chronic arsenic toxicity has a variety of dermatologic manifestations, including hyperpigmentation, brawny desquamation, dermatitis, hyperkeratosis, and Bowen's disease. Some patients develop Aldrich-Mees lines, transverse white bands in the nail beds, that occur approximately 30 to 40 days after initial exposure. Another chronic development largely seen in Taiwan is known as *blackfoot disease*, or gangrene of the feet.

LABORATORY TESTING

Several laboratory studies can be helpful in determining the diagnosis of arsenic intoxication. Although arsenic is initially found in the bloodstream, it is rapidly cleared from the serum within hours. Thus obtaining serum levels is not generally useful. Arsenic is, however, cleared by the kidneys and persists in the urine, making urine studies more useful and predictable. A spot urine level may be helpful, with normal values being below 50 μ/L. The most reliable test is a 24-h quantitative urine collection. Excretion of more than 100 μg/d is considered abnormal. However, it is important to know that consumption of seafood, primarily shellfish, may raise the arsenic levels owing to large quantities of organically bound arsenic. This can result in misleadingly high levels of arsenic being reported in 24-h and spot urine levels. Thus, it is recommended that laboratory speciation be done. Speciation distinguishes the organic from the inorganic form. Other helpful tests include a complete blood count with peripheral smear looking for basophilic stippling, urinalysis, electrolytes with blood urea nitrogen and creatinine, liver function tests, and an electrocardiogram. Although arsenic is radiopaque, it is rapidly absorbed from the GI tract, so radiographs may not be helpful. Arsenic can also be found in hair within 30 hours of exposure; however, external contamination may render the measurement of arsenic in hair unreliable.

MANAGEMENT

The management of acute arsenic poisoning involves the basic principles of decontamination, supportive care, and the possible use of chelation therapy. If ingestion is recent, gastric lavage should be considered. This can be followed by orally administered activated charcoal with a mixed ingestion. However, because charcoal does not efficiently adsorb arsenic, the use of activated charcoal may be of limited value. Consideration should be given to the use of whole bowel irrigation with polyethylene glycol in cases of acute ingestion, particularly if there is radiographic evidence of exposure, as with iron and lead poisoning. Meticulous supportive care is essential and should include careful attention to adequate hydration to maintain urine output, correction of electrolyte imbalances, and the identification and treatment of cardiac dysrhythmias. Serum alkalinization using bicarbonate is recommended to prevent renal dysfunction resulting from myoglobinuria. The use of hemodialysis in the acute treatment of arsenic intoxication is currently an area of controversy. It should be strongly considered in the setting of renal failure.

The definitive treatment for acute arsenic poisoning involves the administration of chelation therapy. Chelating agents incorporate arsenic into a stable heterocyclic ring structure, making it water soluble and easily excreted by the kidneys. According to Cullen and associates, chelation is indicated for symptomatic patients or in those with significant urinary arsenic excretion of over 200 μg/L. BAL or 2, 3-dimercaptopropanol is the chelating agent of choice in cases of acute arsenic intoxication. It is recommended that 3 mg/kg be given IM every 4 hours for up 2 days; then every 12 hours for an additional 7 to 10 days, if necessary. Contraindications to BAL include pregnancy, G6PD deficiency, and peanut allergy because the drug is suspended in peanut oil. In the setting of renal failure, BAL may need to be supplemented with hemodialysis. BAL may be associated with various side effects, including painful injection site, seizures, central nervous system depression, hypertension, fever, nausea and vomiting. Headache, abdominal pain, and chest pain can occur.

Oral analogs of BAL include 2,3 dimercaptosuccinic acid (DMSA or succimer), and 2,3-dimercaptopropane-1 sulfonate (DMPS), which are both water-soluble agents. DMSA is administered orally and current dosing recommendations are 10 mg/kg every 8 hours for 5 days, then every 12 hours. Renal failure is a contraindication to DMSA. Side effects can include hypersensitivity reactions, elevation of transaminase enzymes, GI symptoms, and leukopenia. However, it is important to note that side effects from these drugs tend to be substantially less severe than BAL side effects. DMPS is not currently readily available in the United States. Another chelating agent that has been recommended for treating arsenic intoxication in the past is D-penicillamine. However, this drug is no longer recommended owing to its poor efficacy when compared to BAL and DMSA, as well as a substantial side effect profile. Chelation is administered until the 24-h urinary arsenic level is less than 50 µg/L. Consequently, it is important to carefully monitor the urinary arsenic levels throughout chelation therapy.

Arsine gas poisoning requires different management because acute exposure may cause hemolysis, renal failure, and death when present in high concentrations. Chelators are usually ineffective because they do little to prevent hemolysis. Exchange transfusions and hemodialysis for renal failure may be necessary.

DISPOSITION

Disposition is determined based on the clinical findings. Symptomatic children are admitted to the hospital, preferably to an intensive care setting. BAL is started and a 24-h urine arsenic level sent. Asymptomatic children living with a responsible adult can be discharged to home with instructions for a 24-h urine collection, and follow-up with a knowledgeable pediatrician or medical toxicologist in 24 hours.

CASE OUTCOME

The spot urine arsenic level was reported as 200 µg/L. The 24-h urine collection revealed an arsenic level of 5400 µg/L, 100% of which was found to be inorganic based on specimen speciation. BAL was continued for 2 days while the patient improved. At this time she was started on DMSA 10 mg/kg orally and the BAL stopped. She was discharged to home 3 days later and the DMSA continued until the 24-h urine arsenic level was less than 50 µg/L. There were no posttreatment sequelae.

SUGGESTED READINGS

Agency for Toxic Substances and Disease Registry (ATSDR): *ATSDR Case Studies in Environmental Medicine*. Atlanta: ATSDR; 1990.

Calderon J, Navarro ME, Jimenez-Capdeville ME: Exposure to arsenic and lead and neuropsychological development in Mexican children. *Environmental Research Section* 85:69–76, 2001.

Campbell JP, Alvarez JA: Acute arsenic intoxication. *Am Fam Physician* 40:93–97, 1989.

Chakraborti D, Mukherjee SC, Pati S, et al: Arsenic groundwater contamination in middle Ganga Plain, Bihar, India: A future danger? *Environ Health Perspect* 111:1194–2001, 2003.

Concha G, Vogler G, Nermell B, et al: Low-level arsenic excretion in breast milk of native Andean women exposed to high levels of arsenic in the drinking water. *Int Arch Occup Environ Health* 71:42–46, 1998.

Cullen NM, Wolf LR, St. Clair D: Pediatric Arsenic Ingestion. *Am J Emerg Med* 13:432–435, 1995.

Dulout FN, Grillo CA, Seoane AI, et al: Chromosomal aberrations in peripheral blood lymphocytes from native Andean women and children from northwestern Argentina exposed to arsenic in drinking water. *Mutat Res* 370:151–158, 1996.

Fields S: Caution—Children at play: How dangerous is CCA? *Environ Health Perspect* 109:274–276, 2001.

Gorby MS: Arsenic poisoning [clinical conference]. *West J Med* 149:308–315, 1988.

Graeme KA, Pollack CV: Heavy metal toxicity, part 1: Arsenic and mercury. *J Emerg Med* 16:45–56, 1997.

Hall AH: Chronic arsenic poisoning. *Toxicol Lett* 128:69–72, 2002.

Hsueh YM, Hsu MK, Chiou, HY, et al: Urinary arsenic speciation in subjects with or without restriction from seafood dietary intake. *Toxicol Lett* 133:83–91, 2002.

Jennings FW, Rodgers J, Bradley B, et al: Human African trypanosomiasis: Potential therapeutic benefits of alternative suramin and melarsoprol regimen. *Parasitol Int* 51:381–388, 2002.

Litovitz TL, Klein-Schwartz W, Rodgers GC: 2001 annual report of the American Association of Poison Control Centers Toxic Exposure Surveillance System. *Am J Emerg Med* 20:391–452, 2002.

Miller JL: Arsenic compound approved as cancer chemotherapy agent. *Am J Health Syst Pharm* 57:1940–1942, 2000.

Smith AE: Arsenic exposure in the U.S.: Well water, wood treatment, and residential fertilizers. North American Congress of Clinical Toxicology 2002 Symposium.

Tseng CH, Tseng CP, Chiou HY, et al: Epidemiologic evidence of diabetogenic effect of arsenic. *Toxicol Lett* 133:69–76, 2002.

Wang CH, Jeng JS, Yip PK, et al: Biological gradient between long-term arsenic exposure and carotid atherosclerosis. *Circulation* 105:1804–1809, 2002.

Zheng Y, Wu J, Ng JC: The absorption and excretion of fluoride and arsenic in humans. *Toxicol Lett* 133:77–82, 2002

67
Button Batteries
Toby L. Litovitz

CASE PRESENTATION

The father of an 18-month-old girl replaced the 20-mm lithium battery in his calculator and discarded the discharged cell. Two days later his daughter began complaining of a sore throat and developed a fever. Antibiotics and cough syrup were prescribed. No improvement was evident after several days on this regimen, and a second physician evaluated the patient and obtained a chest x-ray. Despite the absence of a history of ingestion, the presence of the battery in the esophagus was immediately evident and endoscopic removal was performed.

INTRODUCTION AND EPIDEMIOLOGY

In 2002, 2611 button battery exposures were reported to the American Association of Poison Control Centers Toxic Exposure Surveillance System, including 1465 ingestions in children younger than 6 years of age. According to data compiled in 2002 by the National Button Battery Ingestion Hotline, the most commonly ingested batteries were intended for use in hearing aids (49%) and toys and games (17%). Although manufacturers have been responsive to pleas to secure battery compartments in these sources, they continue to be the major sources of ingested button cells. There are a myriad of other potential sources for button battery exposures including watches, calculators, key chains, recording devices, digital thermometers, and cameras.

Fifty-three percent of ingested aids were loose or discarded just prior to the ingestion; another 35% were removed directly from the product and ingested. Seven percent were obtained directly from the original battery package. Modern hearing aids may be so small that the entire aid including the battery may be inadvertently ingested (5% of ingestion cases).

Multiple batteries are ingested in 8% to 13% of cases. The most common sizes of ingested cells are 11.6 mm diameter (50%) and 7.9 mm diameter (36%). Larger cells (15 to 23 mm diameter) are ingested less frequently (9% of ingestions), but account for the majority of poor outcomes.

DEVELOPMENTAL CONSIDERATIONS

Children suffer more severe consequences of battery ingestion than adults. Larger diameter cells are more often implicated in ingestions with severe outcomes. This is especially true in small children, where the ratio of the battery diameter to the esophageal diameter is greatest. Battery lodgment in the esophagus is a major predictor of poor outcome.

Common ingestion scenarios vary with age. Ingestions in infants may only be noted when the battery is discovered in the diaper. Toddlers may ingest batteries thinking the cell is candy or food. Teens and adults may hold batteries in the mouth to test the battery's residual charge, which is not an effective test. Teens and adults also ingest cells in suicide attempts. Older adults may mistake batteries for pills.

PATHOPHYSIOLOGY

Battery-induced tissue injury requires battery lodgment with either leakage of an alkaline electrolyte or generation of an external current. Batteries that do not remain in one place for at least a few hours do not cause clinically significant injury. Although lodgment must occur for injury to occur, batteries may also lodge in the gut for days or even years without causing injury.

Esophageal lodgment is usually associated with the ingestion of cells 20 to 23 mm in diameter. Most of these cells are lithium batteries, and are 3.0 volt rather than the standard 1.5 volt button cells. The combination of the larger diameter and greater voltage makes lithium button batteries the most hazardous when ingested.

Leakage may be a cause of injury following button cell lodgment. Many button batteries contain potassium or sodium hydroxide, in concentrations up to 45%. Corrosion of the battery may occur, especially in the stomach. Corrosion facilitates leakage, possibly causing alkaline damage to adjacent tissue.

Generation of an external current is a second possible cause of injury following button cell lodgment. The external current flows between the battery cathode and anode, passing through adjacent tissue and hydrolyzing the electrolyte-rich tissue fluids. As a result, hydroxides are formed locally, leading to alkaline damage of the tissue in contact with the battery. This occurs even in the absence of battery leakage. Discharged (spent) cells would be expected to produce less injury via this mechanism. However, batteries that are apparently dead and unable to power a product still have considerable residual charge, and can be associated with clinically significant injury.

Pressure necrosis, such as that seen following ingestion of coins, may contribute to injury following battery ingestion. However, leakage and the generation of an external current are more significant factors in battery-induced injury.

Heavy metal poisoning is unlikely following battery ingestion. Despite tens of thousands of button cell ingestions, symptomatic cases of heavy metal poisoning following battery ingestion have not been reported. Four patients developed modest elevations of blood mercury concentrations after ingested mercuric oxide button batteries split open in the GI tract; however, none of these patients developed clinical findings consistent with mercury poisoning. The absence of significant mercury poisoning following ingestion of these cells is likely attributable to the reduction of mercuric oxide to the less toxic elemental mercury in the presence of gastric acid and iron released from the corroding steel battery canister. Ingestion of mercuric oxide button cells is now a rare event following enactment of the Mercury-Containing and Rechargeable Battery Management Act in 1996. This legislation banned the sale of mercuric oxide button cells in the United States, and the use of more than 0.025% mercury in batteries manufactured with other chemical systems.

CLINICAL FINDINGS

The vast majority of button battery ingestions are benign. One study revealed that only 0.08% of 2382 ingestion cases demonstrated a life-threatening or disabling effect. Clinical effects are reported in only 10% of battery ingestion cases, and most commonly involve vomiting (2.4%), abdominal pain and cramps (2.0%), dark, discolored, or bloody stools (1.7%), fever (1.3%), and diarrhea (1.3%). Rashes, often diffuse, are noted in 1.2% of battery ingestion cases, and are likely manifestations of nickel hypersensitivity, because many button cells are nickel plated.

Esophageal lodgment causes the most serious complications of battery ingestion. It may manifest with vomiting, fever, dysphagia, odynophagia, tachypnea, anorexia, and irritability. Although esophageal lodgment is usually associated with 20- to 23-mm diameter cells, these larger cells may pass to the stomach without consequence, and cells as small as 11.6 mm may lodge.

Esophageal burns may occur within 4 to 6 hours of the ingestion. Esophageal rupture has occurred after a battery lodged for just 6 hours. Identification of battery position must be made as soon as possible by radiographic localization. Batteries in the esophagus require urgent endoscopic removal. Failure to promptly remove ingested batteries from the esophagus may lead to esophageal stenosis requiring repeated dilatation or surgical repair, tracheoesophageal fistula, tension pneumothorax or hemothorax, perforation through the aortic arch or its branches, massive exsanguination, and/or cardiac arrest. Two fatal battery ingestion cases have been reported in small children, both involving esophageal lodgment, and both following delays in diagnosis of 24 hours to 4 days. Massive tracheoesophageal fistula and exsanguination occurred in one of these patients, a 2½-year-old boy. The second patient, a 16-month-old girl, experienced esophageal perforation, tension hydropneumothorax, and perforation of the aortic arch.

Most batteries do not lodge in the esophagus. They usually pass spontaneously through the GI tract and do not require endoscopic or surgical removal. Within 72 hours, 78% of ingested cells will pass spontaneously. Longer transit times, in excess of a year, may occur without adverse effects. In general, the transit of larger cells is arrested more proximally; 15- to 23-mm batteries tend to arrest in the esophagus or stomach. Smaller cells tend to arrest more distally; 7.9-mm cells often are found many weeks to months postingestion in the small or large bowel. Only a few cases have been reported with poor outcomes occurring after passage beyond the esophagus, including perforation of a Meckel diverticulum, and localized mucosal damage noted on endoscopic examination. These latter cases generally require no treatment and cause no sequelae despite the evidence of local injury.

Batteries placed in the ear or nose may be associated with severe injury. The initial clinical indication of their presence is either discharge or pain. Prompt removal is absolutely essential, but is often delayed because of failure to make the diagnosis. These cells can cause necrosis of the external ear canal, swelling and erythema of the pinna, perforation or destruction of the tympanic membrane, destruction of the ossicles, hearing impairment, perforation of the nasal septum, saddle deformity of the nose, destruction of the nasal turbinates, paralysis of the facial nerve, chondritis, or atrophic rhinitis.

LABORATORY AND DIAGNOSTIC TESTING

Prompt radiographic localization of the ingested battery is critical (see Figure 24–7A). The presence or absence of symptoms does not serve as a reliable indicator of esophageal lodgment. More than one third of patients with batteries in the esophagus are asymptomatic at the time of initial diagnosis.

Battery passage is best confirmed by inspecting the stools. Repeat radiographs 7 to 14 days postingestion can also be used to confirm passage. More frequent radiographs are generally recommended when a child younger than 6 ingests a large-diameter cell (>15 mm). If these larger cells do not pass through the pylorus of the small child within 48 hours, they are unlikely to pass, and endoscopic removal should be seriously considered.

It can be difficult to accurately determine battery diameter from a radiograph. To more precisely guide therapy and determine the appropriate aggressiveness of intervention, it is helpful to identify the battery diameter and chemical system by checking the imprint code of a duplicate battery, the diameter of the product's battery compartment, or information in the product instructions. The National Button Battery Ingestion Hotline at 202-625-3333 can assist with identification and provide specific treatment guidance. Determining the battery diameter and system is especially helpful because additional monitoring and more careful observation are indicated for lithium batteries and for cells 20 mm or more in diameter.

MANAGEMENT

A nine-step approach to patient management is summarized in Table 67–1. Emergent endoscopic removal of batteries lodged in the esophagus is indicated, ideally within 2 to 4 hours of ingestion. Following removal, patients with endoscopic evidence of tissue injury should be observed and reevaluated for delayed complications. When retrieval is required, endoscopy with direct visualization is preferred to blind removal with a balloon-tipped catheter or to surgical retrieval.

Retrieval of batteries that have passed beyond the esophagus is unnecessary, unless the patient manifests signs or symptoms which suggest significant injury to

Table 67–1. Nine-Step Approach to Button Battery Exposures

1. Consider the diagnosis of button battery exposure in any patient with
   a. Pain and/or discharge in the ear or nose.
   b. Reported "coin" ingestion.
   c. Airway obstruction, wheezing, drooling, or vomiting.
2. If an ingestion is suspected, immediately obtain an x-ray to locate the battery.
3. Promptly remove batteries lodged in the esophagus, nose, or ear.
4. Determine the battery diameter and chemical system from the imprint code. Consult the National Button Battery Ingestion Hotline at 202-625-3333 for assistance in battery identification or patient management.
5. Allow batteries to pass spontaneously if they have passed beyond the esophagus and no clinical indication of significant GI injury is evident. Encourage home management with regular diet and activity.
6. Confirm battery passage by inspecting stools. Consider repeating radiographs to confirm passage if battery passage has not been observed in 7 to 14 days.
7. Closely monitor children younger than 6 who ingest batteries of 15 mm or greater diameter. In these children, repeat the radiograph 48 hours post-ingestion and consider endoscopic removal if the battery has not moved beyond the pylorus in 48 hours.
8. Closely monitor patients who ingest lithium cells, especially if the battery diameter is 20 mm or greater.
9. Avoid
   a. Ipecac administration.
   b. Obtaining blood or urine mercury concentrations.
   c. Chelation therapy.
   d. Endoscopic or surgical removal of batteries, unless there is a clear indication for removal.

the GI tract may have occurred. Patients with hematochezia or abdominal pain with tenderness may require removal. Patients with minor GI symptoms such as transient vomiting, stool discoloration without evidence of blood, or decreased appetite can be observed.

Although no data exist to confirm efficacy, when batteries remain in the stomach for protracted periods, metoclopramide may be recommended to speed gastric passage and an H_2-antagonist given to limit corrosive damage. In the more routine cases, where GI transit is not interrupted, cathartics, metoclopramide, and H_2-antagonists are not used; animal data confirm that these agents do not affect outcome.

Batteries lodged in the ear or nose are removed immediately. Nasal and otic drops are avoided until the battery is removed, because these solutions enhance battery corrosion and leakage and enable generation of an external current. Sedation and direct visualization through an operating microscope may be required for battery removal. Some batteries are magnetic; thus, a magnetized instrument may prove an invaluable asset to removal. Alternately, a 1-mm 90-degree pick can be positioned beyond a button cell in the ear canal, then rotated and retracted.

Ipecac syrup and activated charcoal are ineffective. Clinical evidence of heavy metal poisoning has not been reported; thus, blood or urine mercury concentrations and chelation therapy are not indicated.

DISPOSITION

Urgent removal is required for batteries in the esophagus, nose, or ear. Subsequent management is based on the severity of the local injury. In contrast, most battery ingestion cases are managed as outpatients. When the battery has moved beyond the esophagus and clinical evidence of significant GI injury is absent, the patient should be observed and managed a home.

CASE OUTCOME

The child was discharged after a brief hospitalization but continued to have difficulty swallowing. She was flown to a pediatric referral center where a small tracheoesophageal fistula was diagnosed. The fistula eventually closed without surgical intervention. Three years after the ingestion the child had persistent evidence of an esophageal stricture requiring dietary and food size modifications.

SUGGESTED READINGS

Barber TE, Menke RD: The relationship of ingested iron to the absorption of mercuric oxide. *Am J Emerg Med* 2:500–503, 1984.

Blatnik DS, Toohill RJ, Lehman RH; Fatal complication from an alkaline battery foreign body in the esophagus. *Ann Otol* 86:611–615, 1977.

Kavanagh KT, Litovitz TL: Miniature battery foreign bodies in auditory and nasal cavities. *JAMA* 255:1470–1472, 1986.

Kulig KW, Rumack CM, Rumack BH, et al: Disk battery ingestion. *JAMA* 249:2502–2506, 1983.

Litovitz T, Schmitz BF: Ingestion of cylindrical and button batteries: An analysis of 2,382 cases. *Pediatrics* 89:747–757, 1992.

Litovitz TL, Butterfield AB, Holloway RR: Button battery ingestion: Assessment of therapeutic modalities and battery discharge state. *J Pediatr* 105:868–873, 1984.

Mant TGK, Lewis JL, Mattoo TK, et al: Mercury poisoning after disc-battery ingestion. *Human Toxicol* 6:179–181, 1987.

Mofenson HC, Greensher J, Caraccio TR, et al: Ingestion of small flat disc batteries. *Ann Emerg Med* 12:88–90, 1983.

Shabino CL, Feinberg AN: Esophageal perforation secondary to alkaline battery ingestion. *JACEP* 8:360–362, 1979.

Skinner DW, Chui P: The hazards of "button-sized" batteries as foreign bodies in the nose and ear. *J Laryngol Otol* 100: 1315–1318, 1986.

Watson WA, Litovitz TL, Rodgers GC, et al: 2002 annual report of the American Association of Poison Control Centers Toxic Exposure Surveillance System. *Am J Emerg Med* 21:353–421, 2003.

68

Iron

Steven E. Aks
Milton Tenenbein

CASE PRESENTATION

A 6-year-old boy presents to the emergency department (ED) after ingesting up to 40 sugar-coated 325 mg fer- rous sulfate tablets 4 hours ago. His mother was taking this medication as a prenatal supplement. The child had one episode of spontaneous emesis at home with dark material noted. He reports mild abdominal pain. His past medical history is unremarkable, he currently takes no medications, and has no allergies.

On physical examination he appears slightly pale with a pulse of 135 bpm, a blood pressure of 100/70 mmHg, and a respiratory rate of 24 breaths per minute. The child is afebrile. The capillary refill is 2 seconds. Other than mild epigastric tenderness, the remainder of the physical examination is unremarkable.

Laboratory studies reveal an anion gap of 24, glucose 210 mg/dL, and a WBC of 18 K/mL. A KUB is negative for radiopaque tablets. The serum iron concentration at 4 hours postingestion is 1196 µg/dL. He was started on IV deferoxamine at 15 mg/kg/h.

INTRODUCTION AND EPIDEMIOLOGY

According to 2001 data from the American Association of Poison Control Centers, there were 3550 iron inges- tions. There were 2094 ingestions in children younger than 6 years of age, and 470 ingestions in children 6 to 19 years old. Historically, iron was the most common cause of poisoning death for children under the age of 6. This resulted in the U.S. Food and Drug Administration man- dating unit dose packaging (blister packs) for products containing more than 30 mg elemental iron per tablet. This intervention has resulted in a decreased frequency, severity, and mortality of pediatric iron overdose inci- dents. 1n 1991, 11 pediatric iron deaths were reported to the American Association of Poison Control Centers, ac- counting for 65% of unintentional pediatric overdose deaths. In 2001, no pediatric deaths were reported. In

1991, the iron antidote deferoxamine was administered in 901 patients. In 2001, it was used in only 98 poisoning cases.

DEVELOPMENTAL CONSIDERATIONS

Several factors contribute to iron poisoning in toddlers. Iron is widely available as an over the counter product. In addition, iron-containing products tend to have a sweet taste and a candy-like appearance owing to pharmaceutical sugar coating and bright coloration of tablets and pills. Iron poisoning is also a problem in suicidal adolescents and adults. Pregnant adolescents are a high-risk overdose subgroup owing to the accessibility of iron-containing prenatal supplements that can be used in suicide attempts or as a potential abortifacient.

PATHOPHYSIOLOGY

After absorption, the ferrous (Fe^{2+}) ion is oxidized to its ferric (Fe^{3+}) counterpart in the plasma, and bound to transferrin. The potential for toxicity begins after the transferrin binding capacity is exceeded. Iron is a potent catalyst of free radical generation, which is the chief mechanism of iron toxicity. Targets include the gastrointestinal (GI) epithelium, the liver, the circulatory system, and the heart. Autopsy findings include swelling, fatty degeneration, and necrosis of hepatocytes. Iron deposits can be found in hepatocytes and the reticuloendothelial cells of the liver and spleen. Fatty degeneration occurs in the heart. The lungs may reveal nonspecific congestive changes from cardiovascular collapse. Coagulopathy-induced hemorrhages are frequently found.

TOXICITY AND ESTIMATING RISK

It is important to identify the specific preparation, because content the amount of elemental iron varies (Table 68–1). If the preparation and number of tablets are known, the total dose of elemental iron can be calculated. The potential for toxicity correlates with the ratio of elemental iron to body weight. A dose exceeding 60 mg of elemental iron per kilogram of body weight is associated with life-threatening toxicity.

From a poison control center or office-based perspective, the decision whether a poisoned child can be managed at home or referred to a health care facility is de-

Table 68–1. Iron Preparations

Iron Preparation	Percent Elemental Iron
Ferrous sulfate	20
Ferrous fumarate	33
Ferrous gluconate	12

pendent on the calculation of the amount of elemental iron ingested (Table 68–2). However, if the patient is symptomatic, or if the amount of iron ingested cannot be accurately established, the child should be referred to the nearest health care facility or ED.

CLINICAL PRESENTATION

Patients commonly present to the ED with a history of having ingested iron tablets or vitamins containing iron. If the amount of elemental iron ingested cannot be reasonably determined, always assume that the maximum amount available has been ingested. It is useful to describe iron overdose in terms of the known stages of toxicity. The stages are generally sequential, although there can be overlap.

Stage 1

This stage begins at the time of ingestion and lasts for about 6 hours. Symptoms and signs include vomiting, diarrhea, hematemesis, hematochezia, and the potential for hypovolemic shock from GI fluid and blood loss.

Stage 2

Stage two occurs from about 6 to 12 hours after ingestion, and is known as the stage of relative stability be-

Table 68–2. Treatment Recommendations for Iron Ingestions

Ingested Dose (mg/kg)	Treatment Recommendation
<30	Observe at home
>30–40	If symptomatic, refer to health care facility
>40	Refer to health care facility

cause the patient appears to be improving, or may even be asymptomatic. A meticulous physical assessment looking for evidence of hypovolemia and hypoperfusion is vital in diagnosing a patient in this stage. A blood gas may show evidence of mild metabolic acidosis.

Stage 3

The stage occurs approximately between 12 and 24 hours after ingestion. Patients can develop cardiovascular collapse. The etiology of shock is multifactorial with the primary component being distributive. Other etiologies include hypovolemia from fluid and blood loss from the GI tract, and pump failure owing to the direct effects of iron on the heart. Shock is the most common cause of death in iron poisoning. Acidosis can be profound. Although lactic acidosis from hypoperfusion is a contributor, it is mostly due to the hydration of nontransferrin-bound iron by the reaction $Fe^{3+} + 3H_2O \rightarrow FeOH^3 + 3H^+$. Thus, one ferric ion generates three protons. Altered mental status is secondary to hypoperfusion.

Stage 4

Stage four is the hepatotoxic phase. It is dose dependent and occurs within the first 48 hours of ingestion. Transaminases greater than 2000 to 4000 are an ominous sign, and are associated with significant morbidity and mortality. After shock, hepatic failure is the next most common cause of death in iron poisoning.

Stage 5

This stage results in GI obstruction. It typically occurs 4 to 6 weeks after ingestion. Patients destined to develop this complication often have persistent abdominal pain. The obstruction is a consequence of stricture formation, typically located at the level of the pylorus.

LABORATORY AND DIAGNOSTIC TESTING

Key diagnostic tests are the serum iron concentration and an abdominal radiograph. The iron concentration usually peaks between 2 and 6 hours after ingestion, and serial determinations over this time range are often needed. Iron values greater than 500 μg/dL are typically associated with clinical toxicity, and levels greater than 1000 μg/dL are potentially fatal. The abdominal radiograph directs the initial management. If it is negative and the

patient is asymptomatic, no interventions are indicated. If tablets are seen in the radiograph, GI decontamination is necessary. Arterial blood gas determination is also important. The finding of a metabolic acidosis in a seemingly asymptomatic patient is a marker for the development of shock. Historically, the combination of leukocytosis, hyperglycemia, a positive abdominal radiograph, and the presence of emesis was used to predict an elevated serum iron concentration. However, several studies have demonstrated that these are not valid parameters. Another test no longer recommended test is the TIBC. It was previously used to aid in the decision for initiating chelation therapy; however, this approach has also been shown to lack validity. Other investigations required for the management of significant iron poisoning include a complete blood count, coagulation profile, and renal and hepatic function tests.

MANAGEMENT

Assessment of Risk

Toxicity is related to the ingested dose of elemental iron. Doses less than 40 mg/kg in a child, or 1.5 g in an adolescent, require no interventions; ingestions greater than these require hospital assessment and management. Symptomatic patients, or patients with serum iron concentrations above 500 μg/dL, require admission and IV chelation. A critical care environment should be considered for patients with serum iron concentrations greater than 1000 μg/dL.

GASTROINTESTINAL DECONTAMINATION

The preferred method for the GI decontamination of the iron ingestion patient is whole bowel irrigation (WBI). Ipecac-induced emesis and gastric lavage have not been shown to be effective; activated charcoal does not bind iron. The indication for WBI is a positive abdominal radiograph. In the rare circumstance where an abdominal radiograph is not available, then the ingestion of 40 mg/kg in a child or 1.5 g in an adolescent can be used as criteria for initiating WBI. Polyethylene glycol electrolyte lavage solution is given by nasogastric tube at 25 mL/kg/h in small children and 1.0 to 2.0 L/h in adolescents and adults. The endpoint is a clear rectal effluent. The absence of iron tablets on a subsequent abdominal radiograph can also be used as an endpoint for WBI. Contraindications for WBI include shock, significant GI hemorrhage, ileus, or bowel obstruction.

Historically, interventions aimed at either complexing or chelating iron within the gut were recommended. These included oral deferoxamine, sodium bicarbonate, magnesium, or phosphate. All of these are no longer recommended because they are either ineffective or dangerous.

Specific Therapy and Chelation

Even moderately iron poisoned children require meticulous supportive care to ensure a positive outcome. For patients in shock, large volumes of IV fluids and sodium bicarbonate administration are required to maintain fluid, electrolyte, and acid–base parameters. Severely poisoned patients also require supportive care for hepatic failure and coagulopathy. A critical care environment is required. A Swan-Ganz catheter will assist in determining the etiology of the shock and to monitor response to therapy.

Specific therapy is chelation with deferoxamine (Fig. 68–1). Indications are the presence of significant symptoms as signs of iron poisoning, a serum iron concentration greater than 500 μg/dL, or metabolic acidosis. Historically, the deferoxamine challenge test was used to assist in the decision for chelation therapy. However,

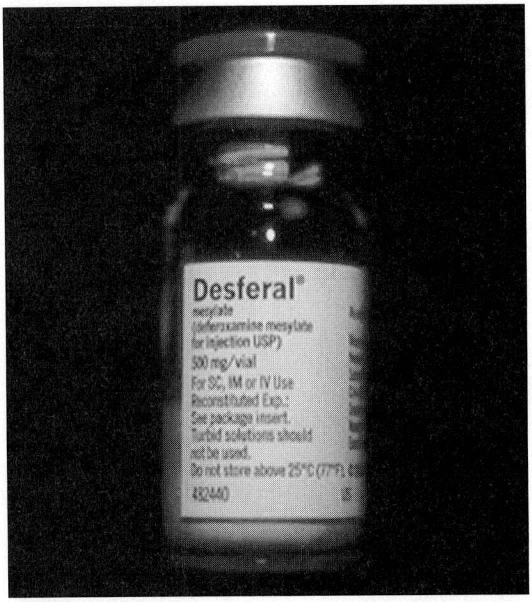

Fig. 68–1. Deferoxamine is the chelating agent of choice for iron poisoning.

neither the test nor the outcome have been validated. Thus, it is no longer recommended.

Deferoxamine should be given IV at a rate of 15 mg/kg/h. The intramuscular route is not recommended because it is less effective. The duration of chelation therapy is variable; there are no reliable endpoints. Serum iron determinations during the course of iron poisoning do not reflect clinical toxicity and they are often unreliable during deferoxamine therapy. Using a return of urine color to normal is not recommended as an endpoint. It has never been validated and pigmentation of urine from the presence of ferrioxamine (traditionally described as *vin rose*) is concentration dependent rather than amount dependent. Using this criterion may result in premature cessation or overly prolonged deferoxamine therapy. A useful criterion for continued chelation is the presence of a metabolic acidosis despite satisfactory perfusion. This indicates the presence of nontransferrin-bound iron in the plasma. Deferoxamine is rarely required beyond the first 24 hours after iron ingestion.

A major complication of deferoxamine includes hypotension if it is given too rapidly by the IV route. Rates in excess of 100 mg/kg/h in dogs are associated with this adverse event. Hypotension has not been reported in humans treated with the recommended dose of 15 mg/kg/h. Another potential complication is acute renal failure if deferoxamine is administered to patients with severe hypovolemia and a contracted intravascular volume. This can be prevented by administering a crystalloid bolus to expand the intravascular volume prior to initiating the deferoxamine infusion. The adult respiratory distress syndrome is a potential fatal complication of continuous deferoxamine infusions of greater than 24 to 48 hours of duration. *Yersinia* infections and transient blindness have also been reported in cases of chronic deferoxamine therapy.

DISPOSITION

A patient with unstable vital signs, shock, or significant metabolic acidosis requires admission to an intensive care unit. After the resolution of metabolic acidosis and other signs and symptoms of toxicity, the patient may be discharged home. For patients who suffer significant toxicity, it is important to arrange close follow-up owing to the potential for persistent abdominal pain and GI obstruction (stage 5 toxicity). Psychiatric evaluation of adolescents with an iron ingestion associated with any suicidal intent is usually indicated.

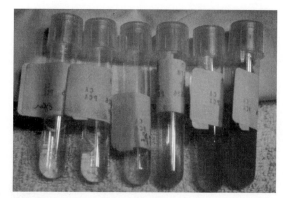

Fig. 68–3. Progression of coloration of vin rose urine over 15 hours.

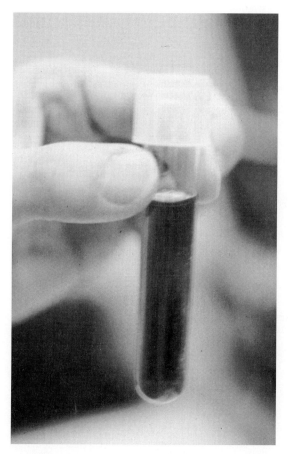

Fig. 68–2. Vin rose colored urine following deferoxamine chelation therapy.

CASE OUTCOME

Deferoxamine chelation therapy is administered for a total of 16 hours at 15 mg/kg/h. The metabolic acidosis completely resolves over this time period. Interestingly, 1 hour after the initiation of the infusion, the child's urine showed the classic vin rose appearance (Figure 68–2). Figure 68–3 shows the progression of urine obtained over the next 15 hours. It is also interesting that the color normalized over this time period. Clinicians should be aware that this finding of vin rose urine coloration is uncommon. Many patients may have significant toxicity without a change in urine color, as discussed. Resolution of acidosis, along with clinical improvement, are the most important signs of successful therapy. This child

did well. He tolerated food 48 hours after admission, and was discharged on the following day. He made a full recovery.

SUGGESTED READINGS

Anderson BD, Turchen SG, Manoguerra AS, et al: Retrospective analysis of ingestions of iron containing products in the United States: Are there differences between chewable vitamins and adult preparations? *J Emerg Med* 19:255–258, 2000.

Burkhart KK, Kulig KW, Hammond KB, et al: The rise in total iron-binding capacity after iron overdose. *Ann Emerg Med* 20:532–535, 1991.

Chyka PA, Brady AY: Assessment of acute iron poisoning by laboratory and clinical observations. *Am J Emerg Med* 11:99–103, 1993.

Klein-Schwartz W, Oderga GM, Gorman RL, et al: Assessment of management guidelines in acute iron ingestion. *Clin Pediatr* 29:316–321, 1990.

Ling LJ, Hornfeldt CS, Winter JP: Absorption of iron after experimental overdose of chewable vitamins. *Am J Emerg Med* 9:24–26, 1991.

Litovitz TL, Holm K, Bailey KM, et al: 1991 annual report of the American Association of Poison Control Centers National Data Collection System. *Am J Emerg Med* 10:452–505, 1992.

Litovitz TL, Klein-Schwartz W, Rodgers GC, et al: 2001 annual report of Poison Control Centers Toxic Exposure Surveillance System. *Am J Emerg Med* 20:391–452, 2002.

Litovitz T, Manoguerra A: Comparison of pediatric poisoning hazards: An analysis of 3.8 million exposure incidents. *Pediatrics* 89:999–1006, 1992.

Morris CC: Pediatric iron poisonings in the United States. *South Med J* 93:352–358, 2000.

Tenenbein M, Kopelow ML, DeSai DJ: Myocardial failure secondary to acute iron poisoning. *Vet Hum Toxicol* 28:491, 1986.

Tenenbein M: Whole bowel irrigation in iron poisoning. *J Pediatr* 111:142–145, 1987.

Tenenbein M: Benefits of parenteral deferoxamine for acute iron poisoning. *J Toxicol Clin Toxicol* 34:485–489, 1996.

Tenenbein M: Hepatotoxicity in acute iron poisoning. *J Toxicol Clin Toxicol* 39:721–726, 2001.

Tenenbein M, Israels SJ: Early coagulopathy in severe iron poisoning. *J Pediatr* 113:695–697, 1988.

Tenenbein M, Kowalski S, Sienko A, et al: Pulmonary toxic effects of continuous desferioxamine administration in acute iron poisoning. *Lancet* 339:699–701, 1992.

69

Lead

Mark Mycyk
Daniel Hryhorczuk
Yona Amitai

HIGH-YIELD FACTS

- Early signs and symptoms of lead poisoning (*plumbism*) are nonspecific and vague.

- Lead poisoning causes multisystem clinical effects: headache, abdominal pain, constipation, vomiting, clumsiness, irritability, and drowsiness.

- Laboratory evaluation can demonstrate anemia, basophilic stippling, elevated erythrocyte protoporphyrin or zinc protoporphyrin (EP/ZPP), or an elevated blood lead level (BLL).

- Management requires identification and removal of the source of exposure.

- Chelation with $CaNa_2EDTA$, British anti-lewisite (BAL), or Succimer is dictated by BLL and severity of symptoms.

CASE PRESENTATION

A 3-year-old girl has undergone four evaluations for constipation and fussiness in several local emergency departments (ED) over the past 2 months. The child was born at 40 weeks gestation, has no medical problems, no allergies, and her immunizations are up to date. Her only medication is a glycerin suppository prescribed for intermittent constipation. Her two older siblings are healthy. A complete blood count at her last ED visit demonstrated microcytic anemia. Despite no clear source of residential lead poisoning, the child's pediatrician ordered a BLL during an office evaluation because of the child's ane-

mia. The BLL is reported to be 92 μg/dL 3 days after the office visit.

INTRODUCTION AND EPIDEMIOLOGY

The average BLL of American children has decreased by more than 80% since the 1970s because of early screening initiatives and hazard reduction. In spite of this progress, several long-term studies have shown an association of lead levels once thought to be nontoxic with impaired growth and delayed neurocognitive development. In 1991, the Centers for Disease Control and Prevention (CDC) revised the 1985 blood lead intervention level of 25 μg/dL downward to 10 μg/dL. However, it is still estimated that 1.7 million children (or 9% of American children) still have some degree of lead poisoning based on the revised CDC lead action level. Lead poisoning affects people of all ages and classes, but the prevalence of lead poisoning remains highest among inner-city underprivileged children.

Sources

Ingestion of leaded paint is the most common and clinically relevant source of lead poisoning in children. Most homes built before 1978 were painted with lead-based paint. A small paint chip containing 50% lead can produce acute lead poisoning in a toddler. Lead poisoning has traditionally been a problem in children living in poorly maintained inner-city buildings. However, renovation of old homes in the last decade and poorly controlled lead abatement have been identified as a significant risk for lead poisoning through inhalation and ingestion of contaminated dust and soil among children of affluent parents. Lead exposure can also occur through ingestion of drinking water contaminated by lead in plumbing. Children living in close proximity to stationary air pollution sources such as lead smelters are at risk for lead poisoning. Other potential sources of toxicity include secondary exposure to lead brought home from work places, drinking from improperly fired lead-glazed pottery, some folk remedies, bullets lodged in joint spaces, and other unusual sources. The phase out of leaded gasoline has had a major impact in reducing exposure to lead.

DEVELOPMENTAL CONSIDERATIONS

Lead is a nonessential metal that can cause toxicity in all age groups. It is particularly hazardous in young children because of the significant delays that lead can impart on neurocognitive development. Children are more susceptible to the hazards of lead than adults for three reasons. First, and most important, human brain development occurs most rapidly from fetal gestation through the second year of life. As neural networks develop and the brain is restructured through cortical synaptogenesis, synaptic pruning, myelin deposition, neurotransmitter development, and voltage-sensitive channel organization, lead's affinity for the nervous system during these critical developmental years may be permanent. Second, the absorption rate of lead through the gastrointestinal (GI) tract in infants and children is about 50%, which is much higher than the 5% to 10% absorption that occurs in adults. Third, children have a greater tendency for pica than adults, thus increasing their exposure to contaminated paint chips and soil.

PHARMACOLOGY AND TOXICOKINETICS

Lead absorption through the GI tract is about 50% in infants and children. The distribution of absorbed lead in the body can be modeled using three compartments: blood, soft tissue, and bone. Under steady-state conditions, 99% of the lead in blood is attached to red blood cells. Under chronic exposure conditions, the bone serves as a storage organ and can release lead back into the blood and soft tissues. Absorbed lead is eliminated primarily in the urine and bile. In adults the elimination of lead is first order and triphasic with elimination half-lives of 1 week, 1 month, and 10 to 20 years. Pediatric data are lacking, but some reports indicate that the biologic half-life of blood lead in 2-year-old children is about 10 months.

PATHOPHYSIOLOGY

The majority of lead exposure in children occurs through the GI tract. Iron deficiency and dietary calcium deficiency increase the absorption of lead in the gut. Lead dust and fumes can also be absorbed through the respiratory tract. Percutaneous absorption of lead is less than 0.1% of the applied quantity. In pregnant females, lead readily crosses the placental barrier, and fetal exposure is cumulative until birth.

Lead toxicity results from interaction of lead with sulfhydryl and other ligands on enzymes and other macromolecules. The major target organs of lead are the bone marrow, central nervous system (CNS), peripheral nervous system, and kidneys. Lead inhibits heme synthesis through inhibition of delta ALA-dehydratase, coproporphyrin utilization, and ferrochelatase, resulting in the build up of aminolevulinic acid, coproporphyrins, and free erythrocyte protoporphyrin (Figure 69–1). Lead also inhibits the enzyme pyrimidine-5′-nucleotidase, thus increasing erythrocyte fragility. Clinically, inhibition of heme synthesis is manifested as anemia. CNS effects result from brain lead interfering with cortical synaptic modeling, myelin deposition, neurotransmitter and neurochemical development, and voltage-sensitive channel organization during postnatal brain development. Lead en-

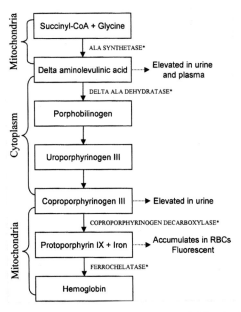

Fig. 69-1. Heme synthesis. (*Source:* Goldfrank LR, Flomenbaum N, Lewin N, et al, eds: *Goldfrank's Toxicologic Emergencies.* 7th ed. New York: McGraw-Hill; 2002:1208.)

cephalopathy is a severe consequence of brain lead accumulation from disrupted calcium-dependent cellular processes that maintain the integrity of the blood–brain barrier. Cell death, tissue necrosis, and vascular damage result in increased cerebrospinal fluid protein and elevated intracranial pressure. Lead can cause demyelination of peripheral nerves; motor neuropathy predominates. Renal damage occurs from precipitation of a lead–protein complex that causes renal dysfunction and hypertension with prolonged exposure.

CLINICAL FINDINGS

Symptoms and signs of lead toxicity are often not noticeable, or may be subtle and nonspecific. With the improvement in preventing childhood lead poisoning in the United States, the most likely cause for ED referral in such children is a high BLL found during a screening program. Because the effects of detrimental lead levels are often clinically silent, emphasis should be placed on periodic screening in preschool children. Symptomatic lead poisoning, on the other hand, is characterized by one or more of the following: decrease in play activity, irritability, drowsiness, anorexia, sporadic vomiting, intermittent abdominal pain, constipation, regression of newly acquired skills (particularly speech), sensorineural hearing loss, clumsiness, and slight attenuation of growth. It is not uncommon for some children to be seen by a health care practitioner several times with these nonspecific symptoms before lead poisoning is even considered. Lead toxicity is grossly correlated with BLL (Table 69–1), but is more pronounced in young children and in those with prolonged exposure to lead. Overt lead encephalopathy may ensue after days or weeks of symptoms and presents with ataxia, forceful vomiting, lethargy, or stupor, and can progress to coma and seizures. Although this is seen less commonly than in the past, it represents a medical emergency. It may occur with a BLL 70 μg/dL, but is generally associated with BLLs in excess of 100 μg/dL. Permanent brain damage can result in 70% to 80% of children with lead encephalopathy, even with optimal treatment. Peripheral neuropathy is rare under the age of 5, and consists mainly of motor weakness in upper and lower limbs. In the upper limbs, weakness can result in wrist drop. Lead nephropathy can result in Fanconi syndrome and acute tubular necrosis, but is rare in children. Mild elevation in liver transaminases can occur. Microcytic anemia frequently coexists with lead poisoning.

Because lead poisoning is so frequent and can present with a variety of signs and symptoms, a high index of sus-

Table 69–1. Clinical Manifestations of Lead Poisoning in Children

Clinical Severity	Typical Blood Lead Levels (μg/dL)
Severe	>70–100
CNS: Encephalopathy (coma, altered sensorium, seizures, bizarre behavior, ataxia, apathy, incoordination, loss of developmental skills; papilledema, cranial nerve palsy, signs of increased ICP)	
GI: Persistent vomiting	
Heme: Pallor (anemia)	
Mild/Moderate (preencephalopathic)	>50–70
CNS: Hyperirritable behavior, intermittent lethargy, decreased interest in play, "difficult" child	
GI: Intermittent vomiting, abdominal pain, anorexia	
Asymptomatic	>10
CNS: Impaired cognition, behavior	
PNS: Impaired fine-motor coordination	
Misc: Impaired hearing, growth	

Abbreviations: CNS, central nervous system; ICP, intracranial pressure; PNS, peripheral nervous system; GI, gastrointestinal; Heme, hematologic; Misc, miscellaneous.

picion is required to make the diagnosis. The differential diagnosis of lead poisoning includes iron deficiency, behavior and emotional disorders, abdominal colic and constipation, mental retardation, afebrile seizures, subdural hematoma, CNS neoplasms, and sickle cell anemia.

LABORATORY AND DIAGNOSTIC TESTING

The definitive diagnosis of lead poisoning and assessment of its severity and chronicity depends on laboratory testing. The most important test is a venous BLL (see Table 69–1). Periodic screening is important in all children aged 6 months to 2 years who live in houses built before 1970, who live near active lead smelters or other lead-related industries, in those who have siblings with lead poisoning, or with parents who have lead-related occupations or hobbies. If screening done on capillary blood indicates a high BLL, a confirmatory venous BLL is obtained because of the potential for lead dust skin contamination in capillary samples. Because 99% of the lead in blood is in the red cells, lead assay is done on whole blood collected in tubes with heparin or EDTA. Definition of lead poisoning classes, the toxic effects of lead at various levels, and the recommended actions are outlined in Table 69–2. Elevation in BLL is followed by a rise in the free EP or ZPP. This occurs because lead inhibits ferrochetolase during heme formation (see Figure 69–1). Because an elevated EP or ZPP reflects inhibited heme synthesis and affects only newly formed RBCs, this effect occurs at BLL 25 µg/dL and lags behind the initial rise in BLL by 2 to 3 weeks. Thus, low EP or ZPP and high BLL suggest recent acute exposure, whereas elevated EP or ZPP with high BLL suggests chronic exposure. An elevated EP/ZPP may also be seen in iron-deficient anemia because of the lack of iron availability for heme synthesis. Because iron-deficient anemia is common with lead poisoning, iron deficiency likely compounds the magnitude of EP/ZPP elevation.

Radiographic evidence of lead poisoning consists of bands of increased density at the metaphyses of long bones that are best seen in radiographs of the distal femur and proximal tibia and fibula (Figure 69–2). The popular term *lead lines* is a misnomer, because the increased radiopacity is caused by abnormal calcification from the disrupted metabolism of bone matrix rather than actual deposition of lead in the metaphysis. The formation of lead lines requires a few months of BLLs above 45 µg/dL, and their width grossly correlates with the duration of lead poisoning. Radiopaque foreign material seen in the intestine on a flat abdominal film suggests a recent (48 hours previously) ingestion of lead-containing paint chips. However, a substantial recent ingestion of small particulate lead may not be seen in a flat abdominal film, such as in the case of lead-laden dust in old homes where renovation or deleading has been done by sanding and dry scraping of painted surfaces. Inner-city adolescents with nonspecific symptoms consistent with plumbism and retained shrapnel noted on radiographs should be evaluated with a BLL, because data suggest that chronic plumbism may be a consequence of slowly leaching lead from retained bullets.

Other essential tests include measurement of hemoglobin and hematocrit, evaluation of the patient's iron status, examination of the blood smear for basophilic stippling of the erythrocytes, and a urinalysis to exclude glycosuria or proteinuria. A spinal tap should be avoided in children with lead encephalopathy owing to the risk for herniation from increased intracranial pressure.

Table 69–2. Pediatric Screening and Followup Guidelines

Screening

Screen
  1. All high-risk children at 1 and 2 y (3–6 y if not previously screened)
  2. Selected low-risk children (any affirmative answer to risk questions) (high-risk community = 12% of young children with elevated BPb, 27% of homes built before 1950; all children enrolled in Medicaid)

Personal Risk Questionnaire
  1. Does your child live in or regularly visit a home built before 1950?
  2. Does your child live in or regularly visit a home built before 1978 undergoing remodeling or renovation (ot has been within 5 mo)?
  3. Specific exposed questions:
    Personal, family history of lead poisoning
    Occupational, industrial, hobby exposures
    Proximity to major roadway
    Hot tap water for consumption
    Cultural exposures (folk remedies, cosmetics, ceramic food containers, trips, residence outside US, international adoptees)
    Migrant farm workers, receipt of poverty assistance
    History of pica for paint chips, dirt
    History of iron deficiency

Followup

BPb (µg/dL)	Recommended Action
<9	Retest in 1 y
10–14	Retest in 3 mo; education
15–19	Retest in 2 mo; education; if 15–19 twice, refer for case management
20–44	Clinical evaluation; education; environmental investigation
45–69	Clinical evaluation and vase management within 48 h; education; environmental investigation; chelation therapy
≥70	Hospitalize child; immediate chelation therapy; education; environmental investigation

BPb, venous blood lead.
Source: Reprinted, with permission, from Centers for Disease Control and Prevention: Screening Young Children for Lead Poisoning: Guidance for State and Local Public Health officials. US Dept of Health and Human Services, Public Health Service, Federal Register, Feb 21, 1997.

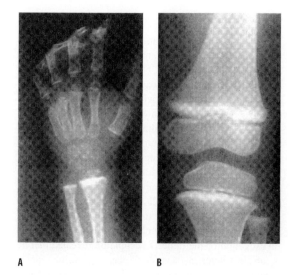

A   B

Fig. 69–2. Lead lines seen on an x-ray. (*Source:* Goldfrank LR, Flomenbaum N, Lewin N, et al, eds: *Goldfrank's Toxicologic Emergencies.* 7th ed. New York: McGraw-Hill; 2002:1201.)

A new method for evaluating the total body lead burden by x-ray fluorometry of bone lead has been introduced in adults and is being studied in children. With further reduction in radiation, this technique may eventually supersede blood lead screening in populations with low blood levels.

MANAGEMENT AND DISPOSITION

The principles of management in lead poisoning include identification and removal of the lead source, correction of dietary deficiencies that enhance lead absorption, pharmacologic chelation, supportive therapy, and long-term follow-up.

For patients with lead levels between 10 and 20 μg/dL, treatment consists of environmental management, nutritional evaluation, and repeated screening. In many cases, this involves removing the child from the home until the source of lead exposure is identified and removed.

Removal of lead-based paint from the home should be done by lead abatement professionals. Nutritional intervention consists of a review of the child's diet and correction of deficiencies of iron, calcium, and zinc. If there is evidence of recent ingestion of lead paint on an abdominal film, cathartics or whole bowel irrigation (WBI) with a polyethylene glycol/electrolyte solution should be considered. WBI at a rate of 500 cc to 2 L/h or 25 cc/kg/h

in small children should be performed until rectal effluent is clear and repeat x-rays are normal. For patients with BLLs between 20 and 44 μg/dL, environmental evaluation and remediation are required. Pharmacologic intervention may be indicated and is accomplished on an outpatient basis if the child is asymptomatic.

Oral dimercaptosuccinic acid (DMSA) is currently the only treatment approved for oral chelation of childhood lead poisoning. DMSA is chemically similar to BAL and produces a lead diuresis comparable to that produced by $CaNa_2EDTA$ without depletion of other metals. It is given 30 mg/kg/d in three divided doses for the first 5 days, then 20 mg/kg/d in two divided doses for 14 more days. It has a bad odor and may cause nausea and vomiting, rashes, and transient elevation of liver enzymes. It is commonly used as an outpatient regimen for patients with lead levels higher than 20 μg/dL, only after environmental and nutritional interventions have also been initiated. Sending a child back to the source of lead exposure while actively on chelation therapy may be detrimental. Even though some authors have questioned the long-term benefits of chelating children with levels between 20 to 44 μg/dL, *considering* the therapeutic option of chelation therapy with oral DMSA is still supported by several health organizations, including the CDC.

Outpatient treatment is also possible with oral D-penicillamine (Cuprimine). Currently it is not approved by the U.S. Food and Drug Administration for the treatment of lead poisoning, but is approved for other uses and has been successful in children not able to tolerate DMSA therapy. Side effects include leukopenia, thrombocytopenia, transient elevation of liver enzymes, vomiting, and, rarely, nephrotoxicity. It must not be given to patients allergic to penicillin. Iron supplements are avoided in patients treated with D-penicillamine, because they can block its absorption.

Children with asymptomatic lead poisoning and BLLs of 45 to 69 μg/dL are admitted to the hospital for chelation therapy with either $CaNa_2EDTA$ or DMSA and aggressive environmental investigation. Children with symptomatic lead poisoning and all patients with BLLs >70 μg/dL should be treated with BAL at a dose of 25 mg/kg/d in six divided doses given by deep intramuscular injection (Figure 69–3). Once the first dose is given and adequate urine flow is established, $CaNa_2EDTA$ is added as a continuous intravenous infusion at 50 mg/kg/d (1500 mg/m²/d) in dextrose or saline. When treating a child with encephalopathy, the intramuscular route for $CaNa_2EDTA$ with procaine 0.5% is preferred to reduce the amount of fluid administered. This combined treatment is given for 2

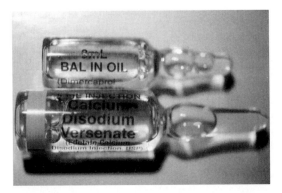

Fig. 69–3. Chelation agents for severe lead poisoning: BAL and calcium EDTA.

to 5 days, with daily monitoring of blood urea nitrogen (BUN), creatinine, liver enzymes, and electrolytes. The child may be transitioned to oral DMSA therapy if symptoms improve and/or the lead level decreases appropriately.

Side effects of CaNa$_2$EDTA include fever and transient renal dysfunction reflected in a rise in BUN, proteinuria, and hematuria. BAL may cause nausea and vomiting, transient hypertension, fever, transient elevation in liver enzymes, and hemolysis in G6PD-deficient patients. Iron can form a toxic complex with BAL and should not be administered simultaneously. BAL is formulated with a peanut oil diluent and should not be administered to patients with a peanut allergy.

Lead encephalopathy should always be considered in young children with mental status changes and no other clinical evidence of infection. Lead encephalopathy is treated with fluid restriction, mechanical hyperventilation, and furosemide or mannitol. Dexamethasone may have a salutary effect in improving vascular integrity. Seizures are controlled with diazepam. Patients with lead encephalopathy are best managed in an intensive care unit.

Lead poisoning is most commonly a consequence of chronic exposure, and a rebound elevation of BLL is expected after each course of chelation therapy as lead is mobilized from body stores. Repeat BLLs 2 weeks after the completion of chelation gives a reasonable peak rebound level. Because successful management of lead poisoning demands environmental, nutritional, and pharmacologic interventions over a prolonged time course, these children should be followed by clinicians who are familiar with the multiple aspects of this disease and who can provide a multidisciplinary team approach. The importance of removing the child from the source of lead exposure cannot be overemphasized.

CASE OUTCOME

The patient's mother is instructed to bring the patient to the hospital for admission and chelation therapy. On arrival, temperature is 98.9°F, blood pressure 90/50 mmHg, heart rate 95 bpm. Clinical examination is remarkable for a healthy-appearing child with pale palpebral conjunctiva. The child's interaction with her mother and the examiner are appropriate. She has no gross neurologic deficits. A screening abdominal radiograph is normal, x-rays of her limbs demonstrate lead lines, and her EP level is elevated. The child is admitted to the hospital and receives 2 days of BAL and CaNa$_2$EDTA parenteral therapy. She responds well and is transitioned to oral DMSA therapy for the next 14 days. Intense environmental investigation of the child's home is unrevealing. Investigation of the father's occupation revealed that he is an instructor at a police academy firing range. Examination of his clothes confirm dust contaminated with lead from the firing range. He is instructed to change his clothes at work before coming home to his family. Follow-up evaluations of the child demonstrate appropriate declines in her BLL, and her constipation and fussiness resolve.

SUGGESTED READINGS

American Academy of Pediatrics, Committee on Drugs: Treatment guidelines for lead exposure in children. *Pediatrics* 96:155–160, 1995.

Angle CR: Childhood lead poisoning and its treatment. *Ann Rev Pharmacol Toxicol* 33:409–434, 1993.

Canfield RL, Henderson CR, Cory-Slechta DA, et al. Intellectual impairment in children with blood lead concentrations below 10 mcg per deciliter. *N Engl J Med* 348:1517–1526, 2003.

Farrell SE, Vandevander P, Schoffstall JM, Lee DC. Blood lead levels in emergency department patients with retained bullets and shrapnel. *Acad Emerg Med* 6:208–212, 1999.

Graef J: Lead poisoning, parts 1–3. *Clin Toxicol Rev* 14:8, 1992.

Henretig FM: Lead. In: Goldfrank LR, Flomenbaum N, Lewin N, et al, eds: *Goldfrank's Toxicologic Emergencies.* 7th Edition. New York: McGraw-Hill; 2002:1200–1227.

Kaufmann RB, Staes CJ, Matte TD: Deaths related to lead poisoning in the United States, 1979–1998. *Environ Res* 91:78–84, 2003.

Lanphear BP, Dietrich KN, Berger O: Prevention of lead toxicity in US children. *Ambul Pediatr* 3:27–36, 2003.

Lidsky TI, Schneider JS: Lead neurotoxicity in children: Basic mechanisms and clinical correlates. *Brain* 126:5–19, 2003.

Liebelt EL, Shannon MW: Oral chelators for childhood poisoning. *Pediatr Ann* 23:616–626, 1994.

Liu X, Dietrich KN, Radcliffe J, et al: Do children with falling lead levels have improved cognition? *Pediatrics* 110:787–791, 2002.

Manton WI, Angle CR, Stanek SL, et al: Acquisition and retention of lead by young children. *Environ Res* 82:60–80, 2000.

Pirkel JL, Brody DJ, Gunter EW, et al: The decline in blood lead levels in the United States—The National Health and Nutrition Examination Surveys (NHANES). *JAMA* 272:284–291, 1994.

Rogan J, Dietrich KN, Ware JH, et al: The effect of chelation therapy with succimer on neuropsychological development in children exposed to lead. *N Engl J Med* 344:1421–1426, 2001.

Shannon M, Graef JW: Lead intoxication in infancy. *Pediatrics* 89:87–90, 1992.

Shannon MW. Severe lead poisoning in pregnancy. *Ambul Pediatr* 3:37–39, 2003.

Su M, Barrueto F, Hoffman RS: Childhood lead poisoning from paint chips: A continuing problem. *J Urban Health* 79:491–501, 2002.

Wright RO, Tsaih SW, Schwartz J, et al: Association between iron deficiency and blood lead level in a longitudinal analysis of children followed in an urban primary care clinic. *J Pediatr* 142:9–14, 2003.

70

Mercury

Charles A. McKay
Alberto Perez
Rachel Goldstein

HIGH-YIELD FACTS

- Mercury may occur in several forms, elemental, inorganic or organic. The absorption of mercury and its toxic effects vary with the form.

- Inhalation of large amounts of elemental mercury causes an acute pneumonitis, then neurologic symptoms of erethism.

- Ingestion of mercury salts causes an erosive gastroenteritis and acute tubular necrosis (ATN).

- Organic mercury (particularly methylmercury) is the major concern for toxicity. Although consumption of fish, particularly larger, predatory species, may result in measurable increases in mercury body burden, acute clinical manifestations of mercury toxicity typically do not occur.

- Daily consumption of methylmercury-containing fish during pregnancy has been associated with decrements in infant neurodevelopment and should therefore be avoided.

CASE PRESENTATION

A mother brings her 5-year-old child to the office for evaluation of an upper respiratory infection. The child has been diagnosed with pervasive development delay, which the mother attributes to his previous vaccinations. The mother is 8 weeks pregnant with another child and is concerned about mercury exposure. She has investigated having her dental amalgams removed, and asks if this would be safe for her unborn child. She is also very upset because she broke a thermometer while measuring her son's temperature and does not know if she cleaned up all the mercury. She knows that "it only takes one thermometer to pollute an entire lake," so wonders if she should have her home cleaned by an environmental clean-up company at a cost of $2500. She has a friend who has received chelation therapy because of fatigue (and a finding of elevated urinary mercury) and is considering the same to flush the toxins from her body before her child is born.

INTRODUCTION

This composite patient represents many of the features encountered in discussions of mercury exposure and toxicity. Although mercury toxicity is not a commonly entertained clinical diagnosis, fear of mercury's effects is very common. Clinicians are unlikely to see a true case of mercury poisoning in a decade; however, they are very likely to be questioned regarding mercury exposure from a variety of sources, including dietary, medicinal, and environmental.

Mercury is an element that has a long history of use in industry, medicine, and dentistry. It is present in all soil and water, and is mined from ore in locations throughout the world. Volcanic activity, erosion, and forest fires have always released mercury into the air and water, but industrial activity over the last century has greatly enhanced this process. Once extracted from ore, it is a liquid in its elemental form. It is heavy, having a density approximately 14 times that of water. It has several valence states $(0, +1, +2)$, meaning that it can exist in its elemental form or bound to other compounds. The toxic effects depend both on the form of mercury present and the route of exposure to the patient. Mercury is biopersistent, meaning that once an organism incorporates the metal, elimination is slow or incomplete. Mercury may be bioconcentrated, bioaccumulated, and biomagnified. Bioconcentration and bioaccumulation are characteristics of all persistent contaminants that are incorporated into organisms low in the food chain, which higher predators then consume. In the case of mercury, aquatic anaerobic bacteria biotransform the elemental form of the metal into organic methylmercury, a potent neurotoxin. The consumption of mercury by organisms higher in the food chain biomagnifies the potential toxic effect of mercury. These features have raised concern regarding the effects of environmental mercury on human health.

This chapter identifies the varied toxicity of the specific mercury compounds (elemental, inorganic, and organic) and highlights the differences between acute and chronic effects from low- and high-level exposures. Table 70–1 summarizes many of the varied aspects of mercury exposure.

EPIDEMIOLOGY

Most common encounters with large amounts of mercury are its elemental form, such as is found in fluorescent lights, switches, sphygmomanometers, thermometers, and other measuring devices. No longer manufactured in the United States, mercury batteries were also a potential source of exposure. Certain cultural practices and folk medicines represent a potentially occult source of mercury exposure. The American Association of Poison Control Centers received over 21,000 calls pertaining to mercury exposures in 2001. More than 80% of these were the result of broken thermometers. Of all the mercury calls, there was only one death, resulting from inhalation of a large volume of mercury fumes released in a small, enclosed space. A review of calls over 38 months between January 1, 2000 and March 31, 2003 identified over 4000 exposures in children younger than 6 years of age, with no major effects. Fifteen moderate effects were noted, the majority of which were related to broken glass.

Historically, pediatric mercury toxicity was associated most commonly with exposure to inorganic mercury salts. The use of calomel (mercurous chloride) as a teething agent exposed large numbers of children to small, repeated doses of mercury salts. Although most clinicians today encounter questions regarding exposures to elemental mercury, such as from broken thermometers,

the driving force behind expressed concerns are fears related to possible effects of organic mercury.

The high-profile neurologic disasters of Minamata Bay and contaminated grain episodes in Iraq serve as stark reminders of the possible neurotoxic effects of large amounts of mercury. This is most applicable to higher-risk groups such as pregnant women and neonates.

DEVELOPMENTAL

Fetal Mercury Exposure

Elemental Mercury

Maternal mercury vapor inhalation is a potential source for systemic elemental mercury exposure. Most of the studies on mercury vapor exposure are epidemiologic, involving dental practitioners and the use of dental amalgams. There are no conclusive reproductive effects on men or women from mercury exposure in this work environment. Studies are underway regarding low-level exposures and their effects on reproduction in both men and women. One investigation documents placental accumulation of mercury and a correlation with increasing numbers of amalgam dental fillings, suggesting elemental mercury as the source. However, both maternal and newborn cord blood mercury measurements were many times less than those associated with toxicity.

Animal studies of offspring exposed in utero to mercury vapor, which is known to penetrate the placental barrier more readily than inorganic mercury, revealed mercury in the brain and kidney. These offspring displayed behavioral changes at a maternal mercury vapor exposure of 0.3 mg/m^3 for 4 h/d, greatly exceeding the occupational Threshold Limit Value, an 8-hour average mercury vapor concentration of 0.025 mg/m^3.

The amount of mercury vapor released in chewing, and the small conversion of mercury to methylmercury by oral bacteria, is insignificant with respect to systemic toxicity.

Organic Mercury

The developing fetus is most sensitive to the neurotoxic effects of methylmercury. Numerous animal studies address fetal incorporation of mercury; human data are largely limited to estimates of exposure following historical mass health disasters.

Large numbers of humans were exposed to methylmercury in two historic events. The 1950s Minamata

Table 70–1. Aspects of Mercury Toxicity Vary With the Specific Form of Mercury Exposure

Mercury Form	Common Name or Sources	Exposure Route of Concern	Primary Target Organs	Relative Toxic (Lethal) Range	Onset of Symptoms With Heavy Exposure	Symptoms and Progression	Biomonitoring or Analytic Tools	Treatment Options
Elemental	Quicksilver; sphygmomanometers, fluorescent light ballast, switches	Inhaled vapors	Pulmonary, CNS	Unlikely if ingested; 1 mg/m^3 chronic inhalation[a]	Hours	Dyspnea progressing to ARDS; delayed onset; neurologic	Timed urinary excretion	Chelation
Salt	Calomel (Hg$^+$) Mercuric chloride (Hg^{+2})	Ingestion	GI, renal	10 mg/kg (Hg$^+$ less toxic than Hg^{+2})	Minutes	Vomiting and voluminous, bloody diarrhea followed by ATN	Timed urinary excretion	Volume resuscitation
Alkyl-	Methyl mercury	Skin, ingestion	CNS	10 mg/kg	Days–weeks	Paresthesias, ataxia, visual field constriction, behavioral, coma	Whole blood measurement	Chelation?
Aryl-	Mercurochrome	Ingestion	CNS	~1/10 as toxic as alkyl	Days	As with alkyl-	As with alkyl-	Chelation?

[a] A cubic meter of air (m^3) is 1000 L, representing approximately 12 hours of ventilation by a 10-kg child.

Abbreviations: ARDS, acute respiratory distress syndrome; ATN, acute tubular necrosis; CNS, central nervous system; GI, gastrointestinal.

Bay, Japan, disaster was traced to a chlor-alkali factory: methylmercury effluent entered the food chain and contaminated fish, a staple of the local diet. The 1970s Iraq disaster occurred when wheat, treated with a methylmercury-containing fungicide in preparation for planting, was used instead to bake bread. Both outbreaks led to widespread poisoning, and children exposed in utero displayed chorea, ataxia, tremors, and seizures. Other severe neurologic deficits among children included cerebral palsy, microcephaly, and psychomotor retardation. Measurements of maternal hair mercury provided estimates of fetal mercury exposure, and correlated with neurologic deficits. Delayed onset to walking was seen with maternal hair mercury concentrations above 20 ppm, and ataxia, dysarthria, deafness, and death were outcomes associated with concentrations progressively above 100 ppm, which correlated with maternal blood concentrations of 400 μg/L. These short-term or high-level exposures may not translate well to the very low-level exposures typically seen in maternal–fetal pairs with low-to-moderate fish consumption.

Epidemiologic studies that attempt to correlate neurodevelopment in children with maternal ingestion of methylmercury have shown conflicting results. This probably reflects the varying amount and intensity of consumption, as well as underlying nutritional and social factors. Studies from the Seychelle Islands indicate that low levels of mercury consumption are actually associated with improved testing results; this has been attributed to the beneficial aspects of fish consumption. Studies from the Faroe Islands, where episodic consumption of pilot whale containing mercury at amounts 10 to 100 times the usual diet (as well as large amounts of polychlorinated biphenyls), suggest minor decrements in some test scores. Based on these studies, a committee of the National Research Council has determined that methylmercury consumption of 0.1 μg/kg body weight per day is a scientifically justified level of methylmercury exposure for maternal–fetal pairs to avoid neurologic injury. This conservative dietary allowance has led to health advisories regarding the consumption of fish during pregnancy and breastfeeding in nearly all states.

Neonatal and Infant Effects

Organic Mercury

The disasters mentioned and other mass mercury exposures in Niigata, Japan, and in Canada, Ghana, and Guatemala provide a uniform picture of the symptomology of methylmercury poisoning. Mental retardation, chronic brain damage, developmental disorders, liver disease, hypertension, and failure to thrive were noted in children and mothers exposed to the contaminated fish. Also, much of the follow-up of the Iraqi grain consumption disaster identified more subtle effects in the form of delayed achievement of developmental milestones and abnormal tendon reflexes in children with prenatal exposure.

Exposure to ethylmercury in the form of thimerosal-containing preservatives in vaccines has generated intense interest. Although exposure to *ethyl*mercury from a full series of childhood vaccines (200 μg) over a period of 6 months could have exceeded the Environmental Protection Agency's conservative reference dose for consumption of *methyl*mercury (0.1 μg/kg/d), this amount is far below the amount of mercury known to cause harm, even for fetal exposure. In addition, the kinetics and toxicity of ethylmercury differ from that of methylmercury. As a precautionary step, vaccine manufacturers essentially eliminated thimerosal from childhood vaccines in the United States by 2002. Although the increasing use of childhood vaccines has been linked to the apparent rise in the incidence of autistic spectrum disorders, most studies have refuted this association, including a recent report analyzing the reported incidence of these disorders in Denmark where thimerosal was removed from vaccines in 1992. The Institute of Medicine has also evaluated the evidence and finds that although developmental effects from ethylmercury are biologically plausible, there is no evidence of causality. Nonetheless, there is still much political and emotional opinion regarding this association. When parents or others present concerns about vaccines, the health care provider can provide information regarding the following:

1. Dose: very small with respect to safety factors considered in vaccine production
2. Dissimilarity of ethylmercury effects to those of methylmercury
3. Significant risks associated with failure to vaccinate

Following the Centers for Disease Control and Prevention/American Academy of Pediatrics advisory, vaccination rates fell, and deaths occurred from vaccine-preventable illnesses.

Aromatic mercury compounds include mercurochrome. Accidental ingestions of this dermal antiseptic agent are nontoxic. Chronic inhalation exposure to phenylmercury-containing fungicides have resulted in cases of acrodynia in the past.

PHARMACOKINETICS AND TOXICOKINETICS

The kinetics of mercury are very much dependent on the class of mercurial compound and thus must be discussed separately.

Elemental

Although oral exposure to elemental mercury is considered nontoxic, the presence of anatomic defects such as a fistula or slow gastrointestinal (GI) transit may be associated with increased absorption. Mercury vapor is absorbed rapidly through the respiratory tract. Once absorbed through the alveolar membrane, mercury has a predilection for the kidneys, liver, spleen, and nervous system. Peak concentrations in the central nervous system (CNS) can be delayed for a few days; nonetheless, intense vapor exposure may rapidly elevate CNS concentrations. The elimination of elemental mercury has a biphasic pattern—an initial rapid decline and a later, slower phase—that yields a biological half-life of approximately 60 days. Mercury is eliminated via the fecal and urinary routes.

Inorganic

Unlike the elemental species, inorganic mercury is absorbed primarily through the GI tract; only 10% of a given dose is absorbed. The most common salt is mercuric chloride (divalent), which requires dissociation before it is absorbed. Calomel (mercurous chloride), a monovalent salt, requires transformation to a divalent compound before it is absorbed. Various case reports of dermal application of calomel-containing ointment or powders document integumentary absorption of inorganic salts. Once absorbed into the blood, inorganic mercury is bound in equal proportions to erythrocytes and plasma proteins. Concentrations drop rapidly in the blood, but rise within the kidneys, affecting primarily the renal tubules. Inorganic mercury is poorly lipophilic and therefore penetrates the CNS only partially; once the blood–brain barrier (BBB) is crossed, the metal accumulates in the cerebral and cerebellar cortices. Excretion of inorganic mercury is primarily fecal, although urinary excretion is observed following chronic exposure.

Organic

Organic mercury exposure is usually by ingestion, although dermal and inhalational absorption may be a concern in some situations. Methylmercury is approximately 90% absorbed through the GI tract. This percentage decreases with longer alkyl chains. Given their lipid solubility, once absorbed, alkyl mercurial compounds readily cross the BBB as well as the placenta. Fetal blood mercury levels are found to be equal to or higher than maternal levels, although the half-life of methylmercury in the child appears shorter. Adult data reveal a half-life of approximately 40 to 50 days. A study of infants following administration of thimerosal-containing vaccines found that the elimination half-life of mercury was approximately 7 days and that the GI tract is a possible mode of elimination of parenterally administered thimerosal. When ingested, methylmercury is primarily (90%) eliminated though feces. Although the CNS effects are diffuse, damage within the cerebellum, calcarine fissure, and precentral gyrus are characteristic. The classic triad of methylmercury toxicity includes dysarthria, ataxia, and constricted visual fields. Perinatal exposure to methylmercury may cause mental retardation and cerebral palsy.

PATHOPHYSIOLOGY

Once absorbed systemically, mercury has a predilection for the kidneys, liver, spleen, and CNS. Short-chain alkylmercurials (methyl- and ethylmercury) penetrate red blood cells and bind to hemoglobin. Methylmercury crosses the BBB, and mercury is sequestered into the lysosomal dense bodies of neurons. Mercurials are attracted to sulfhydryl groups and bind to enzymes and metalloproteins. As one example, mercury combines with the sulfhydryl group of *S*-adenosylmethionine, which is a cofactor for catecholamine-O-methyltransferase (COMT). The inhibition of COMT allows accumulation of norepinephrine, epinephrine, and dopamine; this may account for some of the symptoms seen in acrodynia and erethism.

CLINICAL PRESENTATION

Acute Exposure

Elemental Mercury

Ingestion

The GI absorption of elemental mercury is of negligible clinical significance and considered essentially nontoxic. Thus, caregivers should be reassured that the concern of a broken mercury thermometer in the mouth is the potential for injury from glass.

Inhalation

Inhalation of large amounts of mercury vapor results in an acute, severe illness that may include respiratory distress and noncardiac pulmonary edema. Erosive dermatitis and a characteristic neurologic syndrome called *erethism* may follow should the patient recover from the acute inhalational effects. Patients with erethism often complain of mood swings and exhibit social withdrawal.

Inorganic Mercury

The acute ingestion of mercury salts is very rare, but is seen on occasion following accidental or suicidal ingestion of pesticides containing mercuric chloride. The patient presents with vomiting, abdominal cramps, and diarrhea; volume loss and third spacing lead to cardiovascular collapse. ATN ensues. Immune-mediated glomerulonephritis has also been reported.

Organic Mercury

Symptoms following acute exposures to organic mercurials are often delayed several days. Personality changes, visual field constriction, cerebellar dysfunction, and coma characterize the progressive neurologic deterioration.

Chronic Exposure

Acrodynia (pink disease) is the classic presentation of mercury poisoning in children. Clinical features include an erythematous rash of the extremities that later desquamates, insomnia, personality changes, irritability, profuse sweating, hypertension, and tachycardia. Following the removal from the market of mercury salt-containing teething powders like calomel and phenylmercuric fungicide-containing house paint, cases are rarely seen, but still may occur with inhalational exposure to elemental mercury. Although considered a hypersensitivity reaction to mercury, some of the effects of mercury on enzyme function may also contribute to the symptom complex.

LABORATORY AND DIAGNOSTIC TESTING

Although it is often stated that "one mercury thermometer will pollute an entire lake," this is actually more a commendation of laboratory techniques that are now capable of detecting mercury at concentrations of parts per trillion, than it is a condemnation of mercury health effects (none at this concentration). The diagnosis of mercury poisoning should rest on a combination of clinical and laboratory features. A history of exposure or spectrum of symptoms referable to the particular type of mercury as noted should lead to appropriate laboratory investigation. Of critical importance is modification of dietary intake. There should be no seafood or seaweed-based dietary supplements for several days prior to collection to avoid other potential sources of mercury. Also, appropriate collection container and transport media should be used to avoid external contaminants. In general, a timed urine collection is the most reliable method for determining body burden of elemental or inorganic mercury, and generally reflects exposures over the previous month or two. Diurnal variations of mercury excretion may explain inconsistent spot urine measurements. Nonetheless, they may be useful as screening tests or at the initiation of therapy in a clinically poisoned patient. Although 24-h urine mercury measurements yield the best estimate of mercury excretion, a practical compromise would be a measurement of mercury concentration in a first-void or early morning collection; this would reflect an approximately 8-h collection. Urinary excretion under normal conditions should not exceed 50 μg in 24 hours.

Recent dietary intake affects blood mercury determinations; levels decline quickly following acute exposures to elemental or inorganic mercury. Mercury speciation into organic and inorganic/elemental forms can be helpful, but is not widely available. Whole-blood mercury measurements are more reliable as a measurement of body burden of organic mercury, because this compound is relatively concentrated in the red blood cell. Normal blood mercury levels rarely exceed 1.5 μg/dL, although this level may be elevated several days after consuming certain types of seafood. Hair analysis at a reputable laboratory may be useful for documenting long-term excessive exposure to organic mercury. However, this is generally more a research than a clinical tool. For chronic exposures, concentration of mercury in hair, primarily indicative of methylmercury exposure, is approximately 300 times that from blood. Most of the U.S. population has <1 ppm mercury in hair; maternal measurements for infants showing clinical mercury poisoning were in excess of 100 ppm.

MANAGEMENT

Elemental Mercury Exposure

Ingestion

GI absorption of elemental mercury may become a clinical concern when the mercury is trapped in the appendix and bacterial action creates organic mercurials that are readily absorbed. There is ongoing controversy over the proper management of retained mercury in the appendix. It is reasonable to obtain an abdominal radiograph after a large ingestion (e.g., a ruptured Miller-Abbott tube) and follow urinary excretion if there is residual retained mercury.

Inhalation

Significant symptoms require exposure to amounts of mercury in vapor form greatly in excess of those found immediately after a household mercury spill. The importance of minimizing vaporization after a spill should therefore be emphasized. Protocols for spill management include visualizing mercury droplets with a bright light, scraping together all visible mercury using an adsorbent product if possible, and avoiding dispersion or vaporization by such methods as sweeping or vacuuming. A special mercury vacuum with restricted exhaust is available for larger workplace spills. Assistance should be sought from the state Department of Environmental Protection and the regional poison control center for spills larger than a household clinical thermometer. Efforts to reduce the reliance on mercury measuring devices such as sphygmomanometers and thermometers are worthwhile, given the cost and environmental concern associated with spills from these items.

In the rare circumstance following a significant exposure to elemental mercury when elevated urinary concentrations are documented, chelation therapy may become necessary once the patient is removed from the source of exposure. Developed in World War II, dimercaprol (British anti-lewisite [BAL]) was the mercury chelator of choice for years. Currently, it is reserved for severe mercury poisoning but is not recommended for organic mercury toxicity because of the potential of increasing CNS mercury concentrations secondary to postchelation redistribution. BAL is unstable, and must be administered intramuscularly. BAL is contraindicated in patients with renal dysfunction or peanut allergy because the antidote is contained in a peanut oil diluent.

More recently, less toxic, water-soluble congeners of dimercaprol, meso-2,3-dimercaptosuccinic acid (DMSA) and sodium 2,3-dimercapto-1-propanesulfonate (DMPS), have become available. The dosing of DMSA (Succimer) is 10 mg/kg/dose, TID for 5 days; then BID for 14 days. A 2-week hiatus or drug holiday is recommended for repeat cycles of therapy. The end point of therapy is guided by clinical symptoms and declining mercury levels in the urine.

Inorganic Mercury Exposure

Treatment is focused on volume resuscitation and prevention of ATN and resultant renal failure. Experimental studies indicate that chelators may mobilize mercury from renal tissue, but may then promote entry into motor neurons.

Organic Mercury Exposure

The progression of neurologic dysfunction following organic mercurial exposure is poorly amenable to treatment. Because CNS uptake is very rapid and symptom onset may be delayed for many days, chelation therapy is relatively ineffective. Nonetheless, it is frequently offered. Regimens generally follow those employed for lead treatment, with monitoring of urinary excretion during and after treatment. Recent animal data suggest that *N*-acetylcysteine may have utility in the early (presymptomatic) management of a recognized organic mercury intoxication, but human clinical data are lacking.

CASE OUTCOME

Despite the lack of evidence of any benefit from the steps under consideration, the mother is unconvinced. She thinks there is entirely too much exposure to mercury, and any steps to decrease this must be useful. The possibility that removal of amalgams will actually increase mercury exposure, and the risk of complexing other trace elements with chelation dissuade her from pursuing these steps. A referral to the fish advisory section of the state Department of Public Health is made, in order to obtain information regarding the benefits of fish consumption for her and her unborn child, while still minimizing mercury consumption. She takes the number of the regional poison center to obtain a procedure or referral for appropriate steps to clean up small mercury spills, and agrees to obtain a nonmercury thermometer replacement.

SUGGESTED READINGS

Ball LK, Ball R, Pratt RD: An assessment of thimerosal use in childhood vaccines. *Pediatrics* 107:1147–1154, 2001.

Ballatori N, Lieberman MW, Wang W: *N*-Acetylcysteine as an antidote in methylmercury poisoning. *Environ Health Persp* 106:267–271,1998.

Baum CR: Treatment of mercury intoxication. *Curr Opin Pediatr* 11:265–267, 1999.

Calder IM, Kelman GR, Masin H: Diurnal variations in urinary mercury excretion. *Hum Toxicol* 3:463–467, 1984.

Clarkson TW: The toxicology of mercury—Current exposures and clinical manifestations. *N Engl J Med* 349:1731–1737, 2003.

Clarkson TW, Amin-Zaki L, Al-Tikriti SK: An outbreak of methylmercury poisoning due to consumption of contaminated grain. *Fed Proc* 35:2395–2399, 1976.

Crump KS, Van Landingham C, Shamlaye C, et al: Benchmark concentrations for methylmercury obtained from the Seychelles Child Development Study. *Environ Health Perspect* 108: 257–263, 2000.

Environmental Protection Agency: *EPA Fish Advisories.* Available from http://www.epa.gov/waterscience/presentations/fish/maps_graphics_files/frame.htm. Accessed November 17, 2003.

Graeme KA, Pollack CV: Heavy metal toxicity, part I: arsenic and mercury. *J Emerg Med* 16:45–56, 1998.

Katz SA, Katz RB: Use of hair analysis for evaluating mercury intoxication of the human body: A review. *J Appl Toxicol* 12:79–84, 1992.

Kershaw TG, Clarkson TW, Dhahir PH: The relationship between blood levels and dose of methylmercury in man. *Arch Environ Health* 35:28–35, 1980.

Lewandowski TA, Pierce CH, Pingree SD, et al: Methylmercury distribution in the pregnant rat and embryo during early midbrain organogenesis. *Teratology* 66:235–241, 2002.

Litovitz TL, Klein-Schwartz W, Rodgers GC, et al: 2001 annual report of the American Association of Poison Control Centers—Toxic Exposure Surveillance System. *Am J Emerg Med* 20:391–452, 2002.

Madsen KM, Lauritsen MB, Pedersen CB, et al: Thimerosal and the occurrence of autism: negative ecological evidence from Danish population-based data. *Pediatrics* 112:604–606, 2003.

Mahaffey KR: Recent advances in recognition of low-level methylmercury poisoning. *Curr Opin Neurol* 13:699–707, 2000.

McKay CA, Holland MG, Nelson LS: A call to arms for medical toxicologists: The dose, not the detection, makes the poison [on line]. *Int J Med Toxicol* 6:1, 2003. Available from http://www.ijmt.net/6_1/6_1_1.html. Accessed November 17, 2003.

Phelps RW, Clarkston TW, Kershaw TG, et al: Interrelationship of blood and hair mercury concentrations in a North American population exposed to methylmercury. *Arch Environ Health* 35:161–168,1980.

Pichichero ME, Cernichiari E, Lopreiato J, et al: Mercury concentrations and metabolism in infants receiving vaccines containing thiomersal: A descriptive study. *Lancet* 360:1737–1741, 2002.

Schober SE, Sinks TH, Jones RL, et al: Blood mercury levels in US children and women of childbearing age, 1999–2000. *JAMA* 289:1667–1674, 2003.

Schuurs AH: Reproductive toxicity of occupational mercury. A review of the literature. *J Dent* 27:249–256, 1999.

Shih H, Gartner JC: Weight loss, hypertension, and limb pain in an 11-year-old boy. *J Pediatr* 138:566–569, 2001.

Watson B: Written communication, Bill Watson, PharmD, Associate Director, Toxicosurveillance. AAPCC; April, 2003.

Yoshida M: Placental to fetal transfer of mercury and fetotoxicity. *Tohoku J Exp Med* 196:79–88, 2002.

71

Blood and Cellular Toxins
Christina E. Hantsch

HIGH-YIELD FACTS

• Prevention of oxygen transport to cells is one mechanism by which blood and cellular toxins produce poisoning known as *systemic asphyxiation;* another is disruption of cells' ability to effectively utilize delivered oxygen.

• Methemoglobin-related cyanosis may precede the development of hypoxia-related signs and symptoms. Cyanosis is typically not seen in cases of carbon monoxide and cyanide poisoning.

• Fire victims with smoke inhalation can have poisoning from cyanide in addition to carbon monoxide.

• Exposure to blood and cellular toxins is most often via an inhalational route.

Chapters 72 through 74 cover blood and cellular toxins including two specific agents, carbon monoxide and cyanide, as well as a multitude of agents that produce their toxic effect by precipitating methemoglobinemia. *Methemoglobinemia* is a clinical state in which more than 1% to 2% of total hemoglobin is in the oxidized form known as methemoglobin. Methemoglobin, like carbon monoxide, is incapable of transporting oxygen. Likewise, carboxyhemoglobin is incapable of transporting oxygen. Prevention of oxygen transport to cells is one mechanism by which blood and cellular toxins produce poisoning known as *systemic asphyxiation;* another is disruption of cells' ability to effectively utilize delivered oxygen. Systemic asphyxiation induced by blood

and cellular toxins results in cellular-level hypoxia, even if there is adequate oxygen concentration in the ambient environment and normal pulmonary gas exchange.

Signs and symptoms of poisoning by blood and cellular toxins are first evident in organ systems that are most dependent on adequate oxygen supply. As a result, central nervous system (CNS) and cardiovascular system manifestations are seen early in the clinical course. CNS manifestations may include alterations in level of consciousness, headache, dizziness, confusion, agitation, and seizures. Cardiovascular manifestations include tachycardia, hypotension, and dysrhythmias. Signs and symptoms of oxygen deprivation to other organ system can be seen later in the course of blood and cellular toxin poisoning, or acutely with more severe intoxication. In cases of methemoglobinemia, early findings typically also include dermal cyanosis owing to the bluish appearance of methemoglobin when viewed through the skin. Methemoglobin-related cyanosis may precede the development of hypoxia-related signs and symptoms. Cyanosis is typically not seen in cases of carbon monoxide and cyanide poisoning.

EPIDEMIOLOGY

Blood and cellular toxins are significant causes of poisoning in the United States. Carbon monoxide alone is considered to be the leading cause of poisoning-related mortality in adults and children. In 2002 there were 15,904 cases of carbon monoxide exposure reported to poison centers, which included 4655 children. There were 31 reported fatalities. Despite these high figures, it is likely that many cases went unreported to poison centers. The National Center for Health Statistic death certificate data include more than 2500 fatalities each year attributed to carbon monoxide poisoning. Furthermore, many individuals who sought medical attention after significant carbon monoxide exposure likely presented with nonspecific symptoms, and the responsible etiology went unrecognized.

Cyanide exposures reported to poison centers in 2002 totaled 224, including 27 in children. Additional cases of cyanide poisoning, particularly in children, were reported with exposures to cyanogenic compounds such as acetonitrile in artificial nail remover. Of the 41 total reported cases, 34 involved children. Furthermore, although clear statistical figures are not available, fire victims with smoke inhalation can have poisoning from cyanide in addition to carbon monoxide. Specific epidemiologic information is also lacking on cases of toxin-induced methemoglobinemia, because exposure to multiple substances can precipitate this toxicity.

One important category of methemoglobin-inducing compounds is nitrites. These compounds, in addition to many others, are often abused as inhalants, particularly among adolescents. National and state surveys indicate that 6% of children have tried inhalants by fourth grade, with the incidence of use peaking during the eighth grade at 20%.

DEVELOPMENTAL CONSIDERATIONS

Several factors are important when considering blood and cellular toxin poisoning in children. First, exposure to blood and cellular toxins is most often via an inhalational route. Children have higher metabolic and respiratory rates than adults, which results in an increased toxin dose per body weight during an inhalational exposure. Second, the susceptibility of neonates to development of methemoglobinemia is high. Endogenous reduction of methemoglobin to hemoglobin occurs via the enzyme NADH-cytochrome β5 reductase. This enzyme is not fully active until approximately 4 to 6 months of age. This incomplete enzyme activity increases the susceptibility of neonates to methemoglobinemia. In addition to other factors, such as decreased gastric acid, it is believed that infantile methemoglobinemia is associated with well water nitrate exposure. Finally, the effects of blood and cellular toxins may be more pronounced in neonates. Fetal hemoglobin is present until 6 to 12 months of age. Fetal hemoglobin produces a leftward shift of the oxyhemoglobin dissociation curve and, for a given oxygen tension, tissue oxygenation is decreased. Methemoglobin and carboxyhemoglobin also produce a leftward shift of this curve.

MOST COMMON TOXINS

Carbon monoxide is rapidly absorbed during inhalational exposure. Carbon monoxide is produced by incomplete combustion of any carbon-based fuels. It is one of the main hazards of smoke inhalation during fires. Smoke inhalation is also a significant cause of cyanide exposure because hydrogen cyanide is a byproduct of the combustion of numerous materials including polyurethane, nylon, wool, and cotton. Other common sources of carbon monoxide include home heating systems, gas or wood stoves, and automobile engines. Exposure risk is increased if heating systems are malfunctioning, a furnace flue is blocked, or when automobiles have a malfunctioning exhaust system and are operated in an enclosed space.

Methemoglobinemia can occur after various inhalational exposures. Inhalant abuse of substances such as amyl or butyl nitrite (poppers or snappers), cyclohexyl nitrite (found in room deodorizer), nitrous oxide (found in whipped cream dispensers), or naphthalene (found in some moth balls) can precipitate methemoglobinemia. In addition, several oral and topical exposures, including therapeutic use of some pharmaceutical preparations, are common causes of methemoglobinemia. Cases have been reported after oral use of benzocaine in anesthetic pharyngeal spray or topical teething preparations, and sulfonamides. Likewise, topical use of EMLA cream has resulted in methemoglobinemia.

MOST DANGEROUS TOXINS: SOURCES

An emerging and serious source of carbon monoxide poisoning is houseboats. Life-threatening concentrations of carbon monoxide have been documented both inside the cabin, as well as around the swim decks of these boats despite the appearance of adequate ventilation. Children riding in the back of pickup trucks, or at ice skating arenas near ice cleaning machines, can also be at risk for exposure.

Other dangerous sources of blood and cellular toxins are products associated with delayed onset of poisoning because of metabolism of parent compounds to the responsible toxins. Methylene chloride is a common component of paint removers and other solvents that is readily absorbed after exposure. Metabolism of methylene chloride by the liver generates carbon monoxide. Artificial nail sculpting products may contain toluidine and artificial nail remover may contain acetonitrile. Toluidine has a methemoglobin-inducing metabolite and acetonitrile is metabolized to cyanide. Other methemoglobin-inducing compounds, such as dapsone, may cause have prolonged or recurrent signs and symptoms owing to the contribution of metabolites or due to a prolonged half-life.

CONCLUSION

Blood and cellular toxins are significant causes of poisoning and are potentially fatal. The following chapters provide details on the diagnosis and management of poisoning by blood and cellular toxins in children. Heightened awareness of these dangerous toxins may help to reduce the morbidity and mortality associated with these toxins through prevention of exposure, or early recognition of toxicity so appropriate medical management can be instituted.

SUGGESTED READINGS

Abbruzzi G, Stork AM: Pediatric toxicologic concerns. *Emerg Med Clin North Am* 20:223–247, 2002.

Carbon Monoxide Poisoning—An Invisible Danger on Houseboats. Available from http://www.cdc.gov/nceh/airpollution/carbonmonoxide/spotlight.htm. Accessed January 2004.

Carbon Monoxide Poisoning Fact Sheet. Available from http://www.cdc.gov/nceh/airpollution/carbonmonoxide/cofaq.htm. Accessed January 2004.

Ernst A, Zibrak JD: Current concepts: Carbon monoxide poisoning. *N Engl J Med* 339:1603, 1998.

Mandel J, Schellenberg J, Hales CA: *Smoke inhalation.* Available from: http://www.utdol.com. Accessed January 2004.

National Institute on Drug Abuse: *Research Report Series—Inhalant Abuse.* Available from http://www.nida.nih.gov?researchreports/inhalants/inhalants2.html. Accessed January 2004.

Watson WA, Litovitz TL, Rodgers GC, et al: 2002 Annual report of the American Association of Poison Control Centers Toxic Exposure Surveillance System. *Am J Emerg Med* 21:353, 2003.

72

Carbon Monoxide

Curtis P. Snook

HIGH-YIELD FACTS

- Suspect carbon monoxide (CO) poisoning when multiple patients present from the same scene with flulike symptoms such as headache, weakness, nausea, or vomiting.

- CO exposure in pregnancy has been associated with an increase in short-term complications as well as fetal morbidity and mortality in the absence of significant maternal toxicity.

- CO reduces blood oxygen-carrying capacity and delivery. Histopathologic features suggest reperfusion injury as the mechanism for subsequent neurologic sequelae.

- Deep coma in house fire victims should arouse suspicion of coincident poisoning with cyanide.

- Elevated carboxyhemoglobin levels detect exposure, but often do not correlate with clinical symptoms.

- High-flow oxygen by mask is indicated for CO poisoning to speed toxin elimination and enhance oxygen delivery.

- Hyperbaric oxygen (HBO) treatment is recommended when documented CO exposure occurs in pregnancy or early infancy. It is also suggested in patients with coma, seizures, or syncope.

CASE PRESENTATION

An 8-year-old girl presents to the emergency department (ED) with her parents complaining of headache, nausea, and vomiting. Her parents have also had similar symptoms over the past 24 hours that they ascribe to a viral illness. The child has felt weak, but has had no loss of consciousness. Her past medical history is unremarkable, she currently takes no medications, and has no known allergies.

On physical examination she appears well with a pulse of 95 bpm, blood pressure of 105/72 mmHg, and respiratory rate of 22 breaths per minute. Her oral temperature is 99.8°F. Pupils are equal and reactive to light; extraocular muscles are intact. Her mucous membranes are slightly moist. The cardiac examination is normal, and the lungs are clear to auscultation. The abdominal is soft, nontender, and bowel sounds are normoactive. Her extremities have a full range of motion, with no deformities, and a capillary refill of 2 seconds.

Laboratory studies reveal a carboxyhemoglobin level of 12%. The child is treated with high-flow oxygen by mask.

INTRODUCTION AND EPIDEMIOLOGY

CO is a significant pediatric toxin. It is a common cause of poisoning and has considerable potential for morbidity and mortality. According to the 2001 data from the American Association of Poison Control Centers (AAPCC), there were 17,251 CO exposures, 2181 of which were in children under 6 years of age, and 3101 of which were in children from 6 to 19 years old.

Nine pediatric (<20 years old) CO deaths were reported to the AAPCC, accounting for 4% of unintentional pediatric poisoning deaths among children under 6 years old and 8% of overall poisoning deaths among children under 20 years old.

CO detectors have become widely available for home use, allowing for earlier detection of exposure. There is evidence that their use permits CO detection at lower levels of exposure and symptomatology. It is hoped that their use will reduce morbidity and mortality, given the insidious onset of poisoning from this toxin.

DEVELOPMENTAL CONSIDERATIONS

CO is an airborne toxin produced as a byproduct of combustion by furnaces, heaters, and other fuel-powered devices used in homes It is also a result of house fires. Children of any age, as well as those in utero, can be exposed. Fetal hemoglobin is known to bind CO more avidly than adult hemoglobin, significantly lengthening the half-life of the toxin in the fetus and young infant. CO exposure in pregnancy should always be taken very seriously because it has been associated with an increase in short-term complications as well as fetal morbidity and mortality, even in the absence of significant maternal toxicity. Certain recreational activities associated with adolescence such as riding on the back platform of speedboats, playing around and under the back of houseboats, and riding in the back of pickup trucks, have been associated with CO poisoning.

PHARMACOLOGY AND TOXICOKINETICS

CO has a half-life in the body of 5 hours and 20 minutes in the patient breathing room air. The addition of 100% oxygen by mask (NBO) reduces this half-life to 90 minutes. HBO treatment (100% oxygen at 3 atmospheres) decreases this half-life even further to 23 minutes. The observed kinetics of elimination are also enhanced by hyperbaric conditions, changing from zero order (NBO) to first order (HBO).

PATHOPHYSIOLOGY

CO is in its pure form undetectable—it is colorless, tasteless, odorless, and nonirritating, accounting for the often insidious nature of toxicity. Its specific gravity is 0.97 relative to air permitting easy dispersion without stratification. It is produced as a byproduct of incomplete combustion by fuel-powered devices, in house fires, and endogenously as a product of the metabolism of the furniture stripping solvent methylene chloride. It should be noted that exposure to leaking natural gas without combustion would not be expected to produce CO poisoning. However, this may cause symptoms and pose the risks of asphyxia, fire, and explosion.

Readily absorbed upon inhalation, CO binds avidly to hemoglobin with an affinity 240 times greater than that of oxygen. CO binding to hemoglobin has the effect of increasing the affinity of the remaining binding sites for oxygen (four binding sites total per molecule), thus shifting the oxyhemoglobin dissociation curve to the left. By this mechanism, CO produces a functional anemia by reducing blood oxygen-carrying capacity and delivery (Figure 72–1).

CO also binds other metalloproteins such as myoglobin, cytochrome C oxidase, cytochrome P-450 oxidase, and guanylate cyclase. Myoglobin is important to the uptake of oxygen by skeletal muscle and binds CO with an affinity 40 times that of oxygen. Its dissociation curve is also shifted to the left by CO.

Cellular respiration at the mitochondrial level may also be impaired by CO. Although CO binds to cytochrome C oxidase with an affinity 9 times less than that of oxygen, it is able to compete for binding with the latter under conditions of hypotension or hypoxia. The dissociation rate of CO from cytochrome C oxidase is also very slow. Furthermore, a CO-induced increased production by platelets of free radicals and release of nitric oxide results in increased production of peroxynitrite, which has been demonstrated to inactivate mitochondrial enzymes and impair electron transport.

Two potential mechanistic explanations for the occurrence of CO-induced hypotension are the stimulation of guanylate cyclase, which produces the vasodilator guanosine monophosphate and the displacement of the vasodilator nitrous oxide, also known as endothelial-derived relaxation factor, from its binding sites in platelets.

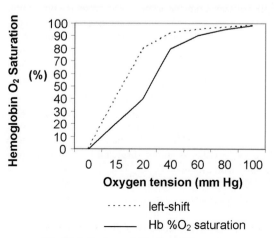

Fig. 72–1. Oxyhemoglobin dissociation curve.

Histopathologic features of CO poisoning in the brain suggest reperfusion injury as the mechanism for subsequent neurologic sequelae. Work by Thom and colleagues suggests the following sequence of events:

1. Disturbance of endothelial homeostasis
2. polymorphonuclear neutrophil (PMN) migration to the site of endothelial hypoxic injury
3. release of protease by adherent PMNs converting xanthine dehydrogenase to xanthine oxidase
4. generation of oxygen radicals by xanthine oxidase followed by further radical formation from lipid peroxidation.

An interesting additional finding of this work was that increased pressure (hyperbaric treatment) interfered with leukocyte adherence at the site of endothelial injury. A reperfusion mechanism like this is compelling in that it would explain the observed lack of correlation between carboxyhemoglobin level and subsequent neurologic toxicity, as well as the therapeutic benefit of hyperbaric over normobaric oxygen treatment that some have observed. In addition, Thom and associates found in their work that a prolonged, low-level exposure to CO (*soaking period*) was needed to initiate signs of reperfusion injury.

CLINICAL PRESENTATION

The diagnosis of CO poisoning is frequently missed because its symptoms and peak incidence in the winter months tend to coincide with influenza epidemics. The key to making the diagnosis is recognizing when multiple patients from the same scene present with similar symptoms and by focused questioning regarding exposure to heating systems or other fuel-burning devices.

Symptoms and signs of CO poisoning range from headache, nausea, vomiting, weakness, decreased mental status to syncope, seizures, coma, and arrhythmias. Severe cases can result in hypoxic end-organ damage. Reversible cardiac damage has been noted in pediatric CO poisoning in the absence of other serious toxicities. Deep coma associated with metabolic acidosis in house fire victims should arouse suspicion of coincident poisoning with cyanide.

CO poisoning is sometimes associated with delayed neurologic sequelae in those patients who survive. In pediatric patients, such delayed sequelae have included chronic headaches, memory difficulties, and decline in school performance.

LABORATORY AND DIAGNOSTIC TESTING

Exposure to CO is detectable in several ways. Use of CO detectors in the home and measurement by fire department rescue personnel at the scene help to detect exposure. In the ED, an elevated carboxyhemoglobin level can also document exposure, although a normal level does not exclude the possibility that exposure occurred followed by a time delay prior to presentation. CO levels are usually measured using arterial blood, although studies have demonstrated that venous blood levels are comparably accurate. Standard pulse oximeters cannot quantify carboxyhemoglobin percentage and typically give normal readings in CO poisoning. Co-oximeters, in contrast, are able to make the distinction between these species and quantify the percentage of carboxyhemoglobin if present.

The detection of CO poisoning in those exposed can be difficult because the symptoms of neuropsychiatric dysfunction are quite subtle, especially in children. It has been demonstrated in adults that a limited battery of neuropsychiatric tests easily administered in the ED setting can distinguish a group of CO-poisoned patients from a comparable group not exposed to CO. Whereas alertness, orientation, and digit span subtests do not successfully make this distinction, more sensitive subtests such as trail making and digit symbol are able to do so. Because there is a normal range of performance on these tests based on a number of factors and there is no gold standard for the diagnosis of poisoning from CO, the positive and negative predictive values of these tests for the individual patient cannot be determined. Furthermore, these tests are only useful in a pediatric population for those patients mature enough to perform them. If a child is too young to understand them and an adult has been poisoned with the child, the results of the adult's testing have been used as an aid in assessing the child's risk of poisoning.

Other baseline laboratory testing in CO poisoning is typically nondiagnostic. A mild metabolic (lactic) acidosis can be present, but there is too much overlap with the normal range for this to be clinically useful in detection of poisoning. A pronounced elevation of serum lactate (above 10 mmol/L) in house fire victims is suggestive of coincident cyanide poisoning.

Because of the high affinity of fetal hemoglobin for CO, fetal poisoning is assumed if documented maternal exposure has occurred. The same degree of caution is appropriate in young infants who still have significant amounts of fetal hemoglobin.

In severely poisoned patients with cerebral injury, computed tomography of the head typically reveals lesions of the basal ganglia and cerebral grey and white matter, which vary in extent according to poisoning severity.

MANAGEMENT

Prehospital

Victims of house fires require prompt evaluation for thermal airway injury and smoke inhalation because early airway management is critical in these patients. The priorities for on-scene management of CO exposure are threefold. The first is the simple recognition of the possibility that CO may be responsible. Multiple victims with flulike symptoms and proximity to a fuel-powered device are valuable clues that should alert first responders to this possibility. The second priority is to remove potential victims from further exposure and ensure appropriate medical evaluation. Finally, the offending fuel-powered device needs to be turned off and its use in future poisoning prevented by appropriate means. Patients should be transported on high-flow oxygen by mask to speed CO elimination and enhance oxygen delivery.

Hospital

Considerable controversy surrounds the treatment of CO poisoning. The primary focus of this controversy is whether HBO is more effective than NBO therapy. Animal data, as discussed, suggests that high ambient pressure in and of itself may offer benefit by arresting reperfusion injury in CO poisoning. The same study also shows, however, that not all CO exposures result in reperfusion injury; certain conditions must be met. Because hyperbaric chambers (Figure 72–2) are not available in all localities, the necessity of patient transport in some cases adds to the cost side of the cost–benefit assessment. At this point in time, no proven or standardized means exist to identify those subsets of patients exposed to CO who will benefit from HBO. The available human trials comparing HBO versus NBO in different populations with different patient selection criteria and methodologies have yielded conflicting results. None of these trials were conducted in pediatric populations.

It is commonly accepted that high-flow oxygen by mask is appropriate in CO poisoning to reduce the half-life of the toxin and correct as soon as possible its detrimental effects on oxygen delivery. To ensure CO elimination, 100% oxygen should be continued for 4 to

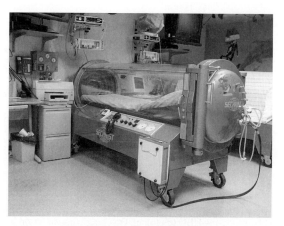

Fig. 72–2. Standard HBO chamber.

6 hours. In the pregnant patient, oxygen therapy should be administered approximately 5 times longer once the mother has normalized, to ensure adequate CO clearance from the fetus.

Asymptomatic children exposed to CO who have no evidence of subtle neuropsychiatric dysfunction by testing would not be considered to have CO poisoning or require treatment.

HBO therapy should be seriously considered for documented CO exposure in pregnancy and early infancy given the long half-life of CO binding to fetal hemoglobin and existing evidence of fetal toxicity in the absence of significant maternal toxicity. HBO should also be considered for children with signs of toxicity from CO exposure—coma, seizure, syncope, neuropsychiatric deficit—in whom cerebral reperfusion injury is possible. Further research is needed to define which patient subsets with CO poisoning require the additional benefits afforded by hyperbaric treatment.

Despite the poor correlation between carboxyhemoglobin levels and symptomatology/toxicity, some sources advocate that HBO therapy be used for patients with documented levels of 40% or greater. Many HBO centers arbitrarily use a more conservative level of 25% as indication for HBO therapy in children, and 15% in pregnant patients. It is important to note that these recommendations are not based on well-designed clinical trials.

DISPOSITION

In terms of poison center triage, any child or pregnant woman who has had either documented exposure to CO as determined by on-scene detectors or symptoms consistent with CO poisoning should be referred to a health care facility for further evaluation.

Children exposed to CO who have low documented levels, are asymptomatic, and are without evidence of subtle neuropsychiatric dysfunction may be discharged home. CO-poisoned patients whose symptoms resolve with either NBO or HBO may be discharged but should be seen in follow-up on an outpatient basis to assess for delayed neuropsychiatric sequelae. Any child with coma, altered mental status, or other evidence of end-organ ischemia should be admitted to the hospital intensive care unit. Obstetric consultation with fetal monitoring is warranted for CO poisoning in late pregnancy when the fetus is viable, following HBO treatment. Psychiatric consultation is required in all cases of intentional CO poisoning.

CASE OUTCOME

High-flow oxygen is administered by mask for a total of 4 hours. The child becomes asymptomatic during this time period. The parents are referred to and treated at a nearby adult hospital and undergo neuropsychiatric testing there, which is within the normal range for their age and educational level. The local fire department is contacted and goes to the home. They detect elevated levels (100 ppm) of CO. A leak is discovered in the exhaust system of the furnace, which is shut down and repaired before the house is reoccupied by the family.

SUGGESTED READINGS

Bartlett R: Carbon monoxide poisoning. In: Haddad LM, Shannon MW, Winchester JF, eds: *Clinical Management of Poisoning and Drug Overdose.* 3rd ed. Philadelphia: Saunders; 1998:885.

Baud FJ, Barriot P, Toffis V, et al: Elevated blood cyanide concentrations in victims of smoke inhalation. *N Engl J Med* 325:1761–1766, 1991.

Brown SD, Piantadosi CA: In vivo binding of carbon monoxide to cytochrome c oxidase in rat brain. *J Appl Physiol* 68:604–610, 1990.

Caravati EM, Adams CJ, Joyce SM: Fetal toxicity associated with maternal carbon monoxide poisoning. *Teratology* 30: 253–257, 1984.

Carbon-monoxide poisoning resulting from exposure to ski-boat exhaust—Georgia, June 2002. *MMWR Morbid Mortal Wkly Rep* 51:829–830, 2002.

Crocker PJ, Walker JS: Pediatric carbon monoxide toxicity. *J Emerg Med* 3:443–448, 1985.

Ducasse JL, Celsis P, Marc-Vergnes JP: Non-comatose patients with acute carbon monoxide poisoning: Hyperbaric or normobaric oxygenation? *Undersea Hyperb Med* 22:9–15, 1995.

Farrow JR, Davis GJ, Roy TM, et al: Fetal death due to nonlethal maternal carbon monoxide poisoning. *JAMA* 261:1039–1043, 1989.

Furchgott RF, Jothianandan D: Endothelium-dependent and -independent vasodilation involving cyclic GMP: Relaxation induced by nitric oxide, carbon monoxide and light. *Blood Vessels* 28:52–61, 1991.

Gandini C, Castoldi AF, Candura SM: Cardiac damage in pediatric carbon monoxide poisoning. *J Toxicol Clin Toxicol* 39: 45–51, 2001.

Hampson NB, Norkool DM: Carbon monoxide poisoning in children riding in the back of pickup trucks. *J Emerg Med* 3:443–448,1985.

Houseboat-associated carbon monoxide poisonings on Lake Powell—Arizona and Utah, 2000. *MMWR Morbid Mortal Wkly Rep* 49:1105–1108, 2000.

Koren G, Sharav T, Pastuszak A, et al: A multicenter, prospective study of fetal outcome following accidental carbon monoxide poisoning in pregnancy. *Neurology* 26:15–23, 1976.

Krenzelok EP, Roth R, Full R: Carbon monoxide. . . The silent killer with an audible solution. *Am J Emerg Med* 14:484–486, 1996.

Messier LD, Myers RA: A neuropsychological screening battery for emergency assessment of carbon-monoxide-poisoned patients. *J Clin Psychol* 47:675–684, 1991.

Radi R, Rodriguez M, Castro L, et al: Inhibition of mitochondrial electron transport by peroxynitrite. *Arch Biochem Biophys* 308:89–95, 1994.

Raphael JC, Elkharrat D, Jars-Guincestre MC, et al: Trial of normobaric and hyperbaric oxygen for acute carbon monoxide intoxication. *Lancet* 1:414–419, 1989.

Scheinkestel CD, Bailey M, Myles PS, et al: Hyperbaric or normobaric oxygen for acute carbon monoxide poisoning: A randomised controlled clinical trial. *Med J Aust* 170:203–210, 1999.

Thom SR, Taber RL, Mendiguren, et al: Delayed neuropsychologic sequelae following carbon monoxide poisoning: Prevention by treatment with hyperbaric oxygen. *Ann Emerg Med* 25:474–480, 1995.

Thom SR, Ohnishi ST, Ischiropoulos H: Nitric oxide released by platelets inhibits neutrophil B2 integrin function following acute carbon monoxide poisoning. *Toxicol Appl Pharmacol* 128:105–110, 1994.

Thom SR: Leukocytes in carbon monoxide-mediated brain oxidative injury. *Toxicol Appl Pharmacol* 123:234–247, 1993.

Thom SR: Smoke inhalation. *Emerg Clin North Am* 7:371–387, 1989.

Tomaszewski C: Carbon monoxide. In: Goldfrank LR, Flomenbaum N, Lewin N, et al, eds: *Goldfrank's Toxicologic Emergencies.* 7th ed. New York: McGraw-Hill; 2002:1478–1491.

Touger M, Gallagher EJ, Tyrell J: Relationship between venous and arterial carboxyhemoglobin levels in patients with suspected carbon monoxide poisoning. *Ann Emerg Med* 25:481–483, 1995.

Utz J, Ullrich V: Carbon monoxide relaxes ileal smooth muscle through activation of guanylate cyclase. *Biochem Pharmacol* 41:1195–1201, 1991.

Van Hoesen KB, Camporesi EM, Moon RE: Should hyperbaric oxygen be used to treat the pregnant patient for acute carbon monoxide poisoning? A case report and literature review. *Ann Emerg Med* 17:714–717, 1988.

Weaver LK, Hopkins RO, Chan KJ, et al: Hyperbaric oxygen for acute carbon monoxide poisoning. *N Engl J Med* 347: 1057–1067, 2002.

Wood EN: Increased incidence of still birth in piglets associated with levels of atmospheric carbon monoxide. *Vet Rec* 104: 283–284, 1979.

73

Cyanide

Mark Mycyk
Anne Krantz

HIGH-YIELD FACTS

- Cyanide poisoning disrupts oxygen utilization and adenosine triphosphate (ATP) production.

- Poisoning causes rapid onset of central nervous system and cardiovascular toxicity.

- Laboratory clues suggestive of cyanide poisoning include lactic acidosis and a diminished arterial-venous O_2 difference.

- Antidotal therapy with nitrites and sodium thiosulfate should be considered early.

- Onset of symptoms may be delayed after oral nitrile ingestion.

CASE PRESENTATION

A 4-year-old boy is brought to the emergency department unconscious. Approximately 6 hours prior to arrival, he ingested an unknown volume of his grandmother's nail care product, which is still at home. He has no medical problems, takes no medications, and has no known allergies. On arrival his heart rate is 60 bpm, blood pressure is unobtainable, respiratory rate is 24 breaths per minute, and pulse oximetry reading is 96%. He is orally intubated and intravenous (IV) fluids are initiated. The arterial blood gas measures a pH 6.85, Pco_2 24 mmHg, and Po_2 169 mmHg. The patient's serum electrolytes show a sodium of 142; potassium 3.9; chloride 108; and bicarbonate 8. An anion gap of 26 is calculated.

INTRODUCTION AND EPIDEMIOLOGY

Cyanide poisoning is unusual in the United States and very rare among children, although its contribution to toxicity and death may be underestimated in victims of smoke inhalation. The American Association for Poison Control Centers reported over 100 pediatric cyanide exposures in the last 5 years. A variety of sources of cyanide exposure occur in the pediatric population. In fires, hydrogen cyanide gas is formed as a combustion product of wool, silk, synthetic fabrics, and building materials. Cyanide exposure by this route is now recognized as a major cause of toxicity among fire victims previously thought to be poisoned by carbon monoxide. Acetonitrile, or methyl cyanide, is found in agents used to remove sculpted nails and is converted in vivo to hydrogen cyanide. Cyanide poisoning owing to acetonitrile ingestion has occurred in children, resulting in at least one reported death. Poisoning has also occurred from accidental ingestion of cyanide-containing metal cleaning solutions imported from Southeast Asia. Amygdalin and other cyanogenic glycosides, found in the seeds and pits of certain plants such as apples, apricots, and peaches, are hydrolyzed in the gut to cyanide (Figure 73–1). Fruit pit ingestion has led to outbreaks of cyanide poisoning in children in Turkey and Gaza. Cassava food products also contain cyanogenic glycosides, and have been frequently implicated in accidental cyanide poisoning in developing countries. Cyanide poisoning can also occur with short-term, high-dose nitroprusside infusions for the treatment of hypertension.

DEVELOPMENTAL CONSIDERATIONS

Cyanide exposure in children is usually unintentional. The most challenging aspect of identifying children with

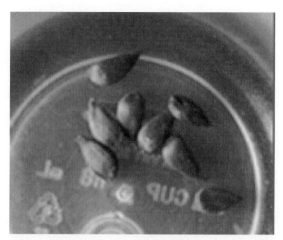

Fig. 73–1. Amygdalin and other cyanogenic glycosides, found in the seeds and pits of certain plants such as apples, apricots, and peaches, are hydrolyzed in the gut to cyanide.

cyanide poisoning is obtaining an accurate exposure history. If cyanide poisoning is confirmed in children younger than 1 year of age, neglect or abuse needs to be considered. Suicidal adolescents can be intentionally exposed to larger doses of cyanide from products obtained from a school laboratory or their work environment.

PHARMACOLOGY AND TOXICOKINETICS

Hydrogen cyanide gas is rapidly absorbed in the lungs and can cause profound toxicity within seconds. Ingested cyanide salts, such as sodium cyanide and potassium cyanide, are also rapidly absorbed across the gastric mucosa and can result in toxicity within minutes. Ingestion of amygdalin and other cyanogenic glycosides requires hydrolysis to release cyanide, so toxicity may be delayed for several hours after ingestion. Acetonitrile appears to release cyanide through oxidative metabolism by the hepatic cytochrome P450 system, thus delaying clinical manifestations of toxicity for 2 to 6 hours from the time of ingestion. There are minimal data on the volume of distribution (V_d) of cyanide in humans. Pharmacokinetic data from one case of potassium cyanide ingestion reported a V_d of 0.41 L/kg. Blood cyanide concentrates in the erythrocytes, with a red blood cell (RBC):plasma ratio of 100:1. Sixty percent of plasma cyanide is protein bound.

Cyanide detoxification and elimination in humans occurs by various endogenous pathways. Approximately 80% of cyanide detoxification is handled by the widely distributed endogenous enzyme rhodanese (sulfotransferase). In the presence of thiosulfate, rhodanese converts cyanide to nontoxic thiocyanate, which is eventually renally excreted. Thiosulfate availability is the rate-limiting factor in this pathway, and significant cyanide poisoning quickly depletes these stores and causes other metabolic derangements, which further impair rhodanese activity. Some cyanide is converted in the presence of hydroxocobalamin to cyanocobalamin, which is also nontoxic. Clinically insignificant amounts of cyanide are excreted in expired air and in sweat. The reported elimination half-life in humans is variable, ranging from 20 minutes to 1 hour in nonlethal exposures to a mean of 3 hours in fire victims treated with antidotes.

Nitroprusside is rapidly hydrolyzed and releases free cyanide, which is converted to thiocyanate by rhodanase enzymes in the liver and blood. Thiocyanate is eliminated by the kidney, but can accumulate in patients with renal compromise.

PATHOPHYSIOLOGY

The primary mechanism of toxicity in cyanide poisoning is disruption of the cytochrome oxidase system, which results in cellular hypoxia. Cyanide has a high affinity for the ferric iron (Fe^{3+}) in cytochrome aa3 of the mitochondrial cytochrome oxidase electron transport chain. Cyanide binding at cytochrome aa3 disrupts oxygen utilization in ATP production. As a result, cells shift to anaerobic metabolism and severe lactic acidosis occurs. Cyanide inhibits a wide variety of other iron- and copper-containing enzymes, although their contribution to clinical toxicity is uncertain. The critical targets of cyanide are those organs most dependent on oxidative phosphorylation, namely the brain and the heart.

CLINICAL FINDINGS

Clinical presentation depends on the route and dose of exposure. Inhalation of cyanide gas causes loss of consciousness within seconds, whereas symptoms from an oral exposure develop anywhere from 30 minutes to several hours from the time of ingestion. Because cyanide poisoning causes profound cellular hypoxia, it makes clinical sense that the central nervous system and the cardiovascular system are affected the earliest. Initial symptoms in victims not experiencing rapid loss of consciousness include headache, anxiety, confusion, blurred vision, palpitations, nausea, and vomiting. With progression of toxicity, patients may experience a feeling of neck constriction, suffocation, and unsteadiness. Early clinical signs of cyanide poisoning are central nervous system stimulation or depression, tachycardia or bradycardia, hypertension, and dilated pupils. Fundoscopy may reveal bright red retinal veins. Late signs of poisoning are seizures, coma, apnea, cardiac arrhythmias, and cardiovascular collapse. The characteristic smell of bitter almonds may be detected in some cases, but the ability to detect this is a genetically determined trait not possessed by every examiner. Although cyanide poisoning causes cellular hypoxia, the presence of cyanosis is a relatively late finding. Oxygen is present, but it is not being used efficiently. Thus, the absence of visible cyanosis in a patient with clinical evidence of severe hypoxia should prompt the healthcare provider to consider the diagnosis of cyanide poisoning.

LABORATORY STUDIES

Whole blood cyanide levels may be obtained, but results are not available emergently. Levels below 0.5 mg/L (<38 μmol/L) are considered nontoxic; levels >1.0 mg/L produce acidosis. Blood gas analysis and serum chemistries may be helpful in the acute setting. Arterial blood gases typically dem-onstrate marked metabolic acidosis. Obtaining a venous blood gas analysis for comparison may demonstrate a diminished arterial-venous O_2 (Ao_2–Vo_2) difference, as tissue extraction of oxygen from the blood is severely impaired. The Ao_2–Vo_2 may approach zero. Serum chemistries demonstrate an elevated anion gap owing to lactic acidosis. Numerous electrocardiographic changes may occur in cyanide toxicity. With continued ATP depletion from untreated poisoning, bradycardia associated with hypotension typically heralds impending death. Thiocyanate levels higher than 50 to 100 mg/L may be associated with delirium and altered mental status after high-dose nitroprusside infusion.

MANAGEMENT

The management of cyanide poisoning requires immediate supportive care as well as specific antidotal therapy. Oxygen is immediately administered and rapid sequence intubation may be necessary. Mouth-to-mouth resuscitation is avoided in primary rescuers because of the theo-

retical risk of secondary cyanide exposure. Fluid resuscitation is initiated in patients with hypotension. Sodium bicarbonate should be considered in profound acidosis. Contaminated clothing should be removed and skin and eyes copiously irrigated. In general, health care personnel do not require decontamination suits. Standard decontamination procedures should be followed to limit any further absorption by the patient, but secondary contamination from cyanide is unlikely, unless the prehospital rescuers are at the scene of cyanide exposure. Gastric decontamination with activated charcoal may be considered only in a patient who arrives with minimal symptoms soon after an oral exposure.

Cyanide Antidotes

Although some victims of cyanide poisoning have survived with supportive care alone, antidotal therapy clearly improves survival and shortens the recovery period. The only antidote currently approved for use in the United States is the Taylor Cyanide Antidote Kit, which contains amyl nitrite perles, sodium nitrite solution, and sodium thiosulfate (Figure 73–2).

The mechanism of action of nitrites in cyanide toxicity is not completely understood. Early evidence suggested that nitrites produce methemoglobin, which has a higher affinity for cyanide than does cytochrome oxidase. This combination of methemoglobin and cyanide forms the relatively nontoxic cyanomethemoglobin. Cyanomethemoglobin production displaces cyanide from cytochrome a3 and allows resumption of oxidative phosphorylation and aerobic metabolism (Figure 73–3). However, more

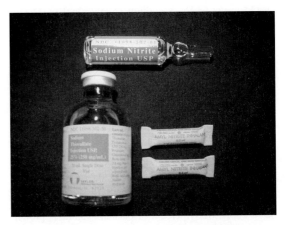

Fig. 73–2. The Taylor/Cyanide Antidote Kit.

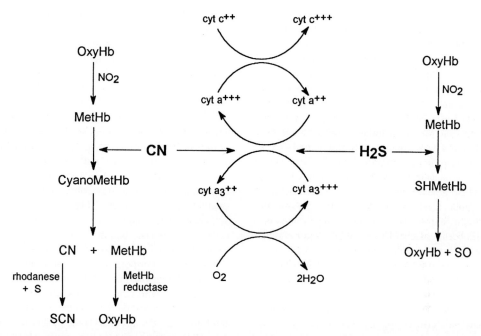

Fig. 73–3. CN pathway diagram. (*Source:* From Goldfrank LR, Flomenbaum N, Lewin N, et al, eds: *Goldfrank's Toxicologic Emergencies.* 7th ed. New York: McGraw-Hill; 2002: Fig 98–2, 1501.)

recent evidence suggests that other mechanisms are relevant. In animals pretreated with methylene blue (so that methemoglobin formation is inhibited), nitrites still effectively reduce cyanide toxicity. Additionally, clinical improvement following nitrite administration occurs within minutes, although peak methemoglobin levels occur later. Some authors suggest that the vasodilatory effect of nitrites allows for greater endothelial enzymatic degradation of cyanide. Indeed, in experimental models, some α-antagonists have also shown antidotal efficacy in cyanide poisoning. Sodium thiosulfate provides a sulfur donor for the rhodanese-mediated conversion of cyanide to thiocyanate. Thiocyanate is minimally toxic and is excreted by the kidneys.

Amyl nitrite perles are administered first. The perles are crushed in gauze and held near the nose and mouth for 30 seconds. Amyl nitrite administration produces a methemoglobin level of 3% to 7%. Once an IV line is established and the sodium nitrite solution prepared, administration of amyl nitrite perles may be discontinued. In critically ill or comatose patients, perles have little utility. In this scenario, only IV antidotes should be administered. Sodium nitrite (see Table 73–1 for pediatric dosing) is administered at a rate of 0.15 to 0.30 mL/kg of a 3% solu-

tion over 5 minutes. In an unstable or hypotensive patient, or when there is concomitant carbon monoxide poisoning, the dose may be given over 30 minutes. With the slower rate of infusion, the methemoglobin level peaks 35 to 70 minutes following administration, and rises to

Table 73–1. Cyanide Management: Pediatric Nitrite Guidelines[a]

Hemoglobin (g)	NaNO$_2$ (mg/kg) (mg/kg)	3%NaNO$_2$ Solution (mL/kg)
7.0	5.8	0.19
8.0	6.6	0.22
9.0	7.5	0.25
10.0	8.3	0.27
11.0	9.1	0.30
12.0	10.0	0.33
13.0	10.8	0.36
14.0	11.6	0.39

[a]Pediatric thiosulfate dose: 1.65 mL/kg of 25% solution.
Source: Reprinted from Goldfrank LR, Flomenbaum NE, Lewin NA, et al., eds: *Goldfrank's Toxicologic Emergencies.* 7th ed. New York: McGraw-Hill; 2002, p 1503.

roughly 10% to 15%. This level is lower than the 25% recommended as a goal of therapy in earlier literature, because it has been shown that lower levels are equally therapeutic and avoid further impairment of tissue oxygen delivery from a high methemoglobin level.

Methemoglobin levels should be monitored periodically after the infusion. Side effects of nitrite administration include headache, blurred vision, nausea, vomiting, and hypotension. Methemoglobin levels of 20% to 30% are associated with symptoms of headache and nausea. Weakness, dyspnea, and tachycardia occur at levels of 30% to 50%, and dysrhythmias, CNS depression, and seizures occur at levels of 50% to 70%. Death occurs at methemoglobin levels around 70%. A fatal methemoglobin level in a child treated with nitrites for cyanide poisoning has been reported. That child received a cumulative dose of 21 mg/kg sodium nitrite.

Following the nitrite administration, sodium thiosulfate is given to enhance clearance of cyanide as thiocyanate. The pediatric dose is 1.65 mL/kg of a 25% solution up to 50 mL (12.5 g). Thiosulfate appears to have few if any side effects. Thiocyanate levels of greater than 10 mg/dL may be associated with nausea, vomiting, arthralgias, and confusion. Because thiocyanate is renally excreted, these symptoms may occur in the setting of renal failure and impaired thiocyanate excretion.

Typically, symptoms and signs of cyanide poisoning begin to respond within minutes of the administration of nitrites. When symptoms recur following antidote administration, both the sodium nitrite and sodium thiosulfate may be given again at half the original doses. Because there is no diagnostic test for cyanide poisoning that can be obtained in a timely manner, the diagnosis in the acute setting needs to be made clinically. In a situation in which cyanide poisoning is being considered but the diagnosis is uncertain, the use of sodium thiosulfate alone may be considered. This approach avoids further compromise of the patient's oxygen-carrying capacity by the nitrites. There are minimal published data on the efficacy of this approach. If cyanide poisoning is confirmed by history or laboratory data, and the patient remains symptomatic despite thiosulfate administration, consider administering a dose of sodium nitrite IV. When a patient is treated with nitrites but shows no clinical response, the diagnosis of acute cyanide toxicity should be reconsidered.

A promising new antidote currently under investigation is hydroxocobalamin (vitamin B_{12a}). Cyanide couples with the cobalt component of hydroxocobalamin, producing cyanocobalamin, which is nontoxic. Concurrent thiosulfate administration enhances cyanide elimi-

nation as thiocyanate. Animal investigations and human case reports from Europe have demonstrated success with hydroxocobalamin without the hypotensive side effects associated with nitrite therapy. Pediatric data are lacking.

Smoke Inhalation

Several studies suggest a correlation between elevated carboxyhemoglobin levels and cyanide levels in smoke inhalation victims. Thus, when an elevated carboxyhemoglobin level is found in a severely ill fire victim, cyanide poisoning is also possible, and treatment for it should be considered early. This is particularly true in a fire victim who requires intubation or has a persistent metabolic acidosis, abnormal mental status, or cardiovascular instability not resolving following treatment for carbon monoxide poisoning. Because nitrite-induced methemoglobinemia may further impair oxygen delivery, a patient with concomitant carbon monoxide and cyanide poisoning should be treated with 100% oxygen and thiosulfate therapy first. If the patient remains critically ill, treatment with sodium nitrite should then be considered. It is administered slowly while the blood pressure is monitored. Some evidence suggests that hyperbaric oxygen therapy conventionally used for severe carbon monoxide poisoning is helpful in the treatment of cyanide toxicity as well.

Nitroprusside

If cyanide poisoning is suspected during administration of a nitroprusside infusion, the drip should be discontinued. If symptoms of toxicity persist, administration of sodium thiosulfate is recommended in standard doses. Sodium nitrate treatment may exacerbate hypotension and should be avoided. Hydroxycobalamin at 25 mg/h IV has also been infused with nitroprusside as a prophylaxis against cyanide poisoning.

DISPOSITION

Patients who are asymptomatic and whose exposure has apparently been minimal are observed for 4 to 6 hours. Those who have ingested cyanogenic glycosides are observed for at least 6 hours for evidence of toxicity. Those ingesting acetonitrile-containing compounds are observed for 12 to 24 hours. Patients requiring antidotal treatment are cared for in an intensive care unit where vital signs, mental status, arterial blood gases, methemoglobin, and carboxyhemoglobin levels can be checked frequently. Following recovery, patients are observed for 24 to 48 hours. Rarely, late neurologic syndromes have been reported following cyanide toxicity, and periodic outpatient follow-up is advised.

CASE OUTCOME

A concomitant arterial and venous blood gas obtained after intubation demonstrates a diminished AO_2–VO_2 difference in the presence of severe metabolic acidosis, with an elevated lactate level. A single dose of IV sodium nitrite is given, followed by a dose of IV sodium thiosulfate. By the time the patient arrives in the intensive care unit, acidosis and mental status have improved. The grandmother's nail care product is identified as an artificial nail remover containing acetonitrile. A confirmatory cyanide level of 43 μmol/L is measured. The patient is extubated and makes a full recovery.

SUGGESTED READINGS

Akintonwa A, Tunwashe OL: Fatal cyanide poisoning from cassava-based meal. *Hum Exp Toxicol* 11:47–49, 1992.

Baud FJ, Barriot P, Toffis V, et al: Elevated blood cyanide concentrations in victims of smoke inhalation. *N Engl J Med* 325:1761–1766, 1991.

Benowitz NL: Nitroprusside. In Olson KR, ed: *Poisoning and Drug Overdose.* New York: Lange Medical & McGraw-Hill; 2002:281–282.

Chin RG, Caldern Y: Acute cyanide poisoning: A case report. *J Emerg Med* 18:441–445, 2000.

Caravati EM, Litovitz TL: Pediatric cyanide intoxication and death from an acetonitrile-containing cosmetic. *JAMA* 260: 3470–3473, 1998.

Clark CJ, Campbell D, Reid WH: Blood carboxyhemoglobin and cyanide levels in fire survivors. *Lancet* 1:1332–1335, 1981.

Delaney KA: Cyanide. In Ford MD, Delaney KA, Ling LJ, et al, eds: *Clinical Toxicology.* Philadelphia: Saunders; 2001:705–711.

Froldi R: A case of suicide by ingestion of sodium nitroprusside. *J Forensic Sci* 46:1504–1506, 2001.

Gonzalez ER: Cyanide evades some noses, overpowers others. *JAMA* 248:2211, 1982.

Hall AH, Linden CH, Kulik KW, et al: Cyanide poisoning from laetrile ingestion: Role of nitrite therapy. *Pediatrics* 78:269–272, 1986.

Hall AH, Rumack BH: Clinical toxicology of cyanide. *Ann Emerg Med* 15:1067–1074, 1986.

Johnson RP, Mellors JW: Arteriolization of venous blood gases: A clue to the diagnosis of cyanide poisoning. *J Emerg Med* 6:401–404, 1988.

Kerns W, Isom G, Kirk M: Cyanide and hydrogen sulfide. In: Goldfrank LR, Flomenbaum N, Lewin N, et al, eds: *Goldfrank's Toxicologic Emergencies.* 7th ed. New York: McGraw-Hill; 2002:1498–1510.

Kirk MA, Gerace R, Kulig KW: Cyanide and methemoglobin kinetics in smoke inhalation victims treated with the cyanide antidote kit. *Ann Emerg Med* 22:1413–1418, 1993.

Kulig KW: Cyanide antidotes and fire toxicology. *N Engl J Med* 325:1801, 1991.

Mannaioni G, Vannacci A, Marzocca C, et al: Acute cyanide intoxication treated with a combination of hydroxycobalamin, sodium nitrite, and sodium thiosulfate. *J Toxicol Clin Toxicol* 40:181–183, 2002.

Ruangkanchanasetr S, Wananukul V, Suwanjutha S: Cyanide poisoning, 2 cases report and treatment review. *J Med Assoc Thai* 82; S162–167, 1999.

Suchard JR, Wallace KL, Gerkin RD: Acute cyanide toxicity caused by apricot kernel ingestion. *Ann Emerg Med* 32:742–744, 1998.

Yen D, Tsai J, Wang LM, et al: The clinical experience of acute cyanide poisoning. *Am J Emerg Med* 13:524–528, 1995.

74

Methemoglobinemia

Kevin C. Osterhoudt

CASE PRESENTATION

A previously healthy 10-day-old infant developed cyanosis, lethargy, and poor feeding. Bleeding had complicated the first trimester of pregnancy, and the mother had been treated for 4 months with progesterone. The mother also received Rhogam for potential maternal–fetal blood type incompatibility. Meconium staining of the amniotic fluid was the only complication at delivery, but the baby had no signs of respiratory illness during his stay in the newborn nursery. The infant appeared well at a religious ceremony at the age of 9 days, and tolerated a circumcision procedure. In the ensuing 24 hours, however, the baby became progressively more cyanotic. No history of diarrhea, fever, cough, or oliguria existed.

On examination in the emergency department, the baby is cyanotic, but respirations are unlabored and movements are vigorous. He is afebrile, heart rate is 180 bpm, respiratory rate is 38 breaths per minute, and pulse oximetry is 87% breathing room air. On auscultation, the lungs are clear and the heart produces no murmur. Peripheral pulses are strong. Samples of blood, urine, and cerebrospinal fluid obtained for a sepsis evaluation are unrevealing. Serum chemistries do not demonstrate metabolic acidosis. An electrocardiogram and a chest radiograph are normal. An echocardiogram, performed to investigate the possibility of structural cyanotic heart disease, is normal. An arterial blood sample, obtained while the infant is breathing room air, demonstrated the following: pH = 7.44, P_{CO_2} = 35 mmHg, P_{O_2} = 75 mmHg (the calculated hemoglobin oxygen saturation equaled 96%). The discordance noted between the calculated and measured hemoglobin oxygen saturation led to the consideration of methemoglobinemia. Fourteen hours after presentation to medical care, co-oximetry reveals a blood methemoglobin concentration of 38.7%.

Table 74–1. Etiology of Methemoglobinemia

Inherited
    Hemoglobin M
    NADH-dependent methemoglobin reductase
      deficiency
    Cytochrome-b_5 deficiency
Acquired
    Illness-associated methemoglobinemia of infancy
    Exposure to an exogenous oxidant drug, chemical,
      or compound

Abbreviation: NADH, nicotine adenine dinucleotide.

Table 74–2. Partial List of Toxins Implicated as Methemoglobin Inducers

Dietary or environmental chemicals
    Chlorates
    Chromates
    Copper sulfate fungicides
    Naphthalene
    Nitrates/nitrites, inorganic
      Contaminated well water
      High-nitrate vegetables
      Meat preservatives
Industrial Chemicals
    Aliphatic nitrates
    Aliphatic nitros
    Aromatic amines
      Aniline compounds
      Toluidine compounds
    Aromatic nitros
      Nitrobenzene and others
    Arsine
    Methyl nitrite
    Nitric oxide
    Nitrosobenzene
    Petroleum octane booster
Drugs
    Acetanilid
    Antimalarials
      Chloroquine
      Primaquine
    Antipyrine
    Chlorhexidine
    Dapsone
    Local anesthetics
      Benzocaine
      Lidocaine
      Prilocaine
    Methylene blue
    Metoclopramide
    Nitrates/nitrites, inorganic
      Bismuth subnitrate
      Nitric oxide
      Nitroprusside
      Silver nitrate
    Nitrates/nitrites, organic
      Amyl nitrite
      Butyl/isobutyl nitrite
      Nitroglycerin
    Phenacetin
    Phenazopyridine
    Resorcinol
    Rifampin
    Sulfonamides
    Vitamin K_3 (menadione)

INTRODUCTION AND EPIDEMIOLOGY

Methemoglobin is a form of hemoglobin in which the deoxygenated heme moiety has been oxidized from the ferrous (Fe^{2+}) to the ferric (Fe^{3+}) state. Deoxygenated hemoglobin must be maintained in the ferrous state to perform the physiologic role of oxygen transport properly. Therefore, methemoglobinemia, which is the accumulation of methemoglobin within the blood, causes decreased efficiency of oxygen delivery to tissues.

Methemoglobinemia may be congenital or acquired (Table 74–1). Acquired forms of methemoglobinemia are often further characterized according to etiology into exogenous or endogenous subgroups. A variety of oxidant drugs, chemicals, and foodstuffs may cause exogenous methemoglobinemia. Acquired cases for which no exogenous oxidant stress is identified are termed *endogenous.* Endogenous cases of methemoglobinemia occur almost exclusively among children younger than 6 months of age, and are most typically associated with diarrheal illness.

Toxicologists are frequently consulted to diagnose and treat methemoglobinemia since most cases result from poisoning. The list of drugs and chemicals implicated in methemoglobin production is vast (Table 74–2). Practitioners continue to express surprise when an infant, ill with diarrhea and acidosis, is noted to have methemoglobinemia, although subclinical methemoglobinemia may be present in as many as two thirds of those with diarrhea. It is important to understand the pathophysiologic differences between toxin-induced methemoglobinemia and transient, illness-associated methemoglobinemia of infancy.

DEVELOPMENTAL CONSIDERATIONS

Susceptibility to methemoglobin formation and tissue vulnerability to reduced oxygen delivery both vary according to development. In addition, inherited or acquired metabolic differences may render some individuals uniquely susceptible to methemoglobin accumulation.

The hemoglobin of infants younger than 6 months of age is more susceptible to oxidant stress than that of older children or adults. The red blood cells of these infants may have less than half of the adult levels of the major physiologic methemoglobin reduction enzyme, reduced nicotine adenine dinucleotide (NADH)-dependent cytochrome b_5 reductase. It has been suggested that fetal hemoglobin may also be more easily oxidized than adult-type hemoglobin. Finally, the microenvironment of the infantile intestinal tract differs from that of the adult in terms of pH, bacterial flora, and immunologic response. These factors may transform relatively inert chemicals into potent methemoglobin formers, and may play a role in diarrhea-associated methemoglobinemia.

In terms of oxygen delivery, fetal hemoglobin possesses a relatively greater affinity for oxygen than that of adult hemoglobin, and is less prone to release oxygen to tissues (the hemoglobin–oxygen dissociation curve is "shifted to the left"). Methemoglobin also causes an increase in oxygen affinity of the normal heme moieties remaining in the heme tetramer, shifting the oxyhemoglobin dissociation curve farther to the left. Methemoglobinemia is typically quantitated as a percentage of total hemoglobin, and hemoglobin concentration varies with age. Hemoglobin concentration is typically highest at birth, reaches a nadir at 2 months of age, and gradually rises to adult levels after adolescence. Cerebral oxygen demand is highest at birth and declines with age. Fortunately, cerebrovascular or coronary artery disease, which can complicate methemoglobinemia, uncommonly affect children.

PATHOPHYSIOLOGY

The principle role of hemoglobin in biological systems is to bind oxygen in the lungs and deliver it to body tissues so that cellular respiration may occur. As discussed, methemoglobin creates an allosteric change in the hemoglobin tetramer that results in reduced oxygen-carrying capacity and diminished oxygen release to tissues. Abnormal increases in methemoglobin occur in several distinct clinical contexts that include (1) congenital abnormalities in hemoglobin structure, (2) inherited deficiencies in methemoglobin reduction enzymes, (3) oxidative hemoglobin injury during infancy in response to illness (usually enteritis), and (4) oxidative hemoglobin injury owing to poisoning.

Toxic Methemoglobinemia

The rate, magnitude, and duration of toxin-induced methemoglobin formation depends on several factors: (1) the rate of entry of the compound into the circulation and red blood cells, (2) the rate of metabolism or biotransformation of the toxin in the body, (3) the rate of excretion of the toxin, and (4) the effectiveness of erythrocyte methemoglobin reduction systems. Some toxins, such as sodium nitrite, oxidize hemoglobin directly and produce methemoglobin rapidly. Other toxins may be considered indirect oxidizers, exerting their effect through generation of oxygen free radicals or H_2O_2. Toxins that undergo biotransformation may delay and prolong methemoglobin formation.

Illness-Associated Methemoglobinemia of Infancy

Transient methemoglobinemia without obvious oxidant drug or chemical exposure is a frequent finding in infants with enteritis and severe acidosis. It has also been reported among infants with diarrhea with no acidosis, acidosis with no diarrhea, bacterial enteritis, dietary protein intolerance, urinary tract infection, renal tubular acidosis, and organic acidurias. Subclinical methemoglobin elevations may be noted in as many as two thirds of young infants with acute diarrhea.

The etiology of illness-associated methemoglobinemia of infancy is likely to be multifactorial, and many physiologic stressors have been implicated in anecdotal and theoretical fashion. Intestinal endothelium produces nitric oxide, and diarrhea-elevated luminal and blood nitrate levels likely promote methemoglobin formation. The presence of acidemia may facilitate methemoglobin accumulation through pH-dependent inhibition of already low levels of reducing enzymes. In addition, the intestinal pH of young infants supports the colonization of bowel flora that facilitates conversion of relatively inert nitrates into powerfully oxidant nitrites. There are reports that many infants with methemoglobinemia are fed soy formula at the time of diagnosis. It is unclear whether this association is coincidental, reflects dietary changes that often are reactionary to infantile enteric symptoms, or is contributory.

Infants poisoned with methemoglobin formers such as benzocaine typically tolerate methemoglobin concentrations in excess of 40% without resultant metabolic acidosis or acidemia. In contrast, infants with illness-associated methemoglobinemia often have profound acidemia at methemoglobin levels less than 10%. Among infants with diarrhea, acidemia, and methemoglobinemia, lactate levels are rarely significantly elevated. Based on these observations, acidosis should be considered a contributing or coexisting factor, rather than a result, of methemoglobinemia among infants with diarrhea.

Congenital Methemoglobinemia

Hemoglobin M is the name given to several rare congenital structural abnormalities of hemoglobin that stabilize heme iron in the ferric state. Hemoglobin M follows an autosomal dominant inheritance pattern, and heterozygotes manifest lifelong cyanosis. Homozygous hemoglobin M is not compatible with life.

Inherited deficiencies in methemoglobin reduction enzymes may also lead to lifelong methemoglobinemia. Congenital deficiency in erythrocyte NADH-dependent cytochrome b_5 methemoglobin reductase is an autosomal recessive disorder that confers clinically apparent cyanosis among homozygotes. A similar enzyme deficiency, when expressed within neural cells, is associated with mental retardation. Heterozygotes for deficiency in NADH-dependent cytochrome b_5 methemoglobin reductase may be undetected, and may have far greater tendencies to develop profound methemoglobinemia during exposure to oxidant drugs and chemicals. Methylene blue therapy would likely be ineffective in the face of another extremely rare inherited disorder, deficiency in NADPH-dependent methemoglobin reductase, but these patients would not be expected to be more susceptible to methemoglobin formation.

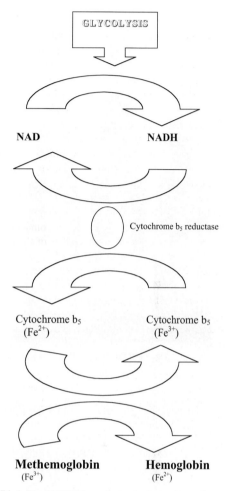

Fig. 74–1. The NADH-dependent cytochrome b_5 methemoglobin reductase pathway responsible for physiologic reduction of methemoglobin. *Abbreviations:* NAD, nicotine adenine dinucleotide; NADH, nicotine adenine dinucleotide (reduced form).

PHARMACOLOGY AND TOXICOKINETICS

Oxidative forces occur naturally within human red blood cells, so methemoglobin formation and reduction is a constant physiologic process. In the presence of intact methemoglobin reduction systems, red blood cells usually contain less than 1.5% methemoglobin. The high-energy compounds responsible for reducing methemoglobin are derived primarily from glycolysis. Under usual physiologic conditions, the enzyme NADH-dependent cytochrome b_5 methemoglobin reductase is almost entirely responsible for methemoglobin reduction (Figure 74–1).

Among normal individuals, the half-life of methemoglobinemia induced by exposure to topical local anesthetics is less than 1 hour. Other cellular antioxidants, such as vitamin C and glutathione, likely play a trivial role in methemoglobin homeostasis. Enzymes such as superoxide dismutase, catalase, and glutathione peroxidase may serve to limit oxidative damage from superoxide radicals.

Antidotal methylene blue (Figure 74–2) serves as a cofactor for an otherwise dormant metabolic system that derives reducing power from the hexose monophosphate shunt. Methylene blue therapy uses reduced nicotine

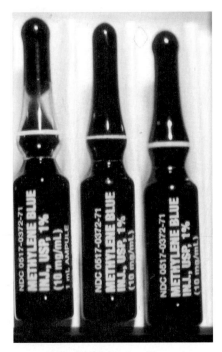

Fig. 74–2. Methylene blue.

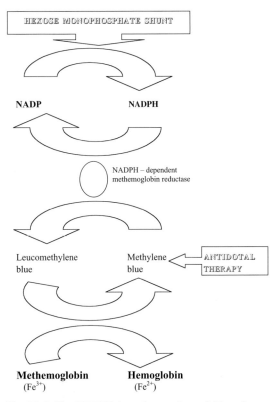

Fig. 74–3. The NADPH-dependent methemoglobin reductase pathway for reduction of methemoglobin after antidotal methylene blue therapy. *Abbreviations:* NADP, nicotine adenine dinucleotide phosphate; NADPH, nicotine adenine dinucleotide phosphate (reduced form).

adenine dinucleotide phosphate (NADPH)-dependent methemoglobin reductase to reduce a large proportion of methemoglobin (Figure 74–3). G-6-PD contributes to the biological production of NADPH, so methylene blue therapy may be ineffective or harmful when administered to patients with severe G-6-PD deficiency.

CLINICAL PRESENTATION

Cyanosis unresponsive to oxygen, despite normal arterial oxygen tension, is the hallmark of methemoglobinemia. Such cyanosis is typically most notable in the skin, lips, and nailbeds, and becomes clinically apparent in the presence of 1.5 g/dL of methemoglobin. A differential diagnosis for cyanosis is listed in Table 74–3, and an algorithm for the evaluation of cyanosis is offered in Figure 74–4. Once an infant is diagnosed with methemoglobinemia, the algorithm in Figure 74–5 may assist in determining its etiology.

A general correlation of methemoglobin level to clinical condition is presented in Table 74–4, but methemoglobin percentages must be interpreted in the contexts of total hemoglobin levels and premorbid health. Rapid

accumulation of methemoglobin will be clinically more severe than a similar degree of methemoglobinemia that developed gradually. In general, the nonanemic patient tolerates the acute accumulation of less than 30% methemoglobin. Neonates and infants often present with nonspecific clinical findings such as tachycardia, poor feeding, vomiting, irritability, excessive crying, and/or excessive sleeping, so the detection of methemoglobinemia in these patients requires a high index of suspicion. Cyanosis, in conjunction with these clinical signs and symptoms, may be easily misinterpreted as a sign of structural heart disease.

Toxic Methemoglobinemia

Children with methemoglobinemia related to xenobiotic oxidative stress typically appear well despite marked

Table 74–3. Differential Diagnosis for Cyanosis

> Deoxygenated hemoglobin
>> Environmental hypoxia
>> Cardiovascular disease
>> Pulmonary disease
> Abnormal hemoglobin
>> Methemoglobinemia
>> Sulfhemoglobinemia
> Factitious
>> Discoloration of skin/mucous membranes

cyanosis at methemoglobin levels near 30%, and tolerate methemoglobin concentrations in excess of 40% without development of acidosis. Toxins responsible for methemoglobin induction often produce other deleterious effects that may complicate the clinical picture. Although oxidant stress affecting the hemoglobin molecule may produce methemoglobin, similar oxidative injury to the cell membrane may lead to hemolysis. Vasodilators such as nitrites may contribute to tachycardia, hypotension, and circulatory inadequacy.

Children with iatrogenic methemoglobinemia may present a particular dilemma for medical practitioners. Many reports exist of abrupt cyanotic methemoglobinemia after topical anesthesia for endoscopy, or after dapsone treatment for heart transplant. Table 74–2 illustrates numerous opportunities for the undesired therapeutic production of methemoglobinemia.

Illness-Associated Methemoglobinemia of Infancy

Infants with diarrhea and methemoglobinemia often suffer from concurrent dehydration and metabolic acidosis. A dusky appearance, abnormal arterial blood color, or lower-than-expected pulse oximetry readings may prompt the astute clinician to consider methemoglobinemia. Although such infants are often profoundly ill and may appear septic, methemoglobinemia should not be considered the proximate cause of such illness. Following methylene blue therapy, diarrhea and acidosis may persist, methemoglobinemia may persist or recur, and hospitalization may be more prolonged than in similarly aged patients with toxic methemoglobinemia.

Congenital Methemoglobinemia

Children with congenital forms of methemoglobinemia appear well yet exhibit lifelong cyanosis. The lack of concurrent illness, and the chronicity of the problem, differentiates these infants from those with acquired methemoglobinemia.

LABORATORY AND DIAGNOSTIC TESTING

Inspection of Blood

The arterial blood of children with methemoglobinemia is classically described as chocolate brown (see Color Plate 16), although comparison of suspect blood to control blood on a white paper towel or filter paper highlights this distinction. In contrast to deoxygenated blood from patients with cardiopulmonary disease, methemoglobin-darkened blood does not redden upon exposure to room air.

Pulse Oximetry

Pulse oximetry assessment of the oxygen saturation of hemoglobin is inaccurate in the setting of methemoglobinemia. Transcutaneous pulse oximetry compares light absorption of oxygenated and deoxygenated hemoglobin to derive hemoglobin oxygen saturation. Methemoglobin has a spectrum of light absorption than differs from that of deoxygenated hemoglobin and thus interferes with this technology. Typically, pulse oximetry underestimates oxygen saturation at low methemoglobin levels, and overestimates oxygen saturation at high levels. Methylene blue therapy may also interfere with pulse oximetry measurements.

Arterial Blood Gas Analysis

Most hospital laboratories do not measure hemoglobin oxygen saturation directly during blood gas analysis, but instead derive it from a nomogram based upon the partial pressure of oxygen (P_{O_2}) within the sample. Because methemoglobinemia affects hemoglobin oxygen saturation, but not P_{O_2}, arterial blood gas analysis overestimates oxygen saturation. A saturation gap suggests the presence of methemoglobin or sulfhemoglobin when the hemoglobin oxygen saturation calculated from blood gas analysis is significantly greater than the measured oxygen saturation.

Co-Oximetry

Multiple-wavelength co-oximetry is the laboratory method of choice for confirming and quantifying methemoglobinemia. Hyperlipidemia or intravenous (IV)

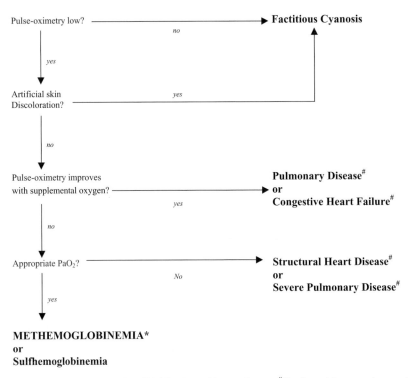

Fig. 74–4. Diagnostic algorithm for the cyanotic child. *Confirm with co-oximetry. #Confirm with appropriate testing. *Abbreviation:* PaO$_2$, arterial partial pressure of oxygen.

administration of methylene blue or other dyes may interfere with this laboratory technique.

Other Ancillary Tests

A complete blood cell count is useful, because methemoglobin percentages must be interpreted in the context of the blood hemoglobin concentration. In addition, hemolysis may complicate the oxidative stress responsible for producing methemoglobinemia. Serum chemistries allow for the assessment of metabolic acidosis. Urine toxicology screens for drugs of abuse are unlikely to uncover causes of methemoglobinemia. Hemoglobin electrophoresis is unnecessary in the evaluation of acquired methemoglobinemia. Quantitation of NADH-dependent cytochrome b$_5$ methemoglobin reductase is not routinely available and is unlikely to alter management. G-6-PD deficiency does not increase susceptibility to methemoglobinemia, so testing is not routinely warranted, unless there are concerns over administration of methylene blue therapy.

MANAGEMENT

In all cases of acquired methemoglobinemia, careful attention should be given to the status of the patient's airway, breathing, circulation, and neurologic function. Cyanosis and transcutaneous pulse oximetry measurements must be interpreted carefully in the presence of methemoglobinemia. Supplemental oxygen should be administered. Supportive care is sufficient therapy for most identified cases of methemoglobinemia.

Antidotal therapy with IV methylene blue should be considered for patients with overt signs of tissue hypoxia, central nervous system depression, or cardiovascular instability. If no contraindications exist, methylene blue therapy is otherwise generally recommended for methemoglobin levels in excess of 30%, or when comorbid conditions limit a patient's tolerance for decreases in oxygen delivery. Methylene blue is administered over 5 minutes at a dose of 1 to 2 mg/kg (0.1 to 0.2 mL/kg) of a 1% solution (Figure 74–2). This dose may be repeated in 1 hour if needed. Persistent or recurrent methemoglobinemia may

Table 74–4. Approximate Correlation of Methemoglobin Concentration to Clinical Symptoms and Signs in a Healthy, Nonanemic Child

Methemoglobin concentration (%)	Clinical Findings
>10	Cyanosis
>30	Malaise, fatigue, dyspnea, tachycardia
>50	Somnolence, tissue ischemia
>70	Potentially lethal

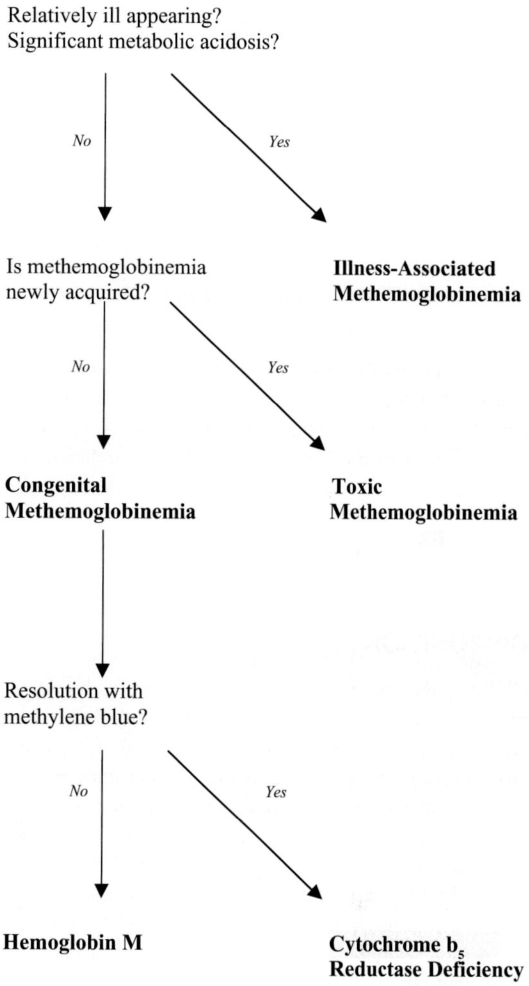

require additional doses, but caution is recommended when the total approaches 4 to 7 mg/kg, because methylene blue itself may become a source of oxidant stress. Methylene blue may discolor skin and interfere with transcutaneous pulse oximetry measurements, so co-oximetry should guide repeat therapy. Continuous infusions of methylene blue, titrated from a starting rate of 0.1 mg/kg/h, have been employed for poisonings expected to produce oxidative injury over a prolonged period.

The kidneys comprise the primary route of elimination for methylene blue, and the urine develops a blue–green discoloration after therapy. Most individuals tolerate methylene blue therapy extremely well, although rapidly administered doses have been associated with side effects such as nausea, chest pain, tachycardia, hypertension, and anxiety. Heinz body hemolytic anemia has been reported in young infants at doses as low as 4 mg/kg. Known or suspected severe G-6-PD deficiency is a relative contraindication to methylene blue therapy, because these patients may have insufficient NADPH to serve as a cofactor for antidotal methemoglobin reduction. In addition, methylene blue may induce hemolysis in patients who are G-6-PD deficient.

If methylene blue therapy is contraindicated, not possible, or ineffective, several other therapies have been proposed. Hyperbaric oxygen therapy and exchange transfusion are heroic measures that have been promoted anecdotally. IV ascorbic acid may increase nonenzymatic reduction of methemoglobin. Despite promising in vitro data, *N*-acetylcysteine has not proven to reduce methemoglobin effectively.

Toxic Methemoglobinemia

A history of drug and chemical exposure should be fully elucidated. An environmental history should include the source of drinking water and the types of baby foods of-

Fig. 74–5. Diagnostic algorithm for the young infant with <40% methemoglobinemia.

fered to the child. The xenobiotic responsible for methemoglobin production should be identified and eliminated. Principles of gastrointestinal decontamination of poisoned children are discussed in Chapter 16. Cimetidine treatment may reduce dapsone-induced methemoglobinemia by inhibiting the drug's bioactivation.

Illness-Associated Methemoglobinemia of Infancy

These infants typically improve clinically with restoration of fluid, electrolyte, and pH balance. Children should be evaluated for possible infection with nitrite-producing bacteria and such infection, if identified, should be treated. Infants with diarrhea-associated methemoglobinemia will continue to produce methemoglobin until their enteritis is healed. In such infants it may be prudent to change to elemental formula until recovery is evident.

Congenital Methemoglobinemia

Despite significant cyanosis, most children with congenital methemoglobinemia are otherwise asymptomatic. Oral methylene blue or ascorbic acid may be used to ameliorate methemoglobin levels, and cosmetic cyanosis, of children with methemoglobin reductase deficiencies. Such therapies do not benefit children with hemoglobin M.

DISPOSITION

Children with acquired methemoglobinemia should remain in a medical supervision until the source of oxidative hemoglobin injury has been removed. Drugs and chemicals that require biotransformation or undergo significant enterohepatic recirculation may lead to recurrence of methemoglobinemia after cessation of methylene blue therapy. The expertise of a toxicologist or regional poison control center may be invaluable in such a scenario. Some infants, such as those fed formula reconstituted with well water, may require environmental investigation.

Infants with illness-associated methemoglobinemia should remain in medical care until the underlying illness has been identified and treated. Consultation with a hematologist should be considered for patients suspected of having inherited either a variant of hemoglobin or a deficiency of methemoglobin reduction enzymes.

CASE OUTCOME

Once methemoglobinemia was implicated as the cause of the baby's cyanosis, the father, a physician, reports that he has been applying a topical 2.5% lidocaine/2.5% prilocaine cream to the circumcision site every few hours. Recognition of the methemoglobinemia by medication history or through consideration of laboratory and examination findings may have obviated the need for medical evaluation for sepsis or congenital heart defect. The infant is treated with methylene blue, 2 mg/kg IV over 5 minutes, with rapid resolution of cyanosis. The pulse oximeter reading decreased to 70% during methylene blue infusion, but rose to 98% within 15 minutes. Use of the topical anesthetic cream is discontinued. The child appears well overnight, returns home the following day, and remains well.

SUGGESTED READINGS

Avner JR, Henretig FM, McAneney CM: Acquired methemoglobinemia: The relationship of cause to course of illness. *Am J Dis Child* 144:1229–1230, 1990.

Bradberry SM, Aw TC, Williams NR, et al: Occupational methaemoglobinaemia. *Occup Environ Med* 58:611–615, 2001.

Dotsch J, Demirakca S, Kratz M, et al: Comparison of methylene blue, riboflavin, and *N*-acetylcysteine for the reduction of nitric oxide-induced methemoglobinemia. *Crit Care Med* 28:958–961, 2000.

Hanokuglu A, Danon PN: Endogenous methemoglobinemia associated with diarrheal disease in infancy. *J Pediatr Gastroenter Nutr* 23:1–7, 1996.

Jaffe ER: Enzymopenic hereditary methemoglobinemia. A clinical/biochemical classification. *Blood Cells* 12:81–90, 1986.

Karim A, Ahmed S, Siddiqui R, et al: Methemoglobinemia complicating topical lidocaine used during endoscopic procedures. *Am J Med* 111:150–153, 2001.

Pollack ES, Pollack CV: Incidence of subclinical methemoglobinemia in infants with diarrhea. *Ann Emerg Med* 24:652–656, 1994.

Wright RO, Lewander WJ, Woolf AD: Methemoglobinemia: Etiology, pharmacology, and clinical management. *Ann Emerg Med* 34:646–656, 1999.

75

Natural and Environmental Toxins

Timothy B. Erickson

HIGH-YIELD FACTS

- Young children are at risk for natural toxin exposure and envenomation owing to their attraction to flowers, leaves, and berries, as well as their innate curiosity toward reptiles, arthropods, and marine creatures.

- Adolescents are at risk for intoxication secondary to recreational use of natural toxins for their euphoric effects, as well as secondary to handling venomous creatures as pets.

- As a result of their small body weight, infants and young children are relatively more vulnerable to severe envenomation and systemic toxicity.

- The most frequent site of a bite or sting is an extremity. Localized tenderness, swelling, and erythema are the most common clinical findings.

- For most environmental bites and stings, local wound care, irrigation, tetanus immunization, wound exploration for foreign bodies, and selected antibiotic coverage are common therapies.

- Antivenoms or antitoxins are available for many environmental and natural poisons including crotalid and coral snakes, black widow spiders, scorpions, stonefish, box jellyfish, cardioglycoside containing plants, and botulinum toxin.

- The majority of plant and mushroom exposures in children are unintentional and involve small quantities. Most patients develop minimal to no symptoms, with gastrointestinal (GI) upset the most common manifestation. For the majority of patients, treatment is supportive.

- Over the past two decades, public fascination with natural foods and traditional medicinal remedies, along with poor federal regulation, have resulted in increased pediatric exposure to herbal products.

- Contrary to public belief, epidemiologic statistics reflect an extremely low case fatality rate associated with environmental and natural toxin exposure in children.

HERBAL PRODUCTS

During the past two decades, public fascination with natural foods and herbal remedies has resulted in increased exposure to herbal products in children. Unfortunately, there is little consumer awareness of the potential harm of most herbal preparations, and federal regulation of these products has been poor.

Epidemiology

According to the 2002 American Association of Poison Control Centers (AAPCC) database, there were 12,616 herbal exposures reported to poison control centers in

2001 in children younger than 20 years of age, with four pediatric deaths.

Developmental Considerations

Parents may give newborns and infants home remedies containing herbal products. Toddlers may be exposed to herbal products through inadvertent ingestions. Adolescents use herbals for their mind-altering properties, as well as their potential aphrodisiac or anabolic effects.

Most Common Toxins

Herbal teas and medications may contain variable amounts of active or poisonous substances. Homeopathic medicines are common and usually very dilute, resulting in minimal toxicity. The most common exposures include Ma huang, Ginkgo biloba, Ginseng, Echinacea, St. John's Wort, creatine, and kava kava.

Most Dangerous Toxins

Naturopathic or steeped teas may be highly concentrated. Commercially packaged products or nutritional supplements may contain toxic plants or dangerous herbal additives. Contamination or adulteration with unlabeled substances may also be present. Herbal products containing heavy metals such as mercury, arsenic, and lead may be inadvertently given to children. Herbal products containing ephedra (Ma huang), salicylates, benzodiazepines, cardiogycosides, corticosteroids, and aphrodisiacs such as yohimbine are also likely to result in more serious toxicity.

FOOD POISONING AND BOTULISM

Increased importation of fresh fruits and meat products have resulted in an increased incidence of food poisoning. Marine foodborne poisonings of note include ciguatoxin, scombrotoxin, paralytic shellfish saxitoxin, and tetrodotoxin. As a result of the wide availability of fresh and frozen fish, there is an increasing frequency of toxic ingestions in North America.

Epidemiology

It is estimated that there are nearly 7 million cases of food poisoning occur in the United States annually, with nearly 10,000 related deaths. However, most cases are unreported. Fewer than half have an etiology determined. Accurate epidemiologic studies are costly and time consuming.

Developmental Considerations

Maternal food poisoning resulting in severe dehydration can have adverse effects on the developing fetus. Although food poisoning is uncommon in breastfed infants; formula-fed infants can suffer GI distress if opened formula is not properly refrigerated. Toddlers being introduced to a variety of solid foods may be prone to poisoning from spoiled products. Adolescents have similar risks to the types of food poisoning as adults, and are susceptible to improperly stored and ill prepared fast foods.

Most Common

Common foodborne poisonings include salmonella, shigella, *Staphylococcus aureus*, *Clostrium perfringes*, and campylobacter.

Ciguatera fish poisoning is a serious health problem in the Caribbean and Indo-Pacific regions. Ciguatoxin is produced by the dinoflagellate *Gambierdiscus toxicus* and concentrated in the food chain of predatory reef fish such as barracuda, red snapper, parrotfish, jacks, jellyfish, and moray eels. When humans ingest contaminated fish, poisoning can cause distinct neurologic and GI symptoms. Classic findings in ciguatera poisoning include circumoral tingling, generalized parethesias, and apparent reversal of hot cold sensations.

Scombroid poisoning is associated with the consumption of certain improperly preserved fish (mostly dark fleshed) such as tuna, bonito, skipjack, mackerel, and mahi-mahi (dolphin fish). These fish have undergone bacterial decontamination owing to poor refrigeration. Scombrotoxin causes a histamine-like or allergic reaction appearing syndrome.

Most Dangerous

Specific neurotoxic species of the dinoflagellate *Gonyaulax* form red tides and concentrate the saxitoxin in bivalve shellfish such as mussels, clams, and scallops. Humans who consume contaminated shellfish can develop paralytic shellfish poisoning, which can result in paresthesias, cranial and peripheral nerve dysfunction, and respiratory failure.

Tetrodotoxin, one of the most potent poisons in nature, results in toxicity after the ingestion of meat from puffer fish, blowfish, balloonfish, and porcupine fish. Other marine animals harboring tetrodotoxin include the eastern salamander, Californian newt, and blue-ringed octopus. Tetrodotoxin can cause death by inducing respiratory paralysis and cardiovascular collapse.

Botulism results from potent neurotoxins elaborated by the bacterium *Clostridium botulinium*, a spore-forming obligate anaerobe. Life-threatening paralytic respiratory illness can result. Several types of botulism exist: foodborne, infantile, and wound botulism. The ingestion of food containing preformed toxin results in the most serious form of botulism. Most cases in the United States occur following the consumption of improperly prepared preserved home canned foods. The incidence of infant botulism is increasing and may be underdiagnosed. Children younger than 1 are most frequently affected. Children from 1 week to 6 months are most susceptible. Although honey is often implicated, a recent association with corn syrup has been made.

MARINE ENVENOMATIONS

As more humans relocate to coastal regions and venture into aquatic environments for recreational activities, the opportunity for children to encounter venomous marine life increases. Also, as more aquarists collect exotic marine life for display in the home, the incidence of bites and stings will rise regardless of the geographic locale.

Epidemiology

According to the AAPCC data collecting system, there were 1287 aquatic bites and envenomations to children reported in the year 2001. The majority of these events (70%) occurred in children between the ages of 7 and 19 years, with 30% in children younger than 6 years of age. Of these marine exposures, the coelenterate group was responsible for over half of the stings reported.

Developmental Considerations

Toddlers are most likely to be envenomed in waters and are typically unable to give a detailed or reliable history. Young children may step on poisonous marine animals or handle them, resulting in extremity stings. Adolescents are more adventurous and frequent deeper waters as surfers, snorklers, and scuba divers; they are also more susceptible to intoxication with ethanol or recreational drugs, impairing their judgment.

Most Common

For most marine stings local wound care, irrigation, tetanus immunization, wound exploration for foreign bodies, and selected antibiotic coverage are common therapies. Coelenterates (phylum *Cnidaria*) include jellyfish, sea anemones, and corals. Jellyfish stings are the most common marine envenomations. Children seem to have a more severe reaction to the numerous fired neumatocysts. Dermatologic irrigation with vinegar, rubbing alcohol, or household ammonia is recommended. Baking soda or papain will neutralize many coelenterate, including jellyfish, envenomations.

There are more than 250 species of venomous fish, consisting mostly of shallow water reef or inshore fish. Stingrays are the most commonly encountered venomous fish, with more than 2000 stings reported annually. Catfish are found in both fresh and salt water. Stings occur from spines contained within an integumentary sheath on their dorsal or pectoral fins. The hands and forearms of fishermen and seafood handlers are the most common sting sites. Hot water soaks are recommended for stingray, scorpion fish, echinoderms, and catfish stings.

Echinoderms are spiny invertebrates that include sea urchins, seastars, starfish, sea cucumbers, and sand dollars. Of these, sea urchins most often cause medically significant envenomations.

Most Dangerous

One of the more feared jellyfish is the Portuguese man'o'war (*Physalia physalis*). This jellyfish is most commonly found in the Gulf of Mexico and off the Florida coasts. Its tentacles can reach up to 30 meters in length. The deadliest and most venomous of the coelenterates is the box jellyfish, or sea wasp of Australia (*Chironex*).

Varieties of scorpion fish include zebrafish and lionfish (*Pterois*), scorpion fish (*Scorpaena*), and the deadly stonefish (*Synanceja*). Lionfish are popular for domestic display as aquarium pets.

Sea snakes of the family *Hydrophiidae* are encountered through the Indo-Pacific region. Sea snakes are air-breathing reptiles with venomous anterior fangs. They are among the deadliest snakes in the world, and may bite without provocation. Most bites are associated with net fishing and inadvertent handling. Antivenoms are available for stonefish, box jellyfish, and sea snake envenomations.

MUSHROOM POISONING

Mushroom poisoning is common, particularly in families who forage or hunt for mushrooms in the wild. Curious young children may take a small bite of a mushroom, usually resulting in minimal to no symptoms.

Epidemiology

There were 8483 mushroom exposures reported to poison control centers in 2001. Ninety percent of the ingestions were inadvertent, with 85% involving children. Significant toxicity was rare, with only 0.3% of patients experiencing a major effect, with no reported deaths.

Developmental Considerations

Mushroom poisonings occur in three different scenarios: inadvertent ingestion by young children, amateur foragers looking for specific mushrooms for eating, and adolescents using mushrooms for their hallucinogenic effects.

Most Common

Most toxic mushroom ingestions are of the GI irritant variety, resulting in gastroenteritis. GI upset that begins within 2 hours of ingestion of a mushroom is almost always self-limited and benign. *Psylocibin* and *Aminita muscaria* mushrooms are often ingested for their hallucinogenic properties.

Most Dangerous

Aminita phalloides and *Aminita virosa* species are extremely hepatotoxic and appear in the fall in the northern hemisphere. Amatoxins are among the most potent toxins known. *Gyromitra* species also contain amatoxins and appear primarily in the spring. GI symptoms that begin more than 6 hours after ingestion may be associated with severe hepatic or renal dysfunction.

A disulfiram-type reaction may occur when consuming alcohol 2 to 72 hours after *Corinus* mushrooms are ingested. *Cortinaris* mushrooms may result in renal toxicity. False morels (*Gyromitra*) mushrooms contain monomethylhydrazine and can cause status epilepticus. Similar to isoniazid toxicity, the antidote of choice is pyridoxine or vitamin B_6.

POISONOUS PLANTS

The majority of plant exposures are unintentional and involve small quantities. Most patients do not develop any symptoms. GI upset is the most common manifestation of symptomatic exposure. For many patients, treatment is supportive.

Epidemiology

Every year, plant ingestions account for 5% of all calls to poison centers in the United States. Nearly 70% of all plant ingestions are by children younger than 6 years. Overall, pediatric ingestion of plants only rarely results in toxicity. Of the 105,560 calls received by poison control centers for plant exposures in 2001, only two deaths were reported.

Developmental Considerations

Plant parts such as flowers, leaves, and berries are most commonly ingested by small children. Two common scenarios exist. Very young children, particularly toddlers, may ingest plant material while exploring their environment. Older children and adolescents may intentionally ingest a certain plant species for its purported psychoactive effect.

Most Common

Chili pepper or *Capsacium* was the most common plant exposure reported to poison control centers in 2001. During the Christmas holidays, children are often exposed to poinsettia, mistletoe, and holly. The majority of these ingestions result in no symptoms, but may cause gastroenteritis. *Diffenbachia* and *Philodendron* are household plants that toddlers tend to ingest and are the most common cause of symptomatic plant ingestions. They can cause oral and pharyngeal pain secondary to injection of insoluble calcium oxalate crystals.

Most Dangerous

Several species of plants contain cardioglycosides. Foxglove, Oleander, and Lily of the Valley may all cause toxicity similar to digitalis intoxication. In severe cases, the use of Digibind may be considered. Water hemlock is easily confused with the wild carrot or Queen Anne's lace. The potential for serious toxicity from ingestion of this plant is significant. Patients may progress to status epilepticus, respiratory distress, rhabdomyolysis, and death.

SNAKE ENVENOMATIONS

Snakebites usually occur when children venture into the snake's natural habitat, but also have been reported in the household environment when the snakes are kept in captivity as pets. Families of venomous snakes indigenous to the United States include *Crotalidae* (pit vipers) and *Elapidae* (coral snakes). Pit viper envenomations result in hematotoxicity; coral snakes cause neurotoxicity.

Prehospital management of snakebites includes immobilization of the bitten extremity, minimization of physical activity, fluid administration, and rapid transport to the nearest health care facility. In addition to supportive care, Crotalid antivenom is the fundamental treatment of pit viper envenomation.

Epidemiology

Over 200 crotalid envenomations are reported every year to poison control centers; many go unreported and the estimated true number may be closer to 8000. Pit vipers account for over 95% of all envenomations and are divided into the genuses *Crotalus* (rattlesnakes), *Agkistrodon* (cotton mouths and copperheads), and *Sistruses* (pigmy rattlesnakes and massasauguas). Coral snakes account for an estimated 1% to 2% of envenomations. According to the 2001 annual report of the AAPCC, 258 children under 20 years of age were bitten by rattlesnakes, 188 by copperheads, 38 by cottonmouths, 15 by coral snakes, and 17 by exotic snakes. One death was reported in a 17-year-old girl from an unknown species of snake. These statistics reflect the low case fatality rate associated with snake envenomations.

Developmental Considerations

Because snakes are defensive animals and rarely attack, they remain immobile or even attempt to retreat if given the opportunity. Bites most commonly occur in small children who are paralyzed with fear or with older children who harass the snake. The severity of envenomation also depends on the location of the bite. As a result of their small body weight, infants and young children are relatively more vulnerable to severe envenomation. In comparison with adults, pediatric patients are given proportionately more antivenom, because children receive a greater amount of venom per kilogram of body weight. More venom may be delivered when a snake is handled or agitated compared with accidentally startling the snake.

Most Common

Most snake bites are from nonvenomous snakes, which usually leave a horseshoe-shaped imprint of multiple teeth marks as opposed to the classic two-fanged puncture wounds associated with rapid extremity edema as suffered with a crotalid bite. The pit vipers (crotalids) ac-

count for the majority of snake envenomations, with copperheads comprising the most common species-specific bite. Approximately 25% of poisonous snakebites may actually be dry bites, resulting in minimal to no toxicity.

Most Dangerous

The prognosis following pit viper envenomation is generally good, with an overall mortality rate of <1% if the antivenom is given in adequate amounts without delay.

Dangerous crotalids include Mojave rattlesnakes, which cause delayed neurologic and respiratory depression several hours after envenomation. Coral snakes are also considered very dangerous owing to neurotoxicity despite the lack of an impressive bite site.

Several bites occur each year from nonindigenous snakes. Dangerous worldwide snakes include the Fierce, Tiger, and Brown snakes of Australia, the sea snake (*Hydrophidae*) commonly found in the Indo-Pacific region, the krait of south east Asia, the king cobra of India (*Elapidae*), and the green and black mamba of Africa. The most common cause of snake bite fatalities worldwide result from the bite of the Russell pit viper.

SPIDER AND ARTHROPOD ENVENOMATIONS

Black widow spiders of the genus *Lactrodectus* are found throughout the temperate and tropical zones of the earth. *Lactrodectus mactans*, the black widow spider of North America, is a shiny black spider with fangs, poison glands, with a characteristic red hourglass mark on the ventral surface of the abdomen. From a toxicologic viewpoint, only the female is venomous to humans. The male spider also has venom, but has small fangs that cannot penetrate human skin. The brown recluse spider, *Loxosceles recluse*, is a brown to fawn-colored spider, with a characteristic violin or fiddle-shaped marking on the dorsal cephalothorax. It is commonly found in the south central regions of the United States.

The scorpion has a pair of anterior legs with pinchers, a segmented body, and a long, mobile tail equipped with a stinger. Although members of the genera *Hadrurus*, *Vejovis*, and *Uroctonus* are capable of inflicting painful wounds, only the southwestern desert scorpion (*Centruroides exilicauda*) poses a serious threat in the United States. The order *Hymenoptera* includes bees, vespids (hornets and wasps), and fire ants.

Epidemiology

According to the annual report of the AAPCC in 2001, 598 children under 20 years of age suffered bites from black widow spiders, and 570 were envenomed by brown recluse spiders. No pediatric deaths were recorded during that time period. In 2001, the same database reported 4023 scorpion stings, 1301 fire ant stings, and 5344 bee, wasp, or hornet stings in children younger than 20 years of age. No deaths were reported.

Most Common

At least 50 species of spiders found in the United States are known to bite humans, although in most cases the diagnosis is not suspected and no treatment is necessary. Spiders causing mild necrotizing bites include the orb-weaver, sac spider, jumping spider, wolf spider, and hobo spider.

Honeybees (*Apis mellifera*) are fuzzy insects with alternating black and tan stripes. Not intrinsically aggressive, they usually sting defensively when stepped on. Like that of other hymenoptera, the honeybee's stinger is a modified ovipositor (only the females sting) that is connected to a venom sac. The most common hornets in the United States are the yellow jackets (*Vespa pennsylvanica*). They are usually seen around garbage cans, beverage containers, and various foods. They are extremely aggressive and sting with little provocation.

Fire ant stings are very common in the southern United States, from Florida to Texas and can cause painful, local skin reactions. Two species of fire ants were imported into the United States: fire ant (*Solenopsis invicta*) and the black fire ant (*Solenopsis richteri*).

Most Dangerous

Black widow spider bites result in painful muscle spasms secondary to neurotoxicity. Although rare (fewer than 5% of cases), death can result from respiratory or cardiac failure. Severe envenomations may be treated with *Lactrodectus*-specific antivenin. Other red and brown species of widow spiders are found in Australia and South Africa. Brown recluse spider bites result in hematotoxicity and manifest locally as skin necrosis. Ounce for ounce, the venom of the *Loxosceles* spider is more potent than that of the rattlesnake and can cause extensive necrosis.

Worldwide, scorpions are responsible for thousands of deaths annually. Some 1500 separate species of scorpion have been identified. Of these, only 25 species are medically important, most of which are in the *Buthidae* family. In the United States, there have been no reported deaths from scorpion stings in more than 25 years. Nevertheless, they remain a public health concern throughout the South and Southwest. Scorpion stings cause severe local pain with occasional systemic effects noted in children. Hyperimmune goat serum antivenom has been used with success for more severe envenomations with potentially life-threatening symptoms.

Bees (*Hymenoptera*) cause one third of all reported envenomations in the United States and an estimated 50 to 150 annual deaths. Although *Hymenoptera* possess intrinsic toxicity, it is their ability to sensitize the victim and cause subsequent reactions that makes them potentially lethal from severe anaphylactic reactions. Systemic reactions occur in approximately 1% of stings. African killer bees (*Apis mellifera scutellata*) were imported into Brazil during the 1960s to improve honey production. Over the years, they evolved into a hybrid species and migrated north into Central America. Recently, they have been sighted in the southern United States. They are very aggressive, attack in swarms, and death has occurred as a result of the large amount of venom injected.

CONCLUSION

As more humans venture and impinge on the outdoor environment, the opportunity for children to encounter venomous wildlife increases. Young children are at risk for natural toxin exposure and envenomation owing to their attraction to flowers, leaves, and berries, as well as their innate curiosity toward reptiles, arthropods, and marine creatures. Despite public belief to the contrary, epidemiologic statistics reflect an extremely low case fatality rate associated with environmental and natural toxin exposure in children. Chapters 76 through 82 discuss each of these natural toxins in greater detail describing their diagnosis, management, and prognosis.

SUGGESTED READINGS

Auerbach P: Envenomation by aquatic animals. In Auerbach PS, ed: *Wilderness Medicine.* 4th ed. St. Louis: Mosby; 2001:1450–1487.

Auerbach PS: Marine envenomations. *N Engl J Med* 325:486–493, 1991.

Banner W: Bites and stings in the pediatric patient. *Curr Probl Pediatr* 18:1–69, 1988.

Biberci E, Altunas Y, Cobanoglu A, et al: Acute respiratory arrest following hemlock (*Conium maculatum*) intoxication. *J Toxicol Clin Toxicol* 40:517–518, 2002.

Clark RF, Wethern-Kestner S, Vance MV, et al: Clinical presentation and treatment of black widow spider envenomation: A review of 163 cases. *Ann Emerg Med* 21:782–787, 1992.

Clark RF: The safety and efficacy of antivenin *Latrodectus mactans*. *Clin Toxicol* 39:125–127, 2001.

Dart RC, McNally J: Efficacy, safety, and use of snake antivenoms in the United States. *Ann Emerg Med* 37:181–188, 2001.

Das S, Nalini P, Antakrishnan S, et al: Cardiac involvement and scorpion envenomation in children. *J Trop Pediatr* 41:338–340, 1995.

Fenner PJ, Williamson JA: Worldwide deaths and severe envenomation from jellyfish stings. *Med J Aust* 165:658, 1996.

Frenner PJ, Williamson JA, Skinner RA: Fatal and nonfatal stingray envenomation. *Med J Aust* 151:621, 1989.

Hughes JM, Potter ME: Scombroid fish poisoning. *N Engl J Med* 324:766–768, 1991.

Jansen PW, Perkin RM, Van Stralen D: Mojave rattlesnake envenomation: prolonged neurotoxicity and rhabdomyolysis. *Ann Emerg Med* 21:322–325, 1992.

Kitchens CS, Van Mierop LH: Envenomation by the eastern coral snake (*Micrurus fulvius fulvius*). A study of 39 victims. *JAMA* 258:1615–1618, 1987.

Krenzelok EP, Jacobsen TD, Aronis J: Hemlock ingestions: The most deadly plant exposures. Abstract. *J Toxicol Clin Toxicol* 601–602, 1996.

Krenzelok EP, Jacobsen TD, Aronis J: Poinsettia exposures have good outcomes. . . Just as we thought. *Am J Emerg Med* 14:671–674, 1996.

Lampe KF, McCann MA: *AMA Handbook of Poisonous and Injurious Plants.* Chicago: American Medical Association; 1985.

Litovitz TL, Klein-Schwartz W, Rodgers GC, et al: 2001 annual report of the American Association of Poison Control Centers Toxic Exposure Surveillance System. *Am J Emerg Med* 20:391–352, 2002.

McInerney J, Shagal P, Bogel M: Scombroid poisoning. *Ann Emerg Med* 8:235, 1996.

Offerman SR, Bush SP, Moynihan JA, et al: Crotaline Fab antivenom for the treatment of children with rattlesnake envenomation. *Pediatrics* 110:968–971, 2002.

Pedaci L, Krenzelok EP, Jacobsen TD, et al: Dieffenbachia species exposures: an evidence-based assessment of symptom presentation. *Vet Hum Toxicol* 41:335–338, 1999.

Rash LD, Hodgson WC: Pharmacology and biochemistry of spider venoms. *Toxicon* 40:225–254, 2002.

Reeves JA, Allison EJ, Goodman PE: Black widow spiderbite in a child. *Am J Emerg Med* 14:469–471, 1996.

Stewert MPM: Ciguatera poisoning: Treatment with intravenous mannitol. *Trop Doctor* 21:54, 1991

Sun K, Wat J, So P: Puffer fish poisoning. *Anaeth Intens Care* 22:307, 1994.

Swift AE, Swift TR: Ciguatera. *Clin Toxicol* 31:1–29, 1993.

Tanen DA, Ruha AM, Graeme KA, et al: Epidemiology and hospital course of rattlesnake envenomations cared for at a tertiary referral center in central Arizona. *Acad Emerg Med* 8:177–182, 2001.

Tomaszewski C: Aquatic envenomations. In: Ford M, DeLaney K, Ling L, et al, eds: *Clinical Toxicology.* Philadelphia: Saunders; 2001:970–984.

Van Hoesen KB, Clark RF: Seafood toxidromes. In Auerbach PS, ed: *Wilderness Medicine.* 4th ed. St. Louis: Mosby; 2001: 1285–1326.

Whitley RE: Conservative treatment of copperhead snakebites without antivenin. *J Trauma* 41:219–221, 1996.

White J: Bites and stings from venomous animals: A global overview. *Ther Drug Monit* 22:65–68, 2000.

Williams RK, Palafox NA: Treatment of pediatric ciguatera fish poisoning. *Am J Dis Child* 144:747–758, 1990.

Woestman R, Perkin R, Van Stralen D: The black widow: is she deadly to children? *Pediatr Emerg Care* 12:360–364, 1996.

76

Herbal Products

Joshua G. Schier
Lewis S. Nelson

CASE PRESENTATION

A 4-year-old Asian girl is brought to the emergency department (ED) because of irritability, inability to sleep, and complaints of headache and abdominal pain. The child has no significant past medical history, does not use any prescription medications, and has no known allergies. During the history, the parents mention that they have been using an herbal skin cream on the child obtained by a relative from China. On physical examination, the child is irritable and inconsolable. Her vital signs reveal a pulse of 110 bpm, blood pressure 100/70 mmHg, and respirations 18 breaths per minute. She is afebrile. The cardiovascular examination is unremarkable. The neurologic examination is normal except for a slight intention tremor. Dermal examination reveals no obvious rash. Laboratory studies demonstrate a normal blood cell count and serum electrolyte profile. A urinalysis shows trace protein; the chest x-ray is normal. Because of concern for symptomatic metal poisoning, a radiograph of the skin cream is obtained, and found to be heterogenously radiopaque. The child is admitted to the hospital for further evaluation and metal testing.

INTRODUCTION

Dietary supplement generally refers to any particular ingredient, usually a vitamin, mineral, herb, amino acid, or other product taken to promote health (Table 76–1). In 1994, the Dietary Supplement Health and Education Act altered the role of the U.S. Food and Drug Administration (FDA) in the approval and overall supervision of the dietary supplement industry. Although new dietary supplements are introduced continually, those ingredients classified as supplements are not subject to the same oversight by the FDA. Supplement manufacturers, marketers, and sellers currently receive little prospective governmental regulation. Unlike prescription drugs, there is no need for the manufacturer to submit evidence of either efficacy or safety prior to marketing a new dietary supplement formulation. The removal of these products from the market by the FDA now occurs only after the product is proven unsafe. The terminology used in classification of these agents can also be confusing, because *alternative*, *complementary*, and *homeopathic* are often used interchangeably.

Table 76–1. Other Dietary Supplements

Supplement	Common Name	Common Uses	Toxicity
Aconite, aconitine	Monkshood, Wolfbane	Topical anesthesia, peripheral edema[a]	GI distress, cardiac dysrhythmias
Carnitine		Hepatoprotective	None reported
Chromium picolinate		Enhanced insulin function and glycogenesis	Hematotoxicity, renal failure, rhabdomyolysis
Garlic	Stinking rose	Antibacterial preparation, hypertension,[a] cancer[a]	GI distress, dermatitis, antiplatelet effects
Ginkgo biloba	Maidenhair or kew tree, tebonin, kaveri	Improve cognitive ability	Increased bleeding risk owing to platelet dysfunction
Goldenseal	Orange or yellow root	Astringent, menstrual therapy	GI distress, paralysis
Jimsonweed	Jamestown weed, thornapple	Asthma,[a] drug of abuse	Anticholinergic effects
Kava	Awa, kava-kava, kew	Relaxation, headaches,[a] wounds,[a] aphrodisiac	Heptatotoxicity, sedation, skin changes, weakness
Khat	Qut, kat, chaat	CNS stimulant, fatigue[a]	Dysphoria, ischemia, infarction
Megavitamins		General health	Varied
Panax ginseng	Ginseng, Ren shen	Health tonic, respiratory illnesses[a]	Ginseng abuse syndrome
Pennyroyal oil	Sqawmint, mosquito plant	Abortifacient, digestive agent, menstrual regulation	Hepatotoxicity
Pokeweed	Inkberry, scoke, pigeon berry	Mistaken for horseradish, other edible plants	GI distress, hematotoxicity
Saw palmetto	Sabal, American dwarf palm tree	Prostatic hypertrophy[a]	GI distress
Sassafras		Stimulant, antispasmodic	Hepatotoxicity
Wormwood	Absinthe	Sedative, analgesic, drug of abuse	Psychosis, hallucinations, seizures
Yohimbine	Yohimbi, yohimbehe	Body building, aphrodisiac	Hypertension, weakness, paralysis

[a] Used in the treatment of this condition.
Abbreviations: CNS, central nervous system; GI, gastrointestinal.

The general population may be falsely reassured by product labels and advertising suggesting a product's safety and efficacy. In addition, there is an often misguided belief that natural products are safe. Clearly, any pharmacologically active product possesses the potential for adverse effects. Furthermore, dietary supplement ingredients may differ in both actual content and amount from that indicated on the product label. Contamination of these products may occur during harvesting, manufacturing, or processing. All of these factors leave the consumer at risk for harm. Patient beliefs about the efficacy of alternative medicines may delay presentation for medical evaluation and treatment. Recently, the United States Pharmacopeia's Dietary Supplement Verification Program has been established to help better regulate the distribution and content of newer herbal and dietary supplement products.

EPIDEMIOLOGY

Data looking specifically at which types of agents are used among which age groups are scarce. Two pediatric ED-based surveys, which found a significant amount of homeopathic, naturopathic, and herbal usage among their alternative therapy user groups, found a mean age in users of 7.0 and 7.4 years. The reasons for use of these products among the pediatric population are undefined, but appear to be significantly higher among children with chronic illnesses. Approximately 75% of teenagers who use complementary and alternative therapies use plant-derived herbal products. Dietary supplements such as weight loss aids (ephedra) and athletic ability enhancers (dehydroepiandrosterone [DHEA] or creatine) appear to be used more commonly among adolescents and teenagers.

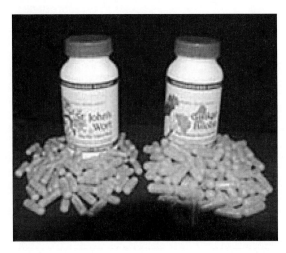

Fig. 76–1. Common herbal products available as OTC preparations include St. John's wort and Ginkgo biloba.

DEVELOPMENTAL CONSIDERATIONS

The effects of herbal products on the growth and development of children are understudied. Unlike pharmaceutical products, herbal substances do not undergo the rigorous testing process maintained by the FDA. The lack of systematic studies of herbal products should provoke caution in health care products as well as patients regarding their uses, especially in children.

Younger children, particularly toddlers and preadolescents may represent a population that lacks the ability to make educated choices regarding the use of nontraditional medications. Parental beliefs and culture may heavily influence treatment choices and result in inappropriate or undocumented herbal therapy in these age groups.

PLANT-DERIVED DIETARY SUPPLEMENTS

St. John's Wort (*Hypericum perforatum*)

This flowering plant is commonly used as an herbal antidepressant (Figure 76–1). Commercial preparations consist of extracts from the above ground portion of the plant. There are at least 10 classes of biologically active detectable compounds in *H. perforatum*. Most preparations are standardized by their hypericin (naphthodianthrone) content, which until recently was thought to be the major active ingredient. Subsequent research suggests that hyperforin (phloroglucinol) significantly inhibits reuptake of serotonin, norepinephrine, and

dopamine in nanomolar concentrations, and is more likely to be responsible for the herb's antidepressant effects.

Toxicity is generally uncommon, but may include mild gastrointestinal (GI) and neurologic symptoms such as fatigue and dizziness. *H. perforatum*'s ability to inhibit biogenic amine reuptake, possibly in conjunction with weak monamine oxidase inhibition, may predispose to the development of the serotonin syndrome when used in conjunction with other serotonergic agonists. Serotonin syndrome results from excessive stimulation of certain serotonin receptors. Signs and symptoms include altered mental status, autonomic instability, and hyperthermia. A more detailed description of serotonin syndrome can be found in Chapter 43.

Other complications of therapy include alterations in serum levels of coadministered drugs. Hypericin is able to induce the 3A4 family of the cytochrome P450 system, thereby lowering levels of drugs metabolized through that pathway. Reported drug interactions include digoxin, cyclosporine, warfarin, indinavir, phenprocoumon, and ethinylestradiol/desogestrel.

Echinacea

The genus *Echinacea* contains nine species of plants, of which three are commonly used medicinally (*E. purpurea*, *E. angustifolia*, and *E. pallida*) for the prevention and treatment of viral upper respiratory infections. Their use is weakly supported by animal models in which *Echinacea* was found to increase circulating white blood cells, cytokine production, and phagocytosis. Most clinical trials looking at outcomes of therapy are methodologically flawed and inconclusive.

There is little reported toxicity associated with *Echinacea*, although rare events include hepatitis, nausea, asthma, and anaphylaxis. Management consists primarily of supportive care.

Ephedra

In April of 2004, the FDA prohibited the sale of any product containing ephedra as a dietary supplement. Manufacturers responded by adding different sympathomimetic amines of unproven safety and efficacy (e.g., synephrine) to their now "ephedra-free" products. Ephedra is discussed because of its historical significance, still relatively easy availability, and only recent removal from the market.

A common component of many previously available over-the-counter central nervous system (CNS) stimulant and weight loss formulations, ephedra alkaloids are extracted from plants of the *Ephedra* genus. They are known in traditional Chinese medicine as *Ma Huang*. The ephedra alkaloids include ephedrine, pseudoephedrine, and methylephedrine. Ephedrine is an indirect acting sympathomimetic alkaloid that affects α_1, β_1, and β_2 adrenergic receptors. This causes vasoconstriction, increased chronotropy, hypertension, mydriasis, headache, and nervousness. It is moderately effective as an appetite suppressant.

The toxicity of ephedra alkaloids, particularly ephedrine, is similar to other sympathomimetic agents. Among the more commonly reported adverse effects are myocardial ischemia and infarction, stroke, seizures, hyperthermia, and rhabdomyolysis. Treatment of toxicity depends on the organ or organ system involved. The general treatment of ephedrine-induced complications consists of supportive care. Benzodiazepines may be used to control psychomotor agitation. Management of cardiovascular or CNS ischemia includes the use of direct-acting vasodilating agents or α-adrenergic receptor-blocking agents, such as phentolamine. A more detailed discussion of the sympathomimetic toxidrome is in Chapter 54.

Ginseng

Ginseng preparations are used for an extremely wide variety of reasons; its reputation as a medicinal panacea accounts for the name of its genus, Panax. Ginseng is commonly used to improve stamina and concentration, relieve stress, and augment general well-being. Historically, ginseng has also been used as an aphrodisiac, an antidepressant, and a diuretic. The most likely pharmacologically active components in Ginseng are the gingenosides, which have a variety of clinical effects. They may cause changes in serum glucose concentration, serum cholesterol levels, hemoglobin production, blood pressure, and heart rate, and they may induce CNS stimulation.

Complications and side effects of usage are variable. Perhaps the most recognized complication of long-term use is a loosely defined collection of findings including hypertension, nervousness, sleeplessness, and morning diarrhea known as the *Ginseng Abuse Syndrome*. Other infrequently reported complications include CNS overstimulation, insomnia, headache, epistaxis, and vomiting. Mastalgia, vaginal bleeding, Stevens–Johnson syndrome, neonatal androgenization from maternal use, and a drug interaction with warfarin resulting in a prolonged international normalized ratio (INR) have also been associated with its use.

Management of side effects associated with ginseng use should begin with the cessation of use. Supportive and symptom focused therapy are the hallmarks of care.

NON–PLANT-DERIVED DIETARY SUPPLEMENTS

Dehydroepiandrosterone

A naturally occurring adrenal precursor to testosterone, DHEA is converted to androstenedione and ultimately testosterone. It is commonly used to increase strength and athletic performance. Banned from prescription sale by the FDA in 1996, it is now marketed as a dietary supplement and therefore available without a prescription. Administration of DHEA and androstenedione is associated with increased serum concentrations of testosterone precursors, testosterone, and estradiol. An overall sense of well-being is commonly reported, which may also occur with chronic administration of anabolic steroids. Most reported toxicity from chronic use of these agents consists of androgenic side effects such as acne and increased body hair. Treatment should start with discontinuation of product use. Supportive care is the mainstay of therapy (see Chapter 55).

Creatine

Athletes wishing to boost athletic ability commonly use creatine-containing preparations. Creatine, in the form of creatine phosphate, is an amino acid that is utilized by the muscle cell to maintain the availability of adenosine triphosphate during times of extreme muscular activity. These preparations frequently include carbohydrates because the combination appears to increase skeletal muscle creatine stores more than creatine alone.

The immense popularity of these agents and overall lack of reported complications suggest that toxicity is limited. However, there are few systematic studies of the toxicity of creatine. Weight gain, water retention, diarrhea, and muscle cramping are among the more commonly reported side effects. There are rare reports of renal complications that were associated with creatine product use, although these may represent exertional rhabomyolysis. Treatment is cessation of product use and provision of supportive care.

CONTAMINANTS

Cardioactive Glycosides

Digoxin-like compounds that share the pharmacologic profile of digoxin are present in numerous preparations marketed as aphrodisiacs (Rock Hard, Love Stone, and Black Stone), herbal remedies for congestive heart failure (Ch'an Su), and contaminants in dietary supplements (Chomper). The aphrodisiacs are topical preparations used for their local anesthetic effects but are not safe to ingest. Ingestion of any cardioactive steroid in a sufficient dose can result in life-threatening digoxin-like toxicity.

Digoxin levels are generally either undetectable or slightly elevated, depending on the particular assay and the cross-reactivity between the cardioactive glycosides and digoxin. Therefore, poisoning may occur with a negative or only mildly elevated digoxin level. Treatment of symptomatic or potentially severe cardioactive steroid poisoning of any kind should begin with 10 to 20 vials of digoxin-specific antibody fragments, regardless of the level measured. A more detailed discussion of digoxin toxicity manifestations, management, and treatment can be found in Chapter 37.

Metals

Some cultures believe in the medicinal value of metals to prevent and treat certain diseases. Thus, although often undisclosed to the consumer, various metals are commonly added to traditional healing preparations. Some of the more common metals implicated in toxicity from topical exposure, as well as products meant for consumption, include lead, mercury, silver, cadmium, arsenic,

and chromium. Lead-containing preparations are among the most commonly reported contaminants among herbal products from around the world. Lead oxide preparations are commonly used in the Mexican/Hispanic culture as digestive tonics (*azarcon*). Lead may also be found in multiple cosmetic preparations used in India (*surma*), the Middle East, and Africa. Arsenic and mercury contamination from hand-rolled mixtures of herbs and honey produced in China has occurred in the United States. Other metals implicated in toxicity include colloidal silver products advertised as antimicrobials and anti-inflammatory agents.

Patients with metal toxicity often have confusing and complex clinical presentations. They may go undiagnosed for long periods of time, see several different clinicians, and may even be given a psychiatric diagnosis. There are often multiple somatic complaints that usually include digestive problems if the agent is being consumed. Serum and urine heavy metal screens assist in diagnosis. Once a specific metal is identified, further quantitation with 24-hour urine collections or by speciation can be performed. Radiography of the product or of the patient's GI tract may reveal radiopaque fragments in a recent ingestion.

LABORATORY AND DIAGNOSTIC TESTING

Laboratory testing is tailored to the individual clinical effects that are identified or by those expected of a known dietary supplement. For example, exposure to ephedrine may warrant troponin and other serum markers of cardiac damage. Cases of suspected cardioactive glycoside steroid poisoning can be confirmed if a serum digoxin level is elevated, although severe toxicity may be present with an undetectable or minimally elevated level.

In most cases, the particular agent will not be known or there will be multiple agents. In these cases, focused screening laboratories such as cell blood counts, serum chemistries, liver function tests, coagulation parameters, and an electrocardiogram should be obtained based on regular clinical indications. Testing of the product is generally not warranted, although occasionally metals may be identified by x-ray of the implicated product or x-ray of the patient.

MANAGEMENT

Most cases of toxicity that result from therapeutic use can be successfully managed with symptom-focused therapy, supportive care, and close follow-up after discharge. Although GI decontamination is not necessary in a patient with a therapeutic misadventure, a patient with an acute, intentional overdose may benefit from a single dose of activated charcoal. These latter patients may need closer monitoring, additional laboratory testing, psychiatric evaluation, and additional GI decontamination. Whole bowel irrigation should be considered for patients who have ingested metal-containing products, because charcoal has limited efficacy in binding to these compounds. Overdoses involving metal-containing products may require treatment with an appropriate chelating agent. An attempt should always be made to identify or classify the agent in order to properly assess risk.

DISPOSITION

Patients can be safely discharged home with exposures to harmless or minimally harmless agents, or if the agent is unknown and the patient is asymptomatic, after a reasonable period of observation in the ED. A follow-up visit within 24 to 72 hours should be arranged in this latter population. Symptomatic patients should be admitted to the hospital for observation and symptomatic treatment, as needed. The decision to admit a symptomatic patient to a monitored or an intensive care unit should be made on an individual basis. If there is any concern that a patient was attempting self-harm, a psychiatric evaluation should be obtained.

Dietary supplement exposures, in the form of a therapeutic error or an intentional suicide attempt, pose unique challenges. The limited information about toxicologic profiles and pharmacokinetics of dietary supplements or their active ingredients often make establishment of causal relationships difficult. Regardless of the cause, sound management begins with discontinuation of the potentially offending agent and provision of supportive and expectant management. Whenever possible, the clinician should educate users and their parents about the potential risks of using these agents and emphasize that natural does not, necessarily, equal safe.

CASE OUTCOME

A serum mercury level was discovered to be 50 µg/L (normal range: <10 µg/L) and a 24-h urine collection was found to contain 176 µg/L (normal range: <20 µg/L). Intramuscular dimercaprol (British anti-Lewisite

[BAL]) along with oral succimer (2,3-dimercaptosuccinic acid) was started. Antidotal therapy was continued for 5 days and the patient improved. Analysis of the cream later revealed 7.7 mg of mercurous chloride per gram of cream. The proper authorities were notified and all family members were appropriately tested and advised to immediately stop use of the cream.

SUGGESTED READINGS

Arlt W, Callies F, van Vlijmen JC, et al: Dehydroepiandrosterone replacement in women with adrenal insufficiency. *N Engl J Med* 341:1073–1074, 1999.

Bose A, Vashishta K, O'Loughlin BJ: Azarcon por empacho—Another cause of lead toxicity. *Pediatrics* 72: 106–110, 1983.

Bouts BA: Images in clinical medicine. Argyria. *N Engl J Med* 340:1554, 1999.

Brubacher JR, Hoffman RS, Bania T, et al: Deaths associated with a purported aphrodisiac—New York City, February 1993–May 1995. *MMWR Morb Mortal Wkly Rep* 44:853–855, 1995.

D'Arcy PF: Adverse reactions and interactions with herbal medicines. Part I. Adverse reactions. *Adverse Drug React Toxicol Rev* 10:189–208, 1991.

Ernst E: Prevalence of complementary/alternative medicine for children: A systematic review. *Eur J Pediatr* 158:7–11, 1999.

Ernst E: The risk-benefit profile of commonly used herbal therapies: Ginkgo, St. John's Wort, Ginseng, Echinacea, Saw Palmetto, and Kava. *Ann Intern Med* 136:42–53, 2002.

Espinoza EO, Mann MJ, Bleasdell B: Arsenic and mercury in traditional Chinese herbal balls [letter]. *N Engl J Med* 333: 803–804, 1995.

Gardiner P, Kemper KJ: Herbs in pediatric and adolescent medicine. *Pediatr Rev* 21:44–57, 2000.

Green AL, Hultman E, Macdonald IA, et al: Carbohydrate ingestion augments skeletal muscle creatine accumulation during creatine supplementation in humans. *Am J Physiol* 271: E821–26, 1996.

Greeson JM, Sanford B, Monti D: St. John's wort (*Hypericum perforatum*): A review of the current pharmacological, toxicological, and clinical literature. *Psychopharmacology* 153: 402–414, 2001.

Haller CA, Benowitz NL: Adverse cardiovascular and central nervous system events associated with dietary supplements containing ephedra alkaloids. *N Engl J Med* 343:1833–1838, 2000.

Hung OL, Lewin NA, Howland MA: Herbal preparations. In: Goldfrank LR, Flomenbaum NE, Lewin NA, et al, eds: *Goldfrank's Toxicologic Emergencies.* 7th ed. New York: McGraw-Hill; 2002:1129–1149.

Juhn MS, O'Kane JW, Vinci DM: Oral creatine supplementation in male collegiate athletes: A survey of dosing habits and side effects. *J Am Diet Assoc* 99:593–595, 1999.

Koren G, Randor S, Martin S, et al: Maternal ginseng use associated with neonatal androgenization. *JAMA* 264:2866, 1990.

Leder BZ, Longcope C, Catlin DH, et al: Oral androstenedione administration and serum testosterone concentrations in young men. *JAMA* 283:779–782, 2000.

Miller LG. Herbal medicinals. *Arch Intern Med* 158:2200–2211, 1998.

O'Hara MA, Kiefer D, Farrell K, et al: A review of 12 commonly used medicinal herbs. *Arch Fam Med* 7:523–536, 1998.

Pitetti R, Singh S, Hornyak D, et al: Complementary and alternative medicine use in children. *Pediatr Emerg Care* 165–169, 2001.

Slifman NR, Obermeyer WR, Musser SM, et al: Contamination of botanical dietary supplements by *Digitalis lanata*. *N Engl J Med* 339:806–811, 1998.

Smith TW, Butler VP, Haber E, et al: Treatment of life-threatening digitalis intoxication with digoxin-specific Fab antibody fragments. *N Engl J Med* 307:1357–1362, 1982.

Tsang WO, McRae A, Leo PJ, et al: The use of alternative medicine by children at an urban community hospital emergency department. *J Altern Complement Med* 7:309–311, 2001.

Vassallo SU: Sports toxicology. In: Goldfrank LR, Flomenbaum NE, Lewin NA, et al, eds: *Goldfrank's Toxicologic Emergencies.* 7th ed. New York: McGraw-Hill; 2002:1699–1712.

White LM, Gardner SF, Gurley BJ, et al: Pharmacokinetics and cardiovascular effects of ma-huang (*Ephedra sinica*) in normotensive adults. *J Clin Pharmacol* 37:116–122, 1997.

77

Food Poisoning and Botulism

Andrea G. Carlson

HIGH-YIELD FACTS

- In the United States, *Salmonella* species, *Campylobacter jejuni*, *Shigella soneii*, and Norwalk-like viruses cause the majority of food poisoning cases.

- Healthy patients with food poisoning recover with supportive care alone. Prevention of dehydration and electrolyte disturbances are the mainstay of therapy.

- Most deaths from food poisoning occur in infants, the elderly, and those with immunocompromise. Such patients require aggressive care, including antibiotic therapy.

- Hemolytic-uremic syndrome (HUS) is a potentially life-threatening complication that most commonly follows enterohemorrhagic *Escherichia coli* O157:H7 infection. Signs of HUS are hemolytic anemia, thrombocytopenia, and renal failure.

- The most common signs of infant botulism are constipation and a weak cry. The presence of a weak suck or gag reflex is the most reliable indicator of need for intubation.

- Botulism trivalent antitoxin will prevent, but not reverse, muscle paralysis. Use of the antitoxin must be considered early, and not delayed for laboratory diagnosis.

- Monosodium glutamate (MSG) is a common flavor enhancer that can cause minor self-limited symptoms in sensitive individuals.

CASE PRESENTATION

A 5-month-old infant is brought to the emergency department by her mother. The child was previously healthy; she recently received her routine immunizations and was advanced from breast milk to solids. According to the mother, the baby had easily adjusted to the change in her diet, which now consists of organic baby food sweetened with honey bought from the same health food store. On the day before presentation, the mother noticed a decrease in appetite and constipation, followed by fussiness, a weak cry, and lethargy. By the following morning the infant would not hold her head up or feed. The mother denied any history of fever, coughing, vomiting, diarrhea, change in urine output, rashes, trauma, or exposure to medications or chemicals. Physical examination is remarkable for poor muscle tone, most notably in the head and neck muscles, loss of facial expression, and a weak gag reflex. Complete blood count, chemistry, and urinalysis are normal. Cerebrospinal fluid analysis is performed, and reveals no abnormalities. Chest and abdominal radiographs, as well as computed tomographic scan of the head, are unremarkable.

INTRODUCTION

Gastroenteritis is a leading cause of morbidity and mortality worldwide. In the United States 76 million people contract foodborne illnesses each year; of these, 325,000 require hospitalization, and nearly 5000 die. Although the majority of foodborne gastrointestinal (GI) illnesses are self-limiting, a subset of patients may experience severe complications and have an increased risk of death (Figure 77–1). The initial differential diagnosis of food poisoning includes bacterial, viral, parasitic, and

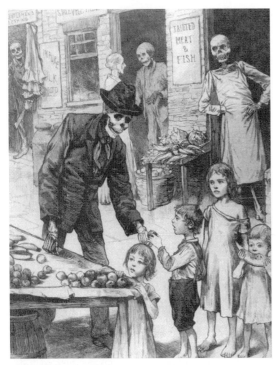

Fig. 77–1. A hint to the Board of Health on how the city invites the cholera (1864). (*Source:* Department of Health, City of New York. Used with permission from the NYC Department of Records, Municipal Archives.)

chemical etiologies. Infectious agents may cause food poisoning syndromes by invasive or toxin-mediated mechanisms. Various food additives may also result in illness when ingested. Other noninfectious etiologies include fishborne (Chapter 78), mushroom (Chapter 79), and plant (Chapter 80) toxins. Poisoning by food contaminated with heavy metals is discussed in Chapter 65.

Owing to the self-limited nature of many types of food poisoning, as well as limitations in speed and availability of laboratory testing, definitive identification of the offending agent may not always be practical or necessary. Historical information, combined with symptoms and signs may adequately guide initial management. However, in severe cases or suspected outbreaks, the local health department or the Centers for Disease Control and Prevention (CDC) should be notified, and appropriate testing should be performed to confirm an etiology. Often the necessary specialized

testing is only accomplished with assistance from these authorities.

EPIDEMIOLOGY

Since 1996, the overall incidence of major foodborne illness has decreased. In 2002, the most commonly reported pathogen was *Salmonella*, followed in order of decreasing frequency by *Campylobacter*, *Shigella*, *E. coli* O157, *Cryptosporidium*, *Yersinia*, *Vibrio*, *Listeria*, and *Cyclospora*.

BACTERIAL ETIOLOGIES

Bacteria cause foodborne illness by one of two mechanisms: bacterial invasion of the GI epithelium, followed by either local cellular toxicity or systemic effects as a result of infection, or elaboration of toxins that exert local and/or systemic effects. In general, the presence of fever, blood, or mucus in the stool, and fecal leukocytes makes the diagnosis of an invasive illness more likely. However, the classic dysentery syndrome of fever, abdominal pain, and stool containing blood, mucus, and sheets of polymorphonuclear leukocytes is present in only 40% of cases of invasive illness, and these findings are occasionally present in toxin-mediated bacterial illnesses as well.

Invasive Illness

Salmonella Species

Clinically relevant strains causing illness include *S. typhimurium*, *S. enteritidis*, and *S. Newport*. *S. typhimurium* remains the most common strain isolated. Illness from *Salmonella* species has been linked to raw or undercooked eggs, raw milk, and contaminated poultry, beef, pork, and alfalfa sprouts. The largest foodborne outbreak ever reported to the CDC occurred in Illinois in 1985 from pasteurized 2% low-fat milk contaminated with *S. typhimurium*; more than 150,000 people were affected. Animals also provide a natural reservoir. Household pets, including chicks, iguanas, and turtles, have been implicated in several cases. *S. typhimurium* secretes an enterotoxin that results in typhoid fever. Young children (<5 years), patients with altered GI function or flora, and immunocompromised patient are at greater risk of serious illness. Ingestion of 1000 or fewer organisms may cause illness. The incubation period for typhoid fever is 1 to 3 weeks, with duration of illness of 3 to 4 weeks.

Nontyphoidal salmonellosis occurs most commonly between July and November. Nontyphoidal salmonellosis has a relatively shorter incubation period (6 to 48 hours) and duration (7 days). Nausea, vomiting, diarrhea, fever, chills, and abdominal pain are commonly present. Bacteremia occurs in 5% to 10% of cases. Fever is present in both typhoidal and nontyphoidal forms, but is short lived in the latter, usually disappearing after 2 days. Illness in otherwise healthy individuals without bacteremia or extraintestinal manifestations should be managed without antibiotics. The use of antibiotics prolongs bacterial shedding, and indiscriminate use in the past may be responsible for the increasing patterns of antibiotic resistance now seen. High-risk patients including neonates, sickle cell patients, and the immunosuppressed, should receive antibiotics without delay. In these patients azithromycin, ceftriaxone, cefotaxime, or ciprofloxacin may be used.

Shigella Species

Shigella sonnei is the most common strain of *Shigella* isolated in the United States. Illness most often occurs during the summer and fall from contaminated vegetables, cheese, and eggs. The bacteria produce an enterotoxin, shigatoxin, which destroys mucosal cells by impairing protein synthesis. Only 10 organisms are needed to cause shigellosis. After a 16- to 72-hour incubation period, patients develop fever, abdominal pain, and diarrhea. The clinical course may be complicated by the development of HUS. Other complications include toxic megacolon, rectal prolapse, protein-losing enteropathy, seizures, and Reiter syndrome. The duration of illness is highly variable, ranging from 1 day to 1 month. Diagnosis can be made by stool or blood culture. Antibiotic therapy is indicated; acceptable agents include azithromycin, trimethoprim/sulfamethoxazole (TMP/SMX), ceftriaxone, or ciprofloxacin.

Campylobacter jejuni

In 1996, *C. jejuni* accounted for 46% of all laboratory confirmed cases of bacterial gastroenteritis. Outbreaks of *Campylobacter* occur in spring and fall; sporadic cases are more common during the summer months. Sources include raw or undercooked poultry, raw milk, and contaminated water. Birds, dogs, and cats can also transmit disease. *Campylobacter* secretes a heat-labile toxin that causes mucosal inflammation, epithelial disruption, and leakage of serosal fluid. Illness occurs most commonly in

children younger than 5 years of age, and young adults. HIV-positive patients also have a higher incidence of disease. Ingestion of 800 organisms can cause illness. Following an incubation period of 1 to 7 days, patients experience a prodrome of fever, headache, and malaise that lasts 12 to 24 hours. Diarrhea (bloody in 50% of cases) and abdominal pain then develop. Vomiting and bacteremia are uncommon. Other complications include lower GI hemorrhage, a typhoid-like syndrome, reactive arthritis, and meningitis. Notably, illness from *Campylobacter* has also been linked to the development of Guillain-Barré syndrome, which complicates 1 in 1000 cases. Because of the fastidious nature of *Campylobacter*, stool culture often does not yield the bacteria. Death from *Campylobacter* food poisoning is rare, occurring primarily in infants, the elderly, and immunocompromised patients. Treatment with azithromycin, erythromycin stearate, or ciprofloxacin is indicated for severe cases. Uncomplicated cases generally resolve within 6 days.

Enterohemorrhagic *E. coli*

Over 20,000 cases of hemorrhagic colitis from Enterohemorrhagic *E. coli* (EHEC) occur annually, resulting in hundreds of deaths. Although multiple EHEC serotypes have been identified, the most commonly reported is serotype O1057:H7. The first outbreak of *E. coli* O157:H7 occurred in 1982 in Oregon and Michigan, and was traced to contaminated hamburgers from a fast food chain. Since then, outbreaks have occurred in nursing homes, schools, and restaurants. Cattle serve as a major reservoir of EHEC, which is part of their normal intestinal flora. Thus, contamination from ground beef and dairy products is most often described. Other reported sources include vegetables, unpasteurized apple cider, and contaminated water. Secondary spread may also occur. The bacteria elaborate a shiga-like toxin, resulting in systemic toxemia. Shiga-toxins directly damage vascular endothelium, causing microangiopathic changes that result in organ ischemia. Illness requires only a small inoculum of less than 100 organisms. Following an incubation of 3 to 4 days, abdominal cramping and watery, nonbloody stools develop. This often progresses to 10 to 14 bloody stools per day, with severe abdominal pain and patchy colonic edema. Blood loss can be substantial. Fecal leukocytes are characteristically absent. Because most patients are afebrile, EHEC infection can be easily mistaken for a lower GI bleed of noninfectious origin. Definitive diagnosis requires sorbitol-MacConkey agar plates for culture, or immunoassays for shiga-toxin. The use of antimicrobials is believed to enhance toxin release and increase the risk of HUS. Antimotility agents should also be avoided. Symptoms resolve after 7 to 8 days of supportive care.

Hemolytic-Uremic Syndrome

HUS is a leading cause of renal failure in children aged 1 to 5 years. Following infection by a shiga-toxin–producing strain of *E. coli*, 5% to 10% of children will develop HUS. Oliguric renal failure develops from a direct effect of shiga-toxin on renal tubular epithelial cells and activation of inflammatory cytokines. Hemolytic anemia and thrombocytopenia develop and can be severe, with decreases in hematocrit of 10% or more. Laboratory evaluation reveals fragmented RBCs on peripheral smear, as well as hyperkalemia and uremia. Treatment requires meticulous supportive care including intravenous (IV) hydration, control of hypertension, transfusions of packed cells or platelets; hemodialysis may be necessary. Secondary complications, such as stroke, coma, acute respiratory distress syndrome, and permanent kidney damage occur in up to 30% of cases. A mortality rate of 5% to 10% has remained unchanged over the last few years. Children with persistent proteinuria 1 year after recovery require long-term nephrology follow-up.

Yersinia enterocolitica

Although the incidence is increasing, infection from *Yersinia* remains relatively rare. Outbreaks peak during winter months. Dogs and pigs are natural reservoirs, and illness has been linked to contaminated milk products and raw pork. Fever, diarrhea, and abdominal pain develop after a variable incubation period of 1 day to more than 1 week. In severe cases, rectal bleeding and ileal perforation may develop. Mesenteric adenitis commonly occurs in children, and may mimic appendicitis. Extraintestinal manifestations include rash, arthritis, pharyngitis, and hepatitis. Mild cases may be treated with TMP/SMX or doxycycline; in more severe cases, ceftriaxone or ciprofloxacin should be given. Recovery occurs within 1 to 3 weeks.

Listeria monocytogenes

Listeriosis is an uncommon foodborne illness, affecting less than 1 in 100,000 adults, and 10 in 100,000 infants. Unpasteurized milk, soft cheeses, undercooked chicken, hot dogs, and deli meats are the most common sources of contamination. After a highly variable incubation period, nonspecific flu-like symptoms combined with nonbloody diarrhea develop. The duration of illness is also highly variable. In high-risk individuals, initial manifestations may progress to bacteremia and meningoencephalitis. Outcome is gravest in fetuses and neonates of women infected during pregnancy. *Listeria* sepsis may lead to chorioamnionitis, preterm delivery, or stillbirth. In surviving neonates, bacterial meningitis may occur 2 to 3 weeks after birth, with a mortality rate of 10%. *Listeria* is the third most common cause meningitis in neonates behind *E. coli* and group B *Streptococcus*. The overall mortality rate in the perinatal period is 50%. Other high-risk groups include the elderly and those with immunocompromise. Treatment with IV ampicillin or TMP/SMX should be instituted promptly.

Vibrio parahaemolyticus and *Vibrio vulnificus*

Outbreaks of *V. parahaemolyticus* occur in costal areas of the United States from eating raw or undercooked shellfish. Incidence peaks in the warmer months of the year. Onset of symptoms occurs 5 to 24 hours after exposure, and is characterized by a sudden, intense inflammatory GI response, with bloody diarrhea, abdominal cramping, fever, and malaise. The duration of illness is short; most cases resolve within 1 to 2 days. For this reason, antibiotics are seldom indicated. *V. vulnificus* may also cause invasive illness, with a higher incidence of septicemia and overall greater mortality than *V. parahaemolyticus*. The presence of hemorrhagic bullous lesions in patients with acute diarrheal illness is suggestive of *V. vulnificus*. First-line therapy consists of doxycycline combined with ceftazidime.

Toxin-Mediated Illnesses

Staphylococcus aureus

Because food contaminated with *S. aureus* often maintains normal appearance, odor, and taste, food poisoning from this agent can result in relatively large outbreaks. The prevalence of pathogenic *S. aureus* carriers, who generally appear healthy, may be as high as 50% in some populations. Dairy and proteinaceous foods are most often implicated, including eggs, mayonnaise-based salads, cream-filled pastries, and gravies. Inadequate refrigeration results in the production of several heat-stable enterotoxins, which have direct toxic effects on the vomiting center in the brain. The incubation period is short, and the onset of illness is characteristically explosive. Within 6 hours of exposure, nausea, vomiting, and diarrhea develop. Affected patients are usually afebrile. Symptoms begin to subside within 5 hours; with supportive care, recovery is usually complete within 24 hours. Stool testing is not useful, and antibiotics are not required.

Bacillus cereus

B. cereus is ubiquitous in soil and raw, dry, and processed foods. *B. cereus* spores produce two distinct toxins. Type I toxin is a preformed heat-stable toxin that causes the emetic form of the disease. Illness from exposure to Type I toxin is clinically indistinguishable from that of staphylococcal food poisoning. After a brief incubation period of 2 to 3 hours, sudden onset of nausea and vomiting occurs. Diarrhea is less prominent, and recovery is generally complete within 10 hours. Improperly prepared and stored fried rice is the prototypical source of exposure for Type I toxin. Type II, the more common toxin, actually consists of three heat labile enterotoxins that result in profuse diarrhea when ingested. Meats and vegetables must be heavily contaminated with *B. cereus* spores, which are then ingested and sporulate within the gut to release Toxin II. Clinical illness mimics that of *E. coli*. Incubation is longer than the emetic form (6 to 14 hours), and both vomiting and fever are uncommon features. Diarrhea usually resolves with 20 to 36 hours. Diagnosis of both forms requires isolation at least 100,000 organisms from stool/g, because *B. cereus* spores are also normally present in healthy people. Owing to its short duration, the emetic form does not require antibiotic therapy. In severe diarrheal forms, use of vancomycin, clindamycin, or a fluoroquinolone may be considered.

Clostridium perfringens

Poisoning from raw meat and poultry contaminated with *C. perfringens* spores is the fourth leading cause of foodborne illness. Several large outbreaks have been reported. Type A spores cause most cases in the United States. These heat-resistant spores can survive cooking and then germinate when food is allowed to cool slowly at room temperature. Once ingested, the spores produce a heat-labile toxin that causes massive GI secretion within 6 to 12 hours. Watery diarrhea and epigastric abdominal cramping last up to 24 hours. Heat-labile Type C spores, rare in the United States, can cause enteritis necroticans, which is characterized by acute onset of severe abdominal pain, vomiting, diarrhea, prostration, and shock. The ensuing hemorrhagic necrotizing enteritis of

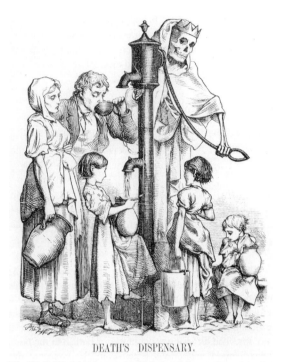

DEATH'S DISPENSARY.

Fig. 77–2. Worldwide, water supplies remain a major source for food poisoning outbreaks (Woodcut 1866). (*Source:* William Helfand Collection, New York: Used with permission.)

jejunum, ileum, and colon may be rapidly fatal. Antibiotics have not proven effective.

Enterotoxigenic *E. coli*

Enterotoxigenic *E. coli* (ETEC) remains a leading cause of traveler's diarrhea worldwide. Most cases occur after ingestion of contaminated vegetables or water (Figure 77–2). The cholera-like illness is attributed to enterotoxins that stimulate secretion in the intestinal brush border cells. Watery diarrhea may be profuse, but vomiting is generally mild or absent. Patients recover within 4 days. Antibiotics are usually not required.

Vibrio cholera

Cholera is relatively rare in the United States. Other than occasional outbreaks in southern coastal regions, most reports involve food transported from tropical countries. As with ETEC, a heat-labile enterotoxin causes GI secretion, occasionally massive enough to result in classic rice water stools. In severe cases, hypovolemic shock, acidosis, and electrolyte disturbances can be seen. Antibiotics have not been shown to shorten the course of disease, and are also limited by widespread resistance. Supportive care with IV hydration and electrolyte replacement has the greatest impact on outcome.

Clostridum botulinum

Botulism is a neuroparalytic disease caused by certain toxigenic *Clostridia* species. Spores from three genetic variants have been reported to cause botulism: *C. botulinum, C. butyricum,* and *C. barati.* These spores are ubiquitous in soil and dust, and are highly resistant to heat. In contrast, the toxins they liberate are heat labile, and easily destroyed by temperatures greater than 80°C. Although eight distinct toxins exist, toxins A, B, and E causes most disease in humans. The toxin binds irreversibly to presynaptic receptors and prevents acetylcholine release.

Nerve endings in the peripheral nervous system and at neuromuscular junctions are affected, which manifests as a symmetric descending paralysis. Recovery requires regeneration of receptors, a process that may take weeks to months. The differential diagnosis of botulism includes stroke, myasthenia gravis, Eaton-Lambert syndrome, the Miller-Fisher variant of Guillain-Barré syndrome, tick paralysis, chemical ingestions, and paralytic shellfish poisoning.

Four syndromes of botulism exist. The most commonly reported type is infant botulism, which accounted for 72% of all cases of botulism reported to the CDC in recent years. Foodborne botulism is the second most common type (24%), followed by wound botulism. Therapeutic botulism is a recently reported phenomenon resulting from the use of botulinum antitoxin for cosmetic and medicinal purposes. Only a few cases of this form have been reported so far. Regardless of type, all forms of botulism should be reported to public health officials. Laboratory confirmation of toxin is performed in some state laboratories and at the CDC.

Infant Botulism

Midura and Arnon first described infant botulism in 1976, after recovering toxin in the stool of four symptomatic infants. With an annual incidence of 2 in 100,000 live births, infant botulism remains the most common form in the United States. On average, 100 cases are reported to the CDC each year. The vast majority of reported cases are sporadic. The disease is endemic to Pennsylvania, Utah, and California. Infant botulism differs from foodborne botulism in that it does not require ingestion of preformed toxin; rather, spores are ingested, which then germinate in vivo to release toxin in the gut. The source of spores is often not found, although some reports have implicated the use of raw honey as a sweetening agent for infant food. Within 18 to 36 hours of exposure, signs of toxicity begin but may initially be subtle. Constipation is often the first complaint, and may precede other symptoms by a few days. Classically, the infant then develops a flaccid descending paralysis of motor and autonomic nerves. Lethargy, floppy head, weak cry, bulbar palsies, and poor feeding may be noted. Weakness worsens, and may progress to impaired respiration and death. Because respiratory compromise is the principal hazard, primary therapy consists of close attention to airway patency and adequacy of ventilation, with mechanically assisted ventilation as necessary. The presence of a weak gag or poor suck is the most reliable indicator of the need for respiratory support. In a recently published series, 37 of 60 children required intubation, with a mean duration of 21 days. Laboratory diagnosis requires detection of botulinum toxin in stool or serum, or isolation of toxigenic *Clostridia* in the stool by culture. Antitoxin has not proven useful owing to the slow release of toxin. However, botulism immune globulin (BIG) has been used with success and clinical experience suggests a decreased overall time to recovery. To avoid delay, therapy may be instituted before laboratory confirmation. If possible, blood, stool, or gastric aspirate specimens should be collected before BIG infusion begins to avoid falsely positive results.

Foodborne Botulism

Foodborne botulism results from ingestion of preformed botulinum toxin in putrefied food. Only 25 cases per year are reported in the United States, and are nearly always sporadic in nature. Home canned fruits vegetables are the most commonly identified source. The incubation period of botulism averages 12 to 36 hours, after which mild GI symptoms occur. Often patients do not seek medical attention at this stage. As the illness progresses, patients develop malaise, fatigue, and small muscle incoordination. This classically manifests as diplopia, dysarthria, or dysphagia. As the descending motor weakness progresses, respiratory compromise occurs, which may require emergent ventilatory support. To date, advances in the management of respiratory failure have had the greatest impact on improving mortality in botulism. Trivalent (A, B, E) equine antitoxin may be useful in foodborne botulism. Recent studies have demonstrated improved mortality and shortened hospital stay. One 10-cc vial

(7500 IU Type A, 5500 IU Type B, 8500 IU Type E) contains an amount of antitoxin that is more than 100-fold greater than that needed to neutralize the largest amount of toxin ever measured at the CDC. Only toxin not yet bound to nerve endings can be neutralized; thus, antitoxin can prevent but not reverse existing paralysis. Hypersensitivity is an important consideration, and the clinician should be prepared to manage anaphylaxis should it occur. Antitoxin has been administered to both children and pregnant women without complications. Within the first 3 days of illness toxin may be isolated from stool or blood; after this time, identification generally requires stool culture. Other diagnostic modalities include electromyogram and pulmonary function testing. With early recognition and appropriate supportive care, death is uncommon (5% to 10%), and usually results from complications of mechanical ventilation. Recovery occurs over weeks to months; residual weakness may persist for years.

Wound Botulism

This rare form of botulism occurs after colonization of a wound by *C. botulinum* and production of toxin. Only 25 cases are reported each year, but numbers are on the rise among IV and subcutaneous illicit drug abusers. Characteristically, the wounds are deep, dirty, or have a significant amount of devitalized tissue. The incubation period of wound botulism is relatively longer, and GI symptoms are absent. Fever is often noted. Surgical debridement and antitoxin administration are the mainstays of therapy. Antibiotic therapy remains controversial.

VIRUSES

Norwalk-like Viruses

Although many viruses have been implicated in foodborne illness, the Norwalk-like viruses account for the majority of reported outbreaks. These small, single-stranded RNA viruses commonly contaminate seafood and drinking and swimming water. Outbreaks have been documented in schools, nursing homes, cruise ships, and camps, and appear to have no seasonal variation. Gastroenteritis begins abruptly 24 to 48 hours after exposure. Low-grade fever, chills, headache, and myalgias may also be experienced. Complications are rare; most cases resolves within 1 to 2 days. Viral shedding may last a week or longer. In most cases, the epidemiologic pattern, rather than laboratory findings, suggest this pathogen.

Hepatitis A

Foodborne illness from hepatitis A most often occurs due to ingestion of fecally contaminated food and water. In the United States, recent outbreaks have been attributed to shellfish from waters polluted by sewage, and contaminated frozen strawberries served in several Michigan schools. Fever, malaise, jaundice, nausea, and abdominal pain develop 15 to 45 days after exposure, and generally resolve after 3 to 4 weeks.

PARASITES

Entamoeba histolytica

This highly contagious waterborne infection occurs most frequently in travelers, and may be indolent, with a variable incubation period and duration of illness, or fulminant with extraintestinal spread. Inflammatory diarrhea occurs and is occasionally accompanied by fever. Mild cases may be treated with oral metronidazole for 10 days, followed by either paromycin or iodoquinol for 7 days. Severe cases require admission and IV therapy with these same agents.

Giardia lamblia

Giardiasis is highly contagious; as few as 10 to 25 cysts can cause infection. Sporadic illness commonly involves travelers or children in daycare centers, and is the most common cause of waterborne diarrhea. Anorexia, bloating, and foul-smelling diarrhea occur 1 to 3 weeks after exposure. Treatment choices include metronidazole or furazolidone. Paromycin should be used in pregnant patients.

Trichinella spiralis

Trichinosis results from ingestion of raw or poorly cooked pork or wild game infested by the roundworm *T. spiralis*. The incidence of trichinosis in the United States has declined significantly owing to emphasis on thorough cooking of pork products. Following a 1- to 2-week incubation, fever, diarrhea, and abdominal pain develop, followed by myositis, eosinophilia, and periorbital edema as larvae invade surrounding tissues and deposit cysts in muscle. Cysts may remain dormant for years, resulting in a persistent carrier state. Diagnosis can be made by serology, and therapy consists of albendazole or mebendazole. Recovery occurs after 3 weeks of treatment.

Cryptosporidium parvum

The largest outbreak of *Cryptosporidium* involved a contaminated water supply in Milwaukee; 400,000 people were affected. Unpasteurized apple cider and chicken salad have also been linked to outbreaks. *Cryptosporidium* is a common cause of diarrhea in daycare centers. On average, illness begins 6 days after exposure. Affected individuals develop fever, chills, diarrhea, abdominal cramps, headache, and myalgias; in most cases, symptoms resolve after 6 days. Patients may intermittently shed cysts, and remain infectious for up to 60 days. Healthy patients will normally recover with supportive care alone; patients with AIDS or other immunocompromise may be treated with nitazoxanide, or a combination of paromycin and azithromycin.

Cyclospora cayetanesis

Since the first outbreak was described in 1990, this coccidian parasite has become an increasingly recognized cause of diarrheal illness in the United States. Before 1996, only three outbreaks were reported in the United States. Most followed exposure to contaminated water. A report of three outbreaks between 1996 and 1998 implicated fresh raspberries imported from Guatemala. Sporadic cases now occur regularly, and usually involve travelers or the immunocompromised. Infestation by the parasite primarily affects the small bowel. Diarrheal illness begins after a 7-day incubation period. In some cases the illness can be quite prolonged, with cyclical diarrhea, weight loss, anorexia, and fatigue lasting weeks. Treatment with TMP/SMX for 1 week may shorten the duration of illness.

CHEMICAL ETIOLOGIES

Monosodium Glutamate

Monosodium glutamate (MSG) is a food additive used worldwide as a flavor enhancer. The estimated average daily MSG intake in industrialized countries is 0.3 to 1.0 g. However, a heavily seasoned restaurant meal may contain as much as 5 g. Sensitivity to MSG has been estimated to occur in less than 1% of the population. Numerous anecdotal reports of the MSG symptom complex exist and encompass a myriad of symptoms. The symptom complex generally occurs when an MSG-containing food is ingested on an empty stomach. Classically, a diffuse burning sensation, facial pressure, head-

ache, flushing, chest pain, nausea and vomiting, and shudder attacks have been described. Potentially life-threatening bronchospasm and angioedema is believed to occur in rare cases. In a double-blind, placebo-controlled randomized study, subjects with self-reported sensitivity to MSG more commonly experienced headache, muscle tightness, numbness/tingling, generalized weakness, and flushing after MSG ingestion than after placebo. A dose–response effect was also demonstrated. No study subject developed rhinoconjunctivitis, asthma, urticaria, angioedema, or anaphylactoid reaction, suggesting that the effects do not appear to be IgE related. Overall, treatment of the MSG symptom complex is supportive; most episodes resolve spontaneously within 1 to 4 hours. Sensitive individuals should be advised to limit MSG intake in the future, particularly on an empty stomach.

CASE OUTCOME

The infant is admitted to the pediatric intensive care unit with a presumptive diagnosis of infantile botulism, attributed to the use of raw honey in her baby food. The patient requires endotracheal intubation and mechanical ventilation for upper airway obstruction. Botulinum toxin Type B is identified in her stool 8 days after illness onset. The patient is treated with BIG-IV. She gradually improves, and is extubated after 15 days. She is discharged after 23 days, and recovers fully.

SUGGESTED READINGS

Altekruse SF, Stern J, Fields PI, et al: Campylobacter jejuni—An emerging foodborne pathogen. *Emerg Infect Dis* 5:28–35, 1999.

Anderson TD, Shah UK, Schreiner MS, et al: Airway complications of infant botulism: Ten-year experience with 60 cases. *Otolaryngol Head Neck Surg* 126:2234–239, 2002.

Armada M, Love S, Barrett E, et al: Foodborne botulism in a six-month-old infant caused by home-canned baby food. *Ann Emerg Med* 42:226–229, 2003.

Bishai WR, Sears CL: Food poisoning syndromes. *Am J Gastroenterol* 22:579–603, 1993.

Bresee JS, Widdowson MA, Monroe SS, et al: Foodborne viral gastroenteritis: Challenges and opportunities. *Clin Infect Dis* 35:748–753, 2002.

Christy C: Foodborne diseases: Fruits and vegetables. *Pediatr Infect Dis J* 18:909–912, 1999.

Daniels NA, Mackinnon L, Rowe SM, et al: Foodborne disease outbreaks in United States schools. *Pediatr Infect Dis J* 21:623–628, 2002.

Foodborne outbreak of Cryptosporidiosis—Spokane, Washington, 1997. *MMWR Morbid Mortal Wkly Rep* 47:565–567, 1998.

Granum PE, Lund T: Bacillus cereus and its food poisoning toxins. *FEMS Microbiol Lett* 157:223–228, 1997.

Helms M, Vastrup P, Gerner-Smidt P, et al: Short and long term mortality associated with foodborne bacterial gastrointestinal infections: Registry based study. *BMJ* 326:357–359, 2003.

Hutin YJ, Pool V, Cramer EH, et al: A multistate, foodborne outbreak of Hepatitis A. *N Engl J Med* 340:595–601, 1999.

Infant botulism—New York City, 2001–2002. *MMWR Morbid Mortal Wkly Rep* 52:21–24, 2002.

Long SS: Infant botulism. *Pediatr Infect Dis J* 20:707–709, 2001.

Lyons AS, Petrucelli RJ: *Medicine: An Illustrated History.* New York: Abradale Books, Harry N. Abrams, Inc; 1987:498–499.

Nauschuetz WN: Emerging foodborne pathogens: Enterohemorrhagic *Escherichia coli. Clin Lab Sci* 11:298–304, 1999.

Outbreaks of Salmonella serotype enteritidis infection associated with eating raw or undercooked shell eggs—United States, 1996–1998. *MMWR Morbid Mortal Wkly Rep* 49:73–79, 2000.

Preliminary FoodNet data on the incidence of foodborne illness—selected sites, United States, 2002. *MMWR Morbid Mortal Wkly Rep* 52:340–343, 2003.

Robinson RF, Nahata MC: Management of botulism. *Ann Pharmacother* 37:127–131, 2003.

Schlech WF: Foodborne listeriosis. *Clin Infect Dis* 31:770–775, 2000.

Shapiro RL, Hatheway C, Swerdlow DL: Botulism in the United States: A clinical and epidemiologic review. *Ann Intern Med* 129:221–227, 1998.

Slutsker L, Altekruse SF, Swerdlow DL: Foodborne diseases: Emerging pathogens and trends. *Emerg Infect Dis* 12:199–215, 1999.

Tanzi MG, Gabay MP: Association between honey consumption and infant botulism. *Pharmacotherapy* 22:1479–1483, 2002.

Trachtman H, Christen E: Pathogenesis, treatment and therapeutic trials in hemolytic uremic syndrome. *Curr Opin Pediatr* 11:162–168, 1999.

Yang WH, Drouin MA, Herbert M, et al: The monosodium glutamate symptom complex: Assessment in a double-blind, placebo-controlled, randomized study. *J Allergy Clin Immunol* 99:757–762, 1997.

78

Marine Envenomations and Seafood Poisoning

Timothy B. Erickson
Paul S. Auerbach

HIGH-YIELD FACTS

- For most marine stings, local wound care, irrigation, tetanus immunization, wound exploration for foreign bodies, and selected, specific antibiotic coverage are common therapies.

- Hot water soaks are recommended for stingray, scorpion fish, echinoderm, and catfish stings.

- Dermatologic irrigation with vinegar, rubbing alcohol, household ammonia, baking soda, or papain will neutralize many coelenterate envenomations, including jellyfish.

- A topical jellyfish sting inhibitor is now commercially available.

- Antivenoms are available for stonefish, box jellyfish, and sea snake envenomations.

- Classic findings in ciguatera poisoning include circumoral tingling, generalized paresthesias, and apparent reversal of hot and cold sensations.

- Scombrotoxin causes a histamine-like or an allergic reaction appearing syndrome.

- Paralytic shellfish poisoning can result in paresthesias, cranial and peripheral nerve dysfunction, and respiratory failure.

- Tetrodotoxin can cause death by inducing respiratory paralysis and cardiovascular collapse.

CASE PRESENTATION

A 5-year-old boy begins to scream with pain while playing in the sand and surf within the Gulf of Mexico. The lifeguard on duty rescues the child and notes whip-like raised erythematous lesions on the child's legs. The lifeguard suspects the sting of a Portuguese man-o'-war as he carries the crying child to the first aid station.

INTRODUCTION

As more humans venture to aquatic environments for recreational activities, vacations, and an improved quality of life, the opportunity for children to encounter venomous marine life increases. Also, as more aquarists collect exotic marine life for display in the home, the incidence of bites and stings will rise regardless of the geographic locale. Hazardous marine life can be classified into four major groups:

- Venomous bites and stings, such as those inflicted by scorpion fish and the Portuguese man-o'-war

- Shock injuries, as from electric eels

- Traumatogenic bites (such as from sharks and barracudas)

- Toxic ingestions or fish poisoning

According to the American Association of Poison Control Centers data collecting system, there were 1287 aquatic bites and envenomations to children reported in 2001. Of these events, 70% occurred in children between the ages of 7 and 19 years, with 30% in children younger than 6 years of age. Of these marine exposures, the coelenterate group was responsible for over half of the stings reported.

DEVELOPMENTAL AND AGE CONSIDERATIONS

Toddlers are most likely to be envenomed in shallow waters and are typically unable to give a detailed or reliable history. Young children may step on poisonous marine animals or handle them, resulting in extremity stings. Adolescents are more adventurous, and frequent deeper waters as surfers, windsurfers, ocean swimmers, snorkelers, and scuba divers. This age group is also more susceptible to intoxication with ethanol or recreational drugs impairing their judgment.

COELENTERATES

Coelenterates (phylum *Cnidaria*) include jellyfish, sea anemones, and corals. Jellyfish stings are the most common marine envenomations, with an estimated 500,000 annual stings occurring in the Chesapeake Bay and 250,000 in Florida (Figure 78–1). A commonly encountered jellyfish is the sea nettle (*Chrysaora quinquecirrha*), which is widely distributed in temperate and tropical waters. One of the more feared jellyfish is the Portuguese man-o'-war (*Physalia physalis*). This jellyfish is most commonly found in the Gulf of Mexico and off the Florida coasts between July and September. Its tentacles can reach up to 30 meters in length. The deadliest and most venomous of coelenterates is the box jellyfish, or sea wasp of Australia.

Pathophysiology

Coelenterates envenomate with organelles called *nematocysts*, which contain venom-bearing threads that reside within specialized epithelial cells on the tentacles. Each nematocyst is a capsule with a folded eversible tubule, carrying a variety of toxins with neurologic, cytolytic, and enzymatic effects. Upon contact or when encountering a change in osmolality, these threads are everted from the nematocysts and thrust into the prey. When a human is stung, the penetration reaches into the innervated and vascular dermis. Both living and dead coelenterates can envenomate, as can fragmented tentacles and unfired nematocysts on the skin. Venoms vary, but generally contain histamine and kinin-like factors capable of causing systemic as well as local tissue effects. The venom in nematocytes is potentially dermatonecrotic, myotoxic, cardiotoxic, neurotoxic, and hemolytic.

Clinical Presentation

Mild coelenterate envenomation from true jellyfish or sea nettles generally causes local pruritis and characteristic linear, spiral, and painful urticarial lesions. The lesions often blister, and there is localized surrounding edema. The pain and stinging sensation occurs instantly, peaks within 60 minutes, and may persist for hours. Systemic symptoms from Portuguese man-o'-war stings may include nausea, vomiting, dysphagia, muscle cramps, myalgias, arthralgias, diaphoresis, and weakness. In addition, hemolysis and renal failure have been described following man-o'-war stings in pediatric patients. Severe systemic symptoms include hemolysis, dysrhythmias, cardiovascular collapse, respiratory distress, paralysis, seizures, coma, and death. Death in a child has been described in the literature following envenomation by the cuboid jellyfish (*Chiropsalmus quadrumanus*), which is found in the Atlantic and Indian Oceans.

Management

Treatment includes reassurance of the victim and immobilization of the injured part. Ice may provide some anal-

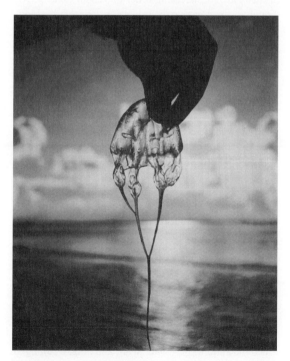

Fig. 78–1. Florida box-type jellyfish, held up at sunset. (Photo by Valeh Levy, MD. Used with permission.)

gesia. The area is rinsed with sterile saline or seawater to maintain a condition isosmolar to seawater, and to wash off unfired nematocysts. Fresh water is not recommended because it is hypoosmolar and often activates unfired nematocysts. As soon as possible apply a topical decontaminant. To inactivate nematocysts remaining on the skin, alter the pH by soaking the wounds with a weak acid like household vinegar (5% acetic acid solution). The inactivated nematocysts are then removed by gentle shaving or scraping. In the absence of a razor and shaving foam, one can also use the edge of a credit card, or something like a popsicle stick or clamshell.

If the victim shows signs and symptoms of anaphylaxis, treat appropriately. In most cases, analgesics and antihistamines are helpful. As a substitute for vinegar, one can apply household ammonia, rubbing alcohol, baking soda paste, or a slurry containing papain, which is commonly found in meat tenderizers. Rubbing sand or pouring ethanol over the wounds has no proven efficacy. Contrary to popular belief, human urine has actually been described as causing massive nematocyst discharge in *Chironex* tentacles. Tetanus immunization is indicated, but prophylactic antibiotics are not.

Sea anemones and corals are sessile creatures that cause local urticarial reactions upon contact. Contact with hard (true) corals may cause lacerations that are treated with vigorous local wound care, topical antiseptics, and tetanus prophylaxis.

For a child envenomed by an Australian box jellyfish, antivenom against *Chironex* is available in Australia and from major U.S. city aquaria and certain theme parks, such as Sea World. The antivenom is ovine in derivation, and has been administered safely in more than 75 episodes of envenomation. One ampule (20,000 U) can be administered IVPB, diluted in 1:5 ratio with crystalloid fluid, or it can be administered intramuscularly according to the manufacturer's instructions.

To prevent coelenterate stings, ocean bathers should wear proper skin protection, such as a neoprene wet suit or Lycra dive skin. Safe Sea jellyfish safe sun block (www.nidaria.com) is a topical sunscreen and jellyfish sting inhibitor combination that can be used to protect skin against stings, and is recommended for anyone who will expose otherwise unprotected skin to jellyfish, fire corals, anemones, or other similar stinging creatures.

Disposition

Mild stings responsive to vinegar can be managed at home after a 3- to 4-hour observation. Children with systemic toxicity or inadequate pain control despite local wound treatment should be kept for observation. Any child envenomed by a box jellyfish should be for observation for 8 hours. Symptomatic patients may require antivenom.

VENOMOUS FISH

There are more than 250 species of venomous fish, consisting mostly of shallow water reef or inshore fish. Stingrays are the most commonly encountered venomous fish, with more than 2000 stings reported annually. Eleven species of stingrays are found in U.S. coastal waters.

On the West coast, the round stingray (*Urolophus halleri*) is most commonly found; on the East coast and in the Caribbean the southern stingray (*Dasyatis americana*) is most frequently encountered. They are flat, round-bodied fish that burrow underneath the sand in shallow waters. When startled or stepped on, the stingray thrusts its spiny tail upward and forward, driving its venom-laden stinging apparatus into the foot or lower extremity of the victim.

Varieties of scorpion-fish include zebrafish and lionfish (*Pterois*), scorpion fish (*Scorpaena*), and stonefish (*Synanceja*), in increasing order of venom toxicity. Although more common in tropical waters of the Indo-Pacific, these fish are found in the shallow water reefs of the Florida Keys, Gulf of Mexico, southern California, and Hawaii. Lionfish are also popular as aquarium pets (Figure 78–2).

Catfish are found in both fresh and salt water. Stings occur from spines contained within an integumentary sheath on their dorsal or pectoral fins. The hands and forearms of fishermen and seafood handlers are the most common sting sites.

Pathophysiology

Stingrays have one to four venomous spines or barbs on the dorsum of a whip-like tail. The spines are retroserrated, so they anchor and may become difficult to remove. As the sting is withdrawn, the sheath surrounding it ruptures and the venom is released. Parts of the sheath may be torn away and remain in the wound. The venom is intensely active, partially heat labile, and causes varying degrees of local tissue necrosis and cardiovascular disturbances. The death of a 12-year-old boy is described in the literature from a stingray spine that directly penetrated the child's chest wall, heart, and lung, resulting in myocardial necrosis and tamponade.

Scorpionfish have venomous spines on the dorsal,

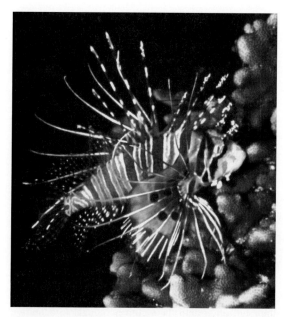

Fig. 78–2. Varieties of scorpion-fish include lionfish (*Pterois*), which are popular as aquarium pets. Envenomations from the spines cause immediate intense pain. (Photo courtesy of Paul Auerbach, MD. Used with permission.)

anal, and pelvic fins. This venom is also partially heat labile. Analysis of stonefish venom reveals several toxic components including hyaluronidase, hemolytic activity, and biogenic amines such as norepinephrine. Cardiotoxicity is primarily from verrucotoxin, a negative chronotropic and ionotropic agent that acts by inhibiting calcium channels.

For catfish spine stings, heat-labile venoms composed of dermatonecrotic, vasoconstrictive, and other bioactive agents produce symptoms similar to those of mild stingray envenomations. A unique parasitic catfish, the Amazonian Candiru (genus *Urinophilus*), may invade its victim by swimming "upstream" into the human urethra. Acute painful hemorrhage may result if forceful extraction of the catfish is attempted.

Clinical Presentation

With stingrays, intense pain out of proportion to the apparent injury is the initial finding, peaking within 1 hour and lasting up to 48 hours. Signs and symptoms are usually limited to the injured area, but weakness, nausea, anxiety, and syncope have been reported.

Envenomations from lionfish, scorpionfish, and stonefish cause immediate and intense pain that peaks within 60 to 90 minutes and persists for up to 12 hours. Local erythema or blanching, edema, and paresthesias may persist for weeks. Systemic findings include nausea, vomiting, weakness, dizziness, and respiratory distress. Although similar to those of the other scorpion fish, stonefish stings are more severe. Stonefish venom, a potent neurotoxin, can cause dyspnea, hypotension, and cardiovascular collapse within 1 hour and death within 6 hours. Local necrosis and severe pain may persist for days.

With catfish stings, burning and throbbing sensation occurs immediately, but usually resolves within 60 to 90 minutes. The discomfort may last up to 48 hours. Systemic symptoms are rarely reported.

Management

Treatment of stingray wounds includes irrigation with sterile saline to dilute the venom and remove sheath fragments. The injured part is immersed in hot water, no warmer than 113°F, for 30 to 90 minutes to inactivate any heat-labile venom components. Analgesics are usually required. Because of the penetrating nature of the - envenomation, wounds are debrided and left open. Tetanus immunization is updated. Treatment with a broad-spectrum prophylactic antibiotic such as trimethoprim-sulfamethoxazole, ciprofloxacin, or a third-generation cephalosporin is recommended because of concern for infection by *Vibrio* species.

Treatment for scorpionfish envenomation is immersion of the affected limb in hot water (113°F) for 30 to 90 minutes, or until pain is relieved. Wounds are irrigated with sterile saline, explored, and cleaned of debris. The wound is left open and treatment with prophylactic antibiotics is initiated.

Local treatment for a stonefish sting is the same as that for envenomations by other scorpion fish, with special attention given to maintaining cardiovascular support. There is a specific stonefish antivenom available in Australia. The antivenom is an equine-derived product and carries the risk for inducing anaphylaxis. One 2-mL ampule of stonefish antivenom is diluted in 50 mL normal saline and given IVPB.

Catfish sting treatment is immediate immersion in hot water (no warmer than 113°F) for pain relief. Catfish spines may penetrate the skin and break off. Sometimes, the spines can be located by routine radiographs. Occasionally, magnetic resonance imaging is necessary to locate a foreign body. The wound should be explored and debrided. Retained catfish spines should be removed by a qualified practitioner. The puncture wound is left open. Treatment with prophylactic broad-spectrum antibiotics and tetanus prophylaxis is indicated.

Disposition

Children with mild stings responsive to hot water soaks may be discharged after observation. Children not responsive to pain management may have a retained foreign body. Children envenomed by stonefish should be monitored in an intensive care setting. If it is available, antivenom administration is indicated in symptomatic patients.

ECHINODERMS

Echinoderms are spiny invertebrates that include sea urchins, seastars, starfish, sand dollars, and sea cucumbers. Of these, sea urchins most often cause medically significant envenomations. They are slow-moving, colorful bottom dwellers found at various ocean depths.

Pathophysiology

The spines or pedicellariae of sea urchins produce painful puncture wounds, swelling, and localized erythema.

Clinical Presentation

The spines can be up to 1 foot long in the needle-spined urchin (genus *Diadema*). They can easily puncture the skin, break off, and be retained. Their venom can cause local pain that may persist for days.

Management

Treatment is immediate immersion in hot water (no warmer than 113°F), careful removal of pedicellariae and spines, and local wound care. Tetanus immunization and/or antibiotic prophylaxis are often indicated.

Disposition

Most sea urchin puncture victims can be discharged home with continued hot water soaks and antibiotic prophylaxis. If there is a retained foreign body, follow-up evaluation is prudent.

SEA SNAKES

Sea snakes of the family *Hydrophiidae* are encountered throughout the Indo-Pacific region. The yellow-bellied sea snake (*Pelamis platurus*) has the widest distribution ranging from the Indo-Pacific to Africa to Central America. Sea snakes are air-breathing reptiles with venomous anterior fangs. They are among the deadliest snakes in the world, and may bite without provocation. Most bites are associated with net fishing and inadvertent handling.

Clinical Presentation

The venom of the sea snake has neurotoxic, myotoxic, and nephrotoxic effects. Most sea snake bites are dry bites with little venom injected. With true envenomations, symptoms usually manifest within 30 minutes to 3 hours. Initial symptoms may include muscle spasms and trismus. Severe envenomations may result in acute neurotoxicity with rapid muscular and respiratory paralysis.

Management

Apply pressure immobilization technique by wrapping the involved extremity with a compression bandage with immobilization until the victim is brought to definitive care. Respiratory support may be required. A polyvalent antivenom from Australia is commercially available. Additionally, a monovalent antivenom designed for the Australian terrestrial tiger snake has been used successfully when the polyvalent sea snake antivenom is unavailable. If antivenom is administered, the patient should be closely monitored for signs of anaphylaxis and given appropriate doses of diphenhydramine, glucocorticoids, and epinephrine as needed.

Disposition

All documented and suspected sea snake envenomation victims should be monitored in an intensive care setting for possible airway management and antivenom administration.

SEAFOOD POISONING

Marine foodborne poisonings of note induce ciguatoxin, scombrotoxin, paralytic shellfish saxitoxin, and tetrodotoxin. As a result of the wide availability of fresh and frozen fish, there is an increasing frequency of toxic ingestions in North America.

Ciguatera

Pathophysiology

Ciguatera fish poisoning is a serious public health problem in the Caribbean and Indo-Pacific regions. Ciguatoxin is produced by a dinoflagellate, *Gambierdiscus toxicus*, and concentrated in the food chain of predatory reef fish such as barracuda, grouper, red snapper, parrotfish, jacks, jellyfish, and moray eels. When humans ingest contaminated fish, poisoning can cause distinct neurologic and gastrointestinal (GI) symptoms.

Clinical Presentation

In nonendemic areas, the diagnosis of ciguatera poisoning is made only with a high index of suspicion combined with a recent history of ingestion of a specific fish. Within hours of ingestion, the patient may complain of neurologic symptoms such as circumoral tingling, headache, tremor, diffuse paresthesias, and classically, apparent reversal of hot and cold sensations. Younger children may only present with discomfort and irritability. Other signs, such as miosis, ptosis, and muscular spasm are more objective, but occur less frequently. The patient also commonly suffers GI symptoms such as watery diarrhea, vomiting, and abdominal cramping, making it difficult to differentiate from typical pediatric gastroenteritis.

Because of their smaller size, children are potentially at a higher risk for greater concentration of the toxin. Potentially fatal cardiovascular manifestations, such as severe bradycardia, hypotension, and respiratory depression, are possible but uncommon. Mortality from poisoning is 0.1%. Neurologic symptoms can persist for weeks to months.

Management

Treatment of ciguatera poisoning is primarily supportive. If the child presents within 1 hour of ingestion of the suspected fish and has not already vomited, decontamination with gastric lavage followed by activated charcoal is indicated. If the patient is already experiencing watery diarrhea, cathartics are not recommended, because they only exacerbate fluid losses and electrolyte disturbances. To date, specific treatment of ciguatera has been limited. Several therapies, such as amitriptyline and nifedipine have been advocated, but are of unproven efficacy. There has been some success with mannitol administration. Its mechanism of action remains speculative, but may be due either to action as an osmotic agent or as a scavenger of hydroxyl radicals from the ciguatoxin-related compounds. Mannitol must be used with caution because it may cause fluid loss and hypotension; its use for ciguatera toxicity in children has not been studied.

Disposition

If the child is experiencing significant fluid losses, electrolyte imbalance, or cardiovascular or neurologic manifestations, admission for supportive therapy is recommended.

Scombrotoxin

Pathophysiology

Scombroid poisoning is associated with the consumption of certain improperly preserved dark-fleshed fish, such as tuna, bonito, skipjack, mackerel, and mahi mahi. These fish have undergone bacterial decomposition owing to poor refrigeration. Although the symptoms of scombroid poisoning resemble an allergic reaction, this is a toxic pseudo-allergic phenomenon, because symptoms are a response to exogenous histamine rather than mast cell degranulation.

Clinical Presentation

Within minutes to hours following ingestion of a fish containing scombrotoxin, the patient experiences a histaminergic syndrome with diffuse erythema, pruritus, urticaria, dysphagia, and headache. Palpitations and dysrhythmias have been reported, but are rare. Other uncommon symptoms include bronchospasm, angioedema, and anaphylaxis. The symptoms usually last about 4 hours, and occasionally may persist for 1 or 2 days.

Management

Although scombroid poisoning is typically self-limited, supportive measures and fluid resuscitation may be necessary. Gastric decontamination may be considered if the ingestion was recent. Antihistamines such as diphenhydramine have been reported to shorten the duration of symptoms, but the benefit is not absolute, suggesting that the syndrome may be mediated by more than histamine alone. Intravenous infusion of a histamine H_2-receptor antagonist, such as cimetidine, has proven effective in patients with inadequate responses to diphenhydramine.

Disposition

If the vital signs are stable and there is good response to antihistamines, patients can be safely discharged home to take diphenhydramine and oral cimetidine for 2 to 3 days. If there is immediate threat of anaphylaxis or angioneurotic edema, aggressive therapy, including proper airway management, fluid resuscitation, and admission, is recommended.

Paralytic Shellfish Poisoning

Pathophysiology

Specific species of the dinoflagellate *Gonyaulax* form red or other colored tides and concentrate the neurotoxin saxitoxin in bivalve shellfish such as mussels, clams, and scallops. Humans who consume contaminated shellfish can develop profound muscle weakness or even paralysis via a curare-like effect mediated through blockage of sodium channels. Another type of neurotoxic shellfish poisoning is caused by brevetoxins, which cause muscle weakness without paralysis. Diarrheal shellfish poisoning is induced by dinophysotoxins and causes rapid GI symptoms. Amnesic shellfish poisoning, caused by the heat-stable toxin domoic acid, can cause memory loss, in addition to a variety of GI and other neurologic symptoms.

Clinical Presentation

With paralytic shellfish poisoning, vomiting, diarrhea, and abdominal cramping may develop within minutes to hours after ingestion. Additionally, the patient may experience headache, ataxia, facial paresthesias, and on rare occasions, muscle paralysis resulting in respiratory paralysis up to 12 hours after ingestion.

Management

Supportive measures include fluid resuscitation, and after recent ingestions, gastric decontamination. If paralytic shellfish poisoning is suspected, the patient is admitted for a 24-hour period for observation for respiratory depression.

Tetrodotoxin

Pathophysiology

Tetrodotoxin, one of the most potent poisons in nature, results in toxicity after the ingestion of meat from puffer fish, blowfish, balloonfish, and porcupine fish (Figure 78–3). In Japan, *fugu* is considered a delicacy prepared from pufferfish by specially trained and licensed chefs. As a result, a large number of tetrodotoxin cases are reported from Japan each year. The highest concentration of poison is contained in the fish liver and ovaries. Other marine animals harboring tetrodotoxin include the *Atergatus floridus* crab, eastern salamander, Californian newt,

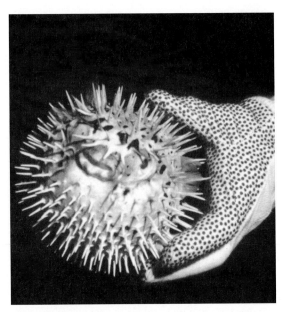

Fig. 78–3. Tetrodotoxin, one of the most potent poisons in nature, results in toxicity after the ingestion of meat from puffer fish, blowfish, balloonfish, and porcupine fish. (Photo by Ken Kizer, MD. Used with permission.)

and the blue-ringed octopus (genus *Hapalochlaena*). The octopus envenoms its victims with a subtle bite from a sharp beak. Intoxication produces profound neurologic symptoms and muscle weakness owing to inhibition of the sodium–potassium pump and subsequent blockade of neuromuscular transmission. In some reports, mortality rates have approached 60%.

Clinical Presentation

Symptoms begin within 30 minutes of ingestion. Early manifestations include circumoral and throat paresthesias, followed by vomiting and abdominal cramps. If the patient has consumed a large amount of toxin, within minutes to hours he may experience a feeling of doom heralding ascending paralysis, respiratory depression, dilated pupils, hypotension, bradycardia, and a classic locked-in or zombie-like syndrome. Death results from respiratory paralysis or cardiovascular collapse. Typically, if the victim survives beyond 24 hours, recovery occurs.

Management

Treatment includes rapid stabilization and gastric decontamination with activated charcoal and gastric lavage if the victim presents within 60 minutes of ingestion. Induced vomiting is contraindicated owing to potentially rapid central nervous system and respiratory depression. Atropine has been recommended for bradycardia and hypotension. Edrophonium and neostigmine may be beneficial in restoring motor strength. Most important, the patient's airway and respiratory status should be supported aggressively.

Disposition

Any patient with suspected poisoning from tetrodotoxin is admitted to an intensive care unit for a minimum observation period of 24 hours.

CASE OUTCOME

The child is rushed to the first aid station by the lifeguard on duty. The leg markings inflicted by stings of the Portuguese man of war are irrigated with vinegar, resulting in moderate pain relief. He is taken to the local emergency department, where he demonstrates stable vital signs and no systemic symptoms. After constant irrigation with a vinegar solution, the child experiences adequate pain relief. After 6 hours of observation, the child is discharged home with his parents, who are given local wound care instructions.

SUGGESTED READINGS

Marine Envenomations

Aldred B, Erickson T, Lipscomb J, et al: Lionfish stings in an urban wilderness. *J Wilderness Environ Med* 4:291–296, 1994.

Auerbach P: Envenomation by aquatic animals. In: Auerbach PS, ed: *Wilderness Medicine.* 4th ed. St. Louis: Mosby; 2001: 1450–1487.

Auerbach PS: Marine envenomations. *N Engl J Med* 325:486–493, 1991.

Auerbach PS, McKinney HE, Rees RS, et al: Analysis of vesicle fluid following the sting of a lionfish (*Pterosis volitans*). *Toxicon* 25:1350–1353, 1987.

Beadnell CE, Rider TA, Williamson JA, et al: Management of a major box jellyfish (*Chironex fleckeri*) sting. Lessons from the first minutes and hours. *Med J Aust* 156–655, 1992.

Bengston K, Nichols MM, Schnadig V, et al: Sudden death in a child following jellyfish envenomation (*Chriopsalmus quadrumanus*). Case Report and autopsy findings. *JAMA* 266: 1404, 1991.

Breault JL: Candiru: Amazonian parasitic catfish. *J Wilderness Med* 2:304, 1991.

Brown CK, Shepherd SM: Marine trauma, envenomations and intoxications. *Emerg Med Clin North Am* 10:385, 1992.

Exton D, Moran PJ, Williamson J: Phylum echinodermata. In: Williamson JA, Fenner PJ, Burnett JW, et al, eds: *Venomous and Poisonous Marine Animals.* Sydney: University of South Wales; 1999:312–326.

Fenner PJ, Williamson JA: Worldwide deaths and severe envenomation from jellyfish stings. *Med J Aust* 165:658, 1996.

Frenner PJ, Williamson JA, Skinner RA: Fatal and nonfatal stingray envenomation. *Med J Aust* 151:621, 1989.

Guess HA, Saviteer PL, Morris CR: Hemolysis and acute renal failure following a Portuguese man o' war sting. *Pediatrics* 70:979, 1983.

Hartwick R, Callanan V, Williamson J: Disarming the box jellyfish: Nematocyst inhibition in *Chironex fleckeri. Med J Aust* 1:15, 1980.

Kreger AS: Detection of a cytolytic toxin in the venom of stonefish (*Syanceia trachynis*). *Toxicon* 29:733, 1991.

Tomaszewski C: Aquatic envenomations. In: Ford M, DeLaney K, Ling L, et al, eds: *Clinical Toxicology.* Philadelphia: Saunders; 2001:970–984.

Seafood Poisoning

Blythe DG, de Slva DP, Femming LE, et al: Clinical experience with IV mannitol in the treatment of ciguatera. *Bull Soc Pathol Exp* 85:425, 1992.

Cameron J, Capra MF: The basis of the paradoxical disturbance of temperature perception in ciguatera poisoning. *J Toxicol Clin Toxicol* 31:571, 1993.

Centers for Disease Control: Tetrodotoxin poisoning associated with eating puffer fish transported from Japan-California, 1996. *MMWR* 45:389, 1996.

Centers for Disease Control: Paralytic shellfish poisoning—Massachusetts and Alaska, 1990. *MMWR* 40:157, 1991.

Herman TE, McAlister WH: Epiglottic enlargement: Two unusual causes. *Pediatr Radiol* 21:139–140, 1991.

Hughes JM, Potter ME: Scombroid fish poisoning. *N Engl J Med* 324:766–68, 1991.

Kaku N, Meier J: Clinical toxicology of fugu poisoning. In: Meier J, White J, eds: *Handbook of Clinical Toxicology of Animal Venoms and Poisons.* Boca Raton, CRC Press; 1995:75–88.

Lange WR, Snyder FR, Fudala PJ: Travel and ciguatera fish poisoning. *Arch Intern Med* 152:2049, 1992.

McInerney J, Shagal P, Bogel M: Scombroid poisoning. *Ann Emerg Med* 8:235, 1996.

Senecal PE, Osterloh JD: Normal fetal outcome after maternal ciguateric toxin exposure in the second trimester. *Clin Toxicol* 29:473–478, 1991.

Shoff WH, Shepherd SM: Scombroid, ciguatera, and other seafood intoxications. In: Ford M, Delaney K, Ling L, et al, eds: *Clinical Toxicology.* Philadelphia: Saunders; 2001:959–969.

Stewert MPM: Ciguatera poisoning: Treatment with intravenous mannitol. *Trop Doctor* 21:54, 1991.

Sun K, Wat J, So P: Puffer fish poisoning. *Anaeth Intens Care* 22:307, 1994.

Swift AE, Swift TR: Ciguatera. *Clin Toxicol* 31:1–29, 1993.

Van Hoesen KB, Clark RF: Seafood toxidromes. In: Auerbach PS, ed: *Wilderness Medicine.* 4th ed. St. Louis: Mosby; 2001:1285–1326.

Williams RK, Palafox NA: Treatment of pediatric ciguatera fish poisoning. *Am J Dis Child* 144:747–758, 1990.

Zlotnick BA, Hintz S, Park DL, Auerbach PS: Ciguatera poisoning after ingestion of imported jellyfish: Diagnostic application of serum immunology. *Wilderness Environ Med* 6:288, 1995.

79

Mushroom Poisoning

Connie Fischbein
Steven E. Aks
Gregory M. Mueller

HIGH-YIELD FACTS

- Mushrooms need to be ingested for toxicity to occur.
- Most potentially life-threatening mushrooms cause symptoms 6 to 8 hours or longer after ingestion. *Amanita smithiana* is an exception to this rule, and may cause symptoms as early as 2 hours after ingestion.
- Cyclopeptide (*Amanita phalloides*) and Monomethylhydrazine (*Gyromitra* spp.) mushrooms can cause life-threatening hepatotoxicity.
- *Amanita muscaria* mushrooms do not cause significant muscarinic symptoms. They belong to the ibotenic acid/muscimol group, and the name is a misnomer.
- The majority of toxic mushrooms belong to the gastrointestinal (GI) irritant group.
- The Orellanine (*Cortinarius spp.*) and *Amanita smithiana* mushrooms can cause life-threatening renal toxicity.
- *Tricholoma equestre* mushrooms can lead to life-threatening rhabdomyolysis.

CASE PRESENTATIONS

Case 1

A 3-year-old boy is found chewing on a large, white mushroom that was found in the backyard. The patient's mother estimates that he has eaten two to three bites from the mushroom cap. Within 30 minutes, the patient has had three episodes of vomiting and is referred to the nearest emergency department after the mother contacts the regional poison center.

On arrival the patient continues to have frequent episodes of vomiting and is tachycardic with a pulse of 130 bpm. In addition to vomiting, he develops nonbloody diarrhea. After consultation with the poison center, intravenous (IV) fluids are started, and a basic metabolic panel along with liver function tests are drawn.

While the laboratory results are pending, several digital photographs of the mushroom are taken and sent via the Internet to both the regional poison center and an expert mycologist for tentative identification. The mushroom is presumptively identified as *Chlorophyllum molybdites*, a Group VII GI irritant species.

Laboratory studies reveal the patient is mildly dehydrated with a blood urea nitrogen of 30, serum creatinine of 1.0, and a bicarbonate of 18. Liver function tests are within normal limits.

Case 2

A 15-year-old boy presents to the emergency department with suspected mushroom poisoning. Forty-eight hours prior to arrival, he and two friends sampled small pieces of dried mushrooms that they believed were hallucinogenic. Approximately 12 hours later, the patient developed abdominal pain, nausea, vomiting, and diarrhea. His friends experienced similar symptoms, and are being treated at other area hospitals.

The patient's heart rate is 112 bpm, and blood pressure is 130/70 mmHg. The physical examination is remarkable for dry mucous membranes and mild epigastric and right upper quadrant tenderness. There is no rebound or rigidity.

Laboratory studies show elevated liver transaminases (AST = 1279 U/L, ALT = 2410 u/L), a mildly elevated international normalized ratio (1.4 mg/dL), and hypoglycemia (glucose 60 mg/dL). Serum ammonia levels and renal function are within normal parameters.

The patient's symptoms begin to resolve. However, because of the late onset of symptoms and abnormal liver function tests, a potentially hepatotoxic mushroom species is suspected, and the patient is admitted to the intensive care unit. He is started on multiple doses of activated charcoal, IV fluids, lactulose, and vitamin K.

While the patient is being admitted, digital images of the dried mushroom samples are sent via the Internet to an expert mycologist who tentatively identifies them as an amatoxin-containing *Amanita* species. The mycologist positively identifies them the following day as *Amanita virosa*.

INTRODUCTION AND EPIDEMIOLOGY

The diagnosis and clinical management of mushroom poisoning is based on the knowledge that most toxic mushroom species fall into one of nine distinct classifications or groups. These groups contain specific chemical toxins that give rise to distinct clinical syndromes.

In general, the more severely toxic and potentially life-threatening species have a delayed onset of symptoms, usually 6 to 24 hours after ingestion (Groups I, II). Mushrooms belonging to Group VIII may even present with symptoms as late as 24 hours to 2 weeks after ingestion. Less toxic species have a relatively short onset of symptoms, usually 30 minutes to 3 hours after ingestion (Groups III through VII). A recently recognized syndrome, Group IX (*Amanita smithiana*), is associated with a short onset of gastroenteritis, followed by oliguric renal failure within 2 to 5 days.

Although most mushroom poisonings fall into one of these nine groups, other, non–life-threatening illnesses from mushroom ingestion is possible. Examples include gastroenteritis from bacterial contamination, absorption by the mushroom of pesticides or other environmental chemical contaminants, ingestion of raw or undercooked mushrooms, individual sensitivity, or ingestion of large quantities. It is also possible for more than one toxic species to be ingested, which can confuse the clinical picture. In these cases, identification of the involved mushroom species becomes more important. When identification is needed, an expert mycologist may be located by contacting the regional poison control center, many of which have a list of available consultants.

The majority of mushroom exposures occur in children. According to the 2002 American Association of Poison Control Centers Toxic Exposure Surveillance System, there were a total of 8722 mushroom exposures. Of these, 59% were ingested by children younger than 6 years of age. There were a total of five fatalities from mushroom ingestion in 2002, all in adults. A very common ingestion in small children is that of the little brown mushroom growing on the lawn. Most often these involve unidentifiable or nontoxic mushrooms such as species of *Psathyrella* or *Agrocybe*, and the quantities ingested are insignificant. These situations usually do not require aggressive GI decontamination. However, there are some potentially toxic species found on the lawn, such as *Conocybe filaris* (hepatotoxic), *Paneolus foenisecii* (hallucinogenic), or *Chlorophyllum molybdites* (GI irritant). Therefore, it is helpful in these situations to consult with the regional poison center and a mycologist.

Table 1. Mushroom and Time to Onset of Symptoms

	Time to Symptom Onset
Life-Threatening Mushroom	
Cyclopeptide (*Amanita phalloides*)	6–24 h
Monomethylhydrazine (*Gyromitra* spp.)	6–12 h
Orellanine (*Cortinarius* spp.)	24 h–2 weeks
Allenic norleucine (*Amanita smithiana*)	2–12 h
Tricholoma equestre	24–72 h
Non–Life-Threatening Mushroom	
Muscarine (*Clitocybe* spp.)	30 min–2 h
Antabuse (*Coprinus spp.*)	30 min–2 h
Ibotenic acid/Muscimol (*Amanita muscaria*)	30 min–3 h
Hallucinogenic (*Psilocibin* spp.)	20 min
GI irritants (*Chlorophyllum*)	<3 h

DEVELOPMENTAL CONSIDERATIONS

A child is at risk for ingesting a mushroom primarily in the outdoors. It is also possible that a child may be given a toxic mushroom in a meal. Children are more susceptible to severe poisoning by mushrooms than adults, because the relative doses of toxins ingested are usually greater. This is especially apparent in cases of amatoxin-containing species where the mortality rate for children is 50%, versus 10% for adults. Even for the usually benign GI irritant species, hypovolemic shock has been observed in small children after *Chlorphyllum* ingestion.

MUSHROOM GROUPS: PATHOPHYSIOLOGY AND CLINICAL FINDINGS

Historically, mushroom poisonings have been categorized into eight distinct clinical syndromes. It is of the utmost clinical importance to identify which toxin group the ingested mushrooms belongs. Cyclopeptide- (Group I) and monomethylhydrazine- (Group II) containing mushrooms tend to have delayed onset of symptoms, and can lead to fulminant hepatic failure in addition to other toxicities. Groups III through VII can cause significant toxicity, but are generally not life threatening. Mushrooms from these groups tend to have

Table 79–2. Mushroom Groups, Toxins, and Major Clinical Effects

Mushroom	Major Toxic Effect
Cyclopeptide (*Amanita phalloides*)	Hepatotoxicity
Monomethylhydrazine (*Gyromitra* spp.)	Hepatotoxicity, seizures
Muscarine (*Clitocybe* spp.)	Cholinergic excess
Antabuse (*Coprinus* spp.)	Antabuse reaction
Ibotenic acid/Muscimol (*Amanita muscaria*)	CNS excitation or depression
Hallucinogenic (*Psilocibin* spp.)	Hallucinations
GI irritants (*Chlorophyllum*)	GI irritation
Orellanine (*Cortinarius* spp.)	Renal failure
Allenic norleucine (*Amanita smithiana*)	Renal failure
Tricholoma equestre	Rhabdomyolysis

Abbreviation: GI, gastrointestinal.

an early onset of clinical symptoms. Group VIII, primarily certain species of *Cortinarius*, tend to cause a syndrome of delayed-onset renal failure. Although these species are found in the United States, there have not been any reported cases of renal toxicity in North America from this group.

Recently, the toxicity of *Amanita smithiana* has been appreciated, and there have been proposals to categorize these mushrooms in a distinct Group IX. *Amanita smithiana* can also cause delayed-onset renal failure, but unlike the other life-threatening mushroom ingestions, it causes GI symptoms early after ingestion.

Group I: Cyclopeptide-Containing Mushrooms

This is one of the major groups of mushrooms that can lead to life-threatening toxicity. Some examples of mushrooms in this group include *Amanita phalloides*, *Amanita verna*, *Amanita virosa*, *Conocybe filaris*, and certain species of *Galerina* and *Lepiota*.

These mushrooms contain amatoxins, phallatoxins, and virotoxins. Only the amatoxins are considered significant in human poisoning. They are felt to cause toxicity by interfering with RNA polymerase reactions.

Initial toxic effects, which consist primarily of nausea, vomiting, and abdominal pain, are usually delayed 6 to 24 hours postingestion. This is an important clinical distinction from the very large group of GI irritants (Group VII). Other clinical effects include fluid and electrolyte derangement, hypotension, central nervous system (CNS) depression, fulminant hepatic failure, coagulopathy, and, rarely, seizures. After the period of initial GI distress, the patient may seem to improve clinically while having a subclinical deterioration in hepatic status. Fulminant hepatic failure is the most important consequence of cyclopeptide toxicity, and is seen approximately 3 days postingestion.

Treatment generally centers on supportive care and replacement of fluid and electrolytes. Activated charcoal is generally recommended. There are a number of interventions that have been attempted for cyclopeptide poisoning, including hemoperfusion, high-dose penicillin, high-dose cimetidine, *N*-acetylcysteine, silibinin, and thioctic acid. None of these therapies have been subjected to controlled studies in humans, and the data regarding their effectiveness are variable. Liver transplant has been used successfully in cases of cyclopeptide-induced fulminant hepatic failure. Extracorporeal liver assistance methods have been used successfully to avoid transplant in cases of *Amanita phalloides* poisoning. This technique is discussed further in Chapter 18.

Group II: Monomethylhydrazine-Containing Mushrooms

The monomethylhydrazine-containing group can also lead to life-threatening hepatotoxicity. Like the Group I mushrooms, there can be a delay in onset of symptoms for 6 to 12 hours postingestion. This group contains the false morels. The true morel or *Morchella* species is a choice edible mushroom found throughout North America. The *Gyromitra* species of mushrooms can be confused with this delicacy, hence the term *false morel.* Representative examples of these mushrooms are *Gyromitra ambigua, Gyromitra esculenta*, other *Gyromitra* sp., and *Helvella* sp.

These mushrooms contain the toxin gyromitrin which is converted to monomethylhydrazine, and *N*-methyl-*N*-formylhydrazine (MFH). Hydrazines are also used as rocket fuels. The hydrazines act by reacting with pyridoxine and inhibiting pyridoxal phosphate-related enzyme reactions. MFH is also felt to deplete hepatic cytochrome P450.

Nausea, vomiting, diarrhea, and abdominal cramps are commonly seen 6 to 12 hours after the mushroom is ingested. Hepatic failure can occur. Important hematologic effects include hemolysis and methemoglobin production. The mechanism of toxicity of the hydrazine-containing mushrooms is similar to that of isoniazid, which is well known to cause seizures in overdose. Likewise, delirium, altered mental status, and metabolic acidosis can be seen after ingestion.

Treatment is primarily focused on supportive care, with replacement of fluid and electrolytes. Seizures can be managed with vitamin B_6 (pyridoxine). An infusion of 1 g can be initiated in children. In older teenagers and adults, a dose of 5 g can be administered. Benzodiazepines can be used synergistically with vitamin B_6 for seizures. For methemoglobinemia, methylene blue can be utilized for the symptomatic patient.

Group III: Muscarine-Containing Mushrooms

The muscarine-containing mushrooms cause a cholinergic toxidrome. The onset of symptoms is early after ingestion, usually between 30 minutes to 2 hours. A useful mnemonic to recall the clinical effect of muscarinic poisoning is SLUGBAM:

*S*alivation

*L*acrimation

*U*rination

*G*astrointestinal distress

*B*ronchorrhea, bradycardia, bronchospasm

*A*bdominal cramping

*M*iosis

Some muscarine-containing species include *Clitocybe dealbata*, certain other species of *Clitocybe*, and numerous species of *Inocybe.*

Treatment is generally supportive, and usually no specific antidotes need to be administered. Rarely, atropine may be administered for excessive muscarinic effects. Atropine can be given with a test dose of 0.05 mg/kg IV. The dose can be doubled every 5 to 10 minutes until there is clearing of tracheobronchial secretions.

Group IV: *Coprinus* Species (Antabuse)

Several species of *Coprinus* contain the toxins coprine and 1-aminocyclopropanol. The representative mushroom is *Coprinus atramentarius* is also known as the *alcohol inky cap* because it turns into a puddle of inky-like liquid as it decomposes. The toxin acts as an inhibitor of aldehyde dehydrogenase and can therefore lead to an antabuse-like reaction when consumed with alcohol.

Clinically, the onset of symptoms is between 30 minutes to 2 hours postingestion. The duration of effects is typically 6 to 8 hours, but enzyme inhibition may last several days, during which patients should not consume alcohol. Typical symptoms include flushing, nausea, vomiting, abdominal cramps, and diarrhea. Dizziness, headache, and, rarely, seizures can be seen. Hypotension and cardiovascular compromise can occur.

Treatment of toxicity is essentially supportive. Resuscitation with crystalloids may be necessary. If a pressor agent is needed for disulfiram-induced hypotension, norepinephrine is theoretically the pressor of choice. Dopamine β-hydroxylase may be inhibited, which may impair dopamine's efficacy.

Group V: Ibotenic Acid and Muscimol

This category of mushrooms has previously been felt to cause anticholinergic effects. However, more recent information shows that most effects are due to GABA and glutamate effects.

Some representative species of this group include *Amanita gemmata, Amanita muscaria*, and *Amanita pan-*

therina. The specific mechanism of toxicity is related to ibotenic acid, which is structurally similar to glutamic acid, and muscimol, which is related to GABA. Effects of glutamate agonism include CNS excitation; GABA agonist effects include CNS depression. Symptoms of overdose begin as early as 30 minutes and up to 3 hours after ingestion. The patient may exhibit ataxia, hallucinations, hysteria or hyperkinetic behavior, CNS depression, myoclonic jerking, and seizures. Vomiting is rare.

Treatment is focused on supportive care. Benzodiazepines and phenobarbital have been used successfully for hallucinations and CNS excitation symptoms.

Group VI: Hallucinogenic Mushrooms

Clinicians may encounter this group of mushrooms due to recreational use by adolescents. Young adults at rock concerts or at other venues may ingest these for euphoric effects. Hallucinogenic mushrooms may be found either in the wild, or may be purchased in the form of kits that can be cultivated at home.

Some representative examples of these mushrooms include certain species of *Conocybe, Gymnopilus, Panaeolus,* and *Psilocybe.* The toxins are indole alkaloids such as psilocybin and psilocin. These substances have LSD-like effects, and possibly cause some serotonin agonism.

Clinically, patients present with delirium, visual hallucinations, psychosis, and erratic and agitated behavior. On physical examination, the patient may have mydriasis, tachycardia, flushing, vomiting, tremors, and, rarely, seizures.

Treatment is supportive. Keeping a patient in a darkened room with minimal stimuli will help as the effects abate. Benzodiazepines are indicated for very agitated patients. There may be a role for antipsychotic agents for severe agitation and psychotic symptoms.

Group VII: Gastrointestinal Irritants

This comprises the largest group of toxic mushrooms. As stated, most of these mushrooms cause symptoms within 3 hours after ingestion. This property can help to distinguish them from mushrooms in Groups I, II, and VIII. One must take care not to miss the ingestion of *Amanita smithiana* based on this clinical pattern. It is also possible that a specimen of a Group I, II, or VIII mushroom could be ingested along with a GI irritant. This would mask the characteristic delay of onset of symptoms from the potentially deadly toxins. Therefore, it is critically important to obtain identifications of all of the mushrooms consumed if more than one species was potentially ingested.

There is a diverse range of species that are included in this group. *Chlorophyllum molybdites* and *Omphalotus olearius* are two common examples (Figures 79–1 and 79–2). Other Group VII mushrooms include certain species of *Agaricus, Boletus, Gomphus, Hebeloma, Lactarius,* and *Lepiota tricholoma.*

These mushrooms contain a wide variety of irritant chemicals that will lead to nausea, vomiting, and diarrhea. Hypovolemic shock has been reported in a 6-year-old girl after ingesting *Chlorphyllum molybdites.* This was due to severe dehydration. The cornerstone of man-

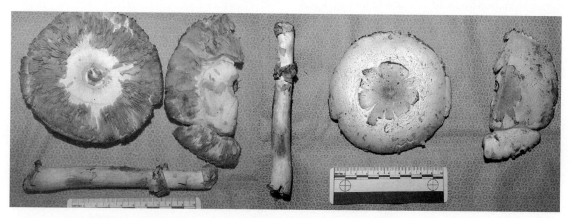

Fig. 79–1. *Chlorophyllum molybdites* (Photo courtesy of St. John's Hospital, Springfield, IL.)

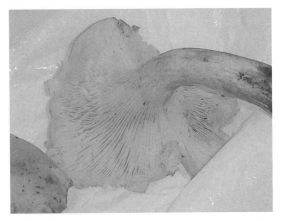

Fig. 79–2. *Omphalotus olearius.* (Photo by Ira Sender, MD, Elmhurst Memorial Hospital, Elmurst, Ill.)

agement is distinguishing this category from the more serious forms of mushroom ingestion. Adequate hydration and maintaining fluid and electrolyte balance are essential.

Groups VIII and IX: Renal Toxins

Two groups of mushrooms are potentially renal toxic, the *Cortinarius orellanus* group and the newly described *Amanita smithiana.*

The *Cortinarius* species include *Cortinarius gentiles,* *Cortinarius orellanus,* and *Cortinarius rainierensis.* These mushrooms contain the toxins orellanine and orelline, which lead to renal toxicity. Like the Group I and II mushrooms, Group VIII species typically cause delayed symptoms and can lead to life-threatening toxicity. Renal failure is estimated to occur in 30% to 45% of these cases. The symptoms from these mushrooms can be delayed 24 hours to 2 weeks after ingestion. Although some of these species are found in the United States, the cases of poisoning have mainly occurred in Europe. No deaths owing to ingestion of these mushrooms have been reported in North America.

A newly appreciated nephrotoxic mushroom is *Amanita smithiana.* This mushroom is found in the Pacific Northwest of the United States. The toxins in this mushroom include allenic norleucine (aminohexadienoic acid) and chlorocrotylglycine. These toxins specifically lead to renal toxicity. In one series the time to onset of symptoms ranged from 20 minutes to 12 hours. Therefore, this species is an exception to the general rule of mushroom

poisoning in that it can cause serious toxicity with an early onset of symptoms.

The treatment for both of these mushroom groups is supportive. Hemodialysis should be instituted for patients developing worsened renal failure.

Miscellaneous

Another mushroom that can cause clinically significant toxicity is *Tricholoma equestre.* This mushroom has been implicated in cases of delayed rhabdomyolysis in France. The mushroom is found throughout the world, and is known as the "Man on Horse" mushroom in the United States. The North American mushroom called *Tricholoma equestre* has been considered as an excellent edible, and there are no reports of toxicity in the United States. It is possible that the North American mushroom is a different species than the mushroom of the same name in France, or the different populations of the fungus may differ in their chemical composition. Currently, it is recommended that health care providers treat ingestions of this mushroom as potentially serious. The toxic constituent has yet to be identified. In the French series, 12 patients became ill and 3 died. Patients reported fatigue, muscle weakness, and myalgias, primarily in the lower extremities, 24 to 72 hours after consuming three consecutive meals containing *Tricholoma equestre.* All of these patients had clinically significant rhabdomyolysis. Treatment for this mushroom ingestion focuses on IV hydration along with management of rhabdomyolysis and its complications.

LABORATORY AND DIAGNOSTIC TESTING

Laboratory testing should be tailored to the type of mushroom ingested. A complete blood count and basic metabolic profiles including renal function and urinalysis can be obtained in patients requiring IV fluids. For potentially hepatotoxic mushroom ingestion, hepatic enzymes and coagulation parameters are recommended. For *Tricholoma equestre* ingestion, creatine phosphokinase should be measured.

To correctly manage mushroom ingestion, it is essential to identify the agent. With the increased availability of the Internet, it is now possible to use digital images sent via the Internet to assist in identifying mushrooms. Although positive identification requires the expertise of a mycologist, it is often possible to rule out potentially deadly species by using this technology. The use of digital images sent over the Internet can serve to facilitate and improve the quality of care provided to the victims of mushroom poisoning.

MANAGEMENT

Gastrointestinal Decontamination

The specifics of management for various mushrooms are listed in the above sections. However, the approach to GI decontamination is the same. Syrup of ipecac has fallen out of favor as a decontaminant for pharmaceutical preparations. Although it may assist in expelling mushrooms fragments that remain in the stomach, it alters the interpretation of the onset of symptoms. For example, if a possible cyclopeptide mushroom ingestion is suspected, one loses the clinical sign of delayed onset of vomiting. Gastric lavage has not been studied in a controlled manner for mushroom ingestions. It can be performed if a patient presents early after ingestion of a potentially life-threatening mushroom. However, in a small child or toddler, the size of the lavage tube limits its efficacy. Thus, activated charcoal is the current GI decontaminant method of choice for patients with acute mushroom ingestion.

DISPOSITION

The disposition of a case depends heavily on the identification of the mushroom. For cases of potentially life-threatening mushroom toxicity such as cyclopeptide, monomethylhydrazine, orellanine-containing mushroom, allenic norleucine-containing mushroom, or *Tricoloma equestre*, the patient should be admitted to monitor for delayed toxicity. For a mushroom that is deemed to be a GI irritant, the child should be hydrated, and observed until adequate oral intake can be ensured.

CASE OUTCOMES

Case 1

The child has a relatively short course of illness. Within 4 hours his symptoms subside. After fluid rehydration overnight, he is discharged the following morning.

The important feature in this case, which aided the diagnosis before a positive identification by the mycologist was obtained, is the short onset of gastroenteritis. The mushroom ingested, *Chlorophyllum molydites*, is the most frequent cause of gastroenteritis secondary to mushroom ingestion in North America. It is also important to note that fluid status should be carefully monitored because there is a risk of severe dehydration and hypovolemic shock.

Case 2

The patient's liver transaminases continue to rise and peak in the 4000 U/L range on day 4. By day 7, liver function tests normalized without evidence of renal injury.

This patient's course of illness is typical of moderate poisoning by amatoxin-containing mushrooms. Key features of poisoning by amatoxin are delayed onset of gastroenteritis (6 to 24 hours postingestion) followed by a phase of remission (48 to 72 hours), which may be followed by recurrent GI symptoms and progressive hepatic or hepatorenal failure. In the case of severe poisoning, symptom onset is usually shorter (6 to 8 hours), indicating a larger ingested dose, and transaminase levels tend to peak earlier and are typically greater than 5000 U/L. Other poor prognostic indicators are a significant rise in prothrombin time in the first 48 hours, metabolic acidosis, persistent hypoglycemia, and elevated ammonia levels.

SUGGESTED READINGS

Bedry R, Baudrimont I, Deffieux G, et al: Wild-mushroom intoxication as a cause of Rhabdomyolysis. *N Engl J Med* 345: 798–802, 2001.

Benjamin DR: Mushroom poisoning in infants and children: The *Amanita pantherina/muscaria* group. *J Toxicol Clin Toxicol* 30:13–22, 1992.

Benjamin DR: *Mushrooms: Poisons and Panaceas, A Handbook for Naturalists, Mycologists, and Physicians.* New York: W.H. Freedman and Company; 1995: 222.

Covic A, Goldsmith DJA, Gusbeth Tatomir P, et al: Successful use of molecular absorbent regenerating system (MARS) dialysis for the treatment of fulminant hepatic failure in children accidentally poisoned by toxic mushroom ingestion. *Liver Int* 23(suppl 3):30–34, 2003.

Erickson TB, Aks SE, Koenigsberg M, et al: Drug use patterns at major rock concert events. *Ann Emerg Med* 28:22–26, 1996.

Fischbein C, Mueller G, Leacock P, et al: Digital imaging: a promising tool for mushroom identification. *Acad Emerg Med* 10:808–811, 2003.

Goldfrank LR: Mushrooms. In Goldrank LR, Flomenbaum NE, Lewin NA, et al, eds: *Goldfrank's Toxicologic Emergencies.* 7th ed. New York: McGraw-Hill; New York; 2002.

Karlson-Stiber C, Persson H: Cytotoxic fungi—An overview. *Toxicon* 42:339–349, 2003.

Klein AS, Hart J, Brems JJ, et al: *Amanita* poisoning: Treatment and the role of liver transplantation. *Am J Med* 86:187–193, 1989.

Leathem AM, Purssell RA, Chan VR, et al: Renal failure caused by mushroom poisoning. *J Toxicol Clin Toxicol* 35:67–75, 1997.

Leikin JB, Paloucek FP, eds: *Approach to Mushroom Poisoning in Poisoning and Toxicology Compendium*. Hudson, OH: Lexi-Comp; 1998.

Lincoff GH: *The Audubon Society Field Guide to North American Mushroom*. New York: Alfred A. Knopf; 1988.

Michelot D: Poisoning by *Coprinus atramentarius*. *Nat Toxins* 2:73–80, 1992.

Miller PL, Gay GR, Ferris KC, et al: Treatment of acute, adverse psychedelic reactions: "I've tripped and I can't get down." *J Psychoactive Drugs* 24:277–279, 1992.

Stenklyft PH, Augenstein WL: *Chlorophyllum molybdites*—Severe mushroom poisoning in a child. *Clin Toxicol* 28:159–168, 1990.

Stolpe HJ, Hentschel H, Hein C, et al: Hepatic injury after ingestion of *Gyromitra esculenta* in children. *J Toxicol Clin Toxicol* 38:260, 2000.

Warden CR, Benjamin DR: Acute renal failure associated with suspected *Amanita smithiana* mushroom ingestions: A case series. *Acad Emerg Med* 8:808–812, 1998.

Watson W, Litovitz T, Rodgers G, et al: The 2002 annual report of the American Association of Poison Control Centers Toxic Exposure Surveillance System. *Am J Emerg Med* 21:353–421, 2003.

80

Poisonous Plants

Andrea G. Carlson
Edward P. Krenzelok

HIGH-YIELD FACTS

- Because the vast majority of plant exposures are unintentional and involve small quantities, most patients do not develop any symptoms.

- Gastrointestinal (GI) upset is the most common manifestation of symptomatic exposure. For most patients, treatment is supportive.

- *Dieffenbachia* and *Philodendron* are houseplants ingested by toddlers and are the most common cause of symptomatic plant ingestions. They can cause oral and pharyngeal pain from ingestion of insoluble calcium oxalate crystals.

- During the Christmas holidays, children are often exposed to *poinsettia*, *mistletoe*, and *holly*. The vast majority of these ingestions results in no symptoms, but may cause mild gastroenteritis.

- *Foxglove*, *oleander*, and *lily of the valley are among* several species of plants that contain cardiac glycosides and may cause toxicity similar to digoxin intoxication. In severe cases, the use of Digibind may be considered.

- *Water hemlock* is easily confused with the wild carrot or Queen Anne's lace. The potential for serious toxicity from ingestion of this plant is significant. Patients may progress to status epilepticus, respiratory distress, rhabdomyolysis, and death.

CASE PRESENTATION

A 3-year-old boy is brought to the emergency department (ED) by his mother. The patient was been playing at the park 30 minutes ago and picked and eaten berries from a vine growing along a fence. The child also reported "tasting" a few leaves from the vine. The patient brought some of the berries to his mother to taste. The mother removed several partially chewed orange-red berries from the child's mouth. The child was unsure exactly how many berries he had eaten. The mother brought a sample of the vine and berries for identification. On the way to the ED the child vomited once, producing two green berries. On examination the patient is awake, alert, and frightened. Vital signs are normal, as is the child's physical examination. Activated charcoal is given, after which the patient has two more bouts of emesis.

INTRODUCTION

Evaluation of a patient with a plant exposure presents several challenges to the health care provider. Significant geographical variation in plant species exists. Historical information regarding the species of plant as well as the amount ingested are often lacking. The degree of toxicity expected may depend on the particular part of the plant structure ingested (e.g., seeds, fruit, stem, root). Plants vary in toxicity during different stages of their growth cycle. Mechanical preparation of the plant material may also affect the overall toxicity. Furthermore, there is considerable overlap in the clinical manifestations of toxicity of many plants. Although the vast majority of plants are nontoxic, a small number are mildly toxic and a few are harmful with even a small exposure.

EPIDEMIOLOGY

Every year, plant ingestions account for 5% of all calls to poison control centers in the United States. Plants are most commonly ingested by children. Two common scenarios exist. Very young children, particularly toddlers, may ingest plant material while exploring their environment. Nearly 70% of plant ingestions are by children younger than 6 years. Older children and adolescents may intentionally ingest a certain plant species for its purported psychoactive effect. Overall, pediatric ingestion of plants only rarely results in toxicity. Of the 105,560 calls received by poison control centers for plant exposures in 2001, only two deaths were reported.

SPECIFIC TOXIC PLANTS

Historical information to be elicited includes whether the plant is an indoor or outdoor variety, a description of the plant's flower, stem, leaves, height, location, and, if possible, name. It is useful to consider certain plants according to the predominant and most serious manifestations of toxicity.

Mucosal Irritants

When ingested, a wide variety of plant species cause mucous membrane irritation owing to microscopic needle-shaped bundles of calcium oxalate (raphides) present throughout the plant structures. Plants containing calcium oxalate include philodendron, dumbcane (*Dieffenbachia*), pothos (*Epipremnum aureum*), caladium, calla lily (*Zantedeschia*), peace lily (*Spathiphyllum* sp.), Jack-in-the-pulpit (*Arisaema atrorubens*), elephant ear (*Colocasia esculenta*), and skunk cabbage (*Symplocarpus foetidus*). When masticated, the rhaphides release the calcium oxalate crystals, which penetrate mucous membranes, and in conjunction with proteolytic enzymes cause immediate burning and inflammation. Symptoms may persist for a week or more. Of the listed species, philodendron and *Dieffenbachia* account for the highest percentage of exposures. Most exposures do not produce toxicity, but based on a recent review of 10,796 *Dieffenbachia* exposures reported to the poison control centers, 34.7% of patients developed symptoms (Figure 80–1). Oral irritation was the most common complaint (18.2%), followed by dermal pain (8.7%), and vomiting (2.6%). Contrary to what is commonly reported in the medical literature, airway obstruction is rare. Treatment is symptomatic, with demulcents such as milk, popsicles,

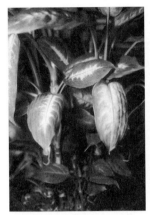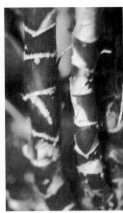

Fig. 80–1. Common household plants like *Diffenbachia* are often ingested by toddlers. These plants can cause severe oral pharyngeal burning from calcium oxylate crystals contained in the leaves and stem.

and cool drinks. Analgesics may be required; pruritus may respond to antihistamines.

Chili pepper or jalapeno (*Capsicum annuum*) was the most common plant exposure reported to the American Association of Poison Control Centers (AAPCC) in 2001. Exposure often occurs by handling or ingesting the pepper, with subsequent mucous membrane contact. Additionally, the toxin responsible for causing symptoms, capsaicin (8-methyl-*N*-vanillyl-6-nonenamide), is the active ingredient in many self-defense sprays. Capsaicin causes release of substance P from sensory nerve endings. Clinical effects consist of intense burning pain, irritation, and erythema. Profuse lacrimation may occur with ocular exposure. Vesication is not seen. Symptoms can persist for hours to days depending on the duration of exposure. A number of remedies have been suggested in the medical literature, including water, vinegar, isopropyl alcohol, antacids, vegetable oil, and 2% lidocaine gel. Immersion or flushing of the exposed area with cool water may bring temporary relief. Washing the affected area with soap and warm water may help to remove some of the residual capsaicin. Exposure does not result in any long-term injury.

Gastrointestinal Irritants

Mistletoe (*Phoradendron* Species)

Reports of significant toxicity from mistletoe involve *Viscum album*, the European variety, which contains a toxin known to cause cardiotoxicity in animal studies. There are a few reports of death owing to this variety, but the toxic effects are not well studied. The common variety found in the United States contains an alkaloid that may cause gastroenteritis. Retrospective review of poison center data suggests that the overall incidence of ingestions causing symptoms is low.

Poinsettia (*Euphorbia pulcherrima*)

The poinsettia was first introduced to the United States in the 1800s. The plant's reputation for toxicity in the early half of 1900s was based on single unconfirmed report of death in a 2-year-old child. Despite no further reports, many published sources and the general public continue to regard this plant as seriously toxic. A review of 22,793 exposures confirmed the relatively benign nature of poinsettia exposures. Most exposures (96.1%) were managed without ED referral and most (92.4%) remained asymptomatic. No fatalities were reported. Management of these exposures requires no more than supportive care; decontamination has not been shown to be of benefit.

Holly (*Ilex* Species)

There are 300 to 350 species of holly, but *Ilex aquifolium* or Christmas holly, is most frequently implicated in plant exposures. The plant produces green berries that mature into red berries that highlight the foliage and are used in holiday decorations. The red berries may be attractive to small children. Both the leaves and berries contain irritants that may produce gastroenteritis, which is usually not severe. Removing plant debris from the child's oral cavity and fluid replacement are sufficient therapy.

Pokeweed (*Phytolacca americana*)

The alkaloid phytolaccine is found in pokeweed. It primarily causes irritation of the skin, mucous membranes, and GI tract. The plant also contains a mitogen that causes mitosis of lymphoid cells and transient lymphocytosis. Careful parboiling can inactivate the toxin; in fact, pokeweed has been prepared as poke salad in the Southeast. As the green berries ripen to purple their toxic content also diminishes. GI symptoms after ingestion of the raw plant or unripe berries can become severe, and admission may be required for supportive care.

Systemic Toxins

Plants Containing Anticholinergic Substances

Jimsonweed (*Datura stramonium, Datura meteloides*); Deadly Nightshade (*Atropa belladonna*); and Black Henbane (*Hyoscyamus niger*)

Jimsonweed, also called *locoweed* and *devil's trumpet*, is a tall plant with a musty odor and spiny seedpods. The plant grows wild throughout the United States, and is thus a common exposure. Jimsonweed and other plants that cause anticholinergic poisoning contain belladona alkaloids, including atropine, hyoscyamine, and scopolamine. Patients with significant ingestion manifest an anticholinergic toxidrome: tachycardia, fever, mydriasis, dry mucous membranes, GI hypomotility, and urinary retention. Central anticholinergic syndrome results in altered mental status, ranging from somnolence to severe agitation. Hallucinations are common. Decontamination with activated charcoal may be considered in the cooperative patient; however, its use in the symptomatic patient is of questionable value. Agitation should be initially treated with benzodiazepines. The use of the antidote physostigmine is reserved for patients with seizures, severe agitation, or arrhythmias. Physostigmine can be given in pediatric doses of 0.02 mg/kg up to 0.5 mg over several minutes. If there is no improvement, readministration after 5 minutes may be attempted, to a total of 2 mg. The dose for adolescents and adults is 1 to 2 mg administered slowly intravenously over several minutes. Because of the short half-life, it may need to be readministered after 30 to 40 minutes. The majority of patients may be adequately managed with supportive care alone. Symptoms of toxicity usually resolve within 24 hours. Other plants with anticholinergic toxicity include deadly nightshade (*Atropa belladonna*) and black henbane (*Hyoscyamus niger*).

Plants Containing Solanine

Plants containing solanaceous alkaloids grow throughout the United States, and include nightshade (*Solanum* spp), tomato (*Lycopersicon esculentum*), nettle (*Solanum* sp.), and Jerusalem cherry (*Solanum tuberosum*). This does not include deadly nightshade (*Atropa belladonna*). Although all parts of the plant are poisonous, many nightshades also produce berries that are most toxic when unripe. Ingestion of green potatoes may also cause illness owing to solanine poisoning, as may ingestion of the sprouts that grow from potato eyes. However, toxicity is unlikely to occur unless the ingestions are significant. The mechanism of toxicity of solanine remains unclear. Small ingestions of these plants generally result in no more than self-limited GI effects. Severe intoxications manifest with central nervous system (CNS) and respiratory depression, as well as heart rate abnormalities, but death is uncommon.

Plants Containing Cardiac Glycosides

Foxglove (*Digitalis purpurea*; Figure 80–2), lily of the valley (*Convallaria majalis*), common oleander (*Nerium oleander*), and yellow oleander (*Thevetia peruviana*) all contain digitalis-like glycosides. Ingestion of yellow oleander results in the most significant degree of toxicity. Of all varieties of oleander, yellow oleander has been responsible for the greatest number of fatal poisonings worldwide. Yellow oleander is a common ornamental shrub found primarily in warmer climates, but not as commonly in the United States. All parts of the plant contain several cardiac glycosides, and can produce a

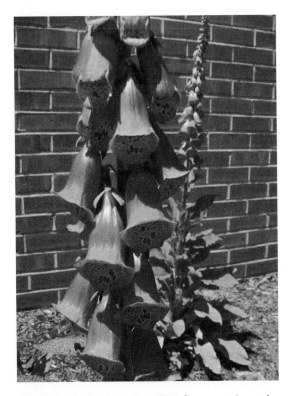

Fig. 80–2. The foxglove plant (*Digitalis purpurea*) contains digitalis-like glycosides.

syndrome similar to digoxin poisoning when ingested. The patient may manifest abdominal pain, nausea, vomiting, and diarrhea, as well as weakness, bradycardia, and atrioventricular block. Because the some of the plant glycosides are structurally similar but not identical to digoxin, a serum digoxin level may not be accurate. Treatment with digoxin immune Fab fragments is safe and effective for significant cardiac arrhythmias. It has been shown to restore sinus rhythm and correct bradycardia and hyperkalemia. The exact dose required is unknown, but a recent randomized, controlled trial suggests that much higher doses may be needed than those used to treat digoxin overdose. Patients with symptomatic ingestions from these plants should be admitted to a monitored setting until toxicity has resolved.

The yew (*Taxus* species) is a short evergreen bush commonly used in landscaping design. Seeds and leaves of the plant contain the toxins taxine A and B. Reported ingestions peak in late summer, probably owing to the appearance of the fleshy red aril surrounding the seed. The aril, although attractive to children, is reportedly nontoxic. Although deaths have been reported in the medical literature, significant toxicity generally requires a large ingestion. A retrospective review of 11,000 yew exposures reported to poison control centers over a 10-year period revealed that the majority of exposures (92.5%) did not develop symptoms, and that no deaths were reported. The most frequently encountered symptoms were GI upset (65.5%), dermal irritation (8.3%), hypotension or arrhythmias (6%), and seizures (6%). Treatment is supportive.

Tobacco (*Nicotiana* Species)

Most deaths from tobacco exposure reported in the literature result from occupational exposure to green tobacco or highly concentrated nicotine preparations. The lethal dose is unknown. Based on a 1928 pharmacology manual and subsequently a 1936 article that appeared in the *Journal of the American Medical Association*, 40 to 60 mg of nicotine has been accepted as lethal, and this has been perpetuated in a number of prominent clinical toxicology reference texts. There are no data that validate the toxic dose. Tobacco products are covered in depth in Chapter 63. Clinical response to nicotine intoxication follows a biphasic course. Initially there is a stimulatory effect at cholinergic receptors in the parasympathetic and sympathetic ganglia, as well as at the neuromuscular junction. Tachycardia, mydriasis, diaphoresis, tremor, and seizures may be seen. The stimulatory phase is then followed by autonomic and neuromuscular blockade from persistent stimulation, resulting in fasiculations and skeletal muscle paralysis. Death is usually due to respiratory arrest or cardiovascular collapse. Treatment is supportive, and many patients may be safely discharged after brief observation. Patients without spontaneous vomiting in the first hour are unlikely to have ingested a toxic amount.

Poison Hemlock (*Conium maculatum*)

Conium can be found throughout the United States. The plant can be identified by the mousy odor that it emits. *Conium* contains coniine, which is structurally similar to nicotine. The concentration of coniine is highly variable, and depends on the age of the plant, geographical location, and time of year. Manifestation of toxicity is also similar to that seen with nicotine, with an initial stimulatory phase that may include tachycardia, diaphoresis, tremor, and seizures, followed by a depressant phase that may involve bradycardia, muscular paralysis, and coma. GI symptoms are also prominent. Although death occurs rarely, and usually results from respiratory arrest, the ingestion of poison hemlock is a potentially significant exposure and mandates 4 to 6 hours of medical observation. Supportive care is the mainstay of treatment.

Water Hemlock (*Cicuta douglasii*)

Water hemlock is easily confused with the wild carrot or water parsnip, and may be mistaken for edible tubers by inexperienced outdoorsmen. The flowering portion of the plant also mimics that of Queen Anne's lace. The plant is often found growing along the borders of freshwater lakes and streams. The plant contains cicutoxin, a potent neurotoxin that is present in highest concentration in the root. A review of 582 cases of *Cicuta* ingestions concluded that these exposures have a higher fatality rate than most plant ingestions—no other plant species has accounted for more fatalities since the AAPCC began collecting data on plant exposure outcomes. Patients may rapidly progress to status epilepticus, respiratory distress, and death. Because there is no available antidote, treatment consists of aggressive supportive care. All patients who ingest water hemlock should be observed for symptoms in a medical setting for 4 to 6 hours. Patients manifesting any symptoms should be admitted to an intensive care setting.

Monkshood (Aconitum napellus)

There are nearly 100 species of monkshood in the United States. Fatality from ingestion of this herbaceous peren-

nial has been reported in the forensic literature as recently as 2002, and is due to the toxin aconite. The mechanism of toxicity of aconite is not well understood. Symptom onset is generally rapid. Cardiovascular symptoms predominate. Bradycardia or atrioventricular block may develop and be responsive to atropine, suggesting a parasympathetic effect. Ectopy manifests as ventricular dysrhythmias. Anti-arrhythmics or cardiac pacing may be needed as part of intensive care support. Respiratory paralysis may ensue, requiring ventilatory support. No antidote exists.

Plants Containing Grayanotoxins

Azalea and Rhododendron (*Rhododendron* Species) *and* Mountain Laurel (*Kalmia latifolia*)

The principle toxins produced by *Rhodendron* are grayanotoxins, which bind to and activate voltage-dependent sodium channels in cell membranes. Not all *Rhododendron* species produce grayanotoxins. Symptoms of exposure are dose dependent, and may include salivation, emesis, and perioral paresthesias. Hypotension, cardiac conduction disturbances, and muscle weakness have also been reported. With adequate supportive care, symptoms generally resolve within 24 hours. Despite the ubiquitous nature of these attractive ornamental plants, *Rhododendron* poisoning in humans is rare, with no published reports since a report of exposure to tainted honey in 1983.

Plants Containing Toxalbumins

Castor Bean (*Ricinus communis*) and Rosary Pea or Jequirty Bean (*Abrus precatorius*)

The toxalbumins of the castor bean (ricin) and the rosary pea (abrin) are some of the most toxic substances known. The bright scarlet and black seed of the rosary pea is very appealing to children, and is used for jewelry and in the making of rattles and maracas in the tropics. Castor beans are used in the production of castor oil, and are cultivated commercially and as garden ornamentals throughout the United States. The seeds have a thick waxy shell, and must be thoroughly chewed to liberate the toxin. Seeds swallowed whole will likely pass through the GI tract without harm. Both toxins inhibit cellular synthesis, affecting cells with rapid turnover (e.g., GI mucosal cells). Additionally, the toxins can cause red blood cell agglutination. Symptoms are commonly delayed, and may include severe vomiting, diarrhea, and life-threatening hemorrhage. Although theoretically beneficial, use of whole bowel irrigation to expedite expulsion of seeds has been studied and not found to be beneficial.

Plants Containing Colchicine

Autumn Crocus (*Colchicum autumnale*) and Glory Lily (*Gloriosa superba*)

Poisoning from these members of the lily family is a rare but serious and potentially fatal event. All parts of the plant contain colchicine, an antimitotic agent used therapeutically in the treatment of gout (see Chapter 36). Acutely, nausea, vomiting, and abdominal pain may result. In more severe intoxications, delayed effects may be seen, including hematologic derangements, liver injury, GI hemorrhage, and disseminated intravascular coagulation. Worldwide, deaths have been reported, and generally occur several days after exposure. Treatment is supportive; there is no effective antidote, although research involving the use of colchicines immune Fab is encouraging, but not commercially feasible.

Rhubarb (*Rheum rhaponticum*)

The stalk of the rhubarb is edible, but the leaves contain high concentrations of soluble oxalate. Once concentrated in the kidneys, theoretically the oxalate could precipitate with calcium and cause renal injury; however, this is unlikely with casual exposures. Symptoms may be delayed up to 24 hours. Because of the precipitation of calcium, patients could develop hypocalcemia, although this has not been commonly reported. Manifestations of hypocalcemia include electrocardiographic changes, paresthesias, tetany, hyperreflexia, muscle twitches, muscle cramps, and seizures. As with most plants, GI symptoms predominate. Serum calcium should be monitored and supplemented with calcium gluconate as needed. Typically, sufficient quantities of leaf material to produce toxicity are not ingested by children. Rhubarb leaf ingestion presents a more significant potential problem for farm animals such as cows.

Ackee (*Blighia sapida*)

Introduced to Jamaica from West Africa, well-ripened ackee fruit is a component of many Caribbean diets. The unripe fruit contains a potent toxin, hypoglycin, which inhibits metabolic pathways and can cause profound hypoglycemia. The illness, which also manifests with severe GI distress and CNS derangements, is also known as *Jamaican vomiting sickness*. The onset of symptoms may be delayed several hours. The clinical impression appears similar to that of Reye syndrome, with liver injury resulting in identical pathologic changes. Fatalities from this exposure are more common among children, possibly owing to lower liver glycogen stores and a greater tendency to hypoglycemia. Treatment requires hospital admission, with careful attention to blood glucose levels as well as hydration status.

Psychoactive Plants

LSD Congeners

Morning Glory (*Ipomea violacea*), Hawaiian Baby Woodrose (*Argyreia nervosa*), and Hawaiian Woodrose (*Merremia tuberosa*)

Seeds from these plants contain amides of lysergic acid, and cause effects similar to LSD. Generally several hundred morning glory seeds must be chewed to achieve a psychogenic effect. In addition to sensory distortion and hallucinations, GI upset may occur. Commercial preparations of the seeds are often sprayed with a noxious chemical, which may increase the likelihood of emesis. Although not life threatening, intoxication may cause discomfort and anxiety. Patients should receive supportive treatment in a quiet, nonthreatening environment (see Chapter 58).

Peyote (*Lopophora williamsii*)

Peyote is a small, fleshy, rounded cactus that grows throughout the southwestern United States and northern Mexico. The tops of the cactus are generally sliced off and dried, forming brown buttons that have a high content of the hallucinogen mescaline. A second toxin, lophophorine, is believed to have weak strychnine-like activity and may account for some of the cactus' GI effects. Shortly after ingestion, peyote produces nausea, vomiting, headache, and abdominal pain, as well as distortion of awareness. Visual hallucinations are common. Symptoms generally subside after a few hours, although the patient may experience disturbing flashbacks and loss of reality for the next several days.

CASE OUTCOME

Via digital photograph, the poison center identifies the plant as *Solanum dulcamara*, or climbing nightshade. The child remains under observation in the ED for several hours. No further signs of toxicity develop, and his GI upset resolves. The patient is discharged home.

SUGGESTED READINGS

Biberci E, Altunas Y, Cobanoglu A, et al: Acute respiratory arrest following hemlock (Conium maculatum) intoxication. *J Toxicol Clin Toxicol* 40:517–518, 2002.

Ceha LJ, Presperin C, Young E, et al: Anticholinergic toxicity from nightshade berry poisoning responsive to physostigmine. *J Emerg Med* 15:65–69, 1997.

Cumpston K, Vogel D, Leikin J, et al: Acute airway compromise requiring emergent tracheostomy following one bite of a diffenbachia stem. *J Toxicol Clin Toxicol* 40:645, 2002.

Danel VC, Wiart JF, Hardy GA, et al: Self-poisoning with Colchicum autumnale L. flowers. *J Toxicol Clin Toxicol* 39:409–411, 2001.

Eddleston M, Rajapakse S, Rajakanthan, et al: Anti-digoxin Fab fragments in cardiotoxicity induced by ingestion of yellow oleander: A randomized controlled trial. *Lancet* 355:967–972, 2000.

Krenzelok EP, Jacobsen TD, Aronis J: American mistletoe exposures. *Am J Emerg Med* 15:516–520, 1997.

Krenzelok EP, Jacobsen TD, Aronis J: Hemlock ingestions: The most deadly plant exposures. Abstract. *J Toxicol Clin Toxicol* 34:601–602, 1996.

Krenzelok EP, Jacobsen TD, Aronis J: Is the yew really poisonous to you? *Clin Toxicol* 36:219–223, 1998.

Krenzelok EP, Jacobsen TD, Aronis J: Poinsettia exposures have good outcomes . . . Just as we thought. *Am J Emerg Med* 14:671–674, 1996.

Lampe KF, McCann MA: *AMA Handbook of Poisonous and Injurious Plants.* Chicago: American Medical Association; 1985.

Litovitz TL, Klein-Schwartz W, Rodgers GC, et al: 2001 annual report of the American Association of Poison Control Centers Toxic Exposure Surveillance System. *Am J Emerg* Med 20:391–352, 2002.

Meda HA, Diallo B, Buchet J, et al: Epidemic of fatal encephalopathy in preschool children in Burkina Faso and consumption of unripe ackee (Blighia sapida) fruit. *Lancet* 353:536–540, 1999.

Pedaci L, Krenzelok EP, Jacobsen TD, et al: Dieffenbachia species exposures: An evidence-based assessment of symptom presentation. *Vet Hum Toxicol* 41:335–338, 1999.

Scharman EJ, Lembersky R, Krenzelok EP: Efficiency of whole bowel irrigation with and without metoclopramide pretreatment. *Am J Emerg Med* 12:302–305, 1994.

Turner NJ, Szczawinski AF: *Common Poisonous Plants and Mushrooms of North America.* Portland: Timber Press, Inc; 1991.

81

Snake Envenomations

William H. Richardson
Steve R. Offerman
Richard F. Clark

HIGH-YIELD FACTS

- Crotaline snakes are responsible for the vast majority of snake envenomations in the United States. Management is the same for all. Identification of exact species is unimportant for treatment.

- Twenty-five percent of crotaline snakebites are nonenvenomated dry bites.

- No first aid technique has ever been proven to improve outcome after envenomation. Rapid transportation to a facility with available antivenom is the most important principle for prehospital care.

- Crotaline Fab antivenom, consisting of highly purified papain-digested antibodies, is the current standard of care for treatment of crotaline snake envenomation.

- Antivenom dosing in pediatric patients is based on potential venom load, not size of the patient in kilograms.

CASE PRESENTATION

A 14-month-old girl is playing in her back yard when she is bitten above the right upper lip by a Southern Pacific rattlesnake (*Crotalus viridis helleri*). Paramedics are contacted, and she is immediately airlifted to a pediatric tertiary care hospital. On arrival to the emergency department (ED), the child has developed respiratory distress with audible stridor. Significant facial edema and ecchymosis involving the perioral, perinasal, and mucous membranes of the oropharyngeal region caused marked respiratory compromise, necessitating emergent orotracheal intubation (Figure 81–1).

Her mother states the toddler has no significant past medical history, no previous envenomations or antivenom therapy, and her immunization status is up to date. Initial vital signs prior to rapid sequence intubation are blood pressure 140/98 mmHg, heart rate 138 bpm, and respiratory rate of 28 breaths per minute with 100% saturations on a nonrebreather oxygen mask. Other significant findings on physical examination include non-bloody chemosis and a small amount of hemorrhage from the oropharynx. Lungs fields are clear except for transmitted upper airway noise; no cyanosis is observed, and the patient grossly moves all extremities symmetrically prior to neuromuscular blockade and intubation. Two vials of Crotalidae Polyvalent Immune Fab (ovine) antivenom (crotaline Fab) and intravenous (IV) fluids are initiated in the ED before transfer to the pediatric intensive care unit (ICU).

Initial laboratory studies reveal a WBC 37.8 K/μL, hemoglobin 11.7 g/dL, hematocrit 33.8%, and platelet count 466 K/μL. Prothrombin time (PT) and partial thromboplastin (PTT) are elevated at 16.1 and 40 seconds, respectively (normal 11.4 to 14.0 and 24 to 38 seconds, respectively). Fibrinogen is decreased at 60 mg/dL (normal 160 to 425 mg/dL). A chemistry panel demonstrates a sodium of 138 mmol/L, potassium 3.3 mmol/L, chloride 114 mmol/L, bicarbonate 17 mmol/L, calcium 7.8 mg/dL, glucose 89 mg/dL, blood urea nitrogen 19 mg/dL, serum creatinine 0.3 mg/dL, serum glutamate pyruvate transaminase 47 U/L, and creatine phosphokinase 177 U/L. Her postintubation venous blood gas reveals a pH 7.31, Pco_2 37 mmHg, and Po_2 34.6 mmHg.

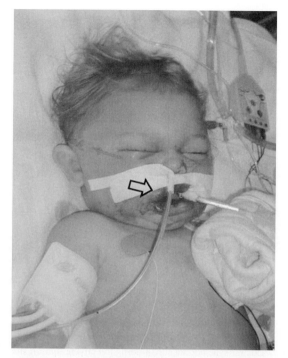

Fig. 81–1. A Southern Pacific rattlesnake bite caused significant facial edema and ecchymosis involving the perioral, perinasal, and mucous membranes of the oropharyngeal region, leading to marked respiratory compromise, necessitating emergent orotracheal intubation in a 14-month-old girl.

In contrast to nonpoisonous snakes, pit vipers have a triangular-shaped head, elliptical pupils, a single row of subcaudal scales below the anal plate, and heat-sensing glands located anteriorly below the eyes. Most indigenous nonvenomous snakes have a rounded contour of the head, circular pupils, and a double row of subcaudal plates. Additionally, the genera *Crotalus* and *Sistrurus* have rattles, but these may be inconspicuous in a very young rattlesnake or absent owing to trauma in adult snakes.

The coral snake (*Micrurus* sp.) is the only elapid found in North America. Clinically significant envenomations by these snakes are infrequent in the United States, probably because of their small size and relatively fewer numbers. Fewer than 70 coral snake bites were reported to the American Association of Poison Control Centers in 2001 as compared to over 2000 crotaline envenomations.

Coral snakes have rounded heads and circular pupils similar to many nonpoisonous species. The coral snake is often mistaken for certain varieties of the nonpoisonous king snake because both have red, yellow, and black rings. The old adage "red on yellow, kill a fellow; red on black, venom lack" helps distinguish the venomous coral snake from the nonpoisonous scarlet king snake. Narrow yellow rings separate larger red and black bands on a coral snake; black rings are adjacent to red bands in the scarlet king snake. These distinguishing patterns are only accurate in North America. Venomous South American coral snakes may have red and black adjacent bands. The much smaller fangs of a coral snake may leave little evidence of envenomation; however, any suspicion of elapid bite warrants medical attention.

INTRODUCTION AND EPIDEMIOLOGY

Excluding Alaska and Hawaii, venomous snakes are found throughout the United States and are classified into two families: Viperidae and Elapidae. Crotalinae is a subfamily of Viperidae collectively known as pit vipers owing to the heat sensing organs on either side of the head. The Crotalinae subfamily includes three genera: *Crotalus* (rattlesnakes), *Agkistrodon* (copperheads and cottonmouths), and *Sistrurus* (massasauguas). Although copperhead (*Agkistrodon contortrix*) and cottonmouth (*Agkistrodon piscivoris*) snakes are primarily located in the southern and eastern United States, 15 species of rattlesnake are found throughout the continental United States. While it is widely assumed that snakebites are extensively underreported, it is estimated that 8000 crotaline envenomations occur in the United States annually. Approximately 20% of these involve patients under 20 years of age.

PATHOPHYSIOLOGY

Because snakes typically hibernate in the winter, snake envenomations are seasonal, occurring primarily between April and October. The majority of bites to humans occur on the arms and hands, providing evidence for a commonly recognized pattern that snakes rarely strike unless provoked or agitated. Crotaline venom is produced by a pair of venom glands located posterior to the eyes that are connected to tubular fangs by venom ducts. These fangs remain folded against the upper jaw when not in use. During a strike, the snake's mouth opens to almost 180 degrees and the fangs rotate down to lie at right angles to the jaw. Usually from a coiled position, the snake lunges to strike its prey from up to a distance of one-half its body length. In humans, approximately 20% to 25% of bites are *dry bites*, which do not manifest signs or symptoms of envenomation. In the vast majority of strikes, the venom is injected subcutaneously in an extremity. The rare death owing to pit viper strikes may be the result of intravascular envenomation or a strike to the head or neck that causes airway compromise.

Crotaline venom contains a complex, heterologous mixture of proteolytic enzymes, lipids, amino acids, DNAase and RNAase enzymes, histamine, leukotrienes, kinins, and metallic ions used to immobilize, kill, and aid in the digestion of prey. The exact content of venom varies based on several factors including the age of the snake, species, geographic region, climate, and diet. The venom effects can primarily be described as local tissue cytotoxicity, hematologic toxicity, and neurotoxic effects.

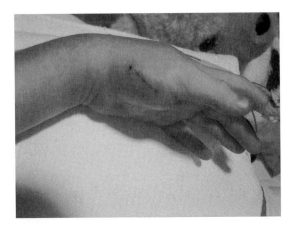

Fig. 81–2. An inconspicuous bite or scratch may make it impossible to identify classic fang marks after pit viper envenomation; a single puncture or complete absence of wounds does not ensure lack of envenomation.

DEVELOPMENTAL CONSIDERATIONS

Rattlesnake envenomation is an unusual poisoning that occurs much more frequently among adults than children. It is estimated that approximately 20% of envenomations in the United States occur in the pediatric age group. Although most children develop a fear of snakes at an early age, it is quite possible that an unknowing toddler or curious preschool-aged child may pursue interaction with a snake. Envenomation is exceedingly rare in children younger than 1 year of age.

It is important to remember that when envenomation occurs, the smaller pediatric patient is generally exposed to a larger milligram per kilogram venom load. Treating physicians should anticipate a higher likelihood of systemic symptoms. However, the basic principles of treatment do not change regardless of age or developmental stage. IV antivenom is always the first-line therapy and dosing should be targeted toward the potential venom load, as opposed to the patient's kilogram weight.

CLINICAL PRESENTATION

Local Effects

After a crotaline strike, venom is deposited most commonly into the subcutaneous tissue. Although potentially more detrimental, subfascial and intravascular venom deposition rarely occurs. Once envenomated, local tissue effects are virtually guaranteed and are initially manifested by significant pain at the bite site. Although it is common to identify classic fang marks after pit viper envenomation, a single puncture or complete absence of wounds does not ensure lack of envenomation. Glancing

strikes and clothing may alter the wound appearance, creating an inconspicuous bite or scratch (Figure 81–2).

Local tissue edema surrounding the envenomation site usually begins within 15 to 30 minutes, but may be delayed in some cases. The rate of edema progression is a useful indicator of the severity of envenomation. Swelling may progress to involve an entire extremity within a few hours after a severe envenomation. Ecchymosis, hemorrhagic blisters, bullae, and tissue necrosis may then develop over the next several hours to days. Patients also commonly report local paresthesias and numbness around the bite site in conjunction with severe pain. Myonecrosis and rhabdomyolysis are unusual, but have been reported following envenomation by certain species of rattlesnake.

Prominent soft tissue edema, pain, and ecchymosis in the affected extremity can mimic the appearance of compartment syndrome. Furthermore, distal extremity pulses may be difficult to palpate once severe edema has developed. Classic compartment syndrome, however, is exceedingly rare following pit viper envenomation, because most strikes are subcutaneous and do not penetrate the fascial compartment. The institution of adequate antivenom therapy is known to increase perfusion pressures and further decreases the risk that a true compartment syndrome will develop. Morbidity associated with fasciotomy is frequently more extensive than that caused by the initial envenomation.

Envenomation by North American crotaline *Agkistrodon* species such as the cottonmouth (*Agkistrodon pis-*

civoris), and in particular the copperhead (*Agkistrodon contortrix*), are generally found to be less severe than rattlesnakes. Although local venom effects do frequently occur, these snakes usually produce only mild to moderate tissue effects. Systemic toxicity is unusual. One series of copperhead envenomations involving 55 patients including 12 children found that 95% of patients developed local swelling and pain, but only 14% developed systemic symptoms. No hematologic toxicity was seen.

Systemic Effects

Diaphoresis, lightheadedness, restlessness, chills, nausea, vomiting, and weakness are often reported by patients after pit viper envenomation. Victims commonly complain of a metallic taste and perioral numbness or tingling. A wide range of systemic symptoms have been reported and are likely a result of the heterogeneous composition of crotaline venom.

Hematologic toxicity is common following crotaline envenomation, and may consist of coagulation abnormalities and thrombocytopenia. In severe cases, findings may mimic disseminated intravascular coagulation (DIC), with elevated prothrombin and partial thromboplastin times, increased fibrin split products and D-dimer, hypofibrinogenemia, and thrombocytopenia. These abnormalities, however, usually do not represent true DIC or carry the same severe bleeding risks. Venom-induced hematologic toxicity is frequently responsive to antivenom therapy. Blood and blood product transfusions are rarely necessary.

Certain species of rattlesnake have been recognized for possessing neurotoxic venom components. For example, Mojave rattlesnake (*C. scutulatus scutulatus*) envenomation is well known to produce neurotoxicity manifesting as reversible cranial nerve dysfunction, obtundation, fasciculations, myokymia, and respiratory paralysis, with minimal local cytotoxicity. Other rattlesnake species may cause neurologic abnormalities and local tissue destruction.

Elapid Envenomation

In contrast to the significant local tissue injury that occurs following most pit viper envenomations, coral snake bites often result in minimal or nonexistent local effects. Neurotoxicity follows approximately 75% of coral snake bites, and one case series of 39 patients bitten by the eastern coral snake reported that neurologic toxicity can be delayed for up to 12 hours. Signs of clinically significant coral snake envenomation include fasciculations, paresthesias, muscle weakness, dysphonia, dysphagia, other cranial nerve abnormalities including ptosis and diplopia, and respiratory difficulty secondary to muscle paralysis. Although these envenomations are extremely rare in children, death can occur and is primarily due to respiratory arrest. With careful supportive care and antivenom therapy, respiratory muscle paralysis is reversible and most patients recover without sequelae.

LABORATORY AND DIAGNOSTIC TESTING

Laboratory studies recommended in the assessment of rattlesnake bites include a complete blood count, prothrombin time or international normalized ratio, PTT, fibrinogen level, and fibrin degradation products. Abnormal hematologic parameters are considered evidence of systemic toxicity and should be incorporated along with clinical examination into the decision to administer antivenom. If initial laboratory testing is normal and minor local tissue swelling and pain are present, it is reasonable to reevaluate these hematologic laboratory values in 2 to 6 hours. If, however, these parameters are abnormal and antivenom has been administered, it may be useful to reexamine these hematologic parameters after completion of antivenom therapy. Halting progression or resolution of systemic toxicity can be assessed by observing trends in the hematologic laboratory parameters.

Other laboratory testing such as chemistry panels, CPK, urinalysis, and electrocardiograms are seldom useful in the acute setting, unless there exists suspicion for the development of rhabdomyolysis, myoglobinuria, and renal insufficiency.

MANAGEMENT

Prehospital Care and First Aid

Throughout the years, many strategies have been advocated for the prehospital management of rattlesnake envenomation. In the past, experts have recommended constriction bands, application of ice, incision, suction, and even electrical shock for the treatment of envenomation wounds. Subsequent studies have shown most of these therapies to be ineffective and some even harmful. The incision and mouth suction of wounds should be strongly discouraged because this may result in damage to underlying structures and introduction of wound infection. No study has ever documented significant venom removal by this technique.

Several snake bite kits, which may be carried and used by victims, are commercially available. Most of these kits have not been studied and there is no factual evidence to support their effectiveness for treatment of North American rattlesnake envenomation. One kit that deserves special mention is the Sawyer Extractor. This device is still widely marketed and has been subjected to experimentation. Early animal data made claims to removal of as much as 34% of venom load. A more recent study used a porcine model to examine the effects of the Sawyer Extractor on local envenomation findings. These authors found no improvement in limb swelling when the extractor was used. In addition, 2 of 10 experimental animals developed localized skin necrosis at the extractor application site.

The prehospital care of the patient following a rattlesnake strike should be directed toward delivery of the patient to the only treatment with any proven efficacy: IV antivenom. Optimal therapy consists of placing the patient at rest with the affected body part raised to the level of the heart. Emergency evacuation should be arranged as quickly as possible for transport to the closest facility with access to antivenom therapy. During transport the wound site should be measured and leading edges marked, so that symptom progression, an important indication for antivenom, can be judged upon hospital arrival. IV access should be obtained if possible and opioid analgesics administered. The prehospital use of crotaline Fab antivenom may be available in the future. At this time, however, this approach is unstudied, and cannot be advocated.

Hospital Care

ABCs

The vast majority of rattlesnake envenomations do not result in life-threatening toxicity. In general these bites represent only a threat to limb function and viability. Two notable exceptions do exist: airway compromise and intravascular envenomation. When envenomation occurs in close proximity to airway structures, massive tissue swelling can pose an imminent threat to airway patency. This is especially true in young pediatric patients. Therefore, envenomation occurring to the face, mouth, or neck should be considered an indication for early airway control. Waiting for obvious signs of respiratory difficulty or to assess the extent of swelling may result in dangerous airway compromise and failure of traditional intubating techniques.

Intravascular envenomation is extremely rare. This entity results in rapid and massive hematologic effects.

Patients sustaining an intravascular strike may develop active bleeding and present in extremis. Many of these patients do not survive to reach hospital care. In these cases, IV fluids, blood products, pressors, and antivenom should be used rapidly and liberally.

Antivenom

Crotaline antivenom should be considered the standard of care for treatment of any rattlesnake strike resulting in envenomation symptoms or significant laboratory abnormalities. For over 50 years, the only available antivenom therapy was an equine (horse serum) preparation consisting of whole IgG antibodies. In an effort to improve antivenom purity and decrease side effects, a new antivenom formulation has recently been developed and is now widely available. *Crotaline Fab antivenom* is an ovine (sheep serum) preparation that is highly purified and consists of only the smaller Fab antibody fragments. Crotaline Fab is as effective and probably safer than the older antivenom product. However, in the event that Fab antivenom is not available, therapy with the traditional equine formulation should not be delayed.

Indications for antivenom therapy are progression of local envenomation symptoms, bite in close proximity to airway structures, active bleeding, platelet count less than 100 K/μL, fibrinogen less than 100 mg/dL, or presence of neurotoxic symptoms. Because as many as 25% of rattlesnake strikes result in a dry or nonenvenomated bite, antivenom should be withheld from patients presenting without symptoms.

Crotaline Fab antivenom is administered IV. It is important to remember that dosing is based on venom load as opposed to the kilogram weight of the patient. Patients with envenomation symptoms should initially receive 4 to 6 vials of crotaline Fab regardless of patient size. Antivenom doses are dissolved in 250 to 500 cc of normal saline and infused over 30 to 60 minutes. The vast majority of pediatric envenomations occur in children who are mobile and therefore heavier than 10 kg. Crotaline Fab doses placed into 250 cc of normal saline for infusion should not be a problem in even the smallest children bitten by snakes. Symptoms should be reassessed hourly and antivenom redosed at 2 to 4 vials until symptoms have stabilized or improved.

Equine-derived crotaline polyvalent antivenom (Antivenin Crotalidae Polyvalent [ACP], Wyeth-Ayerst), an older whole IgG preparation for treatment of rattlesnake envenomation in North and South America, is still available in some hospitals. This antivenom product is thought

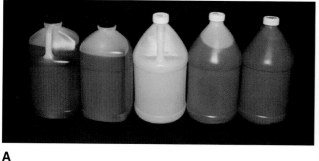

A

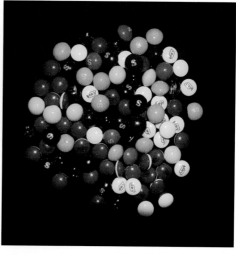

Color Plate 1. A. Ingestion of these colorful methanol-containing products may result in serious toxicity and blindness in children. **B.** Pills can be attractive to children because of their close resemblance to candy. (Photos by Tim Erickson.)

B

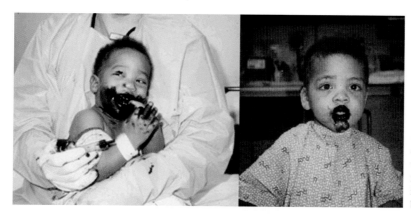

Color Plate 2. Although activated charcoal is the most effective gastrointestinal decontamination agent, its administration can be a challenge in younger pediatric patients. (Photos by Steve Aks and Carl Ferraro.)

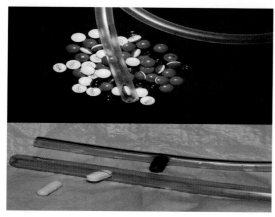

Color Plate 3. Even large-bore gastric lavage tubes may not have sufficient lumen size to aspirate pills and capsules. (Photos by Tim Erickson and Dave Gummin.)

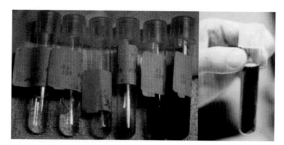

Color Plate 4. Following deferoxamine chelation therapy, children poisoned with iron may demonstrate the urinary color change classically described as *vin rose*. (Photos by Steve Aks and Dan Hryhorczuk.)

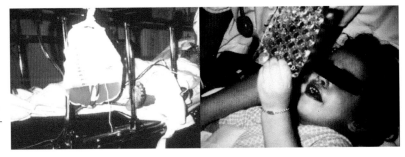

Color Plate 5A. Child with blue urine after ingesting several pills from a blister pack. **B.** Each pill contained a diuretic agent, methyl salicylate, and methylene blue. (Photo by Bonnie McManus.)

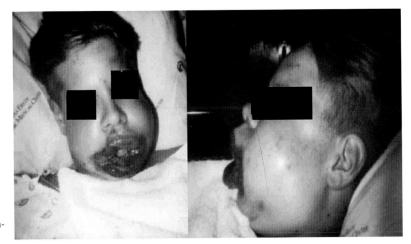

Color Plate 6. Adolescent demonstrating severe oral and facial frostbite with surrounding edema after inhaling or "huffing" freon.

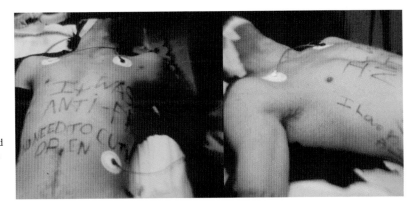

Color Plate 7. This adolescent presented comatose after ingesting antifreeze containing ethylene glycol. He wrote a message on his chest and stomach with the words, "It was antifreeze, no need to cut me open." (Photo by Tim Erickson and Carl Ferraro.)

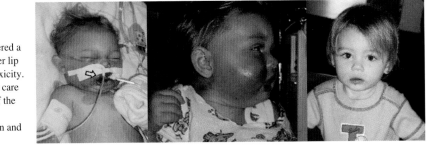

Color Plate 8. This child suffered a rattlesnake envenomation to her lip resulting in severe systemic toxicity. She recovered with aggressive care that included administration of the new Crotaline Fab antivenom. (Photos by William Richardson and Dave Barry.)

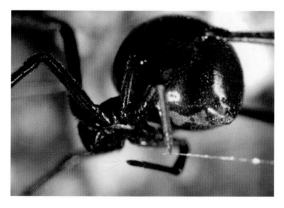

Color Plate 9. *Latrodectus mactans*, or black widow spider, bites can cause severe muscle spasms, abdominal pain, and neurotoxicity. (Photo by Peter Bryant.)

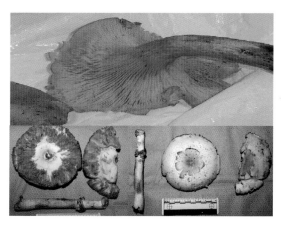

Color Plate 10. Gastrointestinal irritant mushrooms: Jack O'Lantern (*Omphalotusolearius*) and *Chlorophyllum sp*. (Photos by Ira Sender and Anna Moore.)

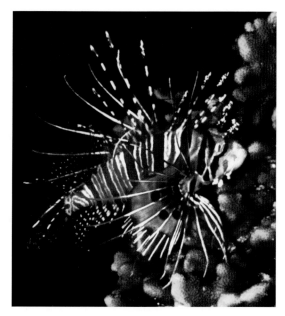

Color Plate 11. Varieties of scorpionfish include lionfish (*Pterois*), which are popular as aquarium pets. Envenomations from the spines cause immediate intense pain. (Photo by Paul Auerbach.)

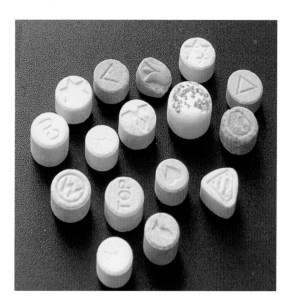

Color Plate 12. Ecstasy abuse among adolescents is on the rise, resulting in severe sympathomimetic toxicity with tachycardia, hypertension, and hyperthermia. (Photo copyright www.streetdrugs.org, used with permission.)

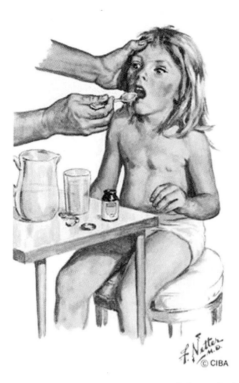

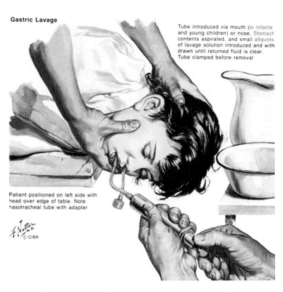

Color Plate 14. Frank Netter drawing depicting pediatric gastric lavage procedure. (Used with permission.)

Color Plate 13. Frank Netter drawing depicting pediatric poisonings: syrup of ipecac administration. (Used with permission.)

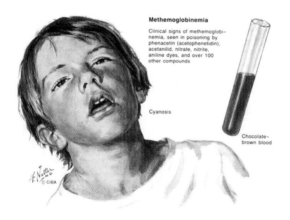

Methemoglobinemia

Clinical signs of methemoglobinemia, seen in poisoning by phenacetin (acetophenetidin), acetanilid, nitrate, nitrite, aniline dyes, and over 100 other compounds

Cyanosis

Chocolate-brown blood

Color Plate 15. Frank Netter drawing depicting pediatric methemoglobinemia resulting in cyanosis and chocolate brown-colored blood. (Used with permission.)

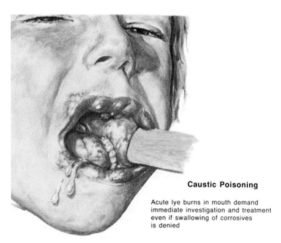

Caustic Poisoning

Acute lye burns in mouth demand immediate investigation and treatment even if swallowing of corrosives is denied

Color Plate 16. Frank Netter drawing depicting pediatric oral caustic burns. (Used with permission.)

to be about 3 to 5 times less potent than the equivalent crotaline Fab antivenom volume. Dosing strategy for ACP is essentially the same as with crotaline Fab except for the number of vials administered. Ten to 20 vials of ACP should be infused initially with subsequent doses of 5 to 10 vials depending on the severity of envenomation and progression of symptoms. Although the predictive value of skin testing for sensitivity to horse serum is unreliable, it is recommended by the ACP package insert to be performed prior to administration owing to risk of allergic reactions. Even in the setting of positive skin test results, the decision to give antivenom should be based on the risk–benefit ratio for the patient. Concurrent treatment with antihistamines, corticosteroids, and epinephrine infusion has reportedly been used to minimize allergic side effects during ACP administration.

Although the severity of acute side effects associated with the new crotaline Fab antivenom appears to be much lower than that of equine-based antivenom, patients should still be observed closely for anaphylactoid reactions. Most of these reactions are easily treated by slowing the infusion rate and administering IV diphenhydramine. The incidence of serum sickness (delayed hypersensitivity) is low when crotaline Fab is used regardless of the number of vials given in the course of treatment.

Crotaline Fab antivenom contains a thimerosal preservative that has raised concern because it contains a small amount of mercury. Although the American Academy of Pediatrics has recommended the removal of thimerosal from pediatric immunizations, there is not yet evidence that exposure to small amounts of thimerosal has caused harm. In any case, the risk associated with rattlesnake envenomation far outweighs that of thimerosal exposure.

Wound Care

Patients presenting after rattlesnake envenomation should be given tetanus prophylaxis when indicated. Affected extremities should be elevated to the level of the heart and previously placed constriction bands or wraps removed. IV access in an unaffected extremity should be established for the delivery of antivenom as well as analgesic medications. The liberal use of pain medications is frequently necessary to control pain. Prophylactic antibiotics are generally not recommended because rattlesnake venom possesses its own bacteriostatic properties. However, evidence of infection or a history of mouth suction to the wound may be indications for wound culture and initiation of a first-generation cephalosporin or amoxicillin-clavulanate.

Although prophylactic fasciotomy and digital dermatomy have been advocated as routine crotaline snakebite treatments in the past, these techniques have been abandoned and should not be performed. Compartment syndrome is rare following rattlesnake envenomation. It is important to remember that rattlesnake strikes generally place venom subcutaneously, not subfascially. The tense edema that is frequently apparent is usually due to swelling and necrosis of the subcutaneous tissues. For this reason, these bitten extremities are not managed like other potential compartment syndromes. The treatment for limb swelling is IV antivenom. Fasciotomy is rarely, if ever, indicated. Surgical therapy should only be considered in cases where elevated compartment pressures have been well documented in the face of aggressive IV antivenom therapy.

Surgical debridement of devitalized tissues or amputation of necrotic digits may become necessary, but should be delayed until the wound appearance is final. Surgical consultation may be withheld until 3 to 5 days after wound stabilization.

Coral Snake Envenomation

The initial management for coral snake envenomation is directed at airway protection and ventilation because neurotoxic venom symptoms usually predominate. Antivenom therapy may help to improve or prevent progression of symptoms. The currently available antivenom preparation is specific for only two species of coral snake: the Eastern coral snake (*Micrurus fulvius fulvius*) and the Texas coral snake (*Micrurus fulvius tenere*). Antivenom should be initiated in any patient with evidence of skin penetration caused by a coral snake bite. Therapy should not be delayed for the development of symptoms, because neurotoxicity may be easier to prevent than reverse. Antivenom therapy preferably within 8 hours of the envenomation is the goal. The current coral snake antivenom preparation is equine derived, and therefore carries a greater risk of both immediate and delayed hypersensitivity reactions than the previously discussed crotaline Fab antivenom. Patients undergoing treatment for coral snake envenomation should be admitted to an intensive care setting where they can be closely monitored for antivenom hypersensitivity or the development of life-threatening neurotoxin-induced respiratory paralysis. If severe neurotoxicity develops, symptoms may be long lived and difficult to reverse. These patients require prolonged ventilatory support.

DISPOSITION

Asymptomatic patients presenting after a rattlesnake strike should be observed for a minimum of 8 hours following injury. If no symptoms or signs of envenomation develop, the patient may be safely discharged with the diagnosis of a dry (nonenvenomated) bite. One exception to this rule includes patients with envenomation by a Mojave rattlesnake (*C. scutulatus scutulatus*). These snakes have been associated with delayed onset of particularly dangerous neurotoxic symptoms. Therefore, patients with presumed Mojave envenomation should be admitted and observed for a minimum of 24 hours.

All patients with symptoms of envenomation require admission for antivenom therapy, wound care, and monitoring. These patients require admission to a setting that allows for frequent wound checks, as well as frequent antivenom and analgesic dosing. This may be accomplished in an ICU or intermediate care unit depending on the particular facility. Wound checks including extremity measurements should be performed hourly during the initial phase of treatment. Once wound symptoms have stabilized for 4 to 6 hours, wound checks may be ordered less frequently.

A phenomenon of recurrent venom effects has been observed following stabilization using crotaline Fab antivenom. It is thought that this effect may be owing to the rapid renal clearance of Fab antivenom in the face of depot venom at the wound site. Therefore, patients should be rechecked for recurrence of local and hematologic venom effects at 48 to 72 hours after stabilization.

This may be accomplished on an inpatient or outpatient basis. Recurrence is generally considered an indication for further antivenom dosing. Some clinicians and the product package insert recommend the administration of two additional vials of crotaline Fab every 6 hours for three doses to patients who develop laboratory evidence of coagulopathy or thrombocytopenia during the course of the envenomation. The efficacy of this extra therapy is unclear.

CASE OUTCOME

The patient receives a total of 16 vials of crotaline Fab over the first 24 hours postenvenomation and the progression of swelling halts. No additional antivenom is required beyond the first day of hospitalization. An initial elevation in PT and PTT to 16.1 and 40.0 seconds, respectively, normalizes after antivenom treatment and remains normal throughout the hospitalization. A fibrino-

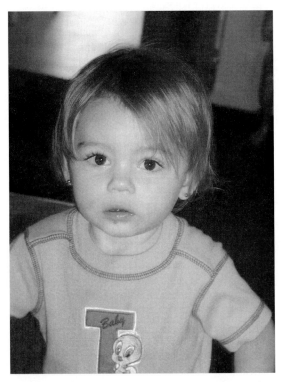

Fig. 81–4. Minimal hyperpigmentation over the right maxillary region is essentially unnoticeable at 3 months' follow up.

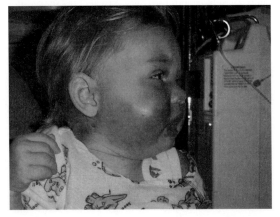

Fig. 81–3. Healing ecchymosis on the face of the 14-month-old girl shown in Figure 81–1.

gen level of 60 mg/dL on admission increases to 154 mg/dL after crotaline Fab treatment and subsequently remains above 200 mg/dL. Despite mild coagulopathy, thrombocytopenia never develops. By hospital day 6, facial and neck swelling have significantly decreased, and the patient is successfully extubated. Although no evidence of tissue necrosis is present, significant healing ecchymosis on the face and neck exist (Figure 81–3). During the next 3 days, the patient's pain becomes manageable with acetaminophen, swelling continues to decrease, and she is able to tolerate a regular diet. She is discharged home on hospital day 8. A 3-month follow-up visit demonstrates minimal hyperpigmentation over the right maxillary region that is essentially unnoticeable (Figure 81–4).

SUGGESTED READINGS

Brent J: Toxicologists and the assessment of risk: The problem with mercury. *Clin Toxicol* 39:707–710, 2001.

Bronstein AC, Russell FE, Sullivan JB: Negative pressure suction in the field treatment of rattlesnake bite victims. *Vet Hum Toxicol* 28:485, 1986.

Burch JM, Agarwal R, Mattox KL, et al: The treatment of crotalid envenomation without antivenin. *J Trauma* 28:35–43, 1988.

Bush SP, Hegewald KG, Green SM, et al: Effects of a negative pressure venom extraction device (extractor) on local tissue injury after artificial rattlesnake envenomation in a porcine model. *Wild Environ Med* 11:180–188, 2000.

Bush SP, Siedenburg E: Neurotoxicity associated with suspected Southern Pacific rattlesnake envenomation. *Wild Environ Med* 10:247–249, 1999.

Carroll RR, Hall EL, Kitchens CS: Canebrake rattlesnake envenomation. *Ann Emerg Med* 30:45–48, 1997.

Clark RF, Selden BS, Furbee B: The incidence of wound infection following crotalid envenomation. *J Emerg Med* 11:583–586, 1993.

Dart RC, McNally J: Efficacy, safety, and use of snake antivenoms in the United States. *Ann Emerg Med* 37:181–188, 2001.

Farstad D, Thomas T, Chow T, et al: Mojave rattlesnake envenomation in southern California: a review of suspected cases. *Wild Environ Med* 8:89–93, 1997.

Glenn JL, Straight RC: Venom characteristics as an indicator of hybridization between *Crotalus viridis viridis* and *Crotalus scutulatus scutulatus* in New Mexico. *Toxicon* 7:857–862, 1990.

Gregory VM, Russell FE, Brewer JR, et al: Seasonal variations in rattlesnake venom proteins. *Proc West Pharmacol Soc* 27:233–236, 1984.

Iyaniwura TT: Snake venom constituents: Biochemistry and toxicology (part 1). *Vet Human Toxicol* 33:468–474, 1991.

Jansen PW, Perkin RM, Van Stralen D: Mojave rattlesnake envenomation: Prolonged neurotoxicity and rhabdomyolysis. *Ann Emerg Med* 21:322–325, 1992.

Kitchens CS, Van Mierop LH: Envenomation by the eastern coral snake (*Micrurus fulvius fulvius*). A study of 39 victims. *JAMA* 258:1615–1618, 1987.

Offerman SR, Bush SP, Moynihan JA, et al: Crotaline Fab antivenom for the treatment of children with rattlesnake envenomation. *Pediatrics* 110:968–971, 2002.

Seifert SA, Boyer LV: Recurrence phenomena after immunoglobulin therapy for snake envenomations: Part I. Pharmacokinetics and pharmacodynamics of immunoglobulin antivenoms and related antibodies. *Ann Emerg Med* 37:189–195, 2001.

Tanen DA, Danish DC, Clark RF: Crotalidae polyvalent immune Fab antivenom limits the decrease in perfusion pressure of the anterior leg compartment in a porcine crotaline envenomation model. *Ann Emerg Med* 41:384–390, 2003.

Tanen DA, Ruha AM, Graeme KA, et al: Epidemiology and hospital course of rattlesnake envenomations cared for at a tertiary referral center in central Arizona. *Acad Emerg Med* 8:177–182, 2001.

Whitley RE: Conservative treatment of copperhead snakebites without antivenin. *J Trauma* 41:219–221, 1996.

Wingert WA, Chan L: Rattlesnake bites in southern California and rationale for recommended treatment. *West J Med* 148:37–44, 1988.

82

Arthropod Bites and Stings

Tri C. Tong
Aaron B. Schneir
Richard F. Clark

HIGH-YIELD FACTS

- Hymenoptera (bees, wasps, ants) are responsible for more adverse outcomes and fatalities in children and adults than any other arthropods.

- Anaphylaxis and airway obstruction are causes of the most severe outcomes in Hymenoptera stings.

- Only spiders that can penetrate the mammalian skin can impart toxicity through bites.

- Antivenom in black widow spider bites is efficacious and safe when infused slowly and diluted, but opioids and benzodiazepines are frequently sufficient for treatment.

- Dapsone offers no proven benefit in the treatment of brown recluse spider bites.

- Hobo spider envenomations can often be mistaken for those of the brown recluse, because of similarity in the course of their envenomations.

- Tarantulas cause most harm by flicking body hairs rather than through envenomation.

- Most scorpion stings in the United States cause only mild to moderate local pain, with the exception of *Centruroides exilicauda*, the bark scorpion.

- Tick paralysis can resemble Guillain-Barré syndrome (GBS), and a thorough search for a tick should precede any diagnosis of GBS.

CASE PRESENTATION

A healthy 7-year-old boy experiences a sudden stinging sensation to his left upper thorax after putting on a shirt. He immediately removes his clothing, but within minutes a burning pain grips his chest and he notes a round area of redness. Within 5 minutes, he develops abdominal cramping and two episodes of nausea and vomiting. Upon inspecting the shirt on the ground, the mother discovers a black spider. She quickly calls 911, and the child, mother, and sacrificed spider are transported to the local emergency department (ED).

In the ED, the child presents in noticeable distress and complains of abdominal pain. Examination reveals a firm abdomen with diffuse tenderness. Initial vital signs include a blood pressure of 162/88 mmHg, a pulse of 104 bpm, respirations of 22 breaths per minute, and a temperature of 97.9°F. The patient's chest is remarkable for an intense, erythematous, round lesion with a lighter center. Upon inspecting the spider, a red-orange hourglass shape is noted on its spherical abdomen, confirming the arthropod as a member of the species *Latrodectus mactans*, commonly known as a black widow spider.

The ED physician considers his therapeutic options and decides to begin with opioid analgesics and a benzodiazepine.

INTRODUCTION AND EPIDEMIOLOGY

The phylum *Arthropoda* is the largest division of the animal kingdom, constituting 95% of the world's living species. Although arthropods are known as nature's joint-legged creatures shrouded in hard exoskeletons, it is their venomous bites and stings that have gained them much notoriety. Many clinicians regard arthropod envenomations as a nuisance rather than a medical problem for humans, but published data suggest otherwise. In 2001, the American Association of Poison Control Centers reported 85,713 cases of exposures to bites and stings in the United States. A significant portion of those exposures was to arthropods, with Hymenoptera stings (bees and wasps) the most common offenders among children.

Bites and stings in children can be problematic for practitioners because of the potential difference in a child's response to envenomation compared to that of an adult. Epidemiologically, it does appear that higher acuity may be observed in children following toxic exposures to arthropods. The presumption has been that children typically receive higher per kilogram doses of toxin than adults because most arthropods that sting or bite do not moderate these functions based on the mass of their victim. Although this belief may be valid, the higher degree of acuity reported in children may also reflect some reporting bias. Minor arthropod bites and stings may go unreported in young children who cannot identify the source of their pain. Thus, pediatric victims of envenomations often present only when acutely ill, and those with minor exposures may go unidentified. Fatalities directly attributable to arthropod envenomations in the United States are rare, although this is likely a function of the limited reporting of deaths resulting from these exposures. Anaphylactic reactions from stings are often not considered toxicologic problems, and may thus not be reported to poison centers.

This chapter focuses on arthropod envenomations common in the pediatric population. Species are examined for their propensity to cause specific organ system toxicity. The potential for arthropods to act as infectious disease vectors through envenomation, although an important issue, does not fall within the scope of this chapter.

HYMENOPTERA (WASPS, BEES, AND ANTS)

Hymenoptera are responsible for more adverse outcomes and fatalities in children and adults than any other arthropod. There are three major, medically important superfamilies or subgroups within this order: (1) *Apidae*, which includes the honeybee and bumblebee, (2) *Vespidae*,

which includes yellow jackets, hornets, and wasps, and (3) *Formicidae*, or ants.

Bees and Wasps (*Apidae* and *Vespidae*)

Apids, such as honeybees and bumblebees, are usually docile, stinging only when provoked. Because bees are not carnivorous, their stinging mechanism has evolved into a primarily defensive weapon. A female honeybee is capable of stinging only once (male bees have no stinger) because its stinger has multiple barbs that cause the sting apparatus to detach from its body, leading to evisceration and inevitable death to the bee. Bumblebees have smoother stingers that do not permanently lodge in mammalian flesh, enabling them to survive for multiple stings.

Africanized honeybees, or so-called killer bees, are now found in Texas, Arizona, California, and most of the temperate southeastern and southwestern states. It is predicted that hives of these Africanized bees eventually will inhabit much of the Southern United States. In the 1950s, African bees were imported into Brazil for breeding experiments designed to improve honey production and disease susceptibility. Some escaped the following year and mated with previously imported European honeybees. These hybrids have since migrated successfully northward along the coasts and temperate regions of the continent. Although the toxicity of their venom is equal to that of their native counterpart, they are far more aggressive. A hive can respond to a perceived threat with more than 10 times the number of bees as its typical native North American counterpart. Massive numbers of stings from an attack of Africanized bees can result in multisystem damage and death from severe venom toxicity.

Most of the allergic reactions reported each year from Hymenoptera exposures occur from vespid (wasp, hornet, and yellow jacket) stings. These arthropods nest in enclosed areas, have volatile tempers, and may be disturbed by activity taking place around their nests. As with bees, only the females have adapted a stinger from the ovipositor on the posterior aspect of the abdomen. Although vespids also possess barbed stingers, they are able to withdraw their stingers following envenomation, thus allowing them to sting multiple times.

Hymenoptera venom contains several components. Histamine was once thought to be the main component responsible for most of the reactions observed following envenomation. Other substances have now been recognized as more important, including mellitin. *Mellitin* is a known membrane-active polypeptide that can cause degranulation of basophils and mast cells. It constitutes over 50% of the dry weight of bee venom. Because all Hymenoptera share many of these components, cross-sensitization may occur in individuals allergic to one species, with perhaps yellow jacket venom being the most potent sensitizer.

Clinical Presentation

The most common response to Hymenoptera venom includes pain, mild erythema, edema, and pruritus at the sting site. In addition to these manifestations, more significant reactions may occur.

Local Reaction

A local reaction consists of urticaria encircling the sting site. There are no systemic signs or symptoms, but a severe local reaction may involve one or more contiguous joints. Local reactions occurring in the mouth or throat can produce swelling that may lead to upper airway obstruction, especially in a young child. Stings around the eye or on the lid may result in the development of an anterior capsule cataract, atrophy of the iris, lens abscess, perforation of the globe, glaucoma, or refractive changes.

Toxic Reaction

A systemic toxic reaction from venom can occur with multiple stings. Africanized bees are notorious for such attacks, but an aggressive native hive may elicit a similar response. Symptoms of a toxic reaction may resemble anaphylaxis, but gastrointestinal manifestations (including nausea, vomiting, and diarrhea) and generalized sensations of light headedness and syncope occur with greater frequency. Headache, fever, drowsiness, involuntary muscle spasms, edema without urticaria, and convulsions may also occur. Although urticaria and bronchospasm are not always present, severe envenomations may lead to respiratory insufficiency and arrest. Hepatic failure also has been reported, as well as rhabdomyolysis and disseminated intravascular coagulation (DIC) in both adult and pediatric victims. Most minor symptoms usually subside within 48 hours, but may last for several days. Toxic reactions are believed to occur from a direct multisystem effect of the venom.

Anaphylactic Reaction

A generalized systemic allergic or anaphylactic reaction may occur after envenomation. Generalized systemic reactions to Hymenoptera venom are thought to occur from an IgE-mediated mechanism, leading to the release of pharmacologically active mediators within mast cells and basophils. Symptoms are often mild, but severe reactions can lead to death within minutes. There is no correlation between systemic allergic reactions and the number of stings. The majority of allergic reactions occur within the first 15 minutes, and nearly all occur within 6 hours. Fatalities that occur within the first hour of the sting usually result from airway obstruction or hypotension. Initial symptoms typically consist of ocular pruritis, facial flushing, generalized urticaria, and dry cough. Symptoms may intensify rapidly with chest or throat constriction, wheezing, dyspnea, abdominal cramping, diarrhea, nausea, vomiting, vertigo, chills and fever, laryngeal stridor, shock, syncope, involuntary bowel or bladder action, and bloody, frothy sputum.

Delayed Reaction

A delayed reaction, appearing 5 to 14 days after a sting, consists of serum sickness-like signs and symptoms of fever, malaise, headache, urticaria, lymphadenopathy, and polyarthritis. This reaction is believed to be immune complex mediated. Frequently, the parents may have forgotten about their child's initial encounter and are perplexed by the sudden appearance of symptoms.

Unusual Reactions

Infrequently, a reaction to Hymenoptera venom produces neurologic, cardiovascular, and urologic symptoms, with signs of encephalopathy, neuritis, vasculitis, and nephrosis. A case of Guillain-Barré syndrome (GBS) has been reported as a possible consequence of a Hymenoptera sting. Transient nephrotic syndrome leading to marked peripheral edema has also been reported in children as a complication following Hymenoptera attack.

Management

Involuntary muscle contraction of the venom gland continues after evisceration and the venom contents are quickly exhausted. Identification and immediate removal of the stinger should thus be the first step in treatment. A scraping technique to minimize additional venom release during the removal of the stinger has been described, but emphasis should be placed on rapidly removing the stinger, rather than the technique. Previous sources recommended cautiously scraping the stinger off with lateral pressure, rather than grasping it, to avoid compression of the venom sac resulting in further release of venom. However, recent studies have demonstrated that this is erroneous, because the venom has likely been completely released within seconds of envenomation.

The sting site should be washed thoroughly with soap and water to minimize the possibility of infection. Although infection is present only in a minority of cases, erythema and swelling may make it difficult rule out cellulitis. For local reactions, swelling and the rate of venom absorption can be limited by intermittently applying local ice packs. Oral antihistamines and analgesics may mitigate discomfort and pruritis. Nonsteroidal anti-inflammatory drugs can be effective in relieving pain, but standard doses of opioid analgesics should also be administered as needed. If edema is significant, elevation and rest of the affected limb should limit swelling unless secondary infection develops.

Initial signs and symptoms of a systemic allergic reaction may be mild, but progression can be rapid. Treatment is similar to that for anaphylaxis, with early consideration of epinephrine (0.3 to 0.5 mg of 1:1000 concentration in adult-sized adolescents and 0.01 mg/kg in children, never more than 0.3 mg). It should be injected subcutaneously or intramuscularly and massaged locally to hasten absorption. The patient should then be observed for several hours to ensure that symptoms do not intensify or recur. Intravenous (IV) administration of standard antihistamines (e.g., diphenhydramine) and H_2 receptor antagonists (e.g., ranitidine) is recommended. Although steroids (e.g., prednisolone) are of little help in stemming the immediate effects of a systemic reaction, their administration tends to limit ongoing urticaria and edema. Bronchospasm is treated with nebulized β-agonists. Hypotension may require massive crystalloid infusion. Persistent hypotension after massive volume replacement can require the use of a vasopressor. The patient who suffers a severe systemic allergic reaction is admitted for observation and further management. Antivenom has been studied for the treatment of massive bee attacks, but is not yet commercially available.

An insect sting kit containing premeasured epinephrine should be considered for each patient who has had a systemic allergic reaction. Physicians must give careful instructions on the use of this device, and should stress that the patient must inject the epinephrine subcutaneously at the first sign of a systemic reaction. Patients who have had severe reactions to insects should consider wearing identification (e.g., Medic Alert tags) concerning their severe allergy. Desensitization therapy is often recommended for patients exhibiting severe reactions to hymenoptera stings.

Ants (*Formicidae*)

There are five known species of fire ants (*Solenopsis*) in the United States. Whereas *S. aurea*, *S. geminata*, and *S. xylon* are native to this country, *S. invicta* and *S. richter* were imported through Mobile, Alabama, in the 1930s. They have now become well established throughout the Gulf Coast states. The fire ant typically inhabits loose dirt and breeds through 9 to 10 months of the year. One mature nest can produce 200,000 ants during a 3-year period, which accounts for the rapid spread of this arthropod through the southwest. The venom of the fire ant is almost entirely an insoluble alkaloid. There is potential cross-reactivity between the venoms of fire ants and other Hymenoptera, and individual stings can produce systemic toxicity in previously sensitized individuals.

Clinical Presentation

Fierce fire ant attacks ensue in response to an alarm pheromone released by one or more individual ants. After swarming upon their victims, a great number of ants may envenomate simultaneously. Because of their limited mobility, small children can become rapidly covered by swarms of these ants, resulting in severe stings or death. Each sting usually results in a papule that becomes a sterile pustule in 6 to 24 hours. Localized necrosis, scarring, and secondary infection can result. Rarely, a systemic reaction manifested by urticaria and angioedema can occur. Fatalities occurring within 20 minutes have been reported in Australia following bites from jumper or red bull ants (*Myrmecia* spp), but those victims were previously sensitized or suffered from preexisting cardiopulmonary disease.

Management

Treatment of fire ant stings consists of local wound care. The usual treatment for anaphylaxis is indicated if there is evidence of a systemic reaction. As with hymenoptera stings, desensitization may be necessary in victims exhibiting potentially life-threatening reactions to these arthropods.

SPIDERS (ARANEAE)

There are over 34,000 species of spiders worldwide, of which only a few dozen produce medically significant envenomations in humans. All spiders are carnivores that utilize venom to paralyze their prey prior to ingestion.

The vast majority of spiders pose little harm to humans, because either their venom injecting fangs are too small to penetrate human skin, the amount of venom injected is too little to produce toxicity even in children, or the toxins in the venom do not affect mammalian cells. Even if a reaction is elicited, it is often local; systemic toxicity is confined to a few specific species.

Widow Spiders (*Latrodectus*)

Latrodectus or widow spiders have a worldwide distribution. In the United States, the black widow is the most well known. Of the five *Latrodectus* species found commonly in the United States, only three (*L. mactans*, *L. various*, and *L. hesperus*) are actually black. Other varieties may be predominantly brown (*L. geometricus*) or red (*L. bishopi*). The classic orange-red hourglass-shaped marking is noted only in *L. mactans* (Figure 82–1). Female spiders are relatively large, with a body size ranging up to 1.5 cm in length and leg spans of 4 to 5 cm. On average, it is three times the size of its male counterpart, which cannot penetrate mammalian skin with its bite. Black widow spiders are found most often in dark, confined areas such as woodpiles, basements, garages, or sheds. *Latrodectus* will aggressively defend her web, particularly when guarding her eggs. Most black widow bites occur between April and October and are usually seen on the hands and forearms. The black widow spider injures its prey with potent venom. The most active component of this venom is α-latrotoxin, a compound that acts through a calcium-mediated mechanism leading to the release of acetylcholine and norepinephrine from nerve terminals.

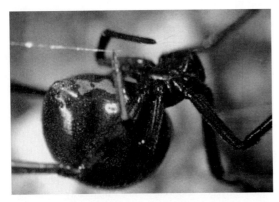

Fig. 82–1. *Latrodectus mactans*, or black widow spider. (Photo courtesy of Peter Bryant.)

Clinical Presentation

Most *Latrodectus* bites are immediately felt as a pinprick sensation at the bite site, followed by increasing local pain that may spread quickly to include the entire bitten extremity. Erythema appears approximately 20 to 60 minutes after the bite. In about one third of cases, the initial wound site may evolve into an erythematous ring surrounding a paler center that is often described as a *target lesion*. Victims frequently complain of cramp-like spasms in large muscle groups. In one review of pediatric black widow spider envenomations over a span of 10 years, all children presented with abdominal pain or rigidity. Such pain often increases progressively, becomes generalized, and can involve the trunk, back, and abdomen. In a young child, symptoms of envenomation may be mistaken as a surgical abdomen because of difficulties in eliciting a history of antecedent exposure. About 60% of all victims develop hypertension, although this is more common and severe in children. Other symptoms include headache, nausea, diarrhea, diaphoresis, photophobia, and dyspnea. Victims of *Latrodectus* envenomation can experience severe pain for 24 hours that can be intermittent or persistent. Rarely, pain may be protracted for several days.

Most adult victims typically see the offending spider because an immediate pinprick sensation is almost always reported with *Latrodectus* bites. In children, however, recovery of an offending spider is rare and diagnosis must be made on clinical grounds. Although confirmatory testing is not available, the presence of a characteristic lesion in association with severe pain and muscle spasms is virtually pathognomonic.

Management

Therapy begins with supportive care of the airway, breathing, and circulation. Cleansing of the bite site is recommended. Pain and muscle spasms can be effectively controlled with liberal doses of opioids and benzodiazepines in about 70% of victims. Although IV calcium has been advocated to relieve symptoms, a retrospective review of 163 patients with *Latrodectus* envenomation found this treatment to be ineffective. For severe envenomations, admission may be required for continued analgesia. The most effective therapies for severe envenomation are parenteral opioids and *Latrodectus* antivenom. Administration of *Latrodectus* antivenom can lead to rapid resolution of symptoms and greatly shorten the course of illness. Even in severely symptomatic cases of *Latrodectus* envenomation, patients can often be discharged from the ED after a short observation period after antivenom is administered. *Latrodectus* antivenom is produced in at least three countries with specificity for indigenous species: Red-Back Spider Antivenom (Commonwealth Serum Laboratories CSL Ltd., Australia), Button Spider Antivenom (South African Vaccine Producers Institute, South Africa), and Antivenin *Latrodectus mactans* (Merck & Co., Inc., United States). Indications, amount, and route of administration vary according to each product. *Latrodectus* antivenom is derived from horse serum and although hypersensitivity reactions are possible, slow administration of diluted Antivenin *Latrodectus mactans* is generally considered safe. One death from anaphylaxis has been reported after administration of Antivenin *Latrodectus mactans* in the United States. That case, however, was confounded by rapid IV infusion of undiluted antivenom and the patient's preexisting asthma and allergies to multiple medications.

Necrotic Arachnidism (*Loxosceles*)

Loxosceles spiders exist in multiple regions throughout the world. Its reputation for producing local necrotic skin lesions and system toxicity is as equally expansive. Three species, *L. reclusa* (true brown recluse), *L. laeta* (corner spider), and *L. arizona* (Arizona brown spider) produce the majority of *Loxosceles* bites in the United States. The brown recluse spider is one of the most common species found in the United States, with an endemic range in the south-central United States from Texas to Georgia and Iowa to Louisiana. These species of spiders have distinct, 1-cm, tan to brown bodies adorned with a violin-shaped mark on its dorsal cephalothorax. *L. reclusa* prefers warm, dry areas such as abandoned buildings, woodpiles, and cellars. Most of the necrotic features of brown recluse bites are related to sphingomyelinase D, an enzyme contained within their venom. Other enzymes including hyaluronidase, alkaline phosphatase, 5′-ribonucleotide phosphohydrolase are also present, but in smaller amounts. After envenomation, neutrophil activation, platelet aggregation, and intravascular thrombosis mediate the dermal necrosis that may ensue.

Clinical Presentation

Bites by *Loxosceles* spiders are initially painless, often prohibiting definitive identification of the spider. Most commonly, a *Loxosceles* bite presents as a mild erythematous lesion that may initially become firm, but then heal with little or no scar over several days to weeks. A more severe local reaction can infrequently occur several hours

after a bite. These severe bites begin with some initial mild to severe pain, and can be followed by erythema, blister formation, and a bluish discoloration within the first 24 hours. Occasionally, this lesion progresses to frank necrosis over the ensuing 3 to 4 days, leading to *Loxosceles*' nefarious reputation. Eschar formation may develop by the end of the first week. These necrotic, slowly healing ulcers may not reach maximum size for many weeks after envenomation, and can result in a significant cosmetic defects.

Systemic effects of *Loxosceles* envenomation appear more often in children than in adults, but are generally infrequent. Effects that may occur 24 to 72 hours after the bite include nausea, vomiting, fever, chills, arthralgias, hemolysis, thrombocytopenia, hemoglobinuria, and renal failure. DIC and death are extraordinarily rare.

Definitively diagnosing a brown recluse envenomation can be challenging. Because the bite is most often initially painless, locating the actual spider is unusual and occurs with even less frequency when pediatric victims are involved. Accurate diagnosis, therefore, typically relies on identifying features of the clinical presentation that are consistent with brown recluse envenomation, and determining whether or not the patient actually resides in an endemic area. Unfortunately, a wide variety of unrelated arthropod species and medical causes can present similarly to a *Loxosceles* envenomation. For this reason, large numbers of wounds are likely incorrectly attributed to the bite of the brown recluse. Currently, a commercial test to aid in diagnosing this bite does not exist, and it remains unclear if one would be beneficial.

Management

Treatment of any possible necrotic spider bite begins with the usual supportive measures. In small children, careful attention must be paid to interpreting secondary signs of pain, and analgesia should be administered as appropriate. Any developing infection is treated with antibiotics, and serial evaluations must be performed to monitor the wound. If ulceration does develop, surgical debridement is delayed until clear margins are established, a process that at times may approach 2 to 3 weeks after the bite. Patients with systemic symptoms following a brown recluse bite merit in-hospital observation.

Many treatments have been advocated for brown spider bites, but none thus far have shown clear benefit. These proposed therapies include hyperbaric oxygen, cyproheptadine, dapsone, steroids, and topical nitroglycerin. Of these, the leukocyte inhibitor dapsone continues to be advocated by some sources. However, a controlled animal study failed to demonstrate benefit with dapsone therapy, and this drug is associated with hemolysis and methemoglobinemia. Antivenom for brown recluse bites is not commercially available at this time.

Hobo Spider (*Tegenaria agrestis*)

Originally from Europe and central Asia, the hobo or Northwestern brown spider now resides in the Pacific Northwest region of the United States and Canada. This spider should be included with *Loxosceles* species when discussing cases of necrotic arachnidism. In fact, similar symptomatology leads many to incorrectly attribute its bite to that of the brown recluse, which lives elsewhere. True to its scientific name, this species exhibits an aggressive nature, biting with minor provocation. Hobo spiders are brown with gray markings, have a 7- to 14-mm body length, and 27- to 45-mm leg span. They live in moist, dark environs such as woodpiles or basements.

Clinical Presentation

As with brown recluse spiders, the initial bite of the hobo spider is often painless, delaying patient presentation until symptoms begin (Table 82–1). Induration surrounded by progressive erythema may occur initially, with blistering, rupture, and necrosis possibly to follow. Healing may take more than 45 days with varying degrees of scarring. Headache is the most common systemic symptom, but nausea, vomiting, and fatigue can also occur. Rare complications include aplastic anemia and death.

Table 82–1. Medically Important Spider Bites by Local Reaction and Systemic Signs

Genus	Local Reaction	Systemic Signs
Loxosceles	• Initially painless. • Most common manifestation a mild firm erythematous lesion heals with little or no scar over several days to weeks. • Occasionally mild to severe pain several hours after the bite followed by erythema and blister formation within 24 hours. • Necrotic lesion develops over the next 3–4 days, with eschar formation by the end of the first week.	• Systemic effects are rare, appear more often in children, and typically occur 24–72 h after the bite. • Nausea, vomiting, fever, chills, arthralgias, hemolysis, thrombocytopenia, hemoglobinuria, and renal failure. • DIC and death are rare.
Tegenaria	• Initial bite is often painless • Induration may initially occur with surrounding erythema, followed by blistering, rupture and necrosis. • Healing may take as long as 45 days and permanent scarring may result.	• Headache is the most common systemic symptom. • Nausea, vomiting, and fatigue can also occur. • Aplastic anemia and death are rare complications.
Latrodectus	• Local pinprick almost always felt. • Immediate mild to moderate pain. • Pain may spread quickly to include the entire extremity. • Erythema appears approximately 20–60 min after the bite. • Erythema evolves into a target lesion 1–2 cm in diameter.	• Muscle cramp-like spasms in large muscle groups • Physical examination of the cramping extremity rarely exhibits rigidity. • Pain increases and becomes generalized, involving the trunk, back, and abdomen. • Pain lasts for 24 hours or more that can be intermittent. • Severe hypertension may occur.

Abbreviation: DIC, disseminated intravascular coagulation.

Management

There are no proven treatments for local or systemic complications following hobo spider envenomation, and there is currently no diagnostic test for its detection. Surgical repair with grafting may be necessary in the long term, but the necrotizing process should be allowed to complete prior to this consideration.

Tarantulas (*Dugesiella, Aphonopelma*, and others)

Tarantulas are large, hairy spiders that have become increasingly popular as pets for children and adults of all ages. These members of the Theraphosidae family detect their victims through vibrations; poor eyesight renders them functionally blind. There are more than 1500 species of tarantulas worldwide, with more than 40 alone in the deserts of the western United States.

Clinical Manifestations

Although tarantulas can bite when provoked or handled roughly, their venom typically has minor effects with the exception of a few tropical species. Local reactions can vary between absent or minimal discomfort to deep, throbbing pain. Erythema and edema may not be present. Local joint stiffness following adjacent bites has been described, but systemic symptoms other than fever are unusual.

More often than biting, tarantulas utilize abdominal hairs in a defensive response to unwanted provocation. In North and South America species, this bed of hairs appears grossly as a velvety abdominal covering. When threatened, tarantulas may flick these hairs a short distance with a rubbing motion from their two hind legs. North American tarantula hairs rarely penetrate mammalian skin, but they can lodge in more vulnerable surfaces. Infiltrating hairs have been found in the conjunctiva and cornea of victims, resulting in inflammation at all levels of the eye, from the conjunctiva to the retina.

Management

Any patient who presents with red eye and pain after handling a tarantula must be examined for evidence of embedded corneal or conjunctival hairs. Hairs may be seen through a slit lamp, but the size of these offending barbs may preclude diagnosis. After identification, therapy includes surgical removal of the hairs and topical steroids to control inflammation. A granulomatous, nodu-

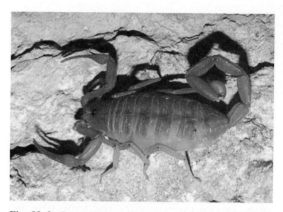

Fig. 82–2. *Centruroides exilicauda*, or bark scorpion. (Photo courtesy of Jim Kalisch).

lar reaction, *ophthalmia nodosa*, can occur in cases of ocular exposure to tarantula hairs. Patients may also develop a diffuse, pruritic, contact dermatitis from indirect hair exposure while cleaning a tarantula cage.

SCORPIONS (SCORPIONIDAE)

Several species of scorpions are found in the warmer parts of the southern United States. All are predominantly nocturnal and capable of stinging humans through a venomous apparatus on their segmented tail called the *telson*. Although the venom of several species worldwide have been associated with serious cardiac and pulmonary toxicity in children and adolescents, most species found in the United States cause little more than localized pain similar to that following Hymenoptera stings. In this country, only *Centruroides exilicauda*, or the bark scorpion, found throughout Arizona, New Mexico, and parts of Texas and California, possesses venom potent enough to cause systemic toxicity. Cytotoxicity or inflammation does not occur from North American scorpion venom, and the exact site of the sting may not be readily apparent.

Clinical Presentation

Venom of the *C. exilicauda* targets excitable neuronal tissue, particularly at the neuromuscular junction, and opens sodium channels. This results in prolonged and excessive depolarization leading to catecholamine release in both the somatic and autonomic nervous systems.

Systemic symptoms from the sting of this scorpion are not common, but they can be severe, particularly in children. Following envenomation, immediate pain and paresthesias in the afflicted region are usually noted and may become generalized. Often, this pain can be exquisitely accentuated by tapping the afflicted region in a diagnostic maneuver often referred to as the *tap test*. In severe cases, cranial nerve and somatic motor dysfunction can develop, resulting in abnormal roving eye movements, blurred vision, pharyngeal muscle incoordination and drooling, occasionally leading to respiratory compromise. Excessive motor activity may present as restlessness or uncontrollable jerking of the extremities, appearing to be seizure-like activity. Nausea, vomiting, tachycardia, and severe agitation can also be present. Symptoms may progress from the moment of envenomation to maximum effect at 5 hours; without antivenom treatment, symptoms may last 24 to 48 hours. Cardiac dysfunction, pulmonary edema, pancreatitis, bleeding disorders, skin necrosis, and occasionally death can be seen with stings from Asian and African scorpions.

Diagnosis of a scorpion sting is strictly clinical. Initially, stings can be confused with other causes of local pain, particularly in children. As the syndrome progresses in moderate to severe cases to include autonomic and motor findings, the diagnosis should become more apparent.

Management

Initial treatment begins with general supportive care of airway, breathing, and circulation; clinicians should be mindful of early administration of analgesics. In young children who manifest severe toxicity, hospitalization should be considered. The severity of the sting directs decisions on antivenom therapy. In the United States, a *Centruroides*-specific, goat-derived antivenom (Antivenom Production Laboratory, Arizona State University) has been available only in the state of Arizona. Production of this antivenom has halted, and supplies will be exhausted within several years. Scorpion antivenom directed against different species has been produced for research or clinical use in over 10 other countries. As with all animal-derived antivenoms, both immediate and delayed allergic reactions including serum sickness are possible. For this reason, *Centruroides*-specific antivenom must be administered judiciously for cases of severe systemic toxicity. Consultation with a toxicologist experienced in scorpion envenomation is recommended before using antivenom. Although one study outside of the United States found no benefit in *routine* administration of an-

tivenom for scorpion stings, one to two vials of antivenom in cases of *severe* toxicity can lead to rapid resolution of symptoms.

CATERPILLARS AND MOTHS (LEPIDOPTERA)

Lepidopterism refers to the adverse effects resulting from contact with butterflies, moths, or their caterpillars. In the mid to late 1990s, American poison centers reported more than 3700 such incidents annually, with greater than 30% of those occurring in children younger than 6 years of age. With the exception of dermatitis from female moths of the *Hylesia* genus found in Central and South America, most symptoms are a result of contact with caterpillars. However, direct contact with an insect or cocoon may not be necessary for injury to occur, because spines that have become detached may also cause envenomation. Oral ingestion is a significant route of exposure in small children.

Clinical Presentation

Caterpillars are the larval stage of moths and use either spines or hairs for protection. Hollow, branching spines are connected to a venom gland. The spines and hairs tend to cause mechanical irritation different from symptoms associated with the venom. The vast majority of caterpillars are harmless to humans. The predominant symptoms following exposure to the hairs and venom is pruritis from localized *caterpillar dermatitis*, and occasionally diffuse urticarial rash. No acute anaphylactic reactions have been reported following lepidopteran stings. Rarely, hairs may become embedded in the eye, resulting in endophthalmitis.

The puss caterpillar (*Megalopyge opercularis*) accounts for most of the serious envenomations in this country, but is found only regionally in the southeastern United States. Typically, after initial contact, patients develop intense local burning pain without pruritus. A uniform pattern of hemorrhagic papules may be seen within 2 to 3 hours of these exposures and may last for several days. Regional lymphadenopathy and considerable limb swelling may develop. Other symptoms include headache, fever, hypotension, and convulsions. No deaths have been reported. Ingestion of the hickory tussock caterpillar (*Lophocampa caryae*), found in the eastern United States, has been reported, with symptoms ranging from drooling to diffuse urticaria (Figure 82–3).

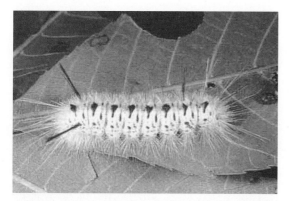

Fig. 82–3. *Lophocampa caryae*, or hickory tussock caterpillar. (Photo courtesy of David Wagner).

Management

No antivenom exists for lepidopterism and treatment is symptomatic and supportive. Spines can be removed by adhesive tape, although individual removal with a microscope may be required. Spines in the oropharynx and the esophagus typically require general anesthesia to facilitate removal. Antihistamines and steroids may be administered for pruritus. For the rare patient with hypotension, IV fluids and subcutaneous epinephrine should be administered.

TICKS (*IXODES, DERMACENTOR, AND OTHERS*)

Tick populations are ubiquitous throughout the world, but concentrate in highest numbers in rural areas. Anatomically, they have a fused abdomen and thorax in an oval shape. Although they may initially be a less than a millimeter in length, they may expand to 50 times their weight when engorged with fluid and blood. Ticks attach to humans painlessly with strong jaws and cement-like biologic adhesive.

Clinical Presentation

Although these obligate, blood-feeding arthropods are second only to mosquitoes in the number of pathogens vectored to humans, their significance to the field of toxicology lies in their venom. Within their venom, certain species of ticks transmit neurotoxins capable of inducing tick paralysis, a symmetric ascending flaccid paralysis associated with loss of deep tendon reflexes. Children are by the far the most common victims of this illness, which can mimic Guillain-Barré syndrome (GBS). In fact, a diagnosis of GBS in a child should not be considered until one has made a thorough search for an engorged tick. Although this neurotoxin's mechanism of action is not clearly understood, there may be some inhibition of acetylcholine release at the neuromuscular junction. Resultant muscle flaccidity can lead to respiratory paralysis. Removal of the tick leads to rapid reversal of symptoms.

Management

Insect repellants and tight-fitting clothing can be helpful in preventing tick bites, and a daily tick check is reasonable in tick-infested areas. Various techniques have been advocated as aids to dislodge a tick so as not to leave its mouth parts beneath the skin surface; none have definitive efficacy. Methods such as applying organic solvents and heat, for instance, have not been proven superior to manual removal. The generally recommended method is a mechanical maneuver to grasp the tick with forceps or fine point tweezers near the point of attachment. The tick should then be pulled straight outward with steady, gentle traction. Because transmission of pathogens and venom is a time-dependent process, prompt removal of ticks is necessary.

BLISTER BEETLES (COLEOPTERA)

Although the order Coleoptera includes a large number and variety of beetles, clinically significant envenomation occurs only from blister beetles. There are approximately 1500 species of blister beetles worldwide, including 200 in the United States. Although not naturally found in the United States, the most well-known blister beetle is the Spanish fly (*Cantharis vesicatoria*).

Clinical Presentation

Blister beetles contain cantharidin, a highly potent vesicant that is exuded from their joints when disturbed or from their body when crushed. Application of these substances in low concentration generates few adverse effects, and in fact, cantharidin-containing preparations are used medicinally in wart removal. However, higher concentrations or prolonged contact with the beetle's venom may cause local inflammation leading to bullae formation. Severe conjunctivitis may also occur if cantharidin contacts the eyes from contaminated hands.

Because of its lipophilicity, high concentrations of cantharidin may result in dermal absorption and systemic toxicity. Systemic toxicity also occurs following ingestion, either of the whole beetle or of cantharidin-containing preparations. Severe vomiting, hematemesis, abdominal pain, and diarrhea may occur, followed by dysuria, hematuria, oliguria, and renal failure as the toxin is concentrated in the kidneys. Death has occurred after large ingestions. Although the exact mechanism by which cantharidin produces systemic toxicity is unknown, the vesicant action may explain much of the symptoms observed. Fortunately, most preparations sold as Spanish fly for purported aphrodisiac properties have very low concentrations of cantharidin. It is thought that the local vascular congestion and urethral inflammation that occurs following ingestion may be interpreted by some as enhanced sexuality.

Management

To avoid significant exposure to cantharidin, the blister beetle should be removed from the skin by blowing or flicking. Treatment of blister beetle toxicity is largely supportive. The skin should be irrigated thoroughly after topical exposure to remove any persistent cantharidin and followed by local wound care. Symptomatic ingestions should be admitted and treated supportively.

CASE OUTCOME

After administering 2 mg of morphine sulfate and 0.5 mg of lorazepam, the young boy's abdominal cramping and distress improve. He is observed in the ED for 4 hours to monitor for relapse, but pain is controlled with standard analgesics. His active tetanus immunity status is confirmed. He is discharged with instructions to administer oral acetaminophen with codeine as needed.

SUGGESTED READINGS

Abroug F, El Atrous S, Nouira S, et al: Serotherapy in scorpion envenomation: A randomized controlled trial. *Lancet* 354: 906–909, 1999.

Banner W: Bites and stings in the pediatric patient. *Curr Probl Pediatr* 18:1–69,1988.

Belyea DA, Tuman DC, Ward TP, et al: The red eye revisited: ophthalmia nodosa due to tarantula hairs. *South Med J* 91:565–567, 1998.

Bucaretchi F, Bacaracat EC, Nogueira RJ, et al: A comparative study of severe scorpion envenomation in children caused by *Tityus bahiensis* and *Tityus serrulatus*. *Rev Inst Trop Sao Paolo* 37:331–336, 1995.

Centers for Disease Control and Prevention: Necrotic arachnidism—Pacific Northwest, 1988–1996. *MMWR* 45:433–436, 1996.

Clark RF: The safety and efficacy of antivenin *Latrodectus mactans*. *Clin Toxicol* 39:125–127, 2001.

Clark RF, Wethern-Kestner S, Vance MV, et al: Clinical presentation and treatment of black widow spider envenomation: A review of 163 cases. *Ann Emerg Med* 21:782–787, 1992.

Das S, Nalini P, Antakrishnan S, et al: Cardiac involvement and scorpion envenomation in children. *J Trop Pediatr* 41:338–340, 1995.

Hamilton RG: Diagnosis of *Hymenoptera* venom sensitivity. *Curr Opin Allergy Clin Immunol* 2:347–351, 2002.

Jones RGA, Corteling RL, To HP, et al: A novel Fab-based antivenom for the treatment of mass bee attacks. *Trop Med Hyg* 61:361–366, 1999.

Kemp SF, deShazo RD, Moffitt JE, et al: Expanding habitat of the imported fire ant (*Solenopsis invicta*): A public health concern. *J Allergy Clin Immunol* 105:683–691, 2000.

Lazoglu AH, Boglioli LR, Taff ML, et al: Serum sickness reaction following multiple insect stings. *Ann Allergy Asthma Immunol* 75:522–523, 1995.

Litovitz TL, Klein-Schwartz W, White S, et al: 2000 Annual report of the American Association of Poison Control Centers Toxic Exposure Surveillance System. *Am J Emerg Med* 20: 391–452, 2002.

McGain F, Winkel KD: Ant sting mortality in Australia. *Toxicon* 40:1095–1100, 2002.

Phillips S, Kohn M, Baker D, et al: Therapy of brown spider envenomation: A controlled trial of hyperbaric oxygen, dapsone, and cyproheptadine. *Ann Emerg Med* 25:363–368, 1995.

Rash LD, Hodgson WC: Pharmacology and biochemistry of spider venoms. *Toxicon* 40:225–254, 2002.

Reeves JA, Allison EJ, Goodman PE: Black widow spiderbite in a child. *Am J Emerg Med* 14:469–471, 1996.

Rhoades R: Stinging ants. *Curr Opin Allergy Clin Immunol* 1:343–348, 2001.

Staub D, Debrunner M, Amsler L, et al: Effectiveness of a repellent containing DEET and EBAAP for preventing tick bites. *Wilderness Environment Med* 13:12–20, 2002.

Tasic V: Nephrotic syndrome in a child after a bee sting. *Pediatr Nephrol* 15:245–247, 2000.

White J: Bites and stings from venomous animals: a global overview. *Ther Drug Monit* 22:65–68, 2000.

Woestman R, Perkin R, Van Stralen D: The black widow: Is she deadly to children? *Pediatr Emerg Care* 12:360–364, 1996.

83

Self-Assessment Questions

Louis Ling
Timothy B. Erickson

1. Which of these methods of decontamination is contraindicated in pregnancy?
   a. Syrup of ipecac
   b. Gastric lavage
   c. Activated charcoal
   d. Whole bowel irrigation

2. Which chelator for lead toxicity is contraindicated in pregnancy?
   a. DMSA
   b. Penicillamine
   c. *N*-acetylcysteine
   d. Deferoxamine

3. Which antidote does not cross the placenta?
   a. *N*-acetylcysteine
   b. Atropine
   c. Oxygen
   d. Deferoxamine

4. What is the most important factor to consider in assessing the risk of a maternal drug to the sucking infant?
   a. Dosing schedule
   b. Protein binding
   c. pka
   d. Corrected age of infant
   e. Volume of milk produced

5. Which of the following drugs are most apt to be a problem in a breast feeding mother?
   a. Antihypertensives
   b. Antidepressants
   c. Drugs of abuse
   d. Herbal teas
   e. Vaccines and serums

6. A patent ductus arteriosus can be responsible for all EXCEPT which of the following findings?
   a. Larger drug volumes of distribution
   b. Increased renal and hepatic drug clearance
   c. Decreased protein binding
   d. Decreased tissue perfusion

7. Which of the following is MOST TRUE regarding APAP administration in premature infants?
   a. Bioavailability of rectally administered acetaminophen is higher in preterm infants than in full-term neonates.
   b. Clearance of acetaminophen is increased compared to term infants.
   c. premature infants require higher doses of rectal acetaminophen to achieve therapeutic serum concentrations.
   d. Premature infants require shorter dosing intervals to maintain acceptable acetaminophen through levels.

8. Which of the following is NOT TRUE regarding protein binding in neonates?
   a. The affinity of albumin for acidic drugs is decreased.
   b. Drugs that are primarily bound to albumin parallel the pharmacologic activity and clearance seen in adults more closely than drugs bound primarily to α_1-acid glycoprotein (AAG).
   c. Fatty acids and bilirubin compete for drug binding sites on protein.
   d. Acidosis and hypoxemia promote increased protein binding.

9. Which of the following statements about the Poison Prevention Packaging Act is TRUE?

a. It mandates that all prescription drugs must be placed in child-resistant packaging unless requested otherwise by the recipient.

b. It defines special packaging as a container that 20% of children cannot open if left alone for 5 minutes but is not difficult for adults age 50 to 70 to open.

c. It does not apply to nonprescription drugs unless they had been prescription drugs previously.

d. It was passed by into law by the U.S Congress in 1945 after WWII.

10. Which of the following statements about Munchausen syndrome by proxy is MOST TRUE?

a. Mortality is estimated to range at 50%.

b. The perpetrator is involved in child's medical care.

c. Peak incidence is in 3- to 5-year old children.

d. Siblings rarely suffer from some form of physical abuse.

11. Significant toxicity could occur in a healthy 10-kg toddler following ingestion of one pill of which drug?

a. Metoprolol

b. Fluoxetine

c. Salicylate

d. Phenylpropanolamine

12. Which of the following has been associated with an increased risk of adolescent addiction?

a. Using drugs or alcohol while alone

b. Riding in a car driven by someone high on drugs or alcohol

c. Poor memory for events happening while on drugs or alcohol

d. Using drugs or alcohol to relax, feel better, and fit in

e. All of the above

13. What percentage of adolescent girls report at least one suicide attempt during high school?

a. 1%

b. 12%

c. 25%

d. 33%

e. 50%

14. A 3-year-old child collapses in a shopping mall. The mother is hysterical and you are only able to make out that the child has a heart problem. What is the most appropriate sequence of actions?

a. Access a nearby automatic external defibrillator, attach it, and follow the instruction provided.

b. Call for EMS, check for a pulse, and initiate CPR.

c. Open the airway, provide rescue breathing, assess for pulse, initiate CPR, and notify EMS.

d. Call for EMS, open the airway, provide rescue breathing, assess for pulse, and initiate CPR.

e. Attempt to ventilate by mouth-to-mouth breathing, ensuring immobilization of the cervical spine before attempting to open the airway.

15. Which of the following is associated with a lower survival rate for cardiac arrest in children?

a. Age >12 months

b. Arrest in the hospital

c. Bradyasystolic arrest

d. Ventricular fibrillation

e. Submersion injury

16. Which of the following statements regarding technique about CPR for a 10-kg infant is most correct?

a. The two-thumb, chest-encircling technique is preferred.

b. The two-finger technique is used with the fingers in the intermammary line.

c. The heel of one hand is placed over the lower third of the sternum.

d. The chest is compressed 1.0 to 1.5 inches with each compression.

e. Ensure adequate padding under the patient before performing CPR.

17. Which of the following characteristics do not affect a child's susceptibility to hazardous materials exposure?

a. High minute ventilation

b. Thinner stratum corneum

c. Smaller blood volume

d. Increased glomerular filtration rate

e. Shorter stature

18. A patient exposed to a hazardous chemical presents with mucous membrane and eye irritation, coughing, and dyspnea. Which toxidrome is most consistent with this presentation?

a. An irritant gas

b. A cholinergic substance

c. A systemic asphyxiant

d. A simple asphyxiant

e. An anticholinergic substance

19. In which setting is human-to-human transmission least likely?
    a. Smallpox disease
    b. Inhalational anthrax
    c. Pneumonic plague
    d. Viral hemorrhagic fever
    e. None of the above

20. Which features help to differentiate smallpox from chickenpox?
    a. Synchronous rash progression with chickenpox
    b. A more centrifugal distribution with smallpox
    c. A more severe prodrome with chickenpox
    d. Absent prodrome with smallpox
    e. A lack of human-to-human transmission with smallpox

21. What is the minimum observation period for an asymptomatic child to rule out toxicity following possible dermal exposure to VX liquid?
    a. 6 hours
    b. 12 hours
    c. 24 hours
    d. 3 days
    e. No observation is period needed.

22. A child presents following an iron overdose with vomiting, acidosis, and multiple pill fragments noted abdominal KUB. Which decontamination method would be most efficacious?
    a. Activated charcoal
    b. Whole bowel irrigation
    c. Cathartic agent
    d. Syrup of ipecac
    e. Gastric lavage

23. Which of the following ingestions would benefit most from multiple doses of activated charcoal?
    a. Iron
    b. Lead paint chips
    c. Acetaminophen
    d. Theophylline
    e. Lithium

24. Which of the following scenarios would benefit the most from gastric lavage?
    a. A 2-year-old child who ingested berries from a bush 2 hours ago and has vomited twice at home.
    b. An adolescent with ingested several "bags" of cocaine while being questioned by the police.

c. A 13-year-old boy who ingested an unknown amount of his mother's amitryptiline 1 hour prior, and is lethargic, intubated, hypotensive, and tachycardic.
    d. A 14-year-old girl who presents 4 hours after ingesting 10 extra-strength acetaminophen tablets following a fight with her boyfriend.
    e. A 3-year-old who presents 30 minutes after ingesting five ibuprofen tablets from her grandparents' medicine cabinet.

25. Which physical characteristic of a drug below is not predictive for effective extracorporeal removal?
    a. High volume of distribution ($V_d > 1$ L/Kg)
    b. Presence of toxin in the central compartment
    c. Low protein binding
    d. Low molecular weight
    e. Water solubility

26. Which of the following drugs or toxins is not commonly removed via extracorporeal therapy?
    a. Salicylates
    b. Methanol
    c. Cyclic antidepressants
    d. Lithium
    e. Barbiturates

27. Which of the following is NOT TRUE regarding hemoperfusion?
    a. Complications include thrombocytopenia, hypotension, and leukopenia.
    b. It is effective for either lipid- or water-soluble drugs.
    c. It is the extracorporeal therapy of choice for salicylate poisoning.
    d. It is effective for drug removal with drug molecular weights up to 40,000 Daltons
    e. Its efficacy can be increased by using standard hemodialyzer and hemoperfusion cartridges in series.

28. Which of the following agents is preferred for intubation of a patient with an unobstructed upper airway?
    a. A depolarizing neuromuscular blocker
    b. A nondepolarizing neuromuscular blocker
    c. A dissociative anesthetic
    d. A benzodiazepine with no other agent

29. Which factor is most likely to limit drug removal for both acute hemodialysis and continuous renal replacement therapies?
    a. Relative renal function
    b. Blood flow rate through the system
    c. Volume of distribution for the toxin
    d. Sieving coefficient of the membrane

30. Which of the following is TRUE regarding laboratory investigations for poisoned patients?
    a. Management of comatose, overdosed patients typically requires rapid availability of toxicology screening results.
    b. Recent data have proven that it is unnecessary to obtain serum acetaminophen levels in children with unintentional acetaminophen ingestions.
    c. The most useful laboratory tests in management of poisoned patients are general tests, such as serum chemistry and glucose.
    d. Diagnosis of carboxyhemoglobinemia (CO poisoning) or methemoglobinemia is best assessed by pulse oximetry.
    e. Absence of an elevated ion gap rules out ingestion of a METALACIDGAP poison.

31. Which of the following regarding toxicology screening tests is MOST TRUE?
    a. Drug of abuse screening is routinely indicated in poisoned patients.
    b. Comprehensive toxicology screening is required for Level I Trauma Center verification.
    c. Drug levels should only be obtained when there is a specific history of exposure to the drug in question.
    d. Drug of abuse screening of teenagers should only be performed after informing the patient of the purpose of the test and their ability to refuse such testing without penalty.
    e. Bedside drug of abuse screening detects date rape drugs.

32. Regarding forensic assays, which of the following is FALSE?
    a. Hair sampling may provide a long-term window with which drug exposure may be detected.
    b. Relative to urine sampling, meconium sampling for drugs of abuse provides a much longer window within which in utero drug exposure can be confirmed.

c. Laboratory assays obtained for forensic purposes may be rendered unhelpful to prosecutors or be ruled inadmissible in court if an appropriate chain of custody is not maintained.
    d. Assays for date rape drugs are readily available in most hospital laboratories.
    e. Any positive drug of abuse screening assay should only be considered definitively positive after confirmation of the result by a second laboratory assay using a different methodology.

33. Elevated anion gap metabolic acidosis is characteristic of intoxication with:
    a. salicylates, methanol, and CO.
    b. acetaminophen, marijuana, and benzodrozepine.
    c. isopropyl alcohol, lead, and cocaine.
    d. pine oil, calcium channel blocker, and ethylene glycol.

34. Which of the following, with regard to toxic ingestion of alcohols, is MOST TRUE?
    a. Hypercalcemia is a hallmark of ethylene glycol toxicity.
    b. An elevated osmolar gap is characteristic of poisoning with methanol, ethanol, ethylene glycol, and isopropyl alcohol.
    c. Methanol toxicity is characterized by hyperchloremic metabolic acidosis.
    d. Hypernatremia is common in ethylene glycol toxicity.

35. Which of the following, with regard to enhancing elimination of toxic substances by alkalinization of the urine, is MOST TRUE?
    a. Ionized drugs diffuse across the renal tubule.
    b. Alkalinization is effective for drugs with a pK of 7.2 to 9.5.
    c. Alkalinization is more effective when hypokalemia is present.
    d. Alkalinization is accomplished by establishing a urine flow of 2 to 5 mL/kg/h and adding sodium bicarbonate to the IV fluids.

36. Which sign or symptom is more common with Neuroleptic Malignant Syndrome than with Central Serotonin Syndrome?
    a. Hypertension
    b. Muscular rigidity
    c. Hyperthermia
    d. Altered mental status
    e. Seizures

37. Which of the following is the classic triad for Malignant Hyperthermia?
  a. Weakness, myoclonus, incoordination
  b. Hyperthermia, diaphoresis, hypertension
  c. Hyperthermia, muscle rigidity, metabolic acidosis
  d. Metabolic alkalosis, vomiting, altered mental status
  e. Hyperthermia, behavior changes, hallucinations

38. Which clue best differentiates sympathomimetic poisoning from anticholinergic toxicity?
  a. Tachycardia
  b. Hyperthermia
  c. Diarrhea
  d. Diaphoretic skin
  e. Ileus

39. Which of the following drug overdoses can increase the QRS duration?
  a. Cocaine
  b. Droperidol
  c. Clonidine
  d. Iron
  e. Phenytoin

40. Acetaminophen toxicity is notorious for causing which of the following injuries?
  a. Zone 1 hepatic injury
  b. Centrilobular necrosis
  c. Steatosis
  d. Ophthalmic injury
  e. Liquefaction necrosis of the GI tract

41. Noncardiogenic pulmonary edema is classically associated with which of the following poisonings?
  a. Acetaminophen
  b. Calcium channel blockers
  c. Opiates
  d. β-Blockers
  e. Monoamine oxidase inhibitors

42. A 2-year-old asymptomatic child is brought to the ED by concerned parents who found the child with an open container of CamphoPhenique. During the observation period in the ED, what specific toxic signs would you be concerned about?
  a. Oropharyngeal burns with upper airway obstruction
  b. Nausea, vomiting, and GI bleeding
  c. Tachypnea and cyanosis poorly responsive to oxygen therapy
  d. Respiratory depression and pinpoint pupils
  e. Sudden onset of seizures

43. Benzocaine is present in many local anesthetic creams and first aid ointments. Ingestion of small quantities of this substance can lead to which of the following?
  a. Respiratory acidosis
  b. Severe hypoxia at the cellular level
  c. Metabolic acidosis
  d. Methemoglobinemia
  e. Salicylism

44. Lomotil is an antidiarrheal preparation that contains a combination of two ingredients that are toxic in very small quantities. These are:
  a. Methylsalicylate and scopolamine
  b. Diphenoxylate and atropine
  c. Metclopromide and hydrocodone
  d. Paregoric and lidocaine
  e. Bismuth subsalicylate and aluminum hydroxide

45. Chloroquine is used in the treatment and prophylaxis of malarial disease. Its primary toxicity is which of the following?
  a. GI bleeding
  b. Cardiac toxicity
  c. Respiratory depression
  d. Neurologic depression
  e. Sever metabolic acidosis

46. An 18-month-old child has ingested about a teaspoon of oil of wintergreen. You advise the parents to do which of the following?
  a. Reassure the parents that this is a nontoxic ingestion that requires no special action.
  b. Observe the child at home for tachypnea or hyperthermia and bring the child to the ED for evaluation if these signs develop.
  c. Administer syrup of ipecac at home and bring the child to the ED for evaluation after vomiting has ceased.
  d. Bring the child to the ED for a measurement of a 6-h salicylate level, anticipating a nontoxic level, and that no further treatment will be necessary.
  e. Bring the child immediately to the ED for gastric evacuation, activated charcoal administration, and evaluation of potential salicylate toxicity.

47. A major feature of benzocaine toxicity involves
    a. pulmonary aspiration.
    b. renal failure.
    c. cyanosis that does not improve with oxygen.
    d. Nystagmus.
    e. oral numbness.

48. Chloroquine toxicity is most likely to present with
    a. hyperkalemia and cardiac arrhythmias.
    b. hypokalemia and cardiac arrhythmias.
    c. methemoglobinemia and cardiac arrhythmias.
    d. methemoglobinemia and hyperkalemia.
    e. hyperchloremic metabolic acidosis.

49. Ingestion of imidazoline decongestants can cause
    a. mydriasis because they are central α_2 agonists.
    b. hypertension because they are central α_2 agonists.
    c. bradycardia only.
    d. CNS depression that usually does not respond to naloxone.
    e. hypotension because they are central α_2 antagonists.

50. In treating lindane-induced seizures, one should avoid
    a. benzodiazepines.
    b. phenobarbital.
    c. phenytoin.
    d. oxygen.
    e. sodium bicarbonate.

51. The toxidrome of cinchonism caused by quinine toxicity includes all of the following EXCEPT:
    a. dermal flushing.
    b. nausea and vomiting.
    c. tinnitus.
    d. dry skin and mucous membranes.
    e. diarrhea.

52. Which of the following histories is consistent with an unintentional exposure?
    a. A 2-month-old girl is found on the bathroom floor with a bar of soap in her mouth.
    b. A 3-year-old girl takes 12 acetaminophen tablets and 8 iron sulfate tablets.
    c. A 4-year-old boy is found with his sister's open makeup bag. There are smudges of several different colors around his mouth.
    d. A 15-year-old girl drinks 6 ounces of household (3%) hydrogen peroxide.
    e. A 16-year-old boy takes 30 tablets of amoxicillin after his girlfriend breaks up with him.

53. Which of the following is an example of a minimally toxic exposure?
    a. A 5-year-old boy has several episodes of vomiting after ingesting an unknown number of iron tablets.
    b. A 4-year-old girl has one episode of vomiting and some diarrhea after ingesting liquid soap.
    c. A 6-year-old girl is asymptomatic after ingesting an unknown amount of rat poison containing brodifacoum.
    d. A 2-year-old boy is irritable, crying and drooling after being found with a bottle of oven cleaner.
    e. A 3-year-old boy is asymptomatic after chewing on a plastic action figure.

54. Which of the following exposures may safely be managed at home?
    a. A 2-year-old girl has several episodes of vomiting and is inconsolable after ingesting leaves from a household plant.
    b. A 15-year-old girl takes all of her birth control pills after being suspended from school.
    c. A 9-year-old boy is asymptomatic after unintentionally drinking an unknown quantity of windshield washer fluid. The 32-oz bottle remains half full.
    d. A 5-year-old girl weighing 20 kg ingests an unknown amount of children's liquid acetaminophen (160 mg/5 mL). Forty milliliters are missing from the bottle.
    e. A 6-week-old boy reportedly ingests 3 oz of household bleach.

55. What are the five most common categories of OTC medications that children ingest?
    a. Aspirin, camphor, diphenhydramine, acetaminophen, and vitamins
    b. Cold medications, vitamins, antacids, aspirin, and acetaminophen
    c. Cold medications, acetaminophen, vitamins, ibuprofen, and diaper rash products
    d. Acetaminophen, diaper rash products, antacids, camphor, and vitamins

56. Which OTC medications are associated with the most morbidity and mortality when ingested?
    a. Camphor and aspirin
    b. Acetaminophen and diphenhydramine
    c. Vitamins and cold medications

d. Ibuprofen and antacids

e. Diaper rash products

57. Which of the following topical OTC medications has the LEAST potential to be toxic when ingested?

a. Wart removers

b. Diaper rash ointment

c. Teething gel

d. Chest rubs

58. Acetaminophen toxicity in children is associated with which of the following?

a. An acute ingestion >140 mg/kg

b. Nomogram indicating an acetaminophen level below the hepatotoxic line

c. A loading dose of *N*-acetylcysteine at 70 mg/kg, followed by 17 subsequent doses at 35 mg/kg

d. Daily doses of acetaminophen greater than 70 mg/kg/d

e. Glucuronide conjugation predominates over sulfate conjugates

59. A 15-year-old girl presents following multiple episodes of emesis 2 days ago. At presentation, she is found to be lethargic. Laboratory testing reveals a bilirubin of 10 mg/dL, glucose of 48 mg/dL, SGOT of 2300, and SGPT of 3400. Which of the following is TRUE regarding this clinical scenario?

a. A normal acetaminophen level will rule out toxicity.

b. Gastric lavage and activated charcoal administration would be very effective in decontaminating this patient.

c. Patients who recover from this condition usually show a dramatic improvement in hepatic-related laboratory parameters within 24 hours.

d. Treatment with urinary alkalinization is recommended.

e. Without aggressive antidote therapy and possible liver transplant, the prognosis for this condition is poor.

60. *N*-acetylcysteine therapy is most effective in acetaminophen poisoning when

a. the initial oral loading dose results in patient vomiting within 15 minutes of administration.

b. the antidote is administered during hemodialysis.

c. the oral loading dose is given within 8 hours of acute ingestion.

d. given in a single dose regimen.

e. given IV 24 hours postingestion.

61. Which of the following tests is unnecessary in patients with altered mental status owing to suspected anticholinergic toxicity?

a. Arterial blood gas

b. Fingerstick glucose

c. ECG

d. CPK concentration

e. Serum acetaminophen concentration

62. Which of the following is MOST TRUE regarding physostigmine?

a. Duration of effect is 3 to 4 hours.

b. It can be given to patients with profound tachycardia.

c. Cyclic antidepressant toxicity is not a contraindication.

d. Toxicity is independent of rate.

e. Historically, it has been used only for anticholinergic toxicity.

63. Which of the following plants does not contain anticholinergic properties?

a. *Atropa belladonna* (deadly nightshade)

b. *Datura stramonium* (jimson weed)

c. *Hyosycamus niger* (black henbane)

d. *Mandragora officinarum* (mandrake)

e. *Amanita muscaria* (fly agaric)

64. Regarding salicylates, which of the following patients can be discharged?

a. The patient has a normal mental status, and a 2-h salicylate level is <30 mg/dL.

b. The patient states he/she only ingested a few aspirin.

c. The patient has nausea and vomiting, but the aspirin bottle is full.

d. Four- and 6-hour salicylate levels are <30 mg/dL.

e. The patient has only nausea and a normal pH.

65. Which statement is MOST TRUE about aspirin toxicity in children?

a. Respiratory alkalosis is typically present before a metabolic acidosis.

b. Acute toxicity tends to be more severe, and patients should be managed more aggressively.

c. Children have a less severe course of aspirin toxicity than adults because the half-life is shorter.

d. Hypoglycemia may develop because of decreased oral intake.

e. Neurologic signs and symptoms are indications of severe toxicity.

66. Which of the following statements is MOST TRUE?
   a. Aspirin's change from first-order to zero-order metabolism occurs near the upper range of therapeutic level.
   b. A positive ferric chloride test reliably quantifies salicylate in the serum.
   c. Multiple-dose activated charcoal is effective in enhancing salicylate excretion.
   d. The goal for urinary alkalinization is to prevent salicylate penetration into the CNS.
   e. Patients in the acute febrile period of Kawasaki disease require decreased salicylate doses to maintain levels in the therapeutic range.

67. Which of the following statements about NSAIDs is TRUE?
   a. Newer NSAIDs known as the coxibs block cyclooxygenase 1.
   b. The coxibs are safe to use in patients with renal impairment.
   c. CNS depression typically associated with acute NSAID overdose.
   d. Acute renal failure can occur from acute use of traditional NSAIDs.
   e. Respiratory alkalosis is seen in NSAID overdose.

68. Which of the following is an induced idiosyncratic reaction with NSAIDs?
   a. Aseptic meningitis
   b. Thrombocytosis
   c. Myoglobinuria
   d. Methemoglobinemia
   e. Polycythemia

69. Which of the following statements regarding NSAID toxicity is TRUE?
   a. Anion gap metabolic acidosis is pathognomonic.
   b. Generally GI toxicity is seen.
   c. Liver toxicity is seen with acute ingestion.
   d. Hypertension and bradycardia are seen in acute overdose.
   e. There is a nomogram for ibuprofen toxicity that has good predictive value for toxicity.

70. Caffeine toxicity most closely resembles which pharmaceutical overdose?
   a. Lithium
   b. Phenthiazines
   c. Digoxin

   d. Theophylline
   e. Phencyclidine

71. Which of the following explains the electrolyte disturbance associated with excessive caffeine intake?
   a. Potassium is excreted exponentially with the intake of caffeine leading to hypokalemia.
   b. Potassium is shifted into the cell by way of a catecholamine-induced mechanism leading to hypokalemia.
   c. Hyponatremia is often seen from a dilutional effect only in caffeinated beverage drinkers.
   d. Hypernatremia is a common finding due to addition of sodium acetate to all caffeinated products sold in the United States.
   e. Caffeine induces an intracellular shift in magnesium leading to hypomagnesemia.

72. Caffeine toxicity may include all of the following EXCEPT
   a. pulmonary edema.
   b. supraventricular and ventricular dysrhythmias.
   c. rhabdomyolysis.
   d. insomnia.
   e. hyperglycemia.

73. Infants may present with failure to thrive from exposure to which of the following vitamins?
   a. Vitamin A
   b. Vitamin B_6
   c. Ascorbic acid
   d. Vitamin D
   e. Niacin

74. Which of the following statements about vitamin A is correct?
   a. Vitamin A is a water-soluble vitamin.
   b. Hypocalcemia may occur as a result of chronic vitamin A intoxication.
   c. An increase in intracranial pressure can be seen with acute and chronic exposures.
   d. Aggressive treatment and hospital admission are often required with overdose.
   e. Plasma vitamin A levels are needed to determine medical management.

75. Which of the following is associated with large chronic oral doses of vitamin C?
   a. Liver failure
   b. Coagulopathy and increased bleeding times

c. Intense cutaneous flushing
d. Nephrolithiasis
e. Peripheral neuropathies

76. Which of the following is NOT indicated in the treatment of calcium channel antagonist toxicity?
    a. Naloxone
    b. Atropine
    c. Calcium chloride
    d. Insulin and dextrose
    e. Glucagon

77. A 3-year-old child presents after ingesting five of her grandfather's clonidine tablets 4 hours prior to presentation. The child has a BP of 50/palp; heart rate of 60 bpm, and respiratory rate of 12 breaths per minute. Which of the following is TRUE regarding this ingestion?
    a. Clonidine is a centrally acting α_2 antagonist that stimulates sympathetic flow.
    b. Calcium gluconate should be administered.
    c. Naloxone administration may benefit this patient.
    d. A temporary pacemaker should be considered.
    e. Glucagon will quickly reverse the clinical effects of clonidine toxicity.

78. Which of the following is an important consideration for the use of digoxin Fab fragments?
    a. Allergic reactions are common.
    b. One should be cautious not to administer too high a dose that can easily lead to toxicity.
    c. One should monitor total digoxin levels at frequent intervals after Fab dosing.
    d. Digoxin Fab fragments are dosed based on either the estimated dose ingested or by serum digoxin concentration.

79. Which of the following is most likely to increase the risk of developing digoxin toxicity?
    a. Salicylates
    b. Hyperkalemia
    c. Antacids
    d. Hypermagnesemia
    e. Hyponatremia

80. Which of the following statements regarding the clinical presentation of digoxin is TRUE?
    a. Calcium and glucagon should be administered in cases of acute digoxin toxicity.
    b. Significant toxicity is frequently noted with digoxin concentration in the therapeutic range.

c. Digoxin concentrations are rarely usefully clinically.
d. Nonspecific signs of illness are a very important clues for chronic digoxin toxicity.

81. In which pattern of theophylline overdose is a serum theophylline concentration most predictive of clinical outcome?
    a. Acute ingestion
    b. Chronic overdose
    c. Acute-overdose-on-chronic
    d. Medication dosing error

82. Which electrolyte disorder is least likely with a theophylline intoxication?
    a. Hyperkalemia
    b. Hypoglycemia
    c. Hypercalcemia
    d. Metabolic acidosis (low serum bicarbonate)

83. Which finding would be the least likely in a theophylline-toxic patient?
    a. Vomiting
    b. Multifocal atrial tachycardia
    c. Hypertension
    d. Seizures

84. Flumazenil would be most appropriate for which of the following scenarios?
    a. A teenager who presents comatose following an unknown drug overdose.
    b. A lethargic child who ingested diazepam and has a history of a seizure disorder.
    c. A child with tuberculosis who presents comatose after an apparent overdose.
    d. A child with respiratory compromise who ingested diazepam 2 hours prior to presentation.

85. Which of the following sedative hypnotic agents may result in cardiotoxicity?
    a. Chloral hydrate
    b. Phenobarbital
    c. GHB
    d. Diazepam

86. A 16-year-old is found at a rave party comatose, with a pulse of 60 bpm, a respiratory rate of 6 breaths per minute, and midrange, minimally reactive pupils. She has no response to IV naloxone and is orally intubated without complications. Four hours later, she suddenly awakens, extubates herself, and sits

upright. Which drugs of abuse is most consistent with this presentation?

a. Heroin
b. Cocaine
c. Ecstasy
d. GHB

87. Which of the following laboratory findings characteristic of exogenous insulin administration?

a. High C-peptide concentration and high insulin concentration
b. Low C-peptide concentration and high insulin concentration
c. High C-peptide concentration and low insulin concentration
d. Low C-peptide concentration and low insulin concentration

88. Which laboratory findings are most characteristic of sulfonylurea ingestion?

a. High C-peptide concentration and high insulin concentration
b. Low C-peptide concentration and high insulin concentration
c. High C-peptide concentration and low insulin concentration
d. Low C-peptide concentration and low insulin concentration

89. Admission is generally unnecessary for unintentional overdose on which of the following drugs?

a. Glipizide
b. Repaglinidec
c. Miglitol
d. Tolbutamide

90. A Native-American teenager is brought by the EMS after taking an overdose of isoniazid of 40 mg/kg. As the treating physician what will be your next course of action?

a. An ECG should be obtained on arrival to search for a prolonged PR.
b. A serum INH level should be drawn on arrival.
c. Activated charcoal, being able to adsorb INH, should be given in all INH overdoses.
d. The patient needs to be observed closely because he is at risk of developing CNS toxicity.

e. Prophylactic pyridoxine should be given IV given the amount ingested.

91. Pyridoxine is also known as

a. Vitamin B_1
b. Vitamin B_6
c. Vitamin B_{12}
d. Vitamin K
e. Vitamin E

92. Which of the following would be most likely in a patient with INH toxicity?

a. pH: 7.3 P_{CO_2}: 30 HCO_3: 12 Anion gap: 8
b. pH: 7.5 P_{CO_2}: 45 HCO_3: 28 Anion gap: 18
c. pH: 6.9 P_{CO_2}: 30 HCO_3: 9   Anion gap: 20
d. pH: 7.2 P_{CO_2}: 50 HCO_3: 14 Anion gap: 10
e. pH: 6.8 P_{CO_2}: 28 HCO_3: 10 Anion gap: 8

93. A 15-year-old girl presents to the ED after ingesting 20 tablets of her uncle's amitryptiline. She is lethargic in the ED with a pulse of 140 bpm, respiratory rate of 8 breaths per minute, blood pressure of 90/60 mmHg, and a temperature of 100.0°F What is the most appropriate course of action?

a. Initiate a dopamine drip.
b. Administer oral activated charcoal and observe.
c. Administer IV physostigmine.
d. Intubate, hyperventilate, and administer IV sodium bicarbonate and a fluid bolus.
e. Administer a loading dose of phenytoin.

94. The cardiovascular toxicity of tricyclic antidepressants is due to which of the following pharmacologic effects?

a. α-Adrenergic effect
b. Qunidine-like effect
c. Norepinephrine reuptake blockade
d. Anticholinergic side effects
e. All of the above

95. Overdose of an SSRI antidepressant agent like fluoxetine generally results in

a. CNS depression.
b. Seizures.
c. Profound hyperthermia and rigidity.
d. Cardiac dysrhythmias.
e. Hallucinations and delirium.

96. Which treatment would be least effective 1 hour after an acute ingestion of a large dose of lithium?

a. Gastric lavage
b. Whole bowel irrigation
c. Hydration
d. Forced diuresis

97. Which of the following drug therapies may increase serum lithium levels?
a. Clarithromycim
b. SSRIs
c. Diuretics
d. Haldol
e. Acetaminophen

98. In which scenario of lithium toxicity is one most likely to see a delay in neurologic symptoms?
a. Acute overdose of lithium
b. Acute overdose in a patient on chronic lithium treatment
c. Chronic overtreatment with lithium
d. After cessation of lithium treatment

99. All of the following statements regarding neuroleptic-induced cardiovascular toxicity are TRUE EXCEPT
a. Piperidine phenothiazines (e.g., thioridazine) pose the greatest risk of cardiac dysrhythmias.
b. Hypotension may be best managed with primarily α-agonists (e.g., norepinephrine) rather than catecholamines with mixed α and β stimulation (e.g., dopamine).
c. Class 1A and 1C antidysrhythmics should be avoided in the management of neuroleptic-induced cardiac toxicity.
d. Cardiac conduction disturbances noted by a very wide QRS complex may be best managed with magnesium sulfate, isoproterenol, or pacemaker.
e. Neuroleptics possess quinidine-like effects; they block sodium and potassium channels in the myocardium.

100. All of the following statements regarding management of neuroleptic malignant syndrome are TRUE EXCEPT:
a. immediately discontinue the offending agent.
b. administer anticholinergic agents (e.g., diphenhydramine or benztropine).
c. aggressive cooling, hydration, and benzodiazepines are the mainstay of therapy.
d. although slow in onset, central dopamine agonists (e.g., bromocriptine) may be considered.

e. 1 to 2 weeks after the NMS has resolved, the patient may be placed on a medication with fewer EPS (i.e., an atypical neuroleptic).

101. All of the following are TRUE with respect to the pharmacology/toxicology of neuroleptics EXCEPT:
a. Dopamine receptor agonism is responsible for both the efficacy and EPS of neuroleptics.
b. Orthostatic hypotension and reflex tachycardia are common features.
c. Either miosis or mydriasis are possible in overdose.
d. Depending on the individual agent, minimal to significant antimuscarinic/antihistaminic symptoms may be noted.
e. Neuroleptics generally undergo extensive hepatic metabolism, are highly protein bound, and are lipophilic with large volumes of distribution.

102. All of the following statements regarding neuroleptic-induced EPS are TRUE EXCEPT:
a. The frequency of EPS is higher among neuroleptics with little anticholinergic activity.
b. Benzodiazepines (e.g., lorazepam) should be used to correct dystonias accompanied by high fever and rigidity rather than anticholinergics.
c. Patients who appear more agitated or restless after neuroleptic dosage increase may be experiencing akathisia.
d. Parkinson-like movements (bradykinesias) are the most common EPS, and respond to dosage adjustments and/or anticholinergic medications.
e. Tardive dyskinesia typically becomes evident when doses of neuroleptics are increased.

103. A 3-year-old child is brought to the ED following ingestion of a generic mouthwash approximately 2 hours ago. A management priority in this child would be which of the following?
a. Syrup of ipecac
b. Urinary toxicology screen
c. Serum glucose
d. Rectal temperature
e. Chest radiograph to rule out aspiration

104. A 15-year-old boy presents to the ED for evaluation of abdominal pain, vomiting, and lethargy after ingesting windshield washer fluid 2 hours prior to presentation. Which of the following would be most helpful in quickly establishing a diagnosis of methanol toxicity?

a. A serum methanol level
b. Respiratory acidosis on ABG
c. Calcium oxalate crystals on the urine
d. Elevated osmolal gap
e. Elevated serum acetone levels

105. You suspect ethylene glycol poisoning in a 4-year-old child brought to the ED. The patient has normal vital signs and laboratory data reveal a mild metabolic acidosis on arterial blood gas. You are informed by the pharmacist that there is no ethanol preparation available for treatment. Which of the following alternative management options would be the most efficacious?
    a. Hemodialysis
    b. Bicarbonate administration
    c. 4-Methylpyrazole
    d. Thiamine
    e. Folate

106. Which of the following are characteristics of caustic ingestions in children?
    a. Most pediatric caustic ingestions occur before 6 years of age.
    b. Caustic injuries are usually more severe in young children.
    c. Preventive legislation has done little to influence pediatric caustic injury in this country.
    d. Toddlers usually ingest large quantities.

107. A 3-year-old child is seen after swallowing some sulfuric acid-containing toilet bowl cleaner 1 hour prior to presentation. On examination, he is drooling, crying, and stridorous. What is the next step in the management of this patient?
    a. Administer activated charcoal.
    b. Give the patient some water in an attempt to dilute the acid.
    c. Gently pass a nasogastric tube in an attempt to lavage and remove the offending acid.
    d. Perform direct laryngoscopy and prepare to intubate the trachea if significant airway injury is present.

108. A 15-month-old child is brought to the ED after being found with a bottle of drain cleaner. Some of the cleaner was found in his mouth, on his lips, and down the front of his shirt. On examination, his vital signs are within normal limits for age, he has some oral burns and drooling, but no respiratory symptoms or stridor. He spontaneously vomits

once in the ED. What should your course of action be for this patient?
    a. Intubate the trachea for airway protection.
    b. Arrange for endoscopy and administer corticosteroids with antibiotics only if third-degree burns are present.
    c. Arrange for endoscopy and give corticosteroids with antibiotics if second-degree esophageal burns are present.
    d. Arrange for endoscopy, but do not give corticosteroids as they have no proven benefit.
    e. Check CBC, administer IV fluids, and observe the patient for 6 hours.

109. The principle concern after most hydrocarbon ingestions is which target organ?
    a. Liver
    b. Intestinal tract
    c. Skin
    d. Lungs
    e. Bone marrow

110. The most important property in determining the risk of aspiration following a hydrocarbon ingestion is
    a. volatility.
    b. surface tension.
    c. molecular weight.
    d. type of hydrocarbon.
    e. viscosity.

111. A 17 year old is brought to the ED in full cardiac arrest. On examination an odor of gasoline or solvents is noted on his clothes. The most likely cause of his arrest is
    a. cardiac dysrhythmia.
    b. hydrocarbon ingestion.
    c. opioid overdose.
    d. pulmonary edema.
    e. intracranial bleed.

112. What is the best therapeutic endpoint for administering atropine to an organophosphate or carbamate poisoned patient?
    a. Pulse >70 bpm
    b. Resolution of muscle weakness
    c. Improvement of oxygenation and ventilation
    d. Resolution of seizures and altered mental status
    e. Resolution of vomiting, diarrhea, and diaphoresis

113. Which of the following statements is most accurate?
    a. Atropine treats only the nicotinic symptoms and does nothing for the muscarinic effects.
    b. Pralidoxime is indicated in severe organochlorine poisoned patients.
    c. There is a risk of masked seizures in organophosphate and carbamate poisoned patients.
    d. Organophosphate and carbamate poisoned patients do not pose a risk to health care workers because of secondary contamination.
    e. The least effective step in decontamination is the removal of the patient's clothing.

114. Lindane is applied multiple times on a small child for a scabies infestation. What would be the important concern?
    a. Lichenification
    b. Urticaria and bronchospasm in those with ragweed allergies
    c. Peripheral neuropathy that resolves after discontinuing the lindane
    d. Phototoxicity
    e. Seizures

For the rodenticides named in questions 115 to 119, match each product with its corresponding clinical effect in the following list:

115. Zinc phosphide

116. Brodifacoum

117. Bromethalin

118. Vacor (PNU)

119. Cholecalciferol
    a. Hypercalcemia
    b. Increased intracranial pressure, myoclonis seizure
    c. Bleeding diathesis
    d. Pulmonary edema, corrosive gastritis, multiorgan failure
    e. Diabetes mellitus, autonomic neuropathy, orthostatic hypotension

120. Which of the following statements regarding vitamin K therapy for super warfarin toxicity is most accurate?
    a. Oral therapy typically lasts for 48 to 72 hours.
    b. IM injection is the safest parenteral route of administration.

    c. Vitamin K_3 (menadione) is ineffective.
    d. Vitamin K activates synthesis of factors III.
    e. The IV route never has anaphylactoid reactions.

121. Which of the following rodenticides is the safest and most likely sold for indoor use?
    a. White phosphorus
    b. Sodium monofluoroacetate
    c. Zinc phosphide
    d. Strychnine
    e. Arsenic

122. Which of the following statements is MOST TRUE regarding anticoagulant rodenticides?
    a. All children should have serial coagulation profiles monitored after a ingesting a warfarin-containing rodenticide.
    b. A single dose of warfarin containing may produce toxicity.
    c. Single large ingestion or repeated small ingestions of super warfarins may produce toxicity.
    d. FFP is unnecessary if adequate vitamin K is given to control active bleeding.
    e. Super warfarins are highly bound in the liver and have very long elimination half-lives.

123. In treating a 16-year-old girl for a laceration on her thigh from falling against a fence, she confides that her menstrual cycles have been irregular and late during the past 3 months. She asks whether she could be pregnant. You learn from her that she is sexually active, takes oral contraceptives, and is an elite tennis athlete. What is a likely scenario to explain her menstrual irregularities?
    a. She is pregnant.
    b. She is modifying her menstrual cycle by stopping and starting her oral contraceptives to avoid premenstrual syndrome before athletic competition.
    c. She is exhibiting part of the spectrum of exercise-related amenorrhea.
    d. She is taking androgenic anabolic steroids or anabolic prohormones, which convert to testosterone to improve her conditioning and strength.
    e. All of the scenarios are possibilities.

124. Which of these adverse effects of androgenic anabolic steroids in adolescents are likely to revert to normal after stopping usage?
    a. Stunted growth
    b. Gynecomastia

c. Increased serum transaminase concentrations

d. Male pattern baldness

e. Low-pitched voice in females

125. During a routine physical exam prior to sports participation of a 14-year-old boy, you observe that he has well-developed muscles, acne, gynecomastia, and apparent testicular atrophy. Which athletic performance-enhancing substances would be most consistent with these findings?
    a. Creatine
    b. Androgenic anabolic steroids
    c. Stimulants such as ephedra or caffeine
    d. Growth hormone
    e. β-Adrenergic agonists

126. In the United Sates what is the estimated number of people trying marijuana for the first time each day?
    a. 300
    b. 3000
    c. 30,000
    d. 3 million

127. The risk of cannabis use in adolescent includes which of the following?
    a. Graduating to using "hard drugs" like cocaine and heroin
    b. Development of schizophrenia
    c. Abusing prescription narcotics as adults
    d. All of the above

128. Which of the following cases may cause a false-positive THC metabolite reading on urine toxicology screening?
    a. Attendee at outdoor hard rock music concert.
    b. A child wearing wet clothing made of hemp.
    c. Propoxyphene has been known to cause false-positive THC metabolites on urine toxicology screening.
    d. Methamphetamine user.
    e. There are no drugs that cause a false-positive THC on urine screening.

129. The clinical effects of cocaine most closely resemble which of the following toxidromes?
    a. Anticholinergic
    b. Cholinergic
    c. Narcotic syndrome
    d. Sympathomimetic
    e. Acute withdrawal toxidrome

130. An 18-year-old boy is brought to the ED by paramedics after being observed to be acting in a threatening and agitated manner. He is uncooperative and admits to smoking "crack" cocaine. His heart rate is 130 bpm; blood pressure is 170/110 mmHg, and respiratory rate is 40 breaths per minute. What is the most appropriate pharmacologic intervention?
    a. Labetalol
    b. Nitroprusside
    c. Haloperidol
    d. Chlorpromazine
    e. Lorazepam

131. A 16-year-old girl presents to the ED with a complaint of sharp chest pain. She admits to "snorting cocaine" 4 hours prior to arrival. Which of the following statements is correct regarding her work up?
    a. A serum level for cocaine should be obtained to document the time of exposure.
    b. ECG has been shown to be an unnecessary test due to the low incidence of true coronary heart disease in this age group.
    c. A chest radiograph may be helpful to exclude pneumothorax or pneumomediastinum.
    d. Elevated serum CPKs in this patient are unlikely to be cardiac in origin and can be attributed solely to muscle breakdown and rhabdomyolysis.

132. Which of the following is considered a potentially dangerous agent to combat cocaine toxicity?
    a. Propranolol
    b. Nitroprusside
    c. Diazepam
    d. Nitroglycerin

133. Which of the following is a recommended treatment for a cocaine body stuffer?
    a. Ipecac
    b. Gastric lavage
    c. Whole bowel irrigation
    d. Endoscopic removal

134. Which of the following signs or symptoms distinguishes a sympathomimetic from an anticholinergic toxidrome?
    a. Diaphoresis
    b. Hypertension
    c. Tachycardia
    d. Mydriasis

135. LSD acts primarily at which receptor?
  a. Adrenergic
  b. 5-HT
  c. Dopaminergic
  d. β-1
  e. GABA

136. LSD can typically cause all of the following EXCEPT
  a. hypertension.
  b. tachycardia.
  c. miosis.
  d. hyperthermia.
  e. synesthesia.

137. The systems primarily affects by mescaline are
  a. pulmonary and neurologic.
  b. pulmonary and GI.
  c. renal and neurologic.
  d. GI and neurologic.
  e. ophthalmologic and renal.

138. Which of the following is described as a unique characteristic of MDMA (Ecstasy) toxicity?
  a. Mydriasis
  b. Persistent neurologic damage even after brief use
  c. Perceptual distortion
  d. Bruxism
  e. Flatulence

139. The urine drug screen may be positive for amphetamine in the presence of
  a. ecstasy.
  b. mescaline.
  c. foxy-methoxy.
  d. LSD.
  e. morning glory seeds.

140. Signs and symptoms of inhalant use may be subtle and tend to vary widely among individuals. Which of the following is most helpful in the diagnosis of inhalant use?
  a. Urine toxicology screen
  b. Routine laboratory tests, including a complete blood count and a standard chemistry panel
  c. Thorough history and physical examination
  d. Chest x-ray and noncontrast head CT
  e. Carboxyhemoglobin and methemoglobin levels

141. Toluene is a hydrocarbon found in glues, spray paints, and paint thinners. What is an important manifestation of toluene-induced toxicity?
  a. Vitamin B_{12}-like peripheral neuropathy
  b. Hypokalemia, muscle weakness, and hyporeflexia
  c. CO poisoning
  d. Methemoglobinemia
  e. Pulmonary fibrosis

142. Diagnostic testing should be guided by the patient's presenting complaints. Which unique diagnostic consideration is most valid?
  a. Methemoglobinemia following inhalation of spray paint
  b. Distal renal tubule acidosis following inhalation of "poppers" or amyl nitrite
  c. Vitamin B_{12}-like peripheral neuropathy following inhalation of "poppers" or amyl nitrite
  d. CO poisoning following inhalation of a paint thinner containing methylene chloride
  e. Hepatitis following inhalation of gasoline

143. Which of the following opioids are at greatest risk for delayed toxicity?
  a. Heroin
  b. Codeine
  c. Morphine
  d. Methadone
  e. Fentanyl

144. Which of the following opioids cause pupillary dilation (mydriasis) as opposed to the classic "pinpoint" or miotic pupils?
  a. Morphine
  b. Heroin
  c. Tramadol
  d. Meperidine
  e. Fentanyl

145. Which of the following opioids causes seizures and cardiac disturbances with an overdose?
  a. Propoxyphene
  b. Methadone
  c. Tramadol
  d. Lomotil
  e. Heroin

146. Which of the following routes are acceptable means of administrating naloxone in the setting of an opioid overdose?

a. IV
b. Subcutaneous
c. Via endotracheal tube
d. Nebulized
e. All of the above

147. Which is the most common drug used in drug facilitated sexual assault?
a. Ethanol
b. GHB
c. Flunitrazepam
d. Ketamine

148. Which of the following statements regarding GHB is correct?
a. It usually causes death from cardiac arrest.
b. It is not associated with seizures.
c. Intubation is required in most cases of overdose.
d. It is believed by the lay public to increase muscle mass by body builders.

149. Which of the following statements regarding flunitrazepam is correct?
a. It is commonly referred to as *Special K.*
b. It is one-tenth the potency of diazepam
c. It will commonly be detected on routine toxicology screens after consumption.
d. It is illegal to distribute or import flunitrazepam in the United States.

150. Phencyclidine has been used as the following:
a. Pain medication
b. Part of the rapid sequence intubation protocol
c. An adjunct for psychotherapy
d. Veterinary tranquilizer

151. Regarding phencyclidine and ketamine, which of the following properties statements is TRUE?
a. Both are used clinically today.
b. Users may exhibit nystagmus, abnormal vital signs, and psychomotor agitation.
c. Laryngospasm and sialorrhea are not seen with phencyclidine.
d. Only rotatory nystagmus is seen with phencyclidine use.

152. All of the following can be used in treating phencyclidine toxicity EXCEPT
a. urinary acidification.
b. benzodiazepines for agitation and dysphoria.

c. activated charcoal if recent ingestion.
d. IV hydration.
e. restraints if the patient becomes a danger to himself or others.

153. All of the following tobacco metabolites are carcinogens EXCEPT
a. 4-(methylnitrosamino)-1-(3-pyridyl)-1-butanone (NNK).
b. cotinine.
c. NNAL (metabolite of NNK).
d. polycyclic aromatic hydrocarbons (PAH).

154. When does a cigarette smoker experiences peak nicotine levels?
a. 10 seconds
b. 1 minute
c. 10 minutes
d. 1 hour

155. Which of the following about smoking is TRUE?
a. Smoking decreases the risk of lung cancer from radon.
b. High school boys prefer smokeless tobacco to cigarettes.
c. Environmental tobacco smoke has been implicated in sudden infant death syndrome.
d. Addiction to smoking may occur after as few as 20 cigarettes.

156. All of the following have been associated with the neonatal abstinence syndrome EXCEPT
a. Heroin.
b. Methadone.
c. Cocaine.
d. Propoxyphene.
e. GHB.

157. All of the following withdrawal syndromes are considered potentially life threatening in a healthy individual EXCEPT
a. GHB.
b. opiates.
c. ethanol.
d. sedative-hypnotics.

158. Withdrawal symptoms can be precipitated by
a. discontinuing the drug.
b. decreasing the dose of the drug.
c. a coexistent medical condition.
d. all of the above.

159. Which of the following forms of arsenic has the greatest potential for causing harmful effects?
    a. Arsenite
    b. Arsenate
    c. Arsine gas
    d. Melarsoprol

160. Which of the following has not been linked to arsenic exposure?
    a. Blackfoot disease
    b. Diabetes mellitus
    c. Leukemia
    d. Bowen disease

161. The chelating agent of choice for an acutely ill child due to arsenic ingestion is
    a. DMPS.
    b. DMSA.
    c. BAL (British Anti-Lewisite agent).
    d. D-penicillamine.

162. What is the most common intended use of an ingested button battery?
    a. Hearing aids
    b. Toys or games
    c. Calculators
    d. Cameras
    e. Watches

163. Which of the following factors is not associated with severe outcomes in battery ingestion cases?
    a. Esophageal lodgment
    b. 20- to 23-mm battery diameter
    c. Lithium battery
    d. Discharged cell
    e. Younger child

164. Which of the following is most helpful following battery ingestion?
    a. Determination of blood mercury concentration
    b. Ipecac syrup
    c. Immediate endoscopic removal if battery is in the stomach
    d. Immediate x-ray localization of battery
    e. Daily x-rays to confirm passage

165. What is the primary reason iron poisoning in children has significantly declined over the past decade?
    a. Childproof safety caps on pill bottles
    b. Blister packaging of iron preparations limiting the total dose dispensed

c. More aggressive deferoxamine therapy
    d. A pharmaceutical market decline in the supply of iron preparations
    e. Increase in the number of pediatric ICUs nationally

166. Which of the following scenarios would gastric decontamination with whole bowel irrigation be most appropriate?
    a. Recent iron ingestion in 2-year-old toddler with bloody vomiting and diarrhea.
    b. Vin rose urine color change following deferoxamine administration.
    c. Recent ingestion of iron tablets in a 14-year-old with evidence of multiple opacities on abdominal radiograph.
    d. Profound iron toxicity resulting in hepatic failure.
    e. Any iron overdose that requires activated charcoal administration.

167. Which of the following are the proper parameters for discontinuing deferoxamine chelation therapy following acute iron poisoning?
    a. Urinary color change to vin rose.
    b. Clearing of iron fragment radiopacities on radiograph.
    c. Rapid decline in demonstrable serum iron levels.
    d. Resolution of metabolic acidosis, improved GI symptoms.
    e. No iron poisoning should be treated beyond 24 hours with deferoxamine therapy.

168. Which of the following laboratory clues is inconsistent with plumbism?
    a. Anemia
    b. Basophilic stippling
    c. Elevated blood lead level
    d. Elevated FEP/ZPP
    e. Hypocalcemia

169. Which of the following oral chelators should be considered first in asymptomatic children with a BLL 50 μg/dL?
    a. BAL
    b. CaNa2EDTA
    c. DMPS
    d. DMSA
    e. D-Penicillamine

170. Which of the following is a consequence of chronic plumbism?
    a. Anemia
    b. Cognitive delays
    c. Hypertension
    d. Nephropathy
    e. All of the above

171. Which is the most important intervention for a child with a lead level of 16 µg/dL,?
    a. Chelation therapy
    b. Environmental assessment
    c. Nutritional assessment
    d. Vitamin supplementation
    e. X-rays of the limbs

172. Which decontamination strategy is best for patients with visible lead chips on x-ray?
    a. Activated charcoal
    b. Gastric lavage
    c. Ipecac
    d. Whole bowel irrigation
    e. Decontamination should not be done; chelation is required

173. Which of the following is MOST TRUE about mercury?
    a. It is toxic in all forms and by all routes of exposure.
    b. It has toxicity that is specific for various organs dependent on both dose and form of mercury.
    c. It is a benign element because it is naturally occurring.
    d. It is unnecessary and should be eliminated from the earth.

174. Neurodevelopmental toxicity is the major concern with mercury and has been demonstrated at concentrations 10 to 100 times those seen in the United States. Currently, neonates in the United States have the greatest exposure from
    a. breastfeeding.
    b. release of elemental mercury from maternal dental amalgams during pregnancy.
    c. maternal consumption of organic mercury from cod and other nonpredatory fish during pregnancy.
    d. application of mercury salts to the umbilical cord.
    e. application of organic mercury compounds to the skin as an antiseptic.

175. A mercury spill has occurred from a household fever thermometer (0.05 mL of elemental mercury) falling to the tile floor. An 8-month-old child is on the floor nearby. What is the best course of action?
    a. To use the edge of a credit card and a bright light to identify and collect mercury globules, scraping them onto a piece of paper or using an eyedropper, making sure that none of the glass or mercury is around or on the child.
    b. Using a vacuum cleaner because mercury globules can be very small.
    c. To cover the area with plastic and call in a hazardous materials cleanup company because mercury is very toxic.
    d. To evacuate the house immediately and have the child tested for mercury exposure, while waiting professional cleanup services.

176. Which of the following is least likely to explain why CO is a common cause of unintentional pediatric poisoning death?
    a. CO is tasteless and odorless.
    b. Symptoms of Co poisoning mimic those of the flu.
    c. A chemical asphyxiant, CO impairs the ability to respond when poisoned.
    d. CO is undetectable in air.
    e. Fetal hemoglobin binds CO more avidly than adult hemoglobin.

177. Which of the following is least likely to be associated with the occurrence of pediatric CO poisoning?
    a. House fire
    b. Houseboat
    c. Pickup trucks
    d. Pregnancy
    e. Natural gas leak

178. Based on current information, which of the following is the best reason for hyperbaric oxygen therapy after CO poisoning?
    a. An elevated COHgb level in an asymptomatic teenager with normal neuropsychiatric testing.
    b. Repeated vomiting in an 8-year-old with prolonged exposure to natural gas.
    c. Confirmed exposure to CO in pregnancy.
    d. Significant elevation of plasma CO level regardless of symptoms.
    e. Increasing airway edema with stridor after smoke inhalation.

179. Cyanide poisoning may occur from ingesting each of the following EXCEPT
    a. apricot pits.
    b. artificial nail remover.
    c. cassava.
    d. fava beans.
    e. peach pits.

180. Which of the following is most consistent with cyanide poisoning?
    a. Arterial-venous O_2 difference is increased.
    b. Arterial-venous O_2 difference is decreased.
    c. Lactate level is low in the setting of severe acidosis.
    d. Diagnosis should await a confirmatory cyanide level.
    e. None of the above.

181. Which of the following is not a part of the Taylor Cyanide Antidote Kit?
    a. Amyl nitrite
    b. Hydroxycobalamin
    c. Sodium nitrite
    d. Sodium thiosulfate
    e. All of the above are contained in the Taylor kit

182. The characteristic smell of _____ may be associated with cyanide poisoning.
    a. apricots
    b. bitter almonds
    c. garlic
    d. freshly mown hay
    e. plastic

183. A 6-year-old boy is administered oxygen for the abrupt onset of cyanosis during an esophagoscopy procedure. Which of the following implicates methemoglobinemia, rather than cardiac or pulmonary disease, as the cause of the cyanosis?
    a. Cyanosis resolves rapidly with mask application of positive pressure ventilation.
    b. Hemoglobin oxygen saturation 87% as measured by pulse oximetry, with Pao_2 <60 torr as measured by arterial blood gas analysis.
    c. Hemoglobin oxygen saturation 87% as measured by pulse oximetry, with Pao_2 >100 torr as measured by arterial blood gas analysis.
    d. Hemoglobin oxygen saturation 100% as measured by pulse oximetry, with Pao_2 <60 torr as measured by arterial blood gas analysis.
    e. Hypotension and poor perfusion.

184. When evaluating drug-induced methemoglobinemia among infants, which of the following statements is MOST TRUE?
    a. Drug-induced methemoglobinemia is associated with more profound metabolic acidosis than enteritis-associated methemoglobinemia.
    b. Fetal hemoglobin cannot be oxidized to methemoglobin.
    c. Infants with methemoglobinemia can be assumed to be G-6-PD deficient.
    d. Infants younger than 6 months of age typically have less efficient endogenous methemoglobin-reducing enzyme systems.
    e. Methylene blue therapy is contraindicated among infants younger than 6 months.

185. Which of the following factors has contributed to the development of toxicity from dietary supplements?
    a. Reduced governmental oversight after the passage of the Dietary Supplement and Health Education Act.
    b. A widespread belief among the general population that natural is safe.
    c. The need to prove a supplement harmful before it can be removed.
    d. Contaminants in a largely unsupervised processing and manufacturing process.
    e. All of the above.

186. Dietary supplements include a wide variety of both plant-derived and nonplant–derived products. Which of the following combinations has the potential to cause severe toxicity?
    a. Dehydroepiandrosterone and a benzodiazepine
    b. Ephedra alkaloids and phentolamine
    c. St. John's Wort and tranylcypromine
    d. Creatine and a potassium-sparing diuretic
    e. Echinacea and a mega multivitamin preparation

187. Diagnosis of the etiologic agent causing toxicity from a dietary supplement exposure may be difficult. Choose the test with the potential to yield the most information and ultimately a diagnosis in a symptomatic patient with an unknown exposure.
    a. A cell blood count
    b. A radiograph of the product or the patient's GI tract
    c. A serum chemistry
    d. A finger stick blood glucose
    e. Coagulation parameters

188. In which of the following conditions would stool culture NOT be essential?
    a. An 8-month-old with suspected *Salmonella* gastroenteritis
    b. Febrile child with bloody diarrhea
    c. Community outbreaks
    d. A 12-month-old with suspected rotovirus
    e. An immunosuppressed child

189. A 4-month-old child presents with lethargy, weak cry, hypotonia, and poor feeding. The mother reports adding honey to the child's formula to "sweeten it up." Which of the following agents is most likely?
    a. Botulism toxin
    b. *Anthrax bacillus*
    c. *Salmonella*
    d. *Shigella*
    e. Methadone

190. Which of the following is TRUE regarding colenterate envenomations from jellyfish, sea anemones, and fire corals?
    a. Dead jellyfish cannot envenom.
    b. They envenom via a stinger that injects venom.
    c. Jellyfish cause the most common marine envenomations.
    d. The Portuguese man-o'-war is a nonvenomous coelenterate.
    e. Treatment consists of immersion in hot water, analgesics, and antibiotics.

191. A 6-year-old boy was stung by a stingray while walking in the shallow waters adjacent to a beach in Florida. Which of the following would be the most appropriate treatment for his injury?
    a. Irrigation with sterile saline, immersion in hot water to tolerance, analgesics, antitetanus prophylaxis, and antibiotics.
    b. Rinsing with vinegar, local wound care, analgesics, and antitetanus prophylaxis.
    c. Surgical debridement to remove the sheath fragments, antibiotics, analgesics, and antitetanus prophylaxis.
    d. Irrigation with sterile saline, analgesics, antitetanus prophylaxis, and antibiotics.
    e. Irrigation with sterile saline, antivenom, and antitetanus prophylaxis.

192. Which of the following is MOST TRUE regarding the treatment of a patient who presents after stepping on a sea urchin spine?

    a. A specific antivenom is available in Australia.
    b. Immersion in hot water, removal of spines, antitetanus prophylaxis, and antibiotics.
    c. Irrigation with sterile saline, rinse with vinegar, removal of spines, antitetanus prophylaxis and antibiotics.
    d. Removal of spines, antitetanus prophylaxis, and antibiotics.
    e. No treatment indicated except local wound care, antitetanus prophylaxis, and antibiotics.

193. Which of the following paired items is correct?
    a. Catfish stings: rinse with vinegar
    b. Sea snake envenomation: local wound care
    c. Sea anemones envenomation: immersion in hot water
    d. Stonefish envenomation: antivenom
    e. Scorpion fish envenomation: rinse with vinegar

194. Which of the following is correct regarding marine envenomations?
    a. Scorpion fish are the most commonly encountered venomous fish.
    b. The stingray uses nematocysts to inject venom.
    c. The box jellyfish typically causes a minor localized urticarial lesion.
    d. Sea snake injuries are common in the southeastern United States.
    e. Catfish stings occur from spines within a sheath on their fins.

195. A 14-year-old patient presents with nonbloody diarrhea and vomiting, with circumoral tingling, and hot/cold temperature reversal after eating at local seafood restaurant. This scenario is most classic for which form of seafood poisoning?
    a. Scombroid poisoning
    b. Ciguatera poisoning
    c. Paralytic shellfish poisoning
    d. Tetrodotoxin poisoning
    e. Shigella food poisoning

196. Which of the following mushrooms causes primarily muscarinic effects?
    a. *Amanita muscaria*
    b. *Clitocybe* spp.
    c. *Coprinus* spp.
    d. The false morel

197. Which of the following statements regarding mushroom poisoning is TRUE?

a. No life-threatening mushroom causes symptoms early after ingestion (<2 to 3 hours).

b. Children <6 years represent the greatest frequency of ingestion of mushrooms.

c. Most mushrooms have a specific antidote.

d. Methemoglobinemia is commonly seen after mushroom ingestion.

198. Which group of mushrooms is responsible for most deaths due to mushroom ingestion in children?
    a. GI irritants
    b. Amatoxin-producing mushrooms such as *Aminita* spp.
    c. *Gyromitrin* mushrooms such as the false morel.
    d. *Coprine* mushrooms, such as the inky cap.
    e. Psychoactive mushrooms.

199. The most commonly encountered toxic mushroom ingestions in children are due to which group of mushrooms?
    a. *Gyromitrin*-producing mushrooms
    b. *Coprine* mushrooms, such as the inky cap
    c. Amatoxin-producing mushrooms
    d. GI irritants
    e. Psychoactive mushrooms

200. Which of the following mushrooms has been known to cause clinically significant renal insufficiency?
    a. *Amanita muscaria*
    b. *Clitocybe* spp.
    c. *Coprinus* spp.
    d. *Amanita smithiana*

201. Diffenbachia and philodendron are common household plants commonly ingested by toddlers. The most common manifestation of toxicity is
    a. nausea, vomiting, and diarrhea.
    b. severe oral and pharyngeal burns.
    c. seizures.
    d. cardiac dysrhythmias.
    e. renal failure.

202. Plants such as foxglove and oleander contain cardiac glycosides and can result in bradydysrhythmias and heart block. In a patient unresponsive to atropine and cardiac pacing, which of the following interventions is indicated?
    a. Phenytoin
    b. Lidocaine
    c. Sodium bicarbonate

d. Digibind Fab fragments

e. Epinephrine

203. Water hemlock ingestion may result in which clinical presentation?
    a. Acute renal failure
    b. Acute hepatic failure
    c. Cardiac arrest
    d. Status epilepticus
    e. Severe dehydration from gastroenteritis and GI bleed

204. What is the occurrence of crotaline dry bites, in which no venom is delivered?
    a. <5%
    b. 5% to 10%
    c. 20% to 25%
    d. 45% to 50%
    e. 75% to 90%

205. Which of the following prehospital treatments have proven to be necessary to avoid detrimental outcomes after snake envenomation?
    a. "Cut and suck" method of venom extraction
    b. Placement of a tourniquet or constricting band
    c. Application of ice
    d. High voltage, electric shock therapy
    e. None of the above therapies has been proven necessary

206. What is the most appropriate method of determining antivenom (CroFab) dosing for pediatric patients after pit viper envenomation?
    a. Based on the venom load and severity of envenomation
    b. Weight (kg)-based dosing
    c. Four to six vials of antivenom every 4 hours until swelling reverses
    d. Four to six vials of antivenom initially, then 4 vials every 8 hours for 48 hours regardless of age or clinical findings
    e. It depends on the species of pit viper identified as causing the envenomation

207. A 6-year-old girl presents with acute-onset abdominal pain with nausea, vomiting, and severe muscle cramps. The child presents to the ED crying and is assuming a fetal position, rocking side to side on the hospital gurney. Which of the following arthropod envenomations is this scenario most consistent with?

a. Brown recluse envenomation
b. Black widow spider bite
c. Scorpion sting
d. Fire ant sting
e. Hymenoptera stings

208. A 5-year-old patient presents with shortness of breath and cyanosis. He was treated for a brown recluse spider bite 2 days prior and is otherwise healthy. What complication is suspected in this case?
a. Hemolytic anemia
b. DIC
c. Methemoglobinemia from pharmaceutical therapy
d. Severe systemic reaction from the spider bite
e. Acute lung injury from the spider venom.

209. Which of the following is TRUE regarding scorpion stings?

a. There is no known antivenom available.
b. Dapsone is indicated for severe necrotic reactions.
c. There have been no pediatric deaths in the United States in the last 25 years.
d. Systemic toxicity from scorpion envenomation classically results in miotic pupils.
e. Hyperbaric oxygen therapy has been shown to be efficacious in severe cases.

210. Which of the following arthropod bites or stings lead to the most pediatric deaths annually?
a. Scorpion stings
b. Black widow spider bites
c. Brown recluse spider bites
d. Hymenoptera stings
e. Fire ant stings

ANSWERS

1. a	(Chapter 4: Maternal-Fetal)
2. b	(Chapter 4)
3. d	(Chapter 4)
4. e	(Chapter 5: Breast Milk)
5. c	(Chapter 5)
6. b	(Chapter 6: Premature Infant)
7. a	(Chapter 6)
8. d	(Chapter 6)
9. c	(Chapter 8: Toddler)
10. b	(Chapter 8)
11. a	(Chapter 8)
12. e	(Chapter 9: Adolescent)
13. b	(Chapter 9)
14. c	(Chapter 13: APLS)
15. c	(Chapter 13)
16. a	(Chapter 13)
17. d	(Chapter 14 Hazardous Materials)
18. a	(Chapter 14)
19. b	(Chapter 15: Weapons of Mass Destruction)
20. b	(Chapter 15)
21. c	(Chapter 15)
22. b	(Chapter 16: GI Decontamination)
23. d	(Chapter 16)
24. c	(Chapter 16)
25. a	(Chapter 18: Extracorporeal Removal)
26. c	(Chapter 18)
27. c	(Chapter 18)
28. b	(Chapter 19: Pediatric Intensive Care Unit)
29. c	(Chapter 19)
30. c	(Chapter 20: Laboratory)
31. d	(Chapter 20)
32. d	(Chapter 20)
33. a	(Chapter 21: Fluid and Electrolytes)
34. b	(Chapter 21)
35. d	(Chapter 21)
36. b	(Chapter 22: Thermoregulatory)
37. c	(Chapter 22)
38. d	(Chapter 22)
39. a	(Chapter 23: Organ Toxicity)
40. b	(Chapter 23)
41. c	(Chapter 23)
42. e	(Chapter 25: Lethal Doses)
43. d	(Chapter 25)
44. b	(Chapter 25)
45. b	(Chapter 25)
46. e	(Chapter 25)
47. c	(Chapter 25)
48. b	(Chapter 25)
49. d	(Chapter 25)

50. c	(Chapter 25)
51. d	(Chapter 25)
52. c	(Chapter 26: Nontoxic Drugs)
53. b	(Chapter 26)
54. d	(Chapter 26)
55. c	(Chapter 27: Over-the-Counter Medications)
56. a	(Chapter 27)
57. b	(Chapter 27)
58. a	(Chapter 28: Acetaminophen)
59. e	(Chapter 28)
60. c	(Chapter 28)
61. a	(Chapter 29: Anticholinergics)
62. b	(Chapter 29)
63. e	(Chapter 29)
64. d	(Chapter 30: Salicylates)
65. e	(Chapter 30)
66. a	(Chapter 30)
67. d	(Chapter 31: NSAIDs)
68. a	(Chapter 31)
69. b	(Chapter 31)
70. d	(Chapter 32: Caffeine)
71. b	(Chapter 32)
72. a	(Chapter 32)
73. d	(Chapter 33: Vitamins)
74. c	(Chapter 33)
75. d	(Chapter 33)
76. a	(Chapter 35: Antihypertensives)
77. c	(Chapter 35)
78. d	(Chapter 37: Digoxin)
79. b	(Chapter 37)
80. d	(Chapter 37)
81. a	(Chapter 38: Theophylline)
82. a	(Chapter 38)
83. c	(Chapter 38)
84. d	(Chapter 39: Sedative-Hypnotics)
85. a	(Chapter 39)
86. d	(Chapter 39)
87. b	(Chapter 40: Insulin/Hypoglycemic Agents)
88. a	(Chapter 40)
89. c	(Chapter 40)
90. d	(Chapter 42: Isoniazid)
91. b	(Chapter 42)
92. c	(Chapter 42)
93. d	(Chapter 43: Antidepressants)
94. e	(Chapter 43)
95. a	(Chapter 43)
96. d	(Chapter 44: Lithium)
97. c	(Chapter 44)
98. a	(Chapter 44)
99. d	(Chapter 45: Neuroleptics)
100. b	(Chapter 45)

101. a   (Chapter 45)
102. e   (Chapter 45)
103. c   (Chapter 47: Toxic Alcohols)
104. d   (Chapter 47)
105. c   (Chapter 47)
106. a   (Chapter 48: Caustics)
107. d   (Chapter 48)
108. c   (Chapter 48)
109. d   (Chapter 49: Hydrocarbons)
110. e   (Chapter 49)
111. a   (Chapter 49)
112. c   (Chapter 51: Insecticides)
113. c   (Chapter 51)
114. e   (Chapter 51)
115. d   (Chapter 52: Rodenticides)
116. c   (Chapter 52)
117. b   (Chapter 52)
118. e   (Chapter 52)
119. a   (Chapter 52)
120. c   (Chapter 52)
121. c   (Chapter 52)
122. c   (Chapter 52)
123. e   (Chapter 55: Steroids)
124. c   (Chapter 55)
125. b   (Chapter 55)
126. b   (Chapter 56: Cannanbinoids)
127. d   (Chapter 56)
128. e   (Chapter 56)
129. d   (Chapter 57: Cocaine)
130. e   (Chapter 57)
131. c   (Chapter 57)
132. a   (Chapter 57)
133. c   (Chapter 57)
134. a   (Chapter 57)
135. b   (Chapter 58: Hallucinogenics)
136. c   (Chapter 58)
137. d   (Chapter 58)
138. d   (Chapter 58)
139. a   (Chapter 58)
140. c   (Chapter 59: Inhalants)
141. b   (Chapter 59)
142. d   (Chapter 59)
143. d   (Chapter 60: Opioids)
144. d   (Chapter 60)
145. a   (Chapter 60)
146. e   (Chapter 60)
147. a   (Chapter 61: Date Rape Drugs)
148. d   (Chapter 61)
149. d   (Chapter 61)
150. d   (Chapter 62: PCP)
151. b   (Chapter 62)

152. a   (Chapter 62)
153. b   (Chapter 63: Tobacco)
154. a   (Chapter 63)
155. c   (Chapter 63)
156. e   (Chapter 64: Withdrawal)
157. b   (Chapter 64)
158. d   (Chapter 64)
159. c   (Chapter 66: Arsenic)
160. c   (Chapter 66)
161. c   (Chapter 66)
162. a   (Chapter 67: Button Batteries)
163. d   (Chapter 67)
164. d   (Chapter 67)
165. b   (Chapter 68: Iron)
166. c   (Chapter 68)
167. d   (Chapter 68)
168. e   (Chapter 68)
169. d   (Chapter 69: Lead)
170. e   (Chapter 69)
171. b   (Chapter 69)
172. d   (Chapter 69)
173. b   (Chapter 70: Mercury)
174. c   (Chapter 70)
175. a   (Chapter 70)
176. d   (Chapter 72: Carbon Monoxide)
177. e   (Chapter 72)
178. c   (Chapter 72)
179. d   (Chapter 73: Cyanide)
180. b   (Chapter 73)
181. b   (Chapter 73)
182. b   (Chapter 73)
183. c   (Chapter 74: Methemoglobin)
184. d   (Chapter 74)
185. e   (Chapter 76: Herbal Agents)
186. b   (Chapter 76)
187. b   (Chapter 76)
188. d   (Chapter 77: Food Poisoning)
189. a   (Chapter 77)
190. c   (Chapter 78: Marine Envenomations)
191. a   (Chapter 78)
192. b   (Chapter 78)
193. d   (Chapter 78)
194. e   (Chapter 78)
195. b   (Chapter 78)
196. b   (Chapter 79: Mushrooms)
197. b   (Chapter 79)
198. b   (Chapter 79)
199. d   (Chapter 79)
200. d   (Chapter 79)
201. b   (Chapter 80: Plants)
202. d   (Chapter 80)

203. d   (Chapter 80)
204. c   (Chapter 81: Snakes)
205. e   (Chapter 81)
206. a   (Chapter 81)

207. b   (Chapter 82: Arthropods)
208. c   (Chapter 82)
209. c   (Chapter 82)
210. d   (Chapter 82)

Index